Ferri's Practical Guide
Fast Facts for Patient Care

Ninth Edition

FRED F. FERRI, MD, FACP

BROWN
Alpert Medical School

Clinical Professor
Alpert Medical School at Brown University
Providence, Rhode Island

Author contact for comments about the book:
fred_ferri@brown.edu

D0503338

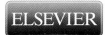
ELSEVIER

ELSEVIER
MOSBY

1600 John F. Kennedy Blvd.
Ste 1800
Philadelphia, PA 19103-2899

FERRI'S PRACTICAL GUIDE: FAST FACTS FOR PATIENT CARE   ISBN:978-1-4557-4459-6

Notices

Knowledge and best practice in this field are constantly changing. As new research and experience broaden our understanding, changes in research methods, professional practices, or medical treatment may become necessary. Practitioners and researchers must always rely on their own experience and knowledge in evaluating and using any information, methods, compounds, or experiments described herein. In using such information or methods they should be mindful of their own safety and the safety of others, including parties for whom they have a professional responsibility.

With respect to any drug or pharmaceutical products identified, readers are advised to check the most current information provided (i) on procedures featured or (ii) by the manufacturer of each product to be administered, to verify the recommended dose or formula, the method and duration of administration, and contraindications. It is the responsibility of practitioners, relying on their own experience and knowledge of their patients, to make diagnoses, to determine dosages and the best treatment for each individual patient, and to take all appropriate safety precautions. To the fullest extent of the law, neither the Publisher nor the authors, contributors, or editors, assume any liability for any injury and/or damage to persons or property as a matter of products liability, negligence or otherwise, or from any use or operation of any methods, products, instructions, or ideas contained in the material herein.

Library of Congress Cataloging-in-Publication Data

Ferri, Fred F., author.
   [Practical guide to the care of the medical patient]
   Ferri's practical guide : fast facts for patient care / Fred F. Ferri. -- Ninth edition.
      p. ; cm.
   Practical guide
   Preceded by Practical guide to the care of the medical patient / Fred F. Ferri. 8th ed. c2011.
   Includes bibliographical references and index.
   ISBN 978-1-4557-4459-6 (pbk.)
   I. Title. II. Title: Practical guide.
   [DNLM: 1. Clinical Medicine--Handbooks. 2. Clinical Laboratory Techniques--Handbooks.
3. Diagnosis, Differential--Handbooks. WB 39]
   RC55
   616--dc23   2013042887

Senior Content Strategist: James Merritt
Content Development Specialist: Maria Holman
Publishing Services Manager: Hemamalini Rajendrababu
Project Manager: Saravanan Thavamani
Senior Book Designer: Lou Forgione
Marketing Manager: Debashis Das

Printed in China

Last digit is the print number: 9 8 7 6 5 4 3 2

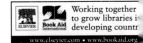

Working together
to grow libraries in
developing countries

www.elsevier.com • www.bookaid.org

Contributors

The author wishes to acknowledge the following physicians who have contributed to this book and to several editions of *Ferri's Clinical Advisor*.

Tanya Ali, MD
Clinical Assistant Professor of
   Medicine
Department of Medicine
Alpert Medical School
Brown University
Providence, Rhode Island

Mel L. Anderson, MD, FACP
Assistant Professor of Medicine
University of Colorado School of
   Medicine
Denver Veterans Affairs Medical Center
Denver, Colorado

Michelle Stozek Anvar, MD
Assistant Professor (Clinical)
Alpert Medical School
Brown University
Providence, Rhode Island

Sudeep Kaur Aulakh, MD, CM, FRCPC
Assistant Professor of Medicine
Tufts University School of Medicine
Baystate Medical Center
Springfield, Massachusetts

Lynn Bowlby, MD, FACP
Medical Director
Duke Outpatient Clinic
Duke Internal Medicine Residency
   Program
Durham, North Carolina

Gaurav Choudhary, MD
Assistant Professor of Medicine
Alpert Medical School
Brown University
Providence, Rhode Island

Alexandra Degenhardt, MD
Director
Multiple Sclerosis Center
New York Methodist Hospital
Brooklyn, New York

Joseph A. Diaz, MD
Associate Professor of Medicine
Division of General Internal Medicine
Memorial Hospital of Rhode Island
Alpert Medical School
Brown University
Providence, Rhode Island

Mark J. Fagan, MD
Director
Medical Primary Care Unit
Rhode Island Hospital
Professor of Medicine
Alpert Medical School
Brown University
Providence, Rhode Island

Timothy W. Farrell, MD
Clinical Assistant Professor
Department of Family Medicine
Alpert Medical School
Brown University
Providence, Rhode Island

Glenn G. Fort, MD, MPH, FACP, FIDSA
Clinical Associate Professor of Medicine
Alpert Medical School
Brown University
Chief
Infectious Diseases
Our Lady of Fatima Hospital
North Providence, Rhode Island

Paul F. George, MD
Assistant Professor
Department of Family Medicine
Alpert Medical School
Brown University
Providence, Rhode Island

Sajeev Handa, MD
Director
Division of Hospitalist Medicine
Rhode Island Hospital
Clinical Assistant Professor
   of Medicine
Alpert Medical School
Brown University
Providence, Rhode Island

Taylor Harrison, MD
Assistant Professor of Neurology
Department of Neurology
Emory University
Atlanta, Georgia

Jennifer Jeremiah, MD
Clinical Associate Professor of Medicine
Alpert Medical School
Brown University
Providence, Rhode Island

v

Powel H. Kazanjian, MD
Professor and Chief
Division of Infectious Disease
Director of HIV Program
University of Michigan Medical Center
Professor of Internal Medicine
University of Michigan Medical School
Ann Arbor, Michigan

Kelly A. McGarry, MD
Program Director
General Internal Medicine Residency
   Program
Rhode Island Hospital
Associate Professor of Medicine
Alpert Medical School
Brown University
Providence, Rhode Island

Lynn McNicoll, MD
Assistant Professor of Medicine
Alpert Medical School
Brown University
Geriatrician
Division of Geriatrics
Rhode Island Hospital
Providence, Rhode Island

Melissa Nothnagle, MD
Assistant Professor of Family Medicine
Alpert Medical School
Brown University
Providence, Rhode Island

Carolyn J. O'Connor, MD
Assistant Clinical Professor
Yale University School of Medicine
Department of Medicine
St. Mary's Hospital
Waterbury, Connecticut

Steven M. Opal, MD
Professor of Medicine
Infectious Disease Division
Alpert Medical School
Brown University
Providence, Rhode Island

Paul A. Pirraglia, MD, MPH
Assistant Professor of Medicine
Alpert Medical School
Brown University
Rhode Island Hospital
Providence, Rhode Island

Harlan G. Rich, MD
Director of Endoscopy
Rhode Island Hospital
Associate Professor of Medicine
Alpert Medical School
Brown University
Providence, Rhode Island

Joanne M. Silvia, MD
Clinical Assistant Professor
Department of Family Medicine
Alpert Medical School
Brown University
Providence, Rhode Island

Dominick Tammaro, MD
Associate Director
Categorical Internal Medicine Residency
Co-Director
Medicine-Pediatrics Residency
Division of General Internal Medicine
Rhode Island Hospital
Associate Professor of Medicine
Alpert Medical School
Brown University
Providence, Rhode Island

Iris Tong, MD
Assistant Professor
Department of Medicine
Alpert Medical School
Brown University Women and Infants
   Hospital
Providence, Rhode Island

Margaret Tryforos, MD
Clinical Assistant Professor
Department of Family Medicine
Alpert Medical School
Brown University
Providence, Rhode Island

Marc S. Weinberg, MD, FACP
Clinical Professor of Medicine
Boston University School of Medicine
Clinical Associate Professor of Medicine
Alpert Medical School
Chief of Nephrology
Roger Williams Medical Center
Providence, Rhode Island

Wen-Chih Wu, MD
Associate Professor of Medicine
Alpert Medical School
Brown University
Cardiologist
Providence VA Medical Center
Providence, Rhode Island

Preface

This manual is a concise reference for the busy clinician in need of immediate medical information. Its purpose is to provide a fast and efficient way to identify important clinical, laboratory, and diagnostic imaging information.

To limit its size to a pocket reference, less emphasis has been placed on pathophysiology and epidemiology, with more emphasis on practical clinical information. Clinical algorithms and tables have been used extensively throughout the manual to simplify difficult topics and to enhance recollection of principal points. It is hoped that its concise style will help the reader, particularly during an active clinical service, when time to read is extremely limited.

The combination of practical clinical information with drug therapeutics, procedures, diagnostic imaging, and laboratory medicine makes this manual unique and useful, not only to medical residents and students but also to practicing physicians and allied health professionals. I wish to thank the many thousands of physicians who have made the prior editions a bestseller in medical publishing and hope that future users will find this edition the most useful medical handbook that they will ever purchase during their training.

Fred F. Ferri, MD, FACP

Pearls of Wisdom in Medicine

1. Common things occur commonly.
2. When you hear hoofbeats, think of horses, not zebras.
3. Place your bets on uncommon manifestations of common conditions, rather than common manifestations of uncommon conditions.
4. If what you are doing is working, keep on doing it.
5. If what you are doing is not working, stop doing it.
6. If you don't know what to do, don't do anything.
7. Above all, never let a surgeon get your patient.

From Matz R: Principles of medicine.
NY State J Med 77:99-101, 1977.

Acknowledgments

I also extend a special thanks to my sons, Dr. Vito F. Ferri and Dr. Christopher A. Ferri for their help in the preparation and review of the manuscript and to the authors and contributors of the following texts who have served as a valuable resource in the development of the ninth edition of this manual:

Goldman L, Schafer AI (eds): Goldman's Cecil Medicine, 24th ed. Philadelphia, Saunders, 2012.

Vincent JL, Abraham E, Moore FA, et al (eds): Textbook of Critical Care, 6th ed. Philadelphia, Saunders, 2011.

Medical Knowledge Self-Assessment Program (MKSAP) 16. Philadelphia, American College of Physicians, 2012.

Gilbert DN, Moellering RC, Eliopoulos GM, et al: The Sanford Guide to Antimicrobial Therapy 2013, 43rd ed. Antimicrobial Therapy, Inc, 2012.

Users of our book are encouraged to use the above noted reference texts for additional information on the topics discussed in this manual.

Fred Ferri, MD

Table of Contents

SECTION **3**

Diseases and Disorders   53

>	Greater than	AML	Acute myelogenous leukemia
<	Less than	AMP	Adenosine monophosphate
+	Positive; plus	ANA	Antinuclear antibody
−	Negative	ANCA	Antineutrophil cytoplasmic antibody
↑	Increase	Ao	Aorta
↓	Decrease	AP	Anteroposterior
AAA	Abdominal aortic aneurysm	APCR	Activated protein C resistance
A-a gradient	Alveolar-arterial gradient	APL	Antiphospholipid antibody
AAT	α₁-antitrypsin deficiency	APS	Antiphospholipid antibody syndrome
Ab	Antibody	APTT	Activated partial thromboplastin time
abd	Abdomen	AR	Aortic regurgitation; autosomal recessive
ABG	Arterial blood gas	ARB	Angiotensin receptor blocker
ABI	Ankle-brachial index	ARDS	Acute respiratory distress syndrome
abnl	Abnormal	ARF	Acute renal failure
abx	Antibiotic	ART	Antiretroviral therapy
ac	Before meals	ARVD	Arrhythmogenic right ventricular dysplasia
ACA	Anticardiolipin antibody	AS	Aortic stenosis
ACC	American College of Cardiology	ASA	Aspirin
ACD	Anemia of chronic disease	ASCA	anti–Saccharomyces cerevisiae antibody
ACE	Angiotensin-converting enzyme	ASD	Atrial septal defect
ACEI	ACE inhibitor	ASLO	Antistreptolysin O
ACL	Anticardiolipin antibody	ASMA	Anti–smooth muscle antibody
ACLS	Advanced cardiac life support	AST	Aspartate aminotransferase
ACS	Acute coronary syndrome	asx	Asymptomatic
ACT	Activated clotting time	ATN	Acute tubular necrosis
ACTH	Adrenocorticotropic hormone	ATRA	All trans-retinoic acid
ACV	Assist-control ventilation	AV	Aortic valve; arteriovenous; atrioventricular
AD	Autosomal dominant	AVM	Arteriovenous malformation
ADA	American Dietetic Association	AVNRT	Atrioventricular nodal reentrant tachycardia
ADH	Antidiuretic hormone	AVRT	Atrioventricular reciprocating tachycardia
ADL	Activities of daily living	BAER	Brainstem auditory evoked response
ADPKD	Autosomal dominant polycystic kidney disease	BAL	Bronchoalveolar lavage
AF	Atrial fibrillation	BBB	Bundle branch block
AFB	Acid-fast bacilli	BCS	Budd-Chiari syndrome
AFP	Alpha-fetoprotein	Benzo	Benzodiazepines
Ag	Antigen	bid	Two times a day
AG	Aminoglycoside; anion gap	bili	Bilirubin
AGN	Acute glomerulonephritis	BiPAP	Bi-level positive airway pressure
AHA	American Heart Association	BM	Bowel movement
AI	Aortic insufficiency	BMI	Body mass index
AIDS	Acquired immunodeficiency syndrome	BMP	Basic metabolic panel
AIHA	Autoimmune hemolytic anemia	BNP	B-type natriuretic peptide; brain natriuretic peptide
AIN	Acute interstitial nephritis	BP	Blood pressure
AKI	Acute kidney injury		
alb	Albumin		
alk phos	Alkaline phosphatase		
ALL	Acute lymphocytic leukemia		
ALT	Alanine aminotransferase		
AMA	Against medical advice		
AMI	Acute myocardial infarction		

BPH	Benign prostatic hypertrophy	CRC	Colorectal cancer
bpm	Beats per minute	CrCl	Creatine clearance
BSA	Body surface area	CRH	Corticotropin-releasing hormone
BUN	Blood urea nitrogen	CRP	C-reactive protein
BW	Body weight	CSD	Cat-scratch disease
bx	Biopsy	CSF	Cerebrospinal fluid
C&S	Culture and sensitivity	CSM	Carotid sinus massage
Ca	Calcium	CST	Cavernous sinus thrombosis
CA-MRSA	Community-acquired methicillin-resistant *Staphylococcus aureus*	CT	Computed tomography
CABG	Coronary artery bypass graft	CTA	Computed tomographic angiography
CAC	Coronary artery calcium	cTnI	Cardiac troponin I
CAD	Coronary artery disease; cold agglutinin disease	cTnT	Cardiac troponin T
cAMP	Cyclic adenosine monophosphate	Cv	Cardiovascular
cath	Catheterization	CVA	Cerebrovascular accident
CBC	Complete blood count	CVD	Cardiovascular disease
CBD	Common bile duct	CVP	Central venous pressure
CC	Chief complaint	CVVHD	Continuous venovenous hemodialysis
CCB	Calcium channel blocker	CXR	Chest x-ray
CCU	Coronary care unit	D&C	Dilation and curettage
CDC	Centers for Disease Control and Prevention	DBP	Diastolic blood pressure
		DBS	Deep brain stimulation
CEA	Carcinoembryonic antigen; carotid endarterectomy	d/c	Discharge; discontinue
		DFA	Direct fluorescent antibody
ceph	Cephalosporin	DI	Diabetes insipidus
CETP	Cholesteryl ester transfer protein	DIC	Disseminated intravascular coagulation
CF	Cystic fibrosis	diff	Differential
CFA	Complement-fixing antibody	DIP	Distal interphalangeal
		DKA	Diabetic ketoacidosis
CHD	Congenital heart disease	DLco	Diffusing capacity of the lung for carbon monoxide
CHF	Congestive heart failure		
CI	Cardiac index	DM	Diabetes mellitus
CIDP	Chronic inflammatory demyelinating polyneuropathy	DMARD	Disease modifying antirheumatic drug
		DNR	Do not resuscitate
CIE	Counterimmunoelectrophoresis	DOT	Directly observed therapy
CK	Creatine kinase	DPAP	Diastolic pulmonary artery pressure
CK-MB	Creatine kinase, myocardial band	DRE	Digital rectal examination
CKD	Chronic kidney disease	DS	Double strength
CLL	Chronic lymphocytic leukemia	DTRs	Deep tendon reflexes
CML	Chronic myelogenous leukemia	DVT	Deep venous thrombosis
		dx	Diagnosis
CMO	Comfort measures only	D_5W	Dextrose (5%) in water
CMP	Comprehensive metabolic panel	$D_{10}W$	Dextrose (10%) in water
		EA	Epidural abscess
CMR	Cardiac magnetic resonance	EBV	Epstein-Barr virus
		EC	Emergency contraception
CMV	Cytomegalovirus; controlled mechanical ventilation	ECF	Extracellular fluid
		ECG	Electrocardiography
		echo	Echocardiography
CNS	Central nervous system	ECM	Erythema chronicum migrans
CO	Cardiac output; carbon monoxide	EDTA	Ethylenediaminetetraacetic acid
COHgb	Carboxyhemoglobin	EEG	Electroencephalography
COPD	Chronic obstructive pulmonary disease	EF	Ejection fraction
		EGD	Esophagogastroduodenoscopy
CP	Chest pain	EIA	Enzyme-linked immunoassay
CPAP	Continuous positive airway pressure		
CPK	Creatine phosphokinase	ELISA	Enzyme-linked immunosorbent assay
CPT	Current Procedural Terminology	EMG	Electromyography
Cr, creat	Creatinine	Epi	Epinephrine

EPS	Electrophysiologic study	GVHD	Graft-versus-host disease
ERCP	Endoscopic retrograde cholangiopancreatography	gyn	Gynecologic
ESA	Erythropoiesis-stimulating agent	H&P	History and physical examination
ESR	Erythrocyte sedimentation rate	HAART	Highly active antiretroviral therapy
ESRD	End-stage renal disease	HA-MRSA	Hospital-acquired methicillin-resistant *Staphylococcus aureus*
ESWL	Extracorporeal shock wave lithotripsy	HAI	Hospital-acquired infection
ET	Essential thrombocythemia	HAV	Hepatitis A virus
EtOH	Alcohol, ethanol	HBA_{1c}	Glycosylated hemoglobin
ETT	Endotracheal tube; exercise tolerance test	HBcAg	Hepatitis B core antigen
EUS	Endoscopic ultrasonography	HBeAG	Hepatitis B e antigen
EVAR	Endovascular aneurysm repair	HBP	High blood pressure
FBS	Fasting blood sugar	HBsAg	Hepatitis B surface antigen
FDP	Fibrin degradation product	HBV	Hepatitis B virus
FENa	Fractional excretion of sodium	HCC	Hepatocellular carcinoma
FEV	Forced expiratory volume	hCG	Human chorionic gonadotropin
FFP	Fresh frozen plasma	HCM	Hypertrophic cardiomyopathy
fhx	Family history	HCO_3^-	Bicarbonate
FiO_2	Inspired oxygen concentration	Hct	Hematocrit
FISH	Fluorescence in situ hybridization	HCV	Hepatitis C virus
FNAB	Fine-needle aspiration biopsy	HDL	High-density lipoprotein
FPG	Fasting plasma glucose	HEENT	Head, eyes, ears, nose, and throat
FQ	Fluoroquinolone	HELLP	Hemolysis, elevated liver enzymes, and low platelet count
FS	Felty's syndrome		
FSH	Follicle-stimulating hormone	Hgb	Hemoglobin
FTA-ABS	Fluorescent treponemal antibody absorbed	HGE	Human granulocytic ehrlichiosis
FTI	Free thyroxine index	HHS	Hyperosmolar hyperglycemic state; hyperosmolar hyperglycemic syndrome
5-FU	5-Fluorouracil		
FUO	Fever of undetermined origin	5-HIAA	5-Hydroxyindoleacetic acid
FVC	Forced vital capacity	HIT	Heparin-induced thrombocytopenia
FVL	Factor V Leiden	HIV	Human immunodeficiency virus
fx	Fracture		
GAS	Group A streptococcus	HJR	Hepatojugular reflux
GBM	Glomerular basement membrane	HLA	Human leukocyte antigen
		HMW	High molecular weight
GBS	Guillain-Barré syndrome	h/o	History of
GCA	Giant cell arteritis	HP	Hypersensitivity pneumonitis
GCS	Glasgow Coma Scale		
GERD	Gastroesophageal reflux disease	HPI	History of present illness
		HPV	Human papillomavirus
GFR	Glomerular filtration rate	hr	Hour
GGT	γ-Glutamyltransferase	HR	Heart rate
GGTP	γ-Glutamyltranspeptidase	H2RA	Histamine H_2 receptor antagonist
GH	Growth hormone	HRCT	High-resolution computed tomography
GHRH	Growth hormone–releasing hormone		
		HRS	Hepatorenal syndrome
GI	Gastrointestinal	HRT	Hormone replacement therapy
GIP	Gastric inhibitory polypeptide		
		hs	Bedtime
GN	Glomerulonephritis	HSP	Henoch-Schönlein purpura
GnRH	Gonadotropin-releasing hormone		
		HSV	Herpes simplex virus
G6PD	Glucose-6 phosphate dehydrogenase	HTLV	Human T-lymphotropic virus
GU	Genitourinary	HTN	Hypertension

HUS	Hemolytic-uremic syndrome	LH	Luteinizing hormone
hx	History	LHRH	Luteinizing hormone–releasing hormone
I&D	Incision and drainage	LLQ	Left lower quadrant
IABP	Intra-aortic balloon pump	LMN	Lower motor neuron
IBD	Inflammatory bowel disease	LMWH	Low-molecular-weight heparin
IBS	Irritable bowel syndrome	LP	Lumbar puncture
ICD	Implantable cardioverter-defibrillator	LPFB	Left posterior fascicular block
ICH	Intracranial hemorrhage	LQTS	Long QT syndrome
ICP	Intracranial pressure	LSB	Left sternal border
ICU	Intensive care unit	LUQ	Left upper quadrant
IEP	Immunoelectrophoresis	LV	Left ventricle
IFA	Immunofluorescence assay	LVEDP	Left ventricle end-diastolic pressure
IGF	Insulin-like growth factor	LVH	Left ventricular hypertrophy
IFN	Interferon	lytes	Electrolytes
IgA	Immunoglobulin A	MAC	*Mycobacterium avium* complex
IHSS	Idiopathic hypertrophic subaortic stenosis	MAOI	Monoamine oxidase inhibitor
ILD	Interstitial lung disease	MAP	Mean arterial pressure
IM	Intramuscular	MAST	Military antishock trousers
IMV	Intermittent mandatory ventilation	MAT	Multifocal atrial tachycardia
INH	Isoniazid	MCH	Mean corpuscular hemoglobin
inpt	Inpatient		
INR	International normalized ratio	MCHC	Mean corpuscular hemoglobin concentration
IPF	Idiopathic pulmonary fibrosis	MCP	Metacarpophalangeal
IRIS	Immune reconstitution inflammatory syndrome	MCTD	Mixed connective tissue disease
IRV	Inverse ratio ventilation	MCV	Mean corpuscular volume
ITP	Immune thrombocytopenic purpura	med	Medication
IV	Intravenous	MEN	Multiple endocrine neoplasia
IVC	Inferior vena cava	mEq	Milliequivalent
IVIG	Intravenous immune globulin	mets	Metastases
		Mg	Magnesium
JNC	Joint National Committee on Prevention, Detection, Evaluation, and Treatment of High Blood Pressure	MG	Myasthenia gravis
		MGUS	Monoclonal gammopathy of uncertain significance
		MI	Myocardial infarction
JVD	Jugular venous distention	MIBG	Metaiodobenzylgua-nidine
JVP	Jugular venous pressure	min	Minute
K+	Potassium	min.	Minimal
KOH	Potassium hydroxide	MINCA	Myocardial infarction with normal coronary arteries
KS	Kaposi's sarcoma		
KUB	Kidneys, ureters, and bladder		
		MM	Multiple myeloma
LA	Left atrium	MMA	Methylmalonic acid
LAD	Left axis deviation; left anterior descending coronary artery	MMEFR	Maximal midexpiratory flow rate
		MMM	Myeloid metaplasia with myelofibrosis
LAFB	Left anterior fascicular block	mo	Month
LAP	Leukocyte alkaline phosphatase	MOM	Milk of magnesia
		MR	Mitral regurgitation
LBBB	Left bundle branch block	MRA	Magnetic resonance angiography
LCR	Ligase chain reaction		
LDH	Lactate dehydrogenase	MRCP	Magnetic resonance cholangiopancreatog-raphy
LDL	Low-density lipoprotein		
LE	Lower extremity	MRI	Magnetic resonance imaging
LES	Lower esophageal sphincter		
LFTs	Liver function tests	MRSA	Methicillin-resistant *Staphylococcus aureus*
LGV	Lymphogranuloma venereum		

MRSE	Methicillin-resistant *Staphylococcus epidermidis*	PAD	Peripheral arterial disease
MS	Mitral stenosis; multiple sclerosis	PADP	Pulmonary artery diastolic pressure
ΔMS	Change in mental status	PAN	Periarteritis nodosa
MSH	Melanocyte-stimulating hormone	p-ANCA	Perinuclear antineutrophil cytoplasmic antibody
MSO_4	Morphine	PAP	Pulmonary artery pressure
MSSA	Methicillin-sensitive *Staphylococcus aureus*	PAS	p-Aminosalicylic acid
MSSE	Methicillin-sensitive *Staphylococcus epidermidis*	PAT	Paroxysmal atrial tachycardia
MTC	Medullary thyroid carcinoma	PAWP	Pulmonary artery wedge pressure
MTX	Methotrexate	PBC	Primary biliary cirrhosis
MVP	Mitral valve prolapse	pc	After meals
$NaHCO_3^-$	Sodium bicarbonate	PCA	Patient-controlled analgesia
NAS	No added sodium		
NCS	Nerve conduction study	PCH	Paroxysmal cold hemoglobinuria
NCV	Nerve conduction velocity	PCI	Percutaneous coronary intervention
NE	Norepinephrine	PCN	Penicillin
NHL	Non-Hodgkin's lymphoma	Pco_2	Partial pressure of carbon dioxide
NG	Nasogastric	PCP	*Pneumocystis jiroveci* pneumonia
NGU	Nongonococcal urethritis		
NIPPV	Noninvasive positive-pressure ventilation	PCR	Polymerase chain reaction
nl	Normal	PCV	Pressure control ventilation
NMS	Neuroleptic malignant syndrome	PCWP	Pulmonary capillary wedge pressure
NNRTIs	Non-nucleoside reverse transcriptase inhibitors	PD	Parkinson's disease
NPH	Normal-pressure hydrocephalus	PDA	Patent ductus arteriosus
NPO	Nothing by mouth	PE	Pulmonary embolism; physical examination
NPPV	Noninvasive positive-pressure ventilation	PEA	Pulseless electrical activity
nRNP	Nuclear ribonucleoprotein	PEEP	Positive end-expiratory pressure
NRTIs	Nucleoside analogue reverse transcriptase inhibitors	PEFR	Peak expiratory flow rate
		PEG	Percutaneous endoscopic gastrostomy
NS	Normal saline	PES	Programmed electrical stimulation
NSAID	Nonsteroidal anti-inflammatory drug	PET	Positron emission tomography
NSCLC	Non–small cell lung cancer	PFTs	Pulmonary function tests
NSR	Normal sinus rhythm	pheo	Pheochromocytoma
NSTEMI	Non–ST elevation myocardial infarction	PI	Protease inhibitor
		PID	Pelvic inflammatory disease
NTG	Nitroglycerin	PIP	Proximal interphalangeal
N/V	Nausea and/or vomiting	PKD	Polycystic kidney disease
NYHA	New York Heart Association	PL	Phospholipid
O&P	Ova and parasites	Plt	Platelet
OB	Occult blood	pmhx	Past medical history
OCP	Oral contraceptive	PMI	Point of maximum impulse
OD	Overdose		
OGTT	Oral glucose tolerance test	PMN	Polymorphonuclear lymphocyte
osmo	Osmolarity; osmolality	PMR	Polymyalgia rheumatica
OTC	Over-the-counter	PN	Parenteral nutrition
PA	Pulmonary artery; posteroanterior	PND	Paroxysmal nocturnal dyspnea
PAC	Premature atrial contraction	PNH	Paroxysmal nocturnal hemoglobinuria
$Paco_2$	Partial pressure of CO_2 in arterial blood	PNS	Peripheral nervous system
Pao_2	Partial pressure of O_2 in arterial blood	PO	By mouth

Po₂	Partial pressure of oxygen	RPGN	Rapidly progressive glomerulonephritis
PO₄	Phosphate	RR	Respiratory rate
postop	Postoperative	RT	Radiation therapy
PPD	Purified protein derivative	RTA	Renal tubular acidosis
		RUQ	Right upper quadrant
PPH	Pulmonary hypertension, primary	RV	Residual volume; right ventricle
PPI	Proton pump inhibitor	RVH	Right ventricular hypertrophy
PPV	Positive predictive value; positive pressure ventilation		
		Rx	Therapy
		SA	Sinoatrial
PR	Per rectum	SAH	Subarachnoid hemorrhage
PRA	Plasma renin activity		
PRBCs	Packed red blood cells	Sao₂	Oxygen saturation
preop	Preoperative	SBP	Spontaneous bacterial peritonitis; systolic blood pressure
PRN	Pro re nata (as needed)		
PSA	Prostate-specific antigen		
PSC	Primary sclerosing cholangitis	SC	Stress cardiomyopathy; subcutaneous
PSV	Pressure support ventilation	SCLC	Small cell lung cancer
		SCM	Sternocleidomastoid
PSVT	Paroxysmal supraventricular tachycardia	SCT	Stem cell transplantation
		SEA	Spinal epidural abscess
		sec	Second
pt	Patient	sens	Sensitivity
PT	Prothrombin time	shx	Social history
PTCA	Percutaneous transluminal coronary angioplasty	SIAD	Syndrome of inappropriate antidiuresis
		SIADH	Syndrome of inappropriate antidiuretic hormone
PTH	Parathyroid hormone		
PTHrP	Parathyroid hormone–related protein		
PTT	Partial thromboplastin time	SIMV	Synchronized intermittent mandatory ventilation
PUD	Peptic ulcer disease		
PUVA	Psoralen plus ultraviolet A	SIRS	Systemic inflammatory response syndrome
PV	Polycythemia vera	SJS	Stevens-Johnson syndrome
PVC	Premature ventricular contraction	SL	Sublingual
PVD	Peripheral vascular disease	SLE	Systemic lupus erythematosus
PVR	Pulmonary vascular resistance	SMBG	Self-monitoring of blood glucose
q	Every	SNRIs	Serotonin-norepinephrine reuptake inhibitors
qd	Daily		
qid	Four times daily	SOB	Shortness of breath
RA	Rheumatoid arthritis; right atrium	s/p	Status post
		SP	Spontaneous pneumothorax
RAD	Right axis deviation		
RAI	Radioactive iodine	SPAP	Systolic pulmonary artery pressure
RAIU	Radioactive iodine uptake		
		spec	Specificity
RAP	Right arterial pressure	SPECT	Single photon emission computed tomography
RAS	Renal artery stenosis		
RBBB	Right bundle branch block	SPEP	Serum protein immunoelectrophoresis
RBC	Red blood cells		
RCT	Randomized controlled trial	SS	Serotonin syndrome; Sjögren's syndrome
RDW	Red cell distribution width	SSRIs	Selective serotonin reuptake inhibitors
RF	Rheumatoid factor	SSS	Sick sinus syndrome
rhabdo	Rhabdomyolysis	SSEP	Somatosensory evoked potential
RIA	Radioimmunoassay		
RIBA	Recombinant immunoblot assay	staph	Staphylococcus
		STAT	Immediately
RLQ	Right lower quadrant	STD	Sexually transmitted disease
RMSF	Rocky Mountain spotted fever		
		STEMI	ST elevation myocardial infarction
r/o	Rule out		
ROS	Review of systems	STI	Sexually transmitted infection
RP	Raynaud's phenomenon		

strep	Streptococcus	TURP	Transurethral resection of prostate
SV	Stroke volume	U/A	Urinalysis
SVC	Superior vena cava	UA	Unstable angina
SVR	Systemic vascular resistance	UC	Ulcerative colitis
SVT	Supraventricular tachycardia	UE	Upper extremity
		UES	Upper esophageal sphincter
sx	Symptoms	UFH	Unfractionated heparin
T_3	Triiodothyronine	UGI	Upper gastrointestinal tract
T_4	Thyroxine	UMN	Upper motor neuron
TAAD	Thoracic aortic aneurysm/dissection	URI	Upper respiratory infection
TB	Tuberculosis	U/S	Ultrasonography
TBG	Thyroxine-binding globulin	UTI	Urinary tract infection
TBNa	Total body sodium	VAT	Video-assisted thoracoscopy
TBW	Total body water	VATS	Video-assisted thoracoscopic surgery
TD	Tardive dyskinesia	VC	Vital capacity
TEE	Transesophageal echocardiography	VDRL	Venereal Disease Research Laboratory (test for syphilis)
TF	Tissue factor	$\dot{V}_E$	Minute ventilation
TG	Triglyceride	VEP	Visual evoked potential
THBR	Thyroid hormone–binding ratio	VF	Ventricular fibrillation
TIA	Transient ischemic attack	VIP	Vasoactive intestinal peptide
TIBC	Total iron binding capacity	VL	Viral load
tid	Three times daily	V/Q	Ventilation-perfusion scan
TIPS	Transjugular intrahepatic portosystemic shunt	VS	Vital signs
TLC	Total lung capacity	VSD	Ventricular septal defect
TMP-SMZ	Trimethoprim-sulfamethoxazole	VT	Ventricular tachycardia
		Vt	Tidal volume
TNF	Tumor necrosis factor	VTE	Venous thromboembolism
TPA	Tissue plasminogen activator	vWD	von Willebrand disease
TPN	Total parenteral nutrition	vWF	von Willebrand factor
TR	Tricuspid regurgitation	w/	With
TRH	Thyrotropin-releasing hormone	WBC	White blood cell count
TSH	Thyroid-stimulating hormone	WHO	World Health Organization
TSI	Thyroid-stimulating immunoglobulin	wk	Week
TSS	Toxic shock syndrome (alph order)	w/o	Without
		WPW	Wolff-Parkinson-White syndrome
TT	Thrombin time	wt	Weight
TTE	Transthoracic echocardiography	w/up	Workup
TTG	Tissue transglutaminase	w/v	Weight/volume
TTP	Thrombotic thrombocytopenic purpura	ZE	Zollinger-Ellison (syndrome)

A. CHARTING

1 ADMISSION ORDERS

A, Admit to: Indicate ward where pt is being admitted and attending physician (e.g., coronary care unit, Dr. Smith's service).

B, Because: Indicate admitting dx (e.g., chest pain).

C, Condition: Specify pt's general condition (stable, fair, poor, critical).

Code status: Specify DNR, full code, CMO.

Consults:

D, Diet: Specify whether regular, clear liquids, NAS, ADA, low cholesterol, other.

DVT prophylaxis:

A, Allergies: Indicate medications (including OTC medications) and specific food products to which the pt has experienced an allergic reaction.

Activity: Specify bed rest, ad lib, bathroom privileges.

V, Vital signs: Specify frequency (e.g., qid, q4h); also indicate any special nursing orders (e.g., VS and neurologic signs q2h × 24h, then q4h if stable).

I, IV fluids: Specify any IV solutions and rate of infusion.

D, Diagnostic tests: Specify laboratory tests, x-rays, ECG, special tests.

Drugs: Indicate medication, dose, frequency, special restrictions (e.g., atenolol 50 mg PO qd; if HR <50 bpm, hold atenolol and notify house).

2 LAB SHORTHAND NOTATION

See Figure 1-1.

3 DICTATING THE H&P

1. **VS:** BP, pulse, respirations, temperature.
2. **General description:** The pt is a (age, sex) who looks her stated age, is pleasant, appears to be well nourished, and seems in a good state of health.
3. **Skin:** The skin is warm and dry; turgor is adequate; color is nl. No icterus, purpura, rash, or unusual pigmentation is noted. Hair is nl in appearance, distribution, and texture.
4. **Lymph nodes:** There is no cervical, supraclavicular, axillary, epitrochlear, or inguinal adenopathy.
5. **HEENT:**
   a. Head: It is normocephalic and atraumatic; no lesions are noted.
   b. Eyes: Cornea is without lesions, conjunctiva is clear, sclera is white. Pupils are equal, measuring approximately 3 mm in diameter, round, and reactive to light and accommodation. Extraocular movements are within nl limits without any nystagmus or strabismus. Fundi appear benign. Disks are well delineated. There are no hemorrhages or exudates. Visual acuity is 20/20 bilaterally, and visual fields are within nl limits.
   c. Ears: Ears are nl in appearance. Auditory canal appears clean and without lesions. The tympanic membranes are intact. Hearing is adequate.
   d. Nose: Septum appears to be within nl limits and without deviation. Nasal mucosa appears pink and without any abnl discharge. No nasal polyps or other lesions are noted. Frontal and maxillary sinuses are nontender.
   e. Mouth and throat: Lips are without cyanosis or pallor. Buccal mucosa is nl in appearance. Teeth appear to be in good condition. Tongue shows no lesions or tremor. Pharyngeal mucosa is pink and does not reveal any lesions, exudates, erythema, or evidence of inflammation. Gag reflex is intact.
6. **Neck:** Neck is supple. Full range of motion is present. There is no evidence of tracheal deviation, JVD, or lymphadenopathy. Carotid pulses are 2+, equal bilaterally, and without bruits. Carotid upstroke is within nl limits. Thyroid gland is nl in size; its palpation does not reveal any nodules or masses.
7. **Back:** Spinal curvature is nl; no scoliosis, kyphosis, or tenderness is present. Full range of motion is present.
8. **Chest:** Thorax is symmetric. Full expansion is noted bilaterally. Anterior-posterior diameter is within nl limits.

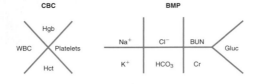

CBC

BMP

COAGS

Others

FIGURE 1-1. Lab shorthand notation.

9. **Lungs:** Fremitus is equal bilaterally. Lung fields are resonant throughout. Breath sounds and voice sounds are nl. There are no rales or rhonchi.

10. **Heart:** Palpation reveals no heaves or thrills. The PMI is medial to the midclavicular line, fourth intercostal space. Auscultation reveals S_1, S_2 of nl intensity. There are no S_3, S_4, rubs, clicks, or other abnl heart sounds. Heart rate is approximately 70 bpm and rhythm is regular.

11. **Breasts** (female pt): Breasts are symmetric and have a nl contour. Skin is of nl color and appearance; there is no edema, ulceration, or erythema. Nipples are of nl size and shape; there is no nipple retraction, ulceration, or discharge. Palpation does not reveal any tenderness or masses.

12. **Abdomen:** Abdomen is of nl size and contour. No capillary dilatations, skin lesions, or surgical scars are noted. Auscultation reveals normoactive bowel sounds and no abdominal bruits. Palpation reveals no abdominal tenderness, guarding, or masses. The liver edge is felt approximately 1 inch below the right costal margin; it is flat, sharp, and smooth. The liver percusses to approximately 8 to 10 cm in total span. The spleen is not palpable.

13. **Rectal examination:** Rectal examination reveals no external anal lesions. Sphincter tone is nl. There are no internal or external hemorrhoids. Rectal mucosa appears nl, and no nodules or masses are present. Stool is brown and (–) for occult blood. Male pt: Prostate is nl in size, no nodules.

14. **Genitalia:** Inspection reveals nl distribution of pubic hair. Female pt: Clitoris and labia are without lesions. Internal examination with speculum reveals nl vaginal wall. The cervical os is well visualized. No lesions or discharges are noted. A specimen was obtained for cervical cytology. Bimanual examination reveals no cervical tenderness or masses. Uterus and ovaries are nontender and of nl size.

15. **Inguinal area:** No lymphadenopathy is noted. Femoral pulses are 2+ and equal bilaterally. Auscultation reveals no femoral bruits.

16. **Extremities:** There is no clubbing, cyanosis, or edema. Brachial, radial, popliteal, dorsalis pedis, and posterior tibialis pulses are 2+ and equal bilaterally. Musculoskeletal examination reveals no joint deformities and full range of motion. No bone, joint, or muscle tenderness is noted.

17. **Neurologic:** Pt is alert and oriented to time, person, and place. Cranial nerves II to XII are within nl limits. Speech, memory, and expression are within nl limits. Muscle strength is 5/5 in both upper and lower extremities. No muscle atrophy or involuntary movement is noted. Testing of cerebellar function reveals nl gait, (–) Romberg test result, and good coordination in finger-to-nose, heel-to-shin,

and alternate motion testing. Sensory is intact to light touch, pain, and vibratory stimuli. No focal motor or sensory deficits are present. Deep tendon reflexes are 2+ and equal bilaterally.

4 PROGRESS (SOAP) NOTE

S, Subjective: observations, pt complaints.

O, Objective: description of physical findings and recording of laboratory, x-ray, or ECG data.

A, Assessment: analysis of data and tentative dx.

P, Plan: diagnostic studies and therapeutic regimen.

5 CONSULT NOTE

- Date/time
- Reason for consult
- HPI
- Current medications
- Physical exam
- Impression
- Recommendations

6 DISCHARGE SUMMARY

The discharge summary should contain only essential information about the investigation and Rx of the pt's illness. It should briefly describe the following:

- Why the pt entered the hospital: a brief statement of the CC, admission dx, and HPI.
- The pertinent laboratory, x-ray, and physical findings; (−) findings may be as pertinent as (+) findings.
- The medical or surgical Rx, including the pt's response, any complications, and consultations; a rationale for what was or was not done.
- The pt's condition when discharged (ambulation, self-care, ability to work).
- Instructions given on continuing care, such as medication by name and specific dosage, diet, type and amount of physical activity, other therapeutic measures, referrals, and appointments.

7 PRONOUNCING DEATH WHILE ON CALL

The legal criteria of death fall within state jurisdiction. One should become familiar with the accepted definition of death in one's own state. When called to pronounce a pt dead, the following steps should be followed:

1. Identify the pt (examine hospital ID tag on the pt's wrist).
2. Examine pt for:
   a. Response to verbal or tactile stimuli (none)
   b. Spontaneous respiration (none)
   c. Heart sounds and pulses (absent)
   d. Pupillary response (pupils fixed and dilated)
3. Document the time the pt was pronounced dead (legal time of death).
4. Notify attending physician (if not already done by the nursing staff) and inquire whether family requests autopsy. Notify the organ bank for possible organ donation, if this is consistent with your hospital's policy.
5. Document findings in pt's chart (e.g., "Called by charge nurse to pronounce Mr. John Smith dead. Pt examined, unresponsive to verbal or tactile stimuli, no spontaneous respiration noted, heart sounds not audible, pulses absent, pupils fixed and dilated. Pt pronounced dead at 11:10 pm. Attending notified. Next of kin to be contacted by attending.") The attending will often not be available, and you will be asked to notify the next of kin.
   a. Familiarize yourself with the pt's medical hx and mode of death.
   b. Identify yourself to the family in a humble and caring manner and inform them that their next of kin has expired. Inform them of the time that the pt was pronounced dead, and always try to comfort them that their relative died peacefully.
   c. If it is not clear from the pt's records, inquire whether the family requests an autopsy.
   d. Ask the next of kin whether the family will be coming to the hospital to view the body before it is transported to the hospital morgue. Notify the charge nurse of their decision.

8 DISCHARGE AGAINST MEDICAL ADVICE (AMA)

1. Discharge AMA, in which a pt chooses to leave the hospital before the treating physician recommends discharge, occurs in 2% of medical admissions.

2. Risk factors are h/o substance or EtOH abuse, lack of insurance, younger age, and male sex.
3. Strategies for preventing AMA discharges include proactively addressing substance abuse issues and recognizing and treating psychological factors. Motivational interviewing, which relies on the principle of pt-centered interviewing and use of nonjudgmental empathetic questioning, is an effective modality in lowering the risk of discharge AMA.
4. If prevention of discharge AMA is not successful, informed consent is a crucial element in managing an AMA discharge. An informed decision means that the decision has been made by the pt in consultation with the physician without being coerced and with a full understanding of the risks, benefits, and alternatives of the decision.
5. The evaluation of the pt being discharged AMA should include the following:
   a. Does the pt understand and appreciate the admission dx, prognosis, and risks and benefits of leaving the hospital? It is important to document that the pt understands the information, terminology, and language (has adequate health literacy).
   b. Is the pt aware of alternative Rxs outside of the hospital and associated risks and benefits?
   c. Is the pt able to make and communicate his/her choice?
   d. Can the pt articulate a reason for the choice that is consistent with his/her choice?
6. If a pt is deemed to be without decision-making capacity and has no surrogate, consultation with a psychiatrist may be helpful to keep the pt in the hospital against his/her will.
7. Managing an AMA discharge also includes ensuring that the discharge is as safe as possible under the circumstances and helping the pt follow up after discharge.

Reference
Alfandre DJ: "I'm going home": Discharges against medical advice, *Mayo Clin Proc* 84:255–260, 2009.

B. EVALUATING THE LABS

This section covers >150 labs. Each test is approached with the following format:
1. Lab test.
2. Normal (nl) range in adult pts.
3. Common abnormalities (e.g., [+] test result, ↑ or ↓ value).
4. Causes of abnl result.

The nl ranges may differ slightly, depending on the laboratory. The reader should be aware of the "nl range" of the particular laboratory performing the test. Every attempt has been made to present current laboratory test data with emphasis on practical considerations. Lab tests do not make diagnoses, physicians do. As such, any lab results should be integrated with the complete clinical picture and radiographic studies (if needed) to make a dx.

ACE LEVEL; SEE ANGIOTENSIN-CONVERTING ENZYME

ACETONE (SERUM OR PLASMA)
Nl: (−)
↑: DKA, starvation, isopropanol ingestion.

ACETYLCHOLINE RECEPTOR (ACHR) ANTIBODY
Nl: <0.03 nmol/L.
↑: myasthenia gravis. Changes in AChR concentration correlate w/the clinical severity of myasthenia gravis after Rx and during Rx w/prednisone and immunosuppressants. False-(+) AChR Ab results may be found in pts w/Eaton-Lambert syndrome.

ACID PHOSPHATASE (SERUM)
Nl range: enzymatic, prostatic, 0-5.5 U/L; enzymatic, total, 2-12 U/L.
↑: carcinoma of prostate, other neoplasms (breast, bone), Paget's disease of bone, hemolysis, MM, osteogenesis imperfecta, malignant invasion of bone, Gaucher's disease, myeloproliferative disorders, prostatic palpation or surgery, hyperparathyroidism, liver disease, chronic renal failure, ITP.

ACTIVATED CLOTTING TIME (ACT)

Nl: This test is used to determine the dose of protamine sulfate to reverse the effect of heparin as an anticoagulant during angioplasty, cardiac surgery, and hemodialysis. The accepted goal during cardiopulmonary bypass surgery is usually 400 to 500 seconds.

ACTIVATED PARTIAL THROMBOPLASTIN TIME (APTT); SEE PARTIAL THROMBOPLASTIN TIME

ADRENOCORTICOTROPIC HORMONE (ACTH)

Nl: 9-52 pg/mL.
↑: Addison's disease, ectopic ACTH-producing tumors, congenital adrenal hyperplasia, Nelson's syndrome, pituitary-dependent Cushing's disease.
↓: secondary adrenocortical insufficiency, hypopituitarism, adrenal adenoma or adrenal carcinoma.

ALANINE AMINOTRANSFERASE (ALT, SGPT)

Nl range: 8-35 U/L (female); 10-40 U/L (male).
↑: liver disease (e.g., hepatitis, cirrhosis, Reye's syndrome), EtOH abuse, drugs (e.g., acetaminophen, statins, NSAIDs, abx, anabolic steroids, narcotics, heparin, labetalol, amiodarone, chlorpromazine, phenytoin), hepatic congestion, infectious mononucleosis, liver mets, MI, myocarditis, severe muscle trauma, dermatomyositis or polymyositis, muscular dystrophy, malignant neoplasms, renal and pulmonary infarction, convulsions, eclampsia, dehydration (relative ↑), Chinese herbs.
↓: azotemia, advanced malnutrition, chronic renal dialysis, chronic alcoholic liver disease, metronidazole therapy.

ALBUMIN (SERUM)

Nl range: 4-6 g/dL.
↑: dehydration (relative), IV alb infusion.
↓: liver disease, nephrotic syndrome, poor nutritional status, rapid IV hydration, protein-losing enteropathies (IBD), severe burns, neoplasia, chronic inflammatory diseases, pregnancy, prolonged immobilization, lymphomas, hypervitaminosis A, chronic GN.

ALDOSTERONE (PLASMA)

Nl: 3-16 ng/dL (adult supine); 7-30 ng/dL (adult upright); 200-800 ng/dL (adrenal vein).
↑: aldosterone-secreting adenoma, bilateral adrenal hyperplasia, secondary aldosteronism (diuretics, CHF, laxatives, nephritic syndrome, cirrhosis w/ascites, Bartter's syndrome, pregnancy, starvation).
↓: Addison's disease, renin deficiency, Turner's syndrome, DM, isolated aldosterone deficiency, post–acute EtOH intoxication (hangover phase).

ALKALINE PHOSPHATASE (SERUM)

Nl range: 30-120 U/L.
↑: biliary obstruction, cirrhosis (particularly PBC), liver disease (hepatitis, infiltrative liver diseases, fatty metamorphosis), Paget's disease of bone, osteitis deformans, rickets, osteomalacia, hypervitaminosis D, hyperparathyroidism, hyperthyroidism, UC, bowel perforation, bone mets, healing fxs, bone neoplasms, acromegaly, infectious mononucleosis, CMV infections, sepsis, pulmonary infarction, hypernephroma, leukemia, myelofibrosis, MM, drugs (estrogens, alb, erythromycin and other abx, cholestasis-producing drugs [phenothiazines]), pregnancy, puberty, postmenopausal women.
↓: hypothyroidism, pernicious anemia, hypophosphatemia, hypervitaminosis D, malnutrition.

ALPHA₁-FETOPROTEIN (SERUM)

Nl range: 0-20 ng/mL.
↑: hepatocellular carcinoma (usually values >1000 ng/mL), germinal neoplasms (testis, ovary, mediastinum, retroperitoneum), liver disease (alcoholic cirrhosis, acute hepatitis, chronic active hepatitis, fetal anencephaly, spina bifida, basal cell carcinoma, breast carcinoma, pancreatic carcinoma, gastric carcinoma, retinoblastoma, esophageal atresia.

ALT; SEE ALANINE AMINOTRANSFERASE

ALUMINUM (SERUM)
Nl range: 0-6 ng/mL.
↑: chronic renal failure on dialysis, parenteral nutrition, industrial exposure.

AMA; SEE MITOCHONDRIAL ANTIBODY

AMMONIA (SERUM)
Nl range: 15-45 μm/dL (adults); 29-70 μm/dL (children).
↑: hepatic failure, hepatic encephalopathy, Reye's syndrome, portacaval shunt, drugs (diuretics, polymyxin B, methicillin).
↓: drugs (neomycin, lactulose), renal failure.

AMYLASE (SERUM)
Nl range: 0-130 U/L.
↑: acute pancreatitis, macroamylasemia, salivary gland inflammation, mumps; pancreatic neoplasm, abscess, pseudocyst, ascites; perforated peptic ulcer; intestinal obstruction, intestinal infarction; acute cholecystitis, appendicitis, ruptured ectopic pregnancy, peritonitis, burns, DKA, renal insufficiency; drugs (morphine); carcinomatosis of lung, esophagus, ovary; acute ethanol ingestion; prostate tumors; after ERCP; bulimia, anorexia nervosa.
↓: advanced chronic pancreatitis, hepatic necrosis, cystic fibrosis.

AMYLASE, URINE; SEE URINE AMYLASE

ANA; SEE ANTINUCLEAR ANTIBODY

ANCA; SEE ANTINEUTROPHIL CYTOPLASMIC ANTIBODY

ANGIOTENSIN II
Nl: 10-60 pg/mL.
↑: HTN, CHF, cirrhosis, renin-secreting renal tumor, volume depletion.
↓: ACEIs, ARB drugs, primary aldosteronism, Cushing's syndrome.

ANGIOTENSIN-CONVERTING ENZYME (ACE LEVEL)
Nl range: <40 nmol/mL/min.
↑: sarcoidosis, PBC, alcoholic liver disease, hyperthyroidism, hyperparathyroidism, DM, amyloidosis, MM, lung disease (asbestosis, silicosis, berylliosis, allergic alveolitis, coccidioidomycosis), Gaucher's disease, leprosy.
↓: ACEI Rx.

ANION GAP
Nl range: 9-14 mEq/L.
↑: lactic acidosis, ketoacidosis (DKA, alcoholic starvation), uremia (chronic renal failure), ingestion of toxins (paraldehyde, methanol, salicylates, ethylene glycol), hyperosmolar nonketotic coma, abx (carbenicillin).
↓: hypoalbuminemia, severe hypermagnesemia, IgG myeloma, lithium toxicity, laboratory error (falsely ↓ Na^+ or overestimation of HCO_3^- or chloride), hypercalcemia of parathyroid origin, abx (e.g., polymyxin).

ANTICARDIOLIPIN ANTIBODY (ACA)
Nl range: (–) Test includes detection of IgG, IgM, and IgA Ab to phospholipid, cardiolipin.
Present in: antiphospholipid Ab syndrome, chronic HCV infection.

ANTICOAGULANT; SEE CIRCULATING ANTICOAGULANT

ANTIDIURETIC HORMONE (ADH)
Nl: 295-300 mOsm/kg; 4-12 pg/mL.
↑: SIADH, antipsychotic meds, ectopic ADH from systemic neoplasm, GBS, CNS infections, brain tumors, nephrogenic diabetes insipidus.
↓: central diabetes insipidus, nephritic syndrome, psychogenic polydipsia, demeclocycline, lithium, phenytoin, EtOH.

ANTI-DNA
6 **Nl range:** absent.
Present in: SLE, chronic active hepatitis, infectious mononucleosis, biliary cirrhosis.

ANTI-DS DNA
Nl: <25 U.
↑: SLE.

ANTI–GLOMERULAR BASEMENT ANTIBODY; SEE GLOMERULAR BASEMENT MEMBRANE ANTIBODY

ANTI-HCV; SEE HEPATITIS C ANTIBODY

ANTIMITOCHONDRIAL ANTIBODY (AMA)
Nl range: <1:20 titer.
↑: PBC (85%-95%), chronic active hepatitis (25%-30%), cryptogenic cirrhosis (25%-30%).

ANTINEUTROPHIL CYTOPLASMIC ANTIBODY (ANCA)
(+) test result:
• **Cytoplasmic pattern (cANCA):** (+) in Wegener's granulomatosis.
• **Perinuclear pattern (pANCA):** (+) in IBD, PBC, PSC, autoimmune chronic active hepatitis, crescentic GN.

ANTINUCLEAR ANTIBODY (ANA)
Nl range: <1:20 titer.
(+) test: SLE (more significant if titer >1:160), drugs (phenytoin, ethosuximide, primidone, methyldopa, hydralazine, carbamazepine, PCN, procainamide, chlorpromazine, griseofulvin, thiazides), chronic active hepatitis, age >60 years (particularly age >80 years), RA, scleroderma, MCTD, necrotizing vasculitis, Sjögren's syndrome.

ANTIPHOSPHOLIPID ANTIBODY; SEE LUPUS ANTICOAGULANT

ANTI-RNP ANTIBODY; SEE EXTRACTABLE NUCLEAR ANTIGEN

ANTI–SCL-70
Nl: absent.
↑: scleroderma.

ANTI-SM (ANTI-SMITH) ANTIBODY; SEE EXTRACTABLE NUCLEAR ANTIGEN

ANTI–SMOOTH MUSCLE ANTIBODY; SEE SMOOTH MUSCLE ANTIBODY

ANTITHROMBIN III
Nl range: 81%-120% of nl activity; 17-30 mg/dL.
↓: hereditary deficiency of antithrombin III, DIC, PE, cirrhosis, thrombolytic Rx, chronic liver failure, postsurgery, third trimester of pregnancy, OCPs, nephrotic syndrome, IV heparin >3 days, sepsis, acute leukemia, carcinoma, thrombophlebitis.
↑: warfarin Rx, after MI.

APOLIPOPROTEIN A-1 (APO A-1)
Nl: recommended > 120 mg/dL.
↑: familial hyperalphalipoproteinemia, statins, niacin, estrogens, weight loss, familial CETP deficiency.
↓: familial hypoalphalipoproteinemia, Tangier disease, diuretics, androgens, cigarette smoking, hepatocellular disorders, chronic renal failure, nephritic syndrome, coronary heart disease, cholestasis.

APOLIPOPROTEIN B (APO B)
Nl: desirable <100 mg/dL; high risk >120 mg/dL.
↑: high-saturated fat diet, high-cholesterol diet, hyperapobetalipoproteinemia, familial combined hyperlipidemia, anabolic steroids, diuretics, β-blockers, corticosteroids, progestins, diabetes, hypothyroidism, chronic renal failure, liver disease, Cushing's syndrome, coronary heart disease.
↓: statins, niacin, low-cholesterol diet, malnutrition, abetalipoproteinemia, hypobetalipoproteinemia, hyperthyroidism.

ARTERIAL BLOOD GASES (ABGS)

Nl range:
- Po_2: 75-100 mm Hg
- Pco_2: 35-45 mm Hg
- HCO_3^-: 24-28 mEq/L
- pH: 7.35-7.45

Abnl values: Refer to individual acid-base disturbances in Chapter 9.

ASPARTATE AMINOTRANSFERASE (AST, SGOT)

Nl range: 0-35 U/L.

↑: liver disease (hepatitis, hemochromatosis, cirrhosis, Reye's syndrome, Wilson's disease), EtOH abuse, drugs (acetaminophen, statins, NSAIDs, ACEIs, heparin, labetalol, phenytoin, amiodarone, chlorpromazine), hepatic congestion, infectious mononucleosis, MI, myocarditis, severe muscle trauma, dermatomyositis and polymyositis, muscular dystrophy, malignant neoplasia, renal and pulmonary infarction, convulsions, eclampsia.

↓: uremia, vitamin B_6 deficiency.

BASOPHIL COUNT

Nl range: 0.4%-1% of total WBCs; 40-100/mm³.

↑: inflammatory processes, leukemia, PV, Hodgkin's lymphoma, hemolytic anemia, after splenectomy, myeloid metaplasia, myxedema.

↓: stress, hypersensitivity reaction, steroids, pregnancy, hyperthyroidism.

BICARBONATE

Nl: 21-28 mEq/L (arterial); 22-29 mEq/L (venous).

↑: metabolic alkalosis, compensated respiratory acidosis, diuretics, corticosteroids, laxative abuse.

↓: metabolic acidosis, compensated respiratory alkalosis; acetazolamide, cyclosporine, cholestyramine, methanol or ethylene glycol poisoning.

BILE ACID BREATH TEST

Nl: The test determines the radioactivity of $^{14}CO_2$ in breath samples at 2 and 4 hr.
- 2 hr after dose: 0.11 ± 0.14
- 4 hr after dose: 0.52 ± 0.09

↑: GI bacterial overgrowth, cimetidine.

BILIRUBIN, DIRECT (CONJUGATED BILIRUBIN)

Nl range: 0-0.2 mg/dL.

↑: hepatocellular disease, biliary obstruction, drug-induced cholestasis, hereditary disorders (Dubin-Johnson syndrome, Rotor's syndrome), advanced neoplastic states.

BILIRUBIN, INDIRECT (UNCONJUGATED BILIRUBIN)

Nl range: 0-1.0 mg/dL.

↑: hemolysis, liver disease (hepatitis, cirrhosis, neoplasm), hepatic congestion caused by CHF, hereditary disorders (Gilbert's disease, Crigler-Najjar syndrome).

BILIRUBIN, TOTAL

Nl range: 0-1.0 mg/dL.

↑: liver disease (hepatitis, cirrhosis, cholangitis, neoplasm, biliary obstruction, infectious mononucleosis), hereditary disorders (Gilbert's disease, Dubin-Johnson syndrome), drugs (steroids, diphenylhydantoin, phenothiazines, PCN, erythromycin, clindamycin, captopril, amphotericin B, sulfonamides, azathioprine, isoniazid, 5-aminosalicylic acid, allopurinol, methyldopa, indomethacin, halothane, OCPs, procainamide, tolbutamide, labetalol), hemolysis, pulmonary embolism or infarct, hepatic congestion resulting from CHF.

BLEEDING TIME (MODIFIED IVY METHOD)

Nl range: 2-9.5 minutes.

↑: thrombocytopenia, capillary wall abnormalities, Plt abnormalities (Bernard-Soulier disease, Glanzmann's disease), drugs (ASA, warfarin, anti-inflammatory medications, streptokinase, urokinase, dextran, β-lactam abx, moxalactam), DIC, cirrhosis, uremia, myeloproliferative disorders, vWD.

Comments: The bleeding time test as a method to evaluate suspected hemostatic incompetence has been replaced in many laboratories by Plt function analysis (PFA-100 assay). The bleeding time test's ability to predict excessive bleeding in clinical situations, such as surgery or invasive diagnostic procedures, is poor. It may play a limited residual role in the evaluation of suspected hereditary disorders of hemostasis.

BNP; SEE B-TYPE NATRIURETIC PEPTIDE

BRCA1, BRCA2

Test involves the detection of carriers of mutations in the genes characterized by predisposition to breast and ovarian cancers. These mutations occur in about 1 in 300 to 500 women in the general population and in about 2% of Ashkenazi Jewish women. Women found to carry the mutation should undergo earlier and more intensive surveillance for breast cancer. Pre-test counseling should be provided before genetic testing. The U.S. Preventive Services Task Force recommends screening in the following:

1. Non-Ashkenazi women:
   a. Two first-degree relatives w/breast or ovarian cancer (including one diagnosed ≤50 years of age).
   b. ≥3 first- or second-degree relatives w/breast cancer.
   c. Both breast cancer and ovarian cancer among first- and second-degree relatives.
   d. A first-degree relative w/bilateral breast cancer.
   e. ≥2 first- or second-degree relatives w/ovarian cancer.
   f. A first- or second-degree relative w/both breast and ovarian cancer.
   g. A male relative w/breast cancer.
2. Ashkenazi women:
   a. Any first-degree relative w/breast or ovarian cancer.
   b. 2 second-degree relatives on the same side of the family w/breast or ovarian cancer.

BREATH HYDROGEN TEST

NI: This test is for bacterial overgrowth H_2 excretion; fasting: 4.6 ± 5.1; after lactulose: early ↑ <12. Lactulose usually results in a colonic response >30 minutes after ingestion.

↑: a high fasting breath H_2 level and an ↑ of at least 12 ppm within 30 minutes after lactulose challenge indicate bacterial overgrowth in the small intestine. The ↑ must precede the colonic response.

False (+): accelerated gastric emptying, laxative use.

False (−): use of abx and pts who are non–hydrogen producers.

B-TYPE NATRIURETIC PEPTIDE (BNP)

NI range: up to 100 μg/L. Natriuretic peptides are secreted to regulate fluid volume, BP, and electrolyte balance. They have activity in the central and peripheral nervous system. In humans, the main source of circulatory BNP is the heart ventricles.

↑: heart failure. This test is useful to differentiate heart failure from COPD manifesting w/dyspnea. Levels are also ↑ in asymptomatic left ventricular dysfunction, arterial and pulmonary HTN, cardiac hypertrophy, valvular heart disease, arrhythmia, and ACS.

BUN; SEE UREA NITROGEN

C3; SEE COMPLEMENT C3

C4; SEE COMPLEMENT C4

CALCITONIN (SERUM)

NI range: <100 pg/mL.

↑: medullary carcinoma of the thyroid (particularly if level >1500 pg/mL), carcinoma of the breast, apudomas, carcinoids, renal failure, thyroiditis.

CALCIUM (SERUM)

NI range: 8.8-10.3 mg/dL.

Abnl values: See "Hypocalcemia" and "Hypercalcemia" in Chapter 5.

CAPTOPRIL STIMULATION TEST

NI: The test is performed by giving 25 mg captopril PO after an overnight fast. The pt should be seated during the test. After captopril, aldosterone <15 ng/dL, renin >2 ng angiotensin I/mL/hr.

Interpretation: In pts w/primary aldosteronism, plasma aldosterone remains high and PRA remains low after captopril.

CARBON DIOXIDE, PARTIAL PRESSURE

NI: 35-48 mm Hg (males); 32-45 mm Hg (females).

↑: respiratory acidosis.

↓: respiratory alkalosis.

CARBON MONOXIDE; SEE CARBOXYHEMOGLOBIN

CARBOXYHEMOGLOBIN

Nl range: saturation of Hgb <2%; smokers <9% (coma, 50%; death, 80%).
↑: smoking, exposure to smoking, exposure to automobile exhaust fumes, malfunctioning gas-burning appliances.

CARCINOEMBRYONIC ANTIGEN (CEA)

Nl range: 0-2.5 ng/mL (nonsmokers); 0-5 ng/mL (smokers).
↑: colorectal carcinomas, pancreatic carcinomas, and metastatic disease usually produce higher elevations (>20 ng/mL); carcinomas of the esophagus, stomach, small intestine, liver, breast, ovary, lung, and thyroid usually produce lesser elevations; benign conditions (smoking, IBD, hypothyroidism, cirrhosis, pancreatitis, infections) usually produce levels <10 ng/mL.

CARDIO CRP; SEE C-REACTIVE PROTEIN

CAROTENE (SERUM)

Nl range: 50-250 µg/dL.
↑: carotenemia, chronic nephritis, DM, hypothyroidism, nephrotic syndrome, hyperlipidemia.
↓: fat malabsorption, steatorrhea, pancreatic insufficiency, lack of carotenoids in diet, high fever, liver disease.

CBC; SEE COMPLETE BLOOD COUNT (CBC)

CD4+ T-LYMPHOCYTE COUNT (CD4+ T CELLS)

Calculated as total WBC × % lymphocytes × % lymphocytes stained w/CD4.

This test is used primarily to evaluate immune dysfunction in HIV infection. It is useful as a prognostic indicator and as a criterion for initiation of prophylaxis for several opportunistic infections that are sequelae of HIV infection. Progressive depletion of CD4+ T lymphocytes is associated w/ ↑ likelihood of clinical complications. Adolescents and adults w/HIV infection are classified as having AIDS if their CD4+ lymphocyte count is <200/µL or if their CD4+ T-lymphocyte percentage is <14%. HIV-infected pts whose CD4+ count is <200/µL and who acquire certain infectious diseases or malignant neoplasms are also classified as having AIDS. Corticosteroids ↓ CD4+ T-cell % and absolute number.

CEA; SEE CARCINOEMBRYONIC ANTIGEN (CEA)

CERULOPLASMIN (SERUM)

Nl range: 20-35 mg/dL.
↑: pregnancy, estrogens, OCPs, neoplastic diseases (leukemias, Hodgkin's lymphoma, carcinomas), inflammatory states, SLE, PBC, RA.
↓: Wilson's disease (values often <10 mg/dL), nephrotic syndrome, advanced liver disease, malabsorption, TPN, Menkes' syndrome.

CHLAMYDIA GROUP ANTIBODY SEROLOGIC TEST

Test description: Acute and convalescent serum samples are drawn 2 to 4 weeks apart. A fourfold ↑ in titer between acute and convalescent sera is necessary for confirmation. A single titer >1:64 is considered indicative of infection.

CHLORIDE (SERUM)

Nl range: 95-105 mEq/L.
↑: dehydration, Na+ loss > chloride loss, respiratory alkalosis, excessive infusion of NS solution, cystic fibrosis, hyperparathyroidism, renal tubular disease, metabolic acidosis, prolonged diarrhea, acetazolamide administration, diabetes insipidus, ureterosigmoidostomy.
↓: vomiting, gastric suction, primary aldosteronism, CHF, SIADH, Addison's disease, salt-losing nephritis, continuous infusion of D_5W, thiazide diuretic administration, diaphoresis, diarrhea, burns, DKA.

CHLORIDE (SWEAT)

Nl: 0-40 mmol/L.
Borderline/indeterminate: 41-60 mmol/L.
Consistent with cystic fibrosis: >60 mmol/L.
False low results: can occur w/edema, excessive sweating, and hypoproteinemia.

CHOLESTEROL, LOW-DENSITY LIPOPROTEIN; SEE LOW-DENSITY LIPOPROTEIN (LDL) CHOLESTEROL

CHOLESTEROL, HIGH-DENSITY LIPOPROTEIN; SEE HIGH-DENSITY LIPOPROTEIN (HDL) CHOLESTEROL

CHOLESTEROL, TOTAL

Nl range: Generally <200 mg/dL.
↑: primary hypercholesterolemia, biliary obstruction, DM, nephrotic syndrome, hypothyroidism, PBC, diet high in cholesterol and total and saturated fat, third trimester of pregnancy, drugs (steroids, phenothiazines, OCPs).
↓: use of lipid-lowering agents (statins, niacin, ezetimibe, cholestyramine, colesevelam); starvation, malabsorption, abetalipoproteinemia, hyperthyroidism; hepatic failure, carcinoma, infection, inflammation.

CHORIONIC GONADOTROPINS, HUMAN (SERUM)

Nl range, serum: <0.8 IU/L (female, premenopausal); <3.3 IU/L (female, postmenopausal); <0.7 IU/L (male).
↑: pregnancy, choriocarcinoma, gestational trophoblastic neoplasia (including molar gestations), placental site trophoblastic tumors; human antimouse antibodies (HAMA) can produce false serum assay for hCG.
The principal use of this test is to diagnose pregnancy. The concentration of hCG ↑ significantly during the initial 6 weeks of pregnancy. Peak values approaching 100,000 IU/L occur 60 to 70 days after implantation
hCG levels generally double every 1 to 3 days. In pts w/concentration <2000 IU/L, an ↑ of serum hCG <66% after 2 days suggests spontaneous abortion or ruptured ectopic gestation.

CHYMOTRYPSIN

Nl: <10 µg/L.
↑: acute pancreatitis, chronic renal failure, PO enzyme preparations, gastric cancer, pancreatic cancer.
↓: chronic pancreatitis, late cystic fibrosis.

CIRCULATING ANTICOAGULANT (ANTIPHOSPHOLIPID ANTIBODY, LUPUS ANTICOAGULANT)

Nl: (−)
Detected in: SLE, drug-induced lupus, long-term phenothiazine Rx, MM, UC, RA, post partum, hemophilia, neoplasms, chronic inflammatory states, AIDS, nephrotic syndrome.
Note: The name is a misnomer because these pts are prone to hypercoagulability and thrombosis.

CK; SEE CREATINE KINASE

CLONIDINE SUPPRESSION TEST

Interpretation: Clonidine inhibits neurogenic catecholamine release and will cause a ↓ in plasma norepinephrine into the reference interval in hypertensive subjects w/o pheochromocytoma. The test is performed by giving 4.3 µg clonidine/kg PO after an overnight fast. Norepinephrine is measured at 3 hr. The result should be within established reference range and ↓ to <50% of baseline concentration. Lack of ↓ in norepinephrine suggests pheochromocytoma.

CLOSTRIDIUM DIFFICILE TOXIN ASSAY (STOOL)

Nl: (−)
Detected in: abx-associated diarrhea and pseudomembranous colitis.

CO; SEE CARBOXYHEMOGLOBIN

COAGULATION FACTORS

Factor reference ranges:
- V: >10%
- VII: >10%
- VIII: 50%-170%
- IX: 60%-136%
- X: >10%
- XI: 50%-150%
- XII: >30%

Figure 1-2 illustrates the blood coagulation pathways.

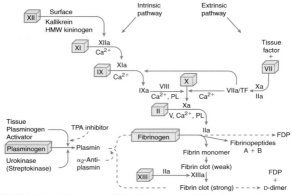

FIGURE 1-2. Coagulation cascade. Fibrin clot formation results from the generation of thrombin, which depends on the sequential interaction of proenzymes and activated coagulation factors in the intrinsic, extrinsic, and common pathways of coagulation. *(From Noble J [ed]: Primary Care Medicine, 3rd ed. St. Louis, Mosby, 2001.)*

COLD AGGLUTININS TITER

Nl range: <1:32.

↑: primary atypical pneumonia (*Mycoplasma* pneumonia), infectious mononucleosis, CMV infection, others (hepatic cirrhosis, acquired hemolytic anemia, frostbite, MM, lymphoma, malaria).

COMPLEMENT (C3, C4)

Nl range:
- C3: 70-160 mg/dL
- C4: 20-40 mg/dL

Abnl values:
- ↓ C3: active SLE, immune complex disease, AGN, inborn C3 deficiency, membranoproliferative GN, infective endocarditis, serum sickness, autoimmune-type chronic active hepatitis.
- ↓ C4: immune complex disease, active SLE, infective endocarditis, inborn C4 deficiency, hereditary angioedema, hypergammaglobulinemic states, cryoglobulinemic vasculitis.

COMPLETE BLOOD COUNT (CBC)

WBCs: 3200-9800/mm^3
RBCs: 4.3-5.9 10^6/mm^3 (male); 3.5-5.0 10^6/mm^3 (female)
Hgb: 13.6-17.7 g/dL (male); 12-15 g/dL (female)
Hct: 39%-49% (male); 33%-43% (female)
MCV: 76-100 μm^3
MCH: 27-33 pg
MCHC: 33-37 g/dL
RDW: 11.5%-14.5%
Plt count: 130-400 × 10^3/mm^3
Diff: 2-6 bands (early mature neutrophils); 60-70 segs (mature neutrophils); 1-4 eosinophils; 0-1 basophils; 2-8 monocytes; 25-40 lymphocytes

CONJUGATED BILIRUBIN; SEE BILIRUBIN, DIRECT

COOMBS, DIRECT (ANTIGLOBULIN TEST, DIRECT, DAT)

Nl: (−)

(+): AIHA, erythroblastosis fetalis, transfusion reactions, drugs (methyldopa, PCNs, tetracycline, sulfonamides, levodopa, cephalosporins, quinidine, insulin).

False (+): may be seen w/cold agglutinins.

COOMBS, INDIRECT

Nl: (−)

(+): acquired hemolytic anemia, incompatible crossmatched blood, anti-Rh antibodies, drugs (methyldopa, mefenamic acid, levodopa).

COPPER (SERUM)

Nl range: 70-140 µg/dL.

↓: Wilson's disease, malabsorption, malnutrition nephrosis, TPN, acute leukemia in remission.

↑: aplastic anemia, biliary cirrhosis, SLE, hemochromatosis, hyperthyroidism, hypothyroidism, infection, iron deficiency anemia, leukemia, lymphoma, OCPs, pernicious anemia, RA.

CORTICOTROPIN-RELEASING HORMONE (CRH) STIMULATION TEST

Nl: A dose of 0.5 mg of dexamethasone is given every 6 hr for 2 days; 2 hr after the last dose, 1 µg/kg CRH is given IV. Samples are drawn after 15 minutes. There is normally a twofold to fourfold ↑ in mean baseline concentration of ACTH or cortisol. Cortisol >1.4 µg/L is virtually 100% specific and 100% diagnostic.

Nl or exaggerated response: pituitary Cushing's disease.

No response: ectopic ACTH-secreting tumor.

A (+) response to CRH or a suppressed response to high-dose dexamethasone has a 97% (+) predictive value for Cushing's disease. However, a lack of response to either test excludes Cushing's disease in only 64% to 78% of pts. When the tests are considered together, (−) responses from both have a 100% predictive value for ectopic ACTH secretion.

CORTISOL (PLASMA)

Nl range: varies w/time of collection (circadian variation):
- 8 am: 4-19 µg/dL
- 4 pm: 2-15 µg/dL

↑: ectopic ACTH production (i.e., oat cell carcinoma of lung), loss of nl diurnal variation, pregnancy, chronic renal failure, iatrogenic, stress, adrenal or pituitary hyperplasia or adenomas.

↓: primary adrenocortical insufficiency, anterior pituitary hypofunction, secondary adrenocortical insufficiency, adrenogenital syndromes.

C-PEPTIDE

Nl range (serum): 0.51-2.70 ng/mL.

↑: insulinoma, sulfonylurea administration, type 2 DM, renal failure.

↓: type 1 DM, factitious insulin administration.

CPK; SEE CREATINE KINASE

C-REACTIVE PROTEIN (CRP)

Nl range: <1 mg/dL. CRP levels are valuable in the clinical assessment of chronic inflammatory disorders such as RA, SLE, vasculitis syndromes, and IBD.

↑: inflammatory and neoplastic diseases, MI, third trimester of pregnancy (acute-phase reactant), OCPs. Moderately high CRP concentrations (3-10 mg/L) predict ↑ risk of MI and stroke. Markedly high levels (>10 mg/L) have been shown to predict CV risk.

Note: High-sensitivity C-reactive protein (hs-CRP, Cardio CRP) is used as a cardiac risk marker. It is ↑ in pts w/silent atherosclerosis for a prolonged period before a CV event and is independent of cholesterol level and other lipoproteins. It can be used to help stratify cardiac risk.

CREATINE KINASE (CK, CPK)

Nl range: 0-130 U/L.

↑: vigorous exercise, IM injections, MI, myocarditis, rhabdo, myositis, crush injury or trauma, polymyositis, dermatomyositis, muscular dystrophy, myxedema, seizures, malignant hyperthermia syndrome, CVA, pulmonary embolism and infarction, acute dissection of aorta.

↓: corticosteroids, ↓ muscle mass, connective tissue disorders, alcoholic liver disease, metastatic neoplasms.

CREATINE KINASE ISOENZYMES

CK-MB

↑: MI, myocarditis, pericarditis, muscular dystrophy, cardiac defibrillation, cardiac surgery, extensive rhabdo, strenuous exercise (e.g., marathon runners), MCTD, cardiomyopathy, hypothermia.

Note: CK-MB exists in the blood in two subforms. MB_2 is released from cardiac cells and converted in the blood to MB_1. Rapid assay of CK-MB subforms can detect MI (CK-MB_2 ≥1.0 U/L, w/a ratio of CK-MB_2/CK-MB_1 ≥1.5) within the first 6 hr of onset of sx.

CK-MM

↑: crush injury, seizures, malignant hyperthermia syndrome, rhabdo, myositis, polymyositis, dermatomyositis, vigorous exercise, muscular dystrophy, IM injections, acute dissection of aorta.

CK-BB

↑: CVA, subarachnoid hemorrhage, neoplasms (prostate, GI tract, brain, ovary, breast, lung), severe shock, bowel infarction, hypothermia, meningitis.

CREATININE (SERUM)

Nl range: 0.6-1.2 mg/dL.

↑: renal insufficiency (acute and chronic), ↓ renal perfusion (hypotension, dehydration, DKA, administration of contrast dyes, ketonemia, drugs (abx [AGs, cephalosporins], ACEIs [in pts w/RAS], diuretics).

Falsely ↑: DKA, administration of some cephalosporins (e.g., cefoxitin, cephalothin).

↓: ↓ muscle mass (including amputees and elderly), pregnancy, prolonged debilitation.

CREATININE CLEARANCE

Nl range: 75-124 mL/min.

↑: pregnancy, exercise.

↓: renal insufficiency, drugs (e.g., cimetidine, procainamide, abx, quinidine), age.

CRYOGLOBULINS (SERUM)

Nl range: not detectable.

Present in: collagen-vascular diseases, chronic active hepatitis, CLL, hemolytic anemias, MM, Waldenström's macroglobulinemia, Hodgkin's disease.

CYSTATIN C

Nl: Cystatin C is a cysteine protease inhibitor that is produced at a constant rate by all nucleated cells. It is freely filtered by the glomerulus and reabsorbed (but not secreted) by the renal tubules w/no extrarenal excretion. Its concentration is not affected by diet, muscle mass, or acute inflammation. Nl range when measured by particle-enhanced nephelometric immunoassay (PENIA) is <0.28 mg/L.

↑: renal disorders; good predictor of the severity of ATN. Cystatin C ↑ more rapidly than Cr in the early stages of GFR impairment. The cystatin C concentration is an independent risk factor for heart failure in older adults and appears to provide a better measure of risk assessment than the serum Cr concentration.

D-DIMER

Nl range: <0.5 µg/mL.

↑: DVT, PE, high levels of RF, activation of coagulation and fibrinolytic systems from any cause.

D-dimer assay by ELISA assists in the dx of DVT and PE. This test has significant limitations because it can be ↑ whenever the coagulation and fibrinolytic systems are activated and can also be falsely ↑ w/high RF levels.

DEXAMETHASONE SUPPRESSION TEST, OVERNIGHT

Nl: Test performed by giving 1 mg dexamethasone PO at 11 pm and measuring serum cortisol at 8 am on the following morning; nl response is cortisol suppression to <3 g/dL. If dose of 4 mg dexamethasone is given, cortisol suppression will be to <50% of baseline.

Interpretation: Cushing's syndrome (>10 µm/dL), endogenous depression (half of pts suppress test values >5 µg/dL). Most pts w/pituitary Cushing's disease demonstrate suppression, whereas pts w/adrenal adenoma, carcinoma, and ectopic ACTH-producing tumors do not.

DIGOXIN
Nl therapeutic range: 0.5-2 ng/mL.
↑: impaired renal function, excessive dosing; corcomitant use of quinidine, amiodarone, verapamil, fluoxetine, nifedipine.

DOPAMINE
Nl range: 0-175 pg/mL.
↑: pheochromocytomas, neuroblastomas, stress vigorous exercise, certain foods (bananas, chocolate, coffee, tea, vanilla).

ELECTROPHORESIS, HEMOGLOBIN; SEE HEMOGLOBIN ELECTROPHORESIS

ELECTROPHORESIS, PROTEIN; SEE PROTEIN ELECTROPHORESIS

ENA COMPLEX; SEE EXTRACTABLE NUCLEAR ANTIGEN

ENDOMYSIAL ANTIBODIES
Nl: not detected.
Present in: celiac disease, dermatitis herpetiformis.

EOSINOPHIL COUNT
Nl range: 1%-4% eosinophils (0-440/mm^3).
↑: allergy, parasitic infestations (trichinosis, aspergillosis, hydatidosis), angioneurotic edema, drug reactions, warfarin sensitivity, collagen-vascular diseases, acute hypereosinophilic syndrome, eosinophilic nonallergic rhinitis, myeloproliferative disorders, Hodgkin's lymphoma, radiation Rx, NHL, L-tryptophan ingestion, urticaria, pernicious anemia, pemphigus, IBD, bronchial asthma.

EPINEPHRINE (PLASMA)
Nl range: 0-90 pg/mL.
↑: pheochromocytomas, neuroblastomas, stress vigorous exercise, certain foods (bananas, chocolate, coffee, tea, vanilla), hypoglycemia.

EPSTEIN-BARR VIRUS SEROLOGY
Nl range:
- IgG anti-VCA <1:10 or (–)
- IgM anti-VCA<1:10 or (–)
- Anti-EBNA <1.5 or (–)

Abn:
- IgG anti-VCA >1:10 or (+) indicates either current or previous infection.
- IgM anti-VCA >1:10 or (+) indicates current or recent infection.
- Anti-EBNA ≥1.5 or (+) indicates previous infection.

ERYTHROCYTE SEDIMENTATION RATE (ESR) (WESTERGREN)
Nl range: 0-15 mm/hr (male); 0-20 mm/hr (female).
↑: inflammatory states (acute-phase reactant), collagen-vascular diseases, infections, MI, neoplasms, hyperthyroidism, hypothyroidism, rouleaux formation, elderly, pregnancy.
Note: Sedimentation rates >100 mm/hr are strongly associated w/serious underlying disease (collagen-vascular, infection, malignant disease). Some clinicians use ESR as a "sickness index"; high rates encountered w/o obvious reason should be repeated rather than pursuing extensive search for occult disease.
↓: sickle cell disease, polycythemia, corticosteroids, spherocytosis, anisocytosis, hypofibrinogenemia, serum viscosity, microcytosis.

ERYTHROPOIETIN
Nl: 3.7-16.0 IU/L by radioimmunoassay. Erythropoietin is a glycoprotein secreted by the kidneys that stimulates RBC production by acting on erythroid committed stem cells.
↑:
- Extremely high: generally seen in pts w/severe anemia (Hct <25, Hgb <7), such as in cases of aplastic anemia, severe hemolytic anemia, hematologic cancers.
- Very high: pts w/mild to moderate anemia (Hct 25-35, Hgb 7-10).
- High: pts w/mild anemia (e.g., AIDS, myelodysplasia).

- Erythropoietin can be inappropriately ↑ in pts w/malignant neoplasms, renal cysts, after renal transplantation, and in meningioma, hemangioblastoma, and leiomyoma.

↓: renal failure, PV, autonomic neuropathy.

ETHANOL (BLOOD)
Nl range: (−) (values <10 mg/dL are considered [−]). Ethanol is metabolized at 10-25 mg/dL/hr. Levels >80 mg/dL are considered evidence of impairment for driving. Fatal blood concentration is considered to be >400 mg/dL, although levels >400 mg/dL may be seen in pts w/chronic alcoholism.

EXTRACTABLE NUCLEAR ANTIGEN (ENA COMPLEX, ANTI-RNP ANTIBODY, ANTI-SM, ANTI-SMITH)
Nl: (−)
Present in: SLE, RA, Sjögren's syndrome, MCTD.

FACTOR V LEIDEN
Test description: PCR test is performed on whole blood or tissue. This single mutation, found in 2% to 8% of the general white population, is the single most common cause of hereditary thrombophilia.

FBS; SEE GLUCOSE, FASTING

FDP; SEE FIBRIN DEGRADATION PRODUCT (FDP)

FECAL FAT, QUALITATIVE; SEE SUDAN III STAIN

FERRITIN (SERUM)
Nl range: 18-300 ng/mL.
↑: inflammatory states, liver disease (ferritin ↑ from necrotic hepatocytes), hyperthyroidism, neoplasms (neuroblastomas, lymphomas, leukemia, breast carcinoma), iron replacement Rx, hemochromatosis, hemosiderosis.
↓: iron deficiency anemia.

FIBRIN DEGRADATION PRODUCT (FDP)
Nl range: <10 μg/mL.
↑: DIC, primary fibrinolysis, PE, severe liver disease.
Note: The presence of RF may cause falsely ↑ FDP.

FIBRINOGEN
Nl range: 200-400 mg/dL.
↑: tissue inflammation or damage (acute-phase protein reactant), OCPs, pregnancy, acute infection, MI.
↓: DIC, hereditary afibrinogenemia, liver disease, primary or secondary fibrinolysis, cachexia.

FLUORESCENT TREPONEMAL ANTIBODY; SEE FTA-ABS (SERUM)

FOLATE (FOLIC ACID)
Nl range:
- Plasma: <3.4 ng/mL (low); >5.4 ng/mL (nl)
- RBC: >280 ng/mL

↓: folic acid deficiency (inadequate intake, malabsorption), alcoholism, drugs (MTX, trimethoprim, phenytoin, OCPs, sulfasalazine), vitamin B_{12} deficiency (defective red cell folate absorption), hemolytic anemia.
↑: folic acid Rx.

FOLLICLE-STIMULATING HORMONE (FSH)
Nl range:
- Female, adult: <40 IU/L (midcycle); <20 IU/L (non-midcycle); 40-160 IU/L (postmenopausal)
- Male, adult: <22 IU/L

↑: primary hypogonadism, gonadal failure, alcoholism, Klinefelter's syndrome, testicular feminization, anorchia, castration.
↓: precocious puberty related to adrenal tumors, congenital adrenal hyperplasia. Nl FSH in an adult nonovulating female pt indicates hypothalamic or pituitary dysfunction.

FREE INSULIN; SEE INSULIN, FREE

FREE T$_4$; SEE T$_4$, FREE

FREE THYROXINE INDEX

Nl range: 1.1-4.3.

Serum free T$_4$ directly measures unbound thyroxine. Free T$_4$ can be measured by equilibrium dialysis (gold standard of free T$_4$ assays) or by immunometric techniques (influenced by serum levels of lipids, proteins, and certain drugs). The FTI can also be easily calculated by multiplying T$_4$ times T$_3$RU and dividing the result by 100; the FTI corrects for any abnl T$_4$ values secondary to protein binding: FTI = T$_4$ xT$_3$RU/100.

FSH; SEE FOLLICLE-STIMULATING HORMONE (FSH)

FTA-ABS (SERUM)

Nl: nonreactive.

Reactive in: syphilis, other treponemal diseases (yaws, pinta, bejel), SLE, pregnancy.

FUROSEMIDE STIMULATION TEST

Nl: The test is performed by giving 60 mg furosemide PO after overnight fast. Pt should be on a nl diet w/o medications the week before the test. Nl results: renin 1-6 ng angiotensin L/ml/hr.

↑: renovascular HTN, Bartter's syndrome, high-renin essential HTN, pheochromocytoma.

No response in: primary aldosteronism, low-renin essential HTN, hyporeninemic hypoaldosteronism.

GAMMA-GLUTAMYLTRANSFERASE (GGT)

Nl range: 0-30 U/L.

↑: chronic alcoholic liver disease, neoplasms (hepatoma, metastatic disease to the liver, carcinoma of the pancreas), nephrotic syndrome, sepsis, cholestasis, drugs (phenytoin, barbiturates).

GASTRIN (SERUM)

Nl range: 0-180 pg/mL.

↑: Zollinger-Ellison syndrome (gastrinoma), use of PPIs, chronic renal failure, gastric ulcer, chronic atrophic gastritis, pyloric obstruction, malignant neoplasms of the stomach, H$_2$ blockers, Ca Rx, UC, RA.

GGT; SEE GAMMA-GLUTAMYLTRANSFERASE (GGT)

GLOMERULAR BASEMENT MEMBRANE ANTIBODY

Nl: (−)

Present in: Goodpasture's syndrome.

GLOMERULAR FILTRATION RATE

Nl:
- Age 20-29: 116 mL/min/1.73 m^2
- Age 30-39: 107 mL/min/1.73 m^2
- Age 40-49: 99 mL/min/1.73 m^2
- Age 50-59: 93 mL/min/1.73 m^2
- Age 60-69: 85 mL/min/1.73 m^2
- Age >70: 75 mL/min/1.73 m^2

↓: renal insufficiency, ↓ renal blood flow.

GLUCAGON

Nl: 20-100 pg/mL.

↑: glucagonoma (900-7800 pg/mL), chronic renal failure, DM, glucocorticoids, insulin, nifedipine, danazol, sympathomimetic amines.

↓: hyperlipoproteinemia (types III, IV), β-blockers, secretin.

GLUCOSE, FASTING (FASTING BLOOD SUGAR, FBS)

Nl range: 60-99 mg/dL.

↑: DM, stress, infections, MI, CVA, Cushing's syndrome, acromegaly, acute pancreatitis, glucagonoma, hemochromatosis, drugs (glucocorticoids, diuretics [thiazides, loop diuretics]), impaired glucose tolerance.

↓: prolonged fasting, excessive dose of insulin or hypoglycemic agents, insulinoma.

GLUCOSE, POSTPRANDIAL

Nl range: <140 mg/dL.
↑: DM, impaired glucose tolerance.
↓: after administration of oral hypoglycemic agents or insulin, after extensive GI resection, in reactive hypoglycemia, hereditary fructose intolerance, galactosemia, leucine sensitivity.

GLUCOSE TOLERANCE TEST

Nl values above fasting:
- 30 minutes: 30-60 mg/dL
- 60 minutes: 20-50 mg/dL
- 120 minutes: 5-15 mg/dL
- 180 minutes: fasting level or below

Abnl in: impaired glucose tolerance, DM, Cushing's syndrome, acromegaly, pheochromocytoma, gestational diabetes.

GLYCOHEMOGLOBIN (HBA1C, GLYCATED HEMOGLOBIN, GLYCOSYLATED HEMOGLOBIN)

Nl range: 4.0%-6.0%.
Diabetes: ≥6.5%
↑: uncontrolled DM (glycated Hgb levels reflect the level of glucose control during the preceding 120 days), lead toxicity, alcoholism, iron deficiency anemia, hypertriglyceridemia.
↓: hemolytic anemias, ↓ RBC survival, pregnancy, acute or chronic blood loss, chronic renal failure, insulinoma, congenital spherocytosis; HbS, HbC, HbD diseases.

HAPTOGLOBIN (SERUM)

Nl range: 50-220 mg/dL.
↑: inflammation (acute-phase reactant), collagen-vascular diseases, infections (acute-phase reactant), drugs (androgens), obstructive liver disease.
↓: hemolysis (intravascular more than extravascular), megaloblastic anemia, severe liver disease, large tissue hematomas, infectious mononucleosis, drugs (oral contraceptives).

HDL; SEE HIGH-DENSITY LIPOPROTEIN (HDL) CHOLESTEROL

HELICOBACTER PYLORI (SEROLOGY, STOOL ANTIGEN)

Nl range: not detected.
Detected in: *H. pylori* infection. (+) serology can indicate current or past infection. (+) stool antigen test result indicates acute infection (sensitivity and specificity >90%). Stool testing should be delayed at least 4 weeks after eradication Rx.

HEMATOCRIT

Nl range: 39%-49% (male); 33%-43% (female).
↑: PV, smoking, COPD, high altitudes, dehydration, hypovolemia.
↓: blood loss (GI, GU), anemia, pregnancy.

HEMOGLOBIN

Nl range: 13.6-17.7 g/dL (male); 12.0-15.0 g/dL (female).
↑: hemoconcentration, dehydration, PV, COPD, high altitudes, false elevations (hyperlipemic plasma, WBCs >50,000 mm^3), stress.
↓: hemorrhage (GI, GU), anemia.

HEMOGLOBIN ELECTROPHORESIS

Nl range:
- HbA$_1$: 95%-98%
- HbA$_2$: 1.5%-3.5%
- HbF: <2%
- HbC: absent
- HbS: absent

HEPARIN-INDUCED THROMBOCYTOPENIA ANTIBODIES

Nl: antigen assay: (–), <0.45; weak, 0.45-1.0; strong, >1.0.
↑: HIT.

HEPATITIS A ANTIBODY

Nl: (–)
Present in: viral hepatitis A; can be IgM or IgG (if IgM, acute hepatitis A; if IgG, previous infection w/hepatitis A).

HEPATITIS B ANTIGEN AND ANTIBODY

NI: (–) These tests are ordered together and should be used only in pts who are chronically HBsAg (+). *The main utility of these tests is to assess response of hepatitis B infection to Rx.*

Present in: Presence of HBeAg implies that infective HBV is present in serum. However, its absence on conversion to anti-HBe does not r/o infectivity, especially in persons infected w/genotypes other than A. Measurement of HBV DNA is useful in persons w/ ↑ ALT but (–) HBeAg.

HEPATITIS B CORE ANTIBODY (HBcAb)

NI: (–)

Present in: hepatitis B. Anti-HBc assay is the first Ab test to become (+) w/exposure to HBV and persists the longest after resolution of acute infection.

HEPATITIS B DNA

NI: (–)

Present in: active hepatitis B infection. It implies infectivity of the serum. Currently used to assess response of hepatitis B to Rx.

HEPATITIS B SURFACE ANTIBODY (HBsAb)

NI: (–)

Present in: after vaccination for hepatitis B (a level >10 U/L for postvaccine testing is the accepted concentration that indicates protection), after infection w/hepatitis B (it generally appears several weeks after disappearance of HBsAg).

HEPATITIS B SURFACE ANTIGEN (HBsAg)

NI: not detected.

Detected in: acute viral hepatitis type B, chronic hepatitis B.

HEPATITIS C ANTIBODY (ANTI-HCV)

NI: (–)

Present in: hepatitis C. CDC guidelines recommend confirmation w/RIBA before reporting of anti-HCV as (+). HCV RNA can also be obtained if there is a high clinical suspicion of HCV despite a (–) anti-HVC, especially in immunosuppressed individuals or in the setting of acute hepatitis. Anti-HCV and the RIBA often do not become (+) during an acute infection; thus, repeated testing several months later is required if HCV RNA is (–).

HEPATITIS C RNA

NI: (–)

↑: hepatitis C. Detection of hepatitis C RNA is used to confirm current infection and to monitor Rx. Quantitative assays (viral load) are needed before Rx to assess response (<2 log ↓ after 12-week Rx indicates lack of response).

HEPATITIS DELTA ANTIGEN AND ANTIBODY

NI: (–)

↑: hepatitis delta. Hepatitis delta is a replication-defective RNA virus that requires the surface coat of hepatitis B (HBsAg) to become an infectious virus. Testing for hepatitis delta is therefore done only in pts (+) for HBsAg. It is useful in pts w/ chronic hepatitis B if there is an exacerbation of stable hepatitis.

HER-2/NEU

NI: (–)

Present in: 25%-30% of primary breast cancers. ↑ can also be found in other epithelial tumors, including lung, hepatocellular, pancreatic, colon, stomach, ovarian, cervical, and bladder cancer. Trastuzumab (Herceptin) is a humanized monoclonal Ab against Her-2/*neu*. The test is useful to identify pts w/metastatic, recurrent, or Rx-refractory unresectable locally advanced breast cancer for trastuzumab Rx.

HFE SCREEN FOR HEREDITARY HEMOCHROMATOSIS

Test description: PCR test can be performed on whole blood or tissue. One mutation (C282Y) and two polymorphisms (H63D, S65C) account for the majority of alleles associated w/this disease.

HIGH-DENSITY LIPOPROTEIN (HDL) CHOLESTEROL

NI range: 45-70 mg/dL (male); 50-90 mg/dL (female).

↑: use of fenofibrates, niacin, estrogens, regular aerobic exercise, mild to moderate (1-oz) daily EtOH intake.

19

↓: familial deficiency of apoproteins, liver disease, sedentary lifestyle, acute MI, CVA, starvation.

Note: A cholesterol/HDL ratio >4.5 is associated w/risk of CAD.

HOMOCYSTEINE (PLASMA)

Nl range:
- 0-30 years: 4.6-8.1 μmol/L
- 30-59 years: 6.3-11.2 μmol/L (males); 4-5-7.9 μmol/L (females)
- >59 years: 5.8-11.9 μmol/L

↑: thrombophilic states; B_6, B_{12}, folic acid, riboflavin deficiency; pregnancy; homocystinuria.

Note: An ↑ homocysteine level is an independent risk factor for atherosclerosis.

hs-CRP; SEE C-REACTIVE PROTEIN (CRP)

HUMAN IMMUNODEFICIENCY VIRUS ANTIBODY, TYPE 1 (HIV-1)

Nl range: not detected.

Abnl result: HIV antibodies usually appear in the blood 1 to 4 months after infection.

Testing sequence:
1. ELISA is the recommended initial screening test. Sensitivity and specificity are >99%. False-(+) ELISA results may occur w/autoimmune disorders, presence of RF, presence of DLA-DR antibodies in multigravida woman, administration of influenza vaccine within 3 months of testing, hemodialysis, (+) plasma reagin test response, and certain medical disorders (hemophilia, hypergammaglobulinemia, alcoholic hepatitis).
2. A (+) ELISA result is confirmed w/Western blot. False-(+) Western blot may be caused by connective tissue disorders, human leukocyte antigen antibodies, polyclonal gammopathies, hyperbilirubinemia, presence of Ab to another human retrovirus, cross-reaction w/other non–virus-derived proteins in healthy persons. Undetermined Western blot may occur in pts w/AIDS w/advanced immunodeficiency (from loss of antibodies) and in recent HIV infections.
3. PCR is used to confirm indeterminate Western blot results or (–) results in persons w/suspected HIV infection.

IMMUNOGLOBULINS

Nl range:
- IgA: 50-350 mg/dL
- IgD: <6 mg/dL
- IgE: <25 μg/dL
- IgG: 800-1500 mg/dL
- IgM: 45-150 mg/dL

↑:
- IgA: lymphoproliferative disorders, Berger's nephropathy, chronic infections, autoimmune disorders, liver disease.
- IgE: allergic disorders, parasitic infections, immunologic disorders, IgE myeloma, AIDS, pemphigoid.
- IgG: chronic granulomatous infections, infectious diseases, inflammation, myeloma, liver disease.
- IgM: PBC, infectious diseases (brucellosis, malaria), Waldenström's macroglobulinemia, liver disease.

↓:
- IgA: nephrotic syndrome, protein-losing enteropathy, congenital deficiency, lymphocytic leukemia, ataxia-telangiectasia, chronic sinopulmonary disease.
- IgE: hypogammaglobulinemia, neoplasm (breast, bronchial, cervical), ataxia-telangiectasia.
- IgG: congenital or acquired deficiency, lymphocytic leukemia, phenytoin, methylprednisolone, nephrotic syndrome, protein-losing enteropathy.
- IgM: congenital deficiency, lymphocytic leukemia, nephrotic syndrome.

INR; SEE INTERNATIONAL NORMALIZED RATIO (INR)

INSULIN AUTOANTIBODIES

Nl: (–)

Present in: exogenous insulin from insulin Rx. The presence of islet cell antibodies indicates ongoing β-cell destruction. This test is useful in the early dx of type 1A DM and in the identification of pts at high risk for type 1A DM.

INSULIN, FREE
Nl: <17 μU/mL.
↑: insulin OD, insulin resistance syndromes, endogenous hyperinsulinemia.
↓: inadequately treated type 1 DM.

INSULIN-LIKE GROWTH FACTOR 1 (IGF-1) (SERUM)
Nl range:
- Age 16-24: 182-780 ng/mL
- Age 25-39: 114-492 ng/mL
- Age 40-54: 90-360 ng/mL
- Age >55: 71-290 ng/mL

↑: adolescence, acromegaly, pregnancy, precocious puberty, obesity.
↓: malnutrition, delayed puberty, DM, hypopituitarism, cirrhosis, old age.

INSULIN-LIKE GROWTH FACTOR 2 (IGF-2)
Nl: 288-736 ng/mL.
↑: hypoglycemia associated w/non-islet cell tumors, hepatoma, and Wilms' tumor.
↓: GH deficiency.

INTERNATIONAL NORMALIZED RATIO (INR)
The INR is a comparative rating of PT ratios. The INR represents the observed PT ratio adjusted by the International Reference Sensitivity Index. INR = PT pt/PT mean. The INR provides a universal result indicative of what the pt's PT result would have been if measured by use of the primary World Health Organization International Reference reagent. For proper interpretation of INR values, the pt should be on stable anticoagulant Rx. Recommended therapeutic INR range: 2-3

INTRINSIC FACTOR ANTIBODIES
Nl: (−)
Present in: pernicious anemia (>50% of pts). Cyanocobalamin may give false-(+) results.

IRON (SERUM)
Nl: 65-175 μg/dL (male); 50-1170 μg/dL (female).
↑: hemochromatosis, excessive iron Rx, repeated transfusions, lead poisoning, hemolytic anemia, aplastic anemia, pernicious anemia.
↓: iron deficiency anemia, hypothyroidism, chronic infection.

IRON-BINDING CAPACITY (TIBC)
Nl range: 250-460 μg/dL.
↑: iron deficiency anemia, pregnancy, polycythemia, hepatitis, weight loss.
↓: anemia of chronic disease, hemochromatosis, chronic liver disease, hemolytic anemias, malnutrition (protein depletion).

IRON SATURATION (% TRANSFERRIN SATURATION)
Nl: 20%-50% (male); 15%-50% (female).
↑: hemochromatosis, excessive iron intake, aplastic anemia, thalassemia, vitamin B_6 deficiency.
↓: hypochromic anemias, GI malignant disease.

LACTATE (BLOOD)
Nl range: 0.5-2.0 mEq/L.
↑: tissue hypoxia (shock, respiratory failure, severe CHF, severe anemia, CO or cyanide poisoning), systemic disorders (liver or renal failure, seizures), abnl intestinal flora (D-lactic acidosis), drugs or toxins (salicylates, ethanol, methanol, ethylene glycol), G6PD deficiency.

LACTATE DEHYDROGENASE (LDH)
Nl range: 50-150 U/L.
↑: infarction of myocardium, lung, kidney; diseases of cardiopulmonary system, liver, collagen, CNS; hemolytic anemias; megaloblastic anemias; transfusions; seizures; muscle trauma; muscular dystrophy; acute pancreatitis; hypotension; shock; infectious mononucleosis; inflammation; neoplasia; intestinal obstruction; hypothyroidism.

LACTATE DEHYDROGENASE ISOENZYMES
Nl range:
- LDH_1: 22%-36% (cardiac, RBCs)
- LDH_2: 35%-46% (cardiac, RBCs)
- LDH_3: 13%-26% (pulmonary)

- LDH$_4$: 3%-10% (striated muscle, liver)
- LDH$_5$: 2%-9% (striated muscle, liver)

Nl range:
- LDH$_1$ < LDH$_2$
- LDH$_5$ < LDH$_4$

Abnl values:
- LDH$_1$ > LDH$_2$: MI (can also be seen w/hemolytic anemias, pernicious anemia, folate deficiency, renal infarct)
- LDH$_5$ > LDH$_4$: liver disease (cirrhosis, hepatitis, hepatic congestion)

LACTOSE TOLERANCE TEST (SERUM)
Nl: The test is performed by giving 2 g/kg BW lactose PO and drawing glucose level at 0, 30, 45, 60, and 90 minutes. Nl response is change in glucose from fasting value to >30 mg/dL. Inconclusive response is of 20 to 30 mg/dL; abnl response is ↑<20 mg/dL.

Abnl in: lactase deficiency.

LAP SCORE; SEE LEUKOCYTE ALKALINE PHOSPHATASE (LAP)

LDH; SEE LACTATE DEHYDROGENASE (LDH)

LDL; SEE LOW-DENSITY LIPOPROTEIN (LDL) CHOLESTEROL

LEAD
Nl: <10 μg/dL (child); <25 μg/dL (adult); <50 μg/dL (acceptable for industrial exposure).
↑: lead exposure, lead poisoning.

LEGIONELLA TITER
Nl: (−)
(+) in: Legionnaires' disease (presumptive, ≥1:256 titer; definitive, fourfold titer ↑ to ≥1:128).

LEUKOCYTE ALKALINE PHOSPHATASE (LAP)
Nl range: 13-100.
↑: leukemoid reactions, neutrophilia resulting from infections (except in sickle cell crisis—no significant ↑ in LAP score), Hodgkin's disease, PV, hairy cell leukemia, aplastic anemia, Down syndrome, myelofibrosis.
↓: acute and chronic granulocytic leukemia, thrombocytopenic purpura, PNH, hypophosphatemia, collagen disorders.

LH; SEE LUTEINIZING HORMONE

LIPASE
Nl range: 0-160 U/L.
↑: acute pancreatitis, perforated peptic ulcer, carcinoma of pancreas (early stage), pancreatic duct obstruction, bowel infarction, intestinal obstruction.

LIPOPROTEIN(A)
Nl: 1.35-19.6 mg/dL (male); 1.24-20.1 mg/dL (female).
↑: CAD, uncontrolled diabetes, hypothyroidism, chronic renal failure, pregnancy, tobacco use, infections, nephritic syndrome.
↓: niacin, omega-3 fatty acids, estrogens, tamoxifen.

LIPOPROTEIN CHOLESTEROL, HIGH DENSITY; SEE HIGH-DENSITY LIPOPROTEIN (HDL) CHOLESTEROL

LIPOPROTEIN CHOLESTEROL, LOW DENSITY; SEE LOW-DENSITY LIPOPROTEIN (LDL) CHOLESTEROL

LIVER-KIDNEY MICROSOME TYPE 1 ANTIBODIES (LKM1)
Nl: <20 U.
↑: autoimmune hepatitis type 2.

LOW-DENSITY LIPOPROTEIN (LDL) CHOLESTEROL
Nl range: <130 mg/dL (<70 mg/dL in diabetics and pts w/CV risk factors).
↑: diet high in saturated fat, familial hyperlipidemia, sedentary lifestyle, poorly controlled DM, nephritic syndrome, hypothyroidism.

↓: use of lipid-lowering agents (statins, niacin, ezetimibe, cholestyramine, colesevelam), starvation, malabsorption, abetalipoproteinemia, hyperthyroidism, hepatic failure, carcinoma, infection, inflammation.

LUPUS ANTICOAGULANT (LA) TEST
Nl: (−)
Present in: antiphospholipid Ab syndrome. False-(+) results may occur w/oral anticoagulant Rx, factor deficiency, specific factor inhibitors.

LUTEINIZING HORMONE (LH) (BLOOD)
Nl range:
- Female, adult: 1.0-18.0 IU/L (follicular phase); 20.0-80.0 IU/L (midcycle phase); 0.5-18.0 IU/L (luteal phase); postmenopausal: 12.0-55.0 IU/L
- Male, adult: 1.0-9.0 IU/L

↑: gonadal failure, anorchia, menopause, testicular feminization syndrome.
↓: primary pituitary or hypothalamic failure.

LYMPHOCYTES
Nl range: 15%-40%.
- Total lymphocyte count: 800-2600/mm³
- Total T lymphocytes: 800-2200/mm³
- CD4 lymphocytes: ≥400/mm³
- CD8 lymphocytes: 200-800/mm³
- Nl CD4/CD8 ratio is 2.0.

↑: chronic infections, infectious mononucleosis and other viral infections, CLL, Hodgkin's disease, UC, hypoadrenalism, ITP.
↓: HIV infection, bone marrow suppression from chemotherapeutic agents or chemoRx, aplastic anemia, neoplasms, steroids, adrenocortical hyperfunction, neurologic disorders (MS, myasthenia gravis, CBS).

CD4 lymphocytes are calculated as total WBCs × % lymphocytes × % lymphocytes stained w/CD4. They are ↓ in AIDS and other forms of immune dysfunction.

MAGNESIUM (SERUM)
Nl range: 1.8-3.0 mg/dL.
Abnl results: Refer to "Hypomagnesemia" and "Hypermagnesemia" in Chapter 9.

MEAN CORPUSCULAR VOLUME (MCV)
Nl range: 76-100 μm³.
↑: EtOH abuse, reticulocytosis, vitamin B_{12} deficiency, folic acid deficiency, liver disease, hypothyroidism, marrow aplasia, myelofibrosis.
↓: iron deficiency, anemia of chronic disease, thalassemia trait or syndrome, other hemoglobinopathies, sideroblastic anemia, chronic renal failure, lead poisoning.

METHYLMALONIC ACID (SERUM)
Nl: <0.2 μmol/L.
↑: vitamin B_{12} deficiency, pregnancy, methylmalonic acidemia.

MITOCHONDRIAL ANTIBODY (AMA ANTIMITOCHONDRIAL ANTIBODY)
Nl: (−)
Present in: PBC (>90% of pts).

MONOCYTE COUNT
Nl range: 2%-8%.
↑: viral diseases, parasites, infections, neoplasms, IBD, monocytic leukemia, lymphomas, myeloma, sarcoidosis.
↓: viral syndrome, glucocorticoid administration, aplastic anemia, lymphocytic leukemia.

NATRIURETIC PEPTIDE; SEE B-TYPE NATRIURETIC PEPTIDE

NEUTROPHIL COUNT
Nl range: 50%-70%.
Subsets:
- Bands (early mature neutrophils): 2%-6%
- Segs (mature neutrophils): 60%-70%

↑: acute bacterial infections, acute MI, stress, neoplasms, myelocytic leukemia.

↓: viral infections, aplastic anemias, immunosuppressive drugs, radiation Rx to bone marrow, agranulocytosis, drugs (abx, antithyroidals), lymphocytic and monocytic leukemias.

NOREPINEPHRINE
NI range: 0-600 pg/mL.
↑: pheochromocytomas, neuroblastomas, stress, vigorous exercise, certain foods (bananas, chocolate, coffee, tea, vanilla).

5′-NUCLEOTIDASE
NI range: 2-16 IU/L.
↑: biliary obstruction, metastatic neoplasms to liver, PBC, renal failure, pancreatic carcinoma, chronic active hepatitis.

OSMOLALITY, SERUM
NI range: 280-300 mOsm/kg. It can also be estimated by the following formula: $2([Na] + [K]) + Glucose/18 + BUN/2.8$.
↑: dehydration, hypernatremia, diabetes insipidus, uremia, hyperglycemia, mannitol Rx, ingestion of toxins (ethylene glycol, methanol, ethanol), hypercalcemia, diuretics.
↓: SIADH, hyponatremia, overhydration, Addison's disease, hypothyroidism.

OSMOTIC FRAGILITY TEST
NI: Hemolysis begins at 0.50, w/v [5.0 g/L] and is complete at 0.30, w/v [3.0 g/L] NaCl.
↑: hereditary spherocytosis, hereditary stomatocytosis, spherocytosis associated w/acquired immune hemolytic anemia.
↓: iron deficiency anemia, thalassemias, liver disease, leptocytosis associated w/ asplenia.

PARATHYROID HORMONE
NI: 10-65 pg/mL (serum, intact molecule); 1.0-5.0 pmol/L (plasma).
↑: hyperparathyroidism (primary or secondary), pseudohypoparathyroidism, anticonvulsants, corticosteroids, lithium, INH, rifampin, phosphates, Zollinger-Ellison syndrome, hereditary vit D def.
↓: hypoparathyroidism, sarcoidosis, cimetidine, β-blockers, hyperthyroidism, hypomagnesemia.

PARIETAL CELL ANTIBODIES
NI: (−)
Present in: pernicious anemia (>90%), atrophic gastritis (up to 50%), thyroiditis (30%), Addison's disease, myasthenia gravis, Sjögren's syndrome, type 1 DM.

PARTIAL THROMBOPLASTIN TIME (PTT), ACTIVATED PARTIAL THROMBOPLASTIN TIME (APTT)
NI range: 25-41 seconds.
↑: heparin Rx, coagulation factor deficiency (I, II, V, VIII, IX, X, XI, XII), liver disease, vitamin K deficiency, DIC, circulating anticoagulant, warfarin Rx, specific factor inhibition (PCN reaction, RA), thrombolytic Rx, nephrotic syndrome.
Note: Useful to evaluate the intrinsic coagulation system.

PFA; SEE PLATELET FUNCTION ANALYSIS (PFA-100 ASSAY)

pH, BLOOD
NI values: 7.35-7.45 (arterial); 7.32-7.42 (venous).

PO₄⁻³ (SERUM)
NI range: 2.5-5 mg/dL.
↑: refer to "Hyperphosphatemia" and "Hypophosphatemia" in Chapter 9.

PLASMINOGEN
NI: immunoassay (antigen), <20 mg/dL.
↑: infection, trauma, neoplasm, MI (acute-phase reactant), pregnancy, bilirubinemia.
↓: DIC, severe liver disease, thrombolytic Rx w/streptokinase or urokinase, alteplase.

PLATELET AGGREGATION
NI: full aggregation (generally >60%) in response to epinephrine, thrombin, ristocetin, ADP, collagen.

↑: heparin, hemolysis, lipemia, nicotine; hereditary and acquired disorders of Plt adhesion, activation, and aggregation.

↓: ASA, some PCNs, chloroquine, chlorpromazine, clofibrate, captopril, Glanzmann's thrombasthenia, Bernard-Soulier syndrome, Wiskott-Aldrich syndrome, cyclooxygenase deficiency. In vWD, there is nl aggregation w/ADP, collagen, and epinephrine but abnl agglutination w/ristocetin.

PLATELET ANTIBODIES

Nl: absent.

Present in: ITP (>90% of pts w/chronic ITP). Pts w/nonimmune thrombocytopenias may have false-(+) results.

PLATELET COUNT

Nl range: 130-400 × 10^3/mm^3.

↑: iron deficiency, after hemorrhage, neoplasms (GI tract), CML, PV, myelofibrosis w/myeloid metaplasia, infections, after splenectomy, post partum, hemophilia, pancreatitis, cirrhosis.

↓: see "Thrombocytopenia" in Chapter 7.

PLATELET FUNCTION ANALYSIS (PFA-100 ASSAY)

Nl: Test is a two-component assay in which blood is aspirated through two capillary tubes, one of which is coated w/collagen and ADP (COL/ADP) and the other w/ collagen and epinephrine (COL/EPI). The test measures the ability of Plts to occlude an aperture in a biologically active membrane treated with COL/ADP and COL/EPI. During the test, the Plts adhere to the surface of the tube and cause blood flow to cease. The closing time refers to the cessation of blood flow and is reported in conjunction w/the Hct and Plt count. Hct count must be >25% and Plt count >50 K/μL for the test to be performed.
- COL/ADP: 70-120 seconds
- COL/EPI: 75-120 seconds

↑: acquired Plt dysfunction, vWD, anemia, thrombocytopenia, use of ASA and NSAIDs.

POTASSIUM (K⁺) (SERUM)

Nl range: 3.5-5 mEq/L.

↑ or ↓: see "Hypokalemia" and "Hyperkalemia" in Chapter 9.

PROGESTERONE (SERUM)

Nl:
- Female: 15-70 ng/dL (follicular phase); 200-2500 ng/dL (luteal phase)
- Male: 15-70 ng/dL

↑: congenital adrenal hyperplasia, clomiphene, corticosterone, 11-deoxycortisol, dihydroprogesterone, molar pregnancy, lipoid ovarian tumor.

↓: primary or secondary hypogonadism, oral contraceptives, ampicillin, threatened abortion.

PROLACTIN

Nl range: <20 ng/mL.

↑: prolactinomas (level >200 highly suggestive), drugs (phenothiazines, cimetidine, tricyclic antidepressants, metoclopramide, estrogens, antihypertensives [methyldopa, verapamil], haloperidol), post partum, stress, hypoglycemia, hypothyroidism.

PROSTATE-SPECIFIC ANTIGEN (PSA)

Nl range: 0-4 ng/mL. There is no PSA level below which prostate cancer can be ruled out and no level above which prostate cancer is certain. The individual's PSA level is only part of the equation. Other risk factors need to be considered, such as age, race, FHx, findings on digital rectal examination, percentage free PSA ratio, and PSA velocity (rate of change from prior PSA measurement).

↑: BPH, carcinoma of prostate, after rectal examination, prostate trauma, androgens, prostatitis, urethral instrumentation.

Note: Measurement of free PSA is useful to assess the probability of prostate cancer in pts w/nl findings on digital rectal examination and total PSA level between 4 and 10 ng/mL. In these pts, the global risk of prostate cancer is 25% to 40%. However, if the free PSA is >25%, the risk of prostate cancer ↓ to 8%; whereas if the free PSA is <10%, the risk of cancer ↑ to 56%. Free PSA is also useful to evaluate the aggressiveness of prostate cancer. A low free PSA percentage generally indicates a high-grade cancer, whereas a high free PSA percentage is generally associated w/a slower growing tumor.

↓: finasteride, dutasteride, bed rest, antiandrogens.

PROSTATIC ACID PHOSPHATASE

NI: 0-0.8 U/L.
↑: prostate cancer (especially in metastatic prostate cancer), BPH, prostatitis, after prostate surgery or manipulation, hemolysis, androgens, clofibrate.
↓: ketoconazole Rx.

PROTEIN (SERUM)

NI range: 6-8 g/dL.
↑: dehydration, sarcoidosis, collagen-vascular diseases, MM, Waldenström's macroglobulinemia.
↓: malnutrition, cirrhosis, nephrosis, low-protein diet, overhydration, malabsorption, pregnancy, severe burns, neoplasms, chronic diseases.

PROTEIN C ASSAY

NI: 70%-140%.
↑: oral contraceptives, stanozolol.
↓: congenital protein C deficiency, warfarin Rx, vitamin K deficiency, renal insufficiency, consumptive coagulopathies.

PROTEIN ELECTROPHORESIS (SERUM)

NI range:
- Alb: 60%-75%; 3.6-5.2 g/dL
- α_1: 1.7%-5%; 0.1-0.4 g/dL
- α_2: 6.7%-12.5%; 0.4-1.0 g/dL
- β: 8.3%-16.3%; 0.5-1.2 g/dL
- Gamma: 10.7%-20%; 0.6-1.6 g/dL

↑:
- Alb: dehydration
- α_1: neoplastic diseases, inflammation
- α_2: neoplasms, inflammation, infection, nephrotic syndrome
- β: hypothyroidism, biliary cirrhosis, DM
- Gamma: see "Immunoglobulins," earlier

↓:
- Alb: malnutrition, chronic liver disease, malabsorption, nephrotic syndrome, burns, SLE
- α_1: emphysema (α_1-antitrypsin deficiency), nephrosis
- α_2: hemolytic anemias (↓ haptoglobin), severe hepatocellular damage
- β: hypocholesterolemia, nephrosis
- Gamma: see "Immunoglobulins," earlier

PROTEIN S ASSAY

NI: 65%-140%.
↑: presence of lupus anticoagulant.
↓: hereditary deficiency, acute thrombotic events, DIC, surgery, oral contraceptives, pregnancy, hormone replacement Rx, L-asparaginase Rx.

PROTHROMBIN TIME (PT)

NI range: 11-13.2 seconds.
Note: The PT is reported as absolute clotting time in seconds and also as a derivative number called the INR. This ratio is derived from the actual PT of the pt divided by the mean PT of a group of healthy subjects. INR should always be used in interpreting PT.
↑: liver disease, oral anticoagulants (warfarin), heparin, factor deficiency (I, II, V, VII, X), DIC, vitamin K deficiency, afibrinogenemia, dysfibrinogenemia, drugs (salicylate, chloral hydrate, diphenylhydantoin, estrogens, antacids, phenylbutazone, quinidine, abx, allopurinol, anabolic steroids).
↓: vitamin K supplementation, thrombophlebitis, drugs (glutethimide, estrogens, griseofulvin, diphenhydramine).

PROTOPORPHYRIN (FREE ERYTHROCYTE)

NI range: 16-36 μg/dL of RBCs.
↑: iron deficiency, lead poisoning, sideroblastic anemias, anemia of chronic disease, hemolytic anemias, erythropoietic protoporphyria.

PSA; SEE PROSTATE-SPECIFIC ANTIGEN (PSA)

PT; SEE PROTHROMBIN TIME (PT)

PTT; SEE PARTIAL THROMBOPLASTIN TIME (PTT)

RDW; SEE RED BLOOD CELL DISTRIBUTION WIDTH (RDW)

RED BLOOD CELL COUNT

Nl range: $4.3-5.9 \times 10^6/mm^3$ (male); $3.5-5.0 \times 10^6/mm^3$ (female).
↑: hemoconcentration and dehydration, stress, PV, smokers, high altitude, CV
  disease, renal cell carcinoma and other erythropoietin-producing neoplasms.
↓: anemias, hemolysis, chronic renal failure, hemorrhage, failure of marrow production.

RED BLOOD CELL DISTRIBUTION WIDTH (RDW)

RDW measures variability of red cell size (anisocytosis)
Nl range: 11.5-14.5.
Nl RDW and:
  • ↑ MCV: aplastic anemia, preleukemia.
  • Nl MCV: nl, anemia of chronic disease, acute blood loss or hemolysis, CLL, CML,
    nonanemic enzymopathy or hemoglobinopathy.
  • ↓ MCV: anemia of chronic disease, heterozygous thalassemia.
↑ RDW and:
  • ↑ MCV: vitamin B_{12} deficiency, folate deficiency, immune hemolytic anemia, cold
    agglutinins, CLL w/high count, liver disease.
  • Nl MCV: early iron deficiency, early vitamin B_{12} deficiency, early folate deficiency,
    anemic globinopathy.
  • ↓ MCV: iron deficiency, RBC fragmentation, HbH disease, thalassemia intermedia.

RED BLOOD CELL FOLATE; SEE FOLATE

RED BLOOD CELL MASS (VOLUME)

Nl range:
  • Male: 20-36 mL/kg of BW ($1.15-1.21$ L/m^2 BSA)
  • Female: 19-31 mL/kg of BW ($0.95-1.00$ L/m^2 BSA)
↑: P vera, hypoxia (smokers, high altitude, CV disease), hemoglobinopathies w/↑O_2
  affinity, erythropoietin-producing tumors (renal cell carcinoma).
↓: hemorrhage, chronic disease, failure of marrow production, anemias, hemolysis.

RENIN (SERUM)

↑: renal HTN, reduced plasma volume, secondary aldosteronism, drugs (thiazides,
  estrogen, minoxidil), chronic renal failure, Bartter's syndrome, pregnancy (nl),
  pheochromocytoma.
↓: primary aldosteronism, adrenocortical HTN, ↑ in plasma volume, drugs
  (propranolol, reserpine, clonidine).

RETICULOCYTE COUNT

Nl range: 0.5%-1.5%.
↑: hemolytic anemia (sickle cell crisis, thalassemia major, autoimmune hemolysis),
  hemorrhage, after anemia Rx (folic acid, ferrous sulfate, vitamin B_{12}), chronic renal
  failure.
↓: aplastic anemia, marrow suppression (sepsis, chemotherapeutic agents, radiation),
  hepatic cirrhosis, blood transfusion, anemias of disordered maturation (iron deficiency
  anemia, megaloblastic anemia, sideroblastic anemia, anemia of chronic disease).

RHEUMATOID FACTOR (RF)

Nl: (−)
Present in titer >1:20: RA, SLE, chronic inflammatory processes, old age, infections,
  liver disease, MM, sarcoidosis, pulmonary fibrosis, Sjögren's syndrome.

RNP; SEE EXTRACTABLE NUCLEAR ANTIGEN

SEDIMENTATION RATE; SEE ERYTHROCYTE SEDIMENTATION RATE

SEMEN ANALYSIS

Nl:
  • Volume: 2-6 mL
  • Sperm density: >20 million/mL
  • Total number of spermatozoa: >80 million/ejaculate
  • Progressive motility score evaluated 2-4 hr after ejaculate: 3-4
  • Live spermatozoa: ≥50% of total
  • Nl spermatozoa: ≥60% of total
  • Immature forms: <4%

↓: cryptorchidism, testicular failure, obstruction of ejaculatory system, after vasectomy, medications (cimetidine, ketoconazole, nitrofurantoin, cancer chemoRx agents, sulfasalazine), testicular radiation.

SGOT; SEE ASPARTATE AMINOTRANSFERASE (AST, SGOT)

SGPT; SEE ALANINE AMINOTRANSFERASE (ALT, SGPT)

SICKLE CELL TEST
Nl: (−)
(+) in: sickle cell anemia, sickle cell trait; combination of Hgb S gene w/other disorders, such as thalassemias.

SMOOTH MUSCLE ANTIBODY
Nl: (−)
Present in: chronic active hepatitis (≥1:80), PBC (≥1:80), infectious mononucleosis.

NA⁺ (SERUM)
Nl range: 135-147 mEq/L.
↑: see "Hypernatremia" in Chapter 9.
↓: see "Hyponatremia" in Chapter 9.

SUDAN III STAIN (QUALITATIVE SCREENING FOR FECAL FAT)
Nl: (−) The test should be preceded by a diet containing 100 to 150 g of dietary fat/day for 1 week, avoidance of high-fiber diet, and avoidance of suppositories or oily material before specimen collection.
(+) in: steatorrhea, use of castor oil or mineral oil droplets.

T₃ (TRIIODOTHYRONINE)
Nl range: 75-220 ng/dL.
Abnl values: see "Hypothyroidism" and "Hyperthyroidism" in Chapter 5.

T₃ RESIN UPTAKE (T₃RU)
Nl range: 25%-35%.
Abnl values: in hyperthyroidism. T_3 resin uptake (T_3RU or RT_3U) measures the percentage of free T_4 (not bound to protein); it does not measure serum T_3 concentration. T_3RU and other tests that reflect thyroid hormone binding to plasma protein are also known as THBR.

T₄, SERUM T₄, AND FREE T₄ (FREE THYROXINE)
Nl range: 0.8-2.8 ng/dL.
Abnl values: see "Hyperthyroidism" in Chapter 5. Serum thyroxine test measures both circulating thyroxine bound to protein (represents >99% of circulating T_4 and unbound [free] thyroxine). Values vary w/protein binding; changes in the concentration of T_4 secondary to changes in TBG can be caused by the following:
• ↑ TBG (↑↑T_4): pregnancy, estrogens, acute infectious hepatitis, oral contraceptives, familial, fluorouracil, clofibrate, heroin, methadone.
• ↓ TBG (↓↑T_4): androgens, glucocorticoids, nephrotic syndrome, cirrhosis, acromegaly, hypoproteinemia, familial, phenytoin, ASA and other NSAIDs, high-dose PCN, asparaginase, chronic debilitating illness.
To eliminate the suspected influence of protein binding on thyroxine values, two additional tests are available: T_3 resin uptake and serum free thyroxine.
Serum free T_4 directly measures unbound thyroxine. Free T_4 can be measured by equilibrium dialysis (gold standard of free T_4 assays) or by immunometric techniques (influenced by serum levels of lipids, proteins, and certain drugs).
The FTI can also be easily calculated by multiplying T_4 times T_3RU and dividing the result by 100; the FTI corrects for any abnl T_4 values secondary to protein binding: $FTI = T_4 \times T_3RU/100$. Nl values equal 1.1 to 4.3.

TESTOSTERONE
Nl range: variable with age and sex.
• Serum/plasma: 170-1000 ng/dL (males); 15-70 ng/dL (females)
• Urine: 50-135 μg/day (males); 2-12 μg/day (females)
↑: adrenogenital syndrome, polycystic ovary disease.
↓: Klinefelter's syndrome, male hypogonadism.

THIAMINE
Nl: 275-675 ng/g.
↑: PV, leukemia, Hodgkin's disease.
↓: alcoholism, dietary deficiency (beriberi), excessive consumption of tea (contains antithiamine factor) or raw fish (contains a microbial thiaminase), chronic illness, prolonged illness, barbiturates.

THROMBIN TIME (TT)
Nl range: 11.3-18.5 seconds.
↑: thrombolytic and heparin Rx, DIC, hypofibrinogenemia, dysfibrinogenemia.

THYROGLOBULIN
Nl: 3-40 ng/mL. Thyroglobulin is a tumor marker for monitoring the status of pts w/ papillary or follicular thyroid cancer after resection.
↑: papillary or follicular thyroid cancer, Hashimoto's thyroiditis, Graves' disease, subacute thyroiditis.

THYROID MICROSOMAL ANTIBODIES
Nl: undetectable. Low titers may be present in 5% to 10% of nl individuals.
↑: Hashimoto's disease, thyroid carcinoma, early hypothyroidism, pernicious anemia.

THYROID-STIMULATING HORMONE (TSH)
Nl: 2-6 U/mL.
↑: see "Hypothyroidism" and "Hyperthyroidism" in Chapter 5.

THYROTROPIN (TSH) RECEPTOR ANTIBODIES
Nl: <130 % of basal activity.
↑: values between 1.3 and 2.0 are found in 10% of pts w/thyroid disease other than Graves' disease. Values >2.8 have been found only in pts w/Graves' disease.

TIBC; SEE IRON-BINDING CAPACITY

TISSUE TRANSGLUTAMINASE ANTIBODY
Nl: (−)
Present in: celiac disease (specificity, 94%-97%; sensitivity, 90%-98%), dermatitis herpetiformis.

TRANSFERRIN
Nl range: 170-370 mg/dL.
↑: iron deficiency anemia, oral contraceptive administration, viral hepatitis, late pregnancy.
↓: nephrotic syndrome, liver disease, hereditary deficiency, protein malnutrition, neoplasms, chronic inflammatory states, chronic illness, thalassemia, hemochromatosis, hemolytic anemia.

TRIGLYCERIDES
Nl range: <150 mg/dL.
↑: hyperlipoproteinemias (types I, IIb, III, IV, V), diet high in saturated fats, hypothyroidism, pregnancy, estrogens, pancreatitis, EtOH intake, nephrotic syndrome, poorly controlled DM, sedentary lifestyle, glycogen storage disease.
↓: malnutrition, vigorous exercise, congenital abetalipoproteinemias, drugs (e.g., gemfibrozil, fenofibrate, nicotinic acid, metformin, clofibrate).

TRIIODOTHYRONINE; SEE T_3 (TRIIODOTHYRONINE)

TROPONINS (SERUM)
Nl range: 0-0.4 ng/mL ([−]). If there is clinical suspicion of evolving acute MI or ischemic episode, repeated testing in 5 to 6 hr is recommended.
Indeterminate: 0.05-0.49 ng/mL. Suggest further tests. In a pt w/unstable angina and this troponin I level, there is an ↑ in risk of a cardiac event in the near future.
High probability of acute MI: ≥0.50 ng/mL.
- cTnT is a highly sensitive marker for myocardial injury for the first 48 hr after MI and for up to 5 to 7 days. It may also be ↑ in renal failure, chronic muscle disease, and trauma.
- cTnI is highly sensitive and specific for myocardial injury (≥CK-MB) in the initial 8 hr, peaks within 24 hr, and lasts up to 7 days. With progressively higher levels of cTnI, the risk of mortality ↑ because the amount of necrosis ↑.

↑: in addition to ACS, many diseases such as sepsis, hypovolemia, AF, CHF, PE, myocarditis, myocardial contusion, and renal failure can be associated w/ an ↑ in troponin level.

TSH; SEE THYROID-STIMULATING HORMONE (TSH)

TT; SEE THROMBIN TIME

UNCONJUGATED BILIRUBIN; SEE BILIRUBIN, INDIRECT

UREA NITROGEN
NI range: 8-18 mg/dL.
↑: dehydration, renal disease (GN, pyelonephritis, diabetic nephropathy), urinary tract obstruction (prostatic hypertrophy), drugs (AGs and other abx, diuretics, lithium, corticosteroids), GI bleeding, ↓ renal blood flow (shock, CHF, MI).
↓: liver disease, malnutrition, third trimester of pregnancy.

URIC ACID (SERUM)
NI range: 2-7 mg/dL.
↑: hereditary enzyme deficiency (hypoxanthine-guanine phosphoribosyltransferase), renal failure, gout, excessive cell lysis (chemotherapeutic agents, radiation Rx, leukemia, lymphoma, hemolytic anemia), acidosis, myeloproliferative disorders, diet high in purines or protein, drugs (diuretics, low doses of ASA, ethambutol, nicotinic acid), lead poisoning, hypothyroidism.
↓: drugs (allopurinol, febuxostat, high doses of ASA, probenecid, warfarin, corticosteroid), deficiency of xanthine oxidase, SIADH, renal tubular deficits (Fanconi's syndrome), alcoholism, liver disease, diet deficient in protein or purines, Wilson's disease, hemochromatosis.

URINALYSIS
NI range:
- Color: light straw
- Appearance: clear
- pH: 4.5-8.0 (average, 6.0)
- Specific gravity: 1.005-1.030
- Protein: absent
- Ketones: absent
- Glucose: absent
- Occult blood: absent

Microscopic examination:
- RBC: 0-5 (high-power field)
- WBC: 0-5 (high-power field)
- Bacteria (spun specimen): absent
- Casts: 0-4 hyaline (low-power field)

URINE AMYLASE
NI range: 35-260 U Somogyi/hr.
↑: pancreatitis, carcinoma of the pancreas.

URINE BILE
NI: absent.
Abn:
- Urine bilirubin: hepatitis (viral, toxic, drug induced), biliary obstruction.
- Urine urobilinogen: hepatitis (viral, toxic, drug induced), hemolytic jaundice, liver cell dysfunction (cirrhosis, infection, mets).

URINE CALCIUM
NI: 6.2 mmol/dL (CF, 0.02495; SMI, 0.1 mmol/dL).
↑: primary hyperparathyroidism, hypervitaminosis D, bone mets, MM, ↑ in Ca intake, steroids, prolonged immobilization, sarcoidosis, Paget's disease, idiopathic hypercalciuria, renal tubular acidosis.
↓: hypoparathyroidism, pseudohypoparathyroidism, vitamin D deficiency, vitamin D–resistant rickets, diet low in Ca, drugs (thiazide diuretics, oral contraceptives), familial hypocalciuric hypercalcemia, renal osteodystrophy, K+ citrate Rx.

URINE cAMP
↑: hypercalciuria, familial hypocalciuric hypercalcemia, primary hyperparathyroidism, pseudohypoparathyroidism, rickets.
↓: vitamin D intoxication, sarcoidosis.

URINE CATECHOLAMINES
Nl range: <100 μg/24 hr (norepinephrine); <10 μg/24 hr (epinephrine).
↑: pheochromocytoma, neuroblastoma, severe stress.

URINE CHLORIDE
Nl range: 110-250 mEq/day.
↑: corticosteroids, Bartter's syndrome, diuretics, metabolic acidosis, severe hypokalemia.
↓: chloride depletion (vomiting), colonic villous adenoma, chronic renal failure, renal tubular acidosis.

URINE CREATININE (24-HOUR)
Nl range: 0.8-1.8 g/day (male); 0.6-1.6 g/day (female).
Note: Useful test as an indicator of completeness of 24-hour urine collection.

URINE CRYSTALS
Uric acid: acid urine, hyperuricosuria, uric acid nephropathy.
Sulfur: abx containing sulfa.
Calcium oxalate: ethylene glycol poisoning, acid urine, hyperoxaluria.
Calcium PO_4^{-3}: alkaline urine.
Cystine: cystinuria.

URINE EOSINOPHILS
Nl: absent.
Present in: interstitial nephritis, ATN, UTI, kidney transplant rejection, HRS.

URINE GLUCOSE (QUALITATIVE)
Nl: absent.
Present in: DM, renal glycosuria (↓ renal threshold for glucose), glucose intolerance.

URINE HEMOGLOBIN, FREE
Nl: absent.
Present in: hemolysis (w/saturation of serum haptoglobin binding capacity and renal threshold for tubular absorption of Hgb).

URINE HEMOSIDERIN
Nl: absent.
Present in: PNH, chronic hemolytic anemia, hemochromatosis, blood transfusion, thalassemias.

URINE 5-HYDROXYINDOLEACETIC ACID (URINE 5-HIAA)
Nl range: 2-8 mg/24 hr.
↑: carcinoid tumors, after ingestion of certain foods (bananas, plums, tomatoes, avocados, pineapples, eggplant, walnuts), drugs (MAOIs, phenacetin, methyldopa, glycerol guaiacolate, acetaminophen, salicylates, phenothiazines, imipramine, methocarbamol, reserpine, methamphetamine).

URINE INDICAN
Nl: absent.
Present in: malabsorption resulting from intestinal bacterial overgrowth.

URINE KETONES (SEMIQUANTITATIVE)
Nl: absent.
Present in: DKA, alcoholic ketoacidosis, starvation, isopropanol ingestion.

URINE METANEPHRINES
Nl range: 0-2.0 mg/24 hr.
↑: pheochromocytoma, neuroblastoma, drugs (caffeine, phenothiazines, MAOIs), stress.

URINE MYOGLOBIN
Nl: absent.
Present in: severe trauma, hyperthermia, polymyositis or dermatomyositis, CO poisoning, drugs (narcotic and amphetamine toxicity), hypothyroidism, muscle ischemia.

URINE NITRITE
Nl: absent.
Present in: UTIs.

31

URINE OCCULT BLOOD

Nl: (−)

(+) in: trauma to urinary tract, renal disease (GN, pyelonephritis), renal or ureteral calculi, bladder lesions (carcinoma, cystitis), prostatitis, prostatic carcinoma, menstrual contamination, hematopoietic disorders (hemophilia, thrombocytopenia), anticoagulants, ASA.

Note: Hematuria w/o erythrocyte casts or significant albuminuria suggests the possibility of renal or bladder cancers.

URINE OSMOLALITY

Nl range: 50-1200 mOsm/kg.

↑: SIADH, dehydration, glycosuria, adrenal insufficiency, high-protein diet.

↓: diabetes insipidus, excessive water intake, IV hydration w/D$_5$W, acute renal insufficiency, GN.

URINE pH

Nl range: 4.6-8.0 (average 6.0).

↑: bacteriuria, vegetarian diet, renal failure w/inability to form ammonia, drugs (abx, NaHCO$_3$, acetazolamide).

↓: acidosis (metabolic, respiratory), drugs (ammonium chloride, methenamine mandelate), DM, starvation, diarrhea.

URINE PO$_4^{-3}$

Nl range: 0.8-2.0 g/24 hr.

↑: ATN (diuretic phase), chronic renal disease, uncontrolled DM, hyperparathyroidism, hypomagnesemia, metabolic acidosis, metabolic alkalosis, neurofibromatosis, adult-onset vitamin D–resistant hypophosphatemic osteomalacia.

↓: acromegaly, ARF, ↓ dietary intake, hypoparathyroidism, respiratory acidosis.

URINE K$^+$

Nl range: 25-100 mEq/24 hr.

↑: aldosteronism (primary, secondary), glucocorticoids, alkalosis, renal tubular acidosis, excessive dietary K$^+$ intake.

↓: ARF, K$^+$-sparing diuretics, diarrhea, hypokalemia.

URINE PROTEIN (QUANTITATIVE)

Nl range: <150 mg/24 hr.

↑: renal disease (glomerular, tubular, interstitial), CHF, HTN, neoplasms of renal pelvis and bladder, MM, Waldenström's macroglobulinemia.

URINE NA$^+$ (QUANTITATIVE)

Nl range: 40-220 mEq/day.

↑: diuretic administration, high Na$^+$ intake, salt-losing nephritis, ATN, vomiting, Addison's disease, SIADH, hypothyroidism, CHF, hepatic failure, chronic renal failure, Bartter's syndrome, glucocorticoid deficiency, interstitial nephritis (caused by analgesic abuse, mannitol, dextran, or glycerol Rx), milk-alkali syndrome, ↓ renin secretion, postobstructive diuresis.

↓: ↑ in aldosterone, glucocorticoid excess, hyponatremia, prerenal azotemia, ↓ salt intake.

URINE SPECIFIC GRAVITY

Nl range: 1.005-1.03.

↑: dehydration, excessive fluid losses (vomiting, diarrhea, fever), x-ray contrast media, DM, CHF, SIADH, adrenal insufficiency, ↓ fluid intake.

↓: diabetes insipidus, renal disease (GN, pyelonephritis), excessive fluid intake or IV hydration.

URINE VANILLYLMANDELIC ACID (VMA)

Nl range: <6.8 mg/24 hr.

↑: pheochromocytoma, neuroblastoma, ganglioblastoma, drugs (isoproterenol, methocarbamol, levodopa, sulfonamides, chlorpromazine), severe stress; after ingestion of bananas, chocolate, vanilla, tea, coffee.

↓: drugs (MAOIs, reserpine, guanethidine, methyldopa).

VASOACTIVE INTESTINAL PEPTIDE (VIP)

Nl: <50 pg/mL.

↑: pancreatic VIPomas, neuroblastoma, pancreatic islet call hyperplasia, liver disease, multiple endocrine neoplasia type I, ganglioneuroma, ganglioneuroblastoma.

VENEREAL DISEASE RESEARCH LABORATORIES (VDRL)

Nl range: (–)

(+) test: syphilis, other treponemal diseases (yaws, pinta, bejel).
Note: A false-(+) test result may be seen in pts w/SLE and other autoimmune diseases, infectious mononucleosis, HIV infection, atypical pneumonia, malaria, leprosy, typhus fever, rat-bite fever, and relapsing fever.

VIP; SEE VASOACTIVE INTESTINAL PEPTIDE (VIP)

VISCOSITY (SERUM)

Nl range: 1.4-1.8 relative to water (1.10-1.22 centipoise).
↑: monoclonal gammopathies (Waldenström's macroglobulinemia, MM), hyperfibrinogenemia, SLE, RA, polycythemia, leukemia.

VITAMIN B$_{12}$

Nl range: 190-900 ng/mL.
↓: pernicious anemia, dietary (strict lacto-ovovegetarians, food faddists), malabsorption (achlorhydria, gastrectomy, ileal resection, Crohn's disease of terminal ileum, pancreatic insufficiency, drugs [omeprazole and other PPIs], metformin, cholestyramine]), chronic alcoholism, *H. pylori* infection.

VITAMIN D, 1,25-DIHYDROXYCHOLECALCIFEROL

Nl: 32-65 pg/mL.
↑: tumor calcinosis, primary hyperparathyroidism, sarcoidosis, tuberculosis, idiopathic hypercalciuria.
↓: postmenopausal osteoporosis, chronic renal failure, hypoparathyroidism, tumor-induced osteomalacia, rickets, ↑ blood lead levels.

VITAMIN K

Nl: 0.10-2.20 ng/mL.
↓: PBC, anticoagulants, abx, cholestyramine, GI disease, pancreatic disease, cystic fibrosis, obstructive jaundice, hypoprothrombinemia, hemorrhagic disease of the newborn.

VON WILLEBRAND FACTOR

Nl: levels vary according to blood type: 50-150 U/dL (blood type O); 90-200 U/dL (blood type non-O).
↓: vWD (however, in type II vWD, the antigen may be nl but the function is impaired).

WBCs; SEE COMPLETE BLOOD COUNT (CBC)

WESTERGREN; SEE ERYTHROCYTE SEDIMENTATION RATE (ESR)

WHITE BLOOD CELL COUNT; SEE COMPLETE BLOOD COUNT (CBC)

D-XYLOSE ABSORPTION

Nl range: 21%-31% excreted in 5 hr.
↓: malabsorption syndrome.

D-XYLOSE ABSORPTION TEST

Nl range:
- Urine: ≥4 g/5 hr (5-hour urine collection in adults ≥12 years; 25-g dose)
- Serum: ≥25 mg/dL (adult, 1 hour, 25-g dose, nl renal function)

Nl results: In pts w/malabsorption, nl results suggest pancreatic disease as a cause of the malabsorption.

Abnl results: celiac disease, Crohn's disease, tropical sprue, surgical bowel resection, AIDS. False-(+) results can occur w/ ↓ renal function, dehydration or hypovolemia, surgical blind loops, ↓ gastric emptying, vomiting.

References

Dhingra R, Gona P, Nam BH, et al: C-reactive protein, inflammatory conditions, and CV disease risk, *Am J Med* 120:1054–1062, 2007.

Jeremias A, Gibson M: Narrative review: Alternative cause for ↑ cardiac troponin levels when acute coronary syndromes are excluded, *Ann Intern Med* 142:786–791, 2005.

Jones JS: Four no more: The PSA cutoff era is over, *Cleve Clin J Med* 75:30–32, 2008.

McKie PM, Burnett JC: B-type natriuretic peptide as a marker beyond heart failure: Speculations and opportunities, *Mayo Clin Proc* 80:1029–1036, 2005.

Pagana KD, Pagana TJ: *Mosby's Diagnostic and Laboratory Test Reference*, ed 8, St. Louis, 2007, Mosby.

Sarnak MJ, Katz R, Stehman-Breen CO, et al: Cystatin C concentration as a risk factor for heart failure in older adults, *Ann Intern Med* 142:497–505, 2005.

Wu AHB: *Tietz Clinical Guide to Laboratory Tests*, Philadelphia, 2006, Saunders.

C. FORMULARY

1 IV DRIPS

See Table 1-1.

TABLE 1-1 ■ IV Drips

Medication	Dose	Indication	Comments and Adverse Effects
Vasopressors			
Dopamine	1-20 µg/kg/min	Cardiogenic, septic shock; low dose can preserve renal blood flow and promote urinary output	May cause tachyarrhythmias, ischemic limb necrosis
Phenylephrine (Neo-Synephrine [Bayer Corporation, West Haven, Ct])	10-200 µg/min	Hypotension	Pure α agonist
Norepinephrine (Levophed [Abbott Laboratories, Abbott Park, Ill])	1-20 µg/min	Septic shock w/hypotension refractory to dopa (low systemic vascular resistance and adequately resuscitated)	Potent α agonist (vasoconstrictor); avoid in cardiogenic shock
Vasopressin	0.01-0.04 unit/min	Refractory vasodilatory shock (late)	Avoid w/CAD
Dobutamine	2-20 µg/kg/min	Severe systolic heart failure	Inotrope and systemic vasodilator
Epinephrine	1-20 µg/min or 30-100 ng/kg/min	Second line for cardiogenic shock	Chronotrope, inotrope, and vasoconstrictor
Antihypertensives			
Nitroprusside (Nipride [Roche Laboratories, Nutley, NJ])	0.5-5 µg/kg/min	Severe HTN (particularly w/low CO)	Potent vasodilator; caution in renal and hepatic failure (cyanide/thiocyanate toxicity); do not use alone in dissection (reflex tachycardia); can ↓ Pao_2 as a result of pulmonary shunting
Nitroglycerine	10-400 µg/min	Augment CO (intermediate dose), angina (low dose, typically 0.3-0.6 mg SL q5min); hypertensive crisis	Predominantly venodilator, mediated by nitric oxide; rapid onset; headache; ↑ ICP; methemoglobinemia; tachyphylaxis
Nicardipine	5-15 mg/hr	HTN, ↓ cerebral vasospasm	Potent CCB, vasodilator; renal clearance
Diltiazem	5-15 mg/hr	HTN, atrial fibrillation	CCB, monitor HR and BP, especially if also on β-blocker
Esmolol	50-300 µg/kg/min	HTN, particularly w/aortic dissection; supraventricular tachycardia	$β_1$-Blocker, short acting
Paralytics			
Vecuronium	0.05-0.1 mg/kg/hr	Paralysis	Monitor muscle twitch (2/4 train-of-four); nondepolarizing; onset 1-2 min; caution w/hepatic failure; caution w/ steroids (including myopathy)
Cisatracurium	0.5-10 µg/kg/min	Paralysis w/renal or hepatic failure	Nondepolarizing, Hoffman elimination
Sedative			
Midazolam (Versed [Roche Laboratories, Nutley, NJ])	1-10 mg/hr	Sedation	Potent, short acting but can result in accumulation

From Nguyen TC, Abilez OJ (eds): Practical Guide to the Care of the Surgical Patient: The Pocket Scalpel. Philadelphia, Mosby, 2009.

The Differential Diagnosis: Zebras or Horses? 2

1 ABDOMINAL DISTENTION

Nonmechanical Obstruction
Excessive intraluminal gas
Intra-abdominal infection
Trauma
Retroperitoneal irritation (renal colic, neoplasms, infections, hemorrhage, ruptured AAA)
Vascular insufficiency (thrombosis, embolism)
Mechanical ventilation
Extra-abdominal infection (sepsis, pneumonia, empyema, osteomyelitis of spine)
Metabolic/toxic abnlities (hypokalemia, uremia, lead poisoning)
Chemical irritation (perforated ulcer, bile, pancreatitis)
Peritoneal inflammation
Severe pain, pain medications
Pseudo-obstruction in the elderly (Ogilvie syndrome)

Mechanical Obstruction
Neoplasm (intraluminal, extraluminal)
Adhesions, endometriosis
Infection (intra-abdominal abscess, diverticulitis)
Gallstones
Foreign body, bezoars
Pregnancy
Hernias
Volvulus
Stenosis at surgical anastomosis, radiation stenosis
Fecaliths
IBD
Gastric outlet obstruction
Hematoma
Other: parasites, superior mesenteric artery syndrome, pneumatosis

2 ABDOMINAL PAIN

Diffuse
Early appendicitis
Aortic aneurysm
Gastroenteritis (crampy pain)
Intestinal obstruction
Diverticulitis
Peritonitis
Mesenteric insufficiency or infarction
Pancreatitis
IBD
Irritable bowel
Mesenteric adenitis
Metabolic: toxins, lead poisoning, uremia, drug OD, DKA, heavy metal poisoning

Sickle cell crisis
Pneumonia (rare)
Trauma
UTI, PID
Other: narcotic withdrawal, acute intermittent porphyria, tabes dorsalis, PAN, Henoch-Schönlein purpura, adrenal insufficiency

Epigastric
Gastric: PUD, gastric outlet obstruction, gastric ulcer
Duodenal: PUD, duodenitis
Biliary: cholecystitis, cholangitis
Hepatic: hepatitis
Pancreatic: pancreatitis
Intestinal: high small bowel obstruction, early appendicitis
Cardiac: angina, MI, pericarditis
Pulmonary: pneumonia, pleurisy, pneumothorax
Subphrenic abscess
Vascular: dissecting aneurysm, mesenteric ischemia

Suprapubic
Intestinal: colon obstruction or gangrene, diverticulitis, appendicitis
Reproductive system: ectopic pregnancy, mittelschmerz, torsion of ovarian cyst, PID, salpingitis, endometriosis, rupture of endometrioma
Urinary system: cystitis, rupture of urinary bladder; bladder distention/urinary outlet obstruction

Right Upper Quadrant
Biliary: calculi, infection, inflammation, neoplasm
Hepatic: hepatitis, abscess, hepatic congestion, neoplasm, trauma
Gastric: PUD, pyloric stenosis, neoplasm, alcoholic gastritis, hiatal hernia
Pancreatic: pancreatitis, neoplasm, stone in pancreatic duct or ampulla
Renal: calculi, infection, inflammation, neoplasm, rupture of kidney
Pulmonary: pneumonia (RLL), pulmonary infarction, right-sided pleurisy
Intestinal: retrocecal appendicitis, intestinal obstruction, high fecal impaction, diverticulitis
Cardiac: myocardial ischemia (particularly involving the inferior wall), pericarditis
Cutaneous: herpes zoster
Trauma

Fitz-Hugh–Curtis syndrome
(perihepatitis)
Hepatic flexure syndrome

Left Upper Quadrant
Gastric: PUD, gastritis, pyloric stenosis, hiatal hernia
Pancreatic: pancreatitis, neoplasm, stone in pancreatic duct or ampulla
Cardiac: MI, angina pectoris
Splenic: splenomegaly, ruptured spleen, splenic abscess, splenic infarction
Renal: calculi, pyelonephritis, neoplasm
Pulmonary: pneumonia, empyema, pulmonary infarction
Vascular: ruptured aortic aneurysm
Cutaneous: herpes zoster
Trauma
Intestinal: high fecal impaction, perforated colon, diverticulitis
Splenic flexure syndrome

Periumbilical
Intestinal: small bowel obstruction or gangrene, early appendicitis
Vascular: mesenteric thrombosis, dissecting aortic aneurysm
Pancreatic: pancreatitis
Metabolic: uremia, DKA
Umbilical hernia, incarcerated
Trauma

Right Lower Quadrant
Intestinal: acute appendicitis, regional enteritis, incarcerated hernia, cecal diverticulitis, intestinal obstruction, perforated ulcer, perforated cecum, Meckel's diverticulitis
Reproductive: ectopic pregnancy, ovarian cyst, torsion of ovarian cyst, salpingitis, tubo-ovarian abscess, mittelschmerz, endometriosis, seminal vesiculitis
Renal: renal and ureteral calculi, neoplasms, pyelonephritis
Vascular: leaking aortic aneurysm
Psoas abscess
Trauma
Cholecystitis

Left Lower Quadrant
Intestinal: diverticulitis, intestinal obstruction, perforated ulcer, IBD, perforated descending colon, inguinal hernia, neoplasm, appendicitis
Reproductive: ectopic pregnancy, ovarian cyst, torsion of ovarian cyst, tubo-ovarian abscess, mittelschmerz, endometriosis, seminal vesiculitis
Renal: renal or ureteral calculi, pyelonephritis, neoplasm
Vascular: leaking aortic aneurysm
Psoas abscess
Trauma

3 ADNEXAL MASS
Ovary (neoplasm, endometriosis, functional cyst)
Fallopian tube (ectopic pregnancy, neoplasm, tubo-ovarian abscess, hydrosalpinx, paratubal cyst)
Uterus (fibroid, neoplasm)
Retroperitoneum (neoplasm, abdominal wall hematoma or abscess)
Urinary tract (pelvic kidney, distended bladder, urachal cyst)
IBD
GI tract neoplasm
Diverticular disease
Appendicitis
Bowel loop w/feces

4 ADRENAL MASSES

Unilateral Adrenal Mass
Functional Lesions
Adrenal adenoma
Adrenal carcinoma
Pheochromocytoma
Primary aldosteronism, adenomatous type
Nonfunctional Lesions
Incidentaloma of adrenal gland
Ganglioneuroma
Myelolipoma
Hematoma
Adenolipoma
Metastasis

Bilateral Adrenal Mass
Functional Lesions
ACTH-dependent Cushing's syndrome
Congenital adrenal hyperplasia
Pheochromocytoma
Conn's syndrome, hyperplastic variety
Micronodular adrenal disease
Idiopathic bilateral adrenal hypertrophy
Nonfunctional Lesions
Infection (tuberculosis, fungi)
Infiltration (leukemia, lymphoma)
Replacement (amyloidosis)
Hemorrhage
Bilateral mets

5 AMENORRHEA
Pregnancy, early menopause
Hypothalamic dysfunction: defective synthesis or release of luteinizing hormone–releasing hormone, anorexia nervosa, stress, exercise
Pituitary dysfunction: neoplasm, postpartum hemorrhage, surgery, radiationRx
Ovarian dysfunction: gonadal dysgenesis, 17α-hydroxylase deficiency, premature ovarian failure, polycystic ovarian disease, gonadal stromal tumors
Uterovaginal abnlities:
   Congenital: imperforate hymen, imperforate cervix, imperforate or absent vagina, müllerian agenesis
   Acquired: destruction of endometrium w/curettage (Asherman's syndrome),

closure of cervix or vagina caused by traumatic injury, hysterectomy
Other: androgen insensitivity (testicular feminization), metabolic diseases (liver, kidney), malnutrition, rapid weight loss, exogenous obesity, endocrine abnlities (Cushing's syndrome, Graves' disease, hypothyroidism)

6 AMNESIA

Degenerative diseases (e.g., Alzheimer's, Huntington's)
CVA (especially when involving thalamus, basal forebrain, and hippocampus)
Head trauma
Postsurgical (e.g., mammillary body surgery, bilateral temporal lobectomy)
Infections (herpes simplex encephalitis, meningitis)
Wernicke-Korsakoff syndrome
Cerebral hypoxia
Hypoglycemia
CNS neoplasms
Creutzfeldt-Jakob disease
Medications (e.g., midazolam and other benzos)
Psychosis
Malingering

7 ANISOCORIA

Mydriatic or miotic drugs
Prosthetic eye
Inflammation (keratitis, iridocyclitis)
Infections (herpes zoster, syphilis, meningitis, encephalitis, diphtheria, botulism)
Subdural hemorrhage
Cavernous sinus thrombosis
Intracranial neoplasm
Cerebral aneurysm
Glaucoma
CNS degenerative diseases
Internal carotid ischemia
Toxic polyneuritis (alcohol, lead)
Adie's syndrome
Horner's syndrome
DM
Trauma
Congenital

8 ARTHRITIS AND RASH

Chronic urticaria
Vasculitic urticaria
SLE
Dermatomyositis
Polymyositis
Psoriatic arthritis
Reactive arthritis
Chronic sarcoidosis
Serum sickness
Sweet's syndrome
Leprosy
Juvenile RA
Rubella
Erythema nodosum

9 BACK PAIN

Trauma: injury to bone, joint, or ligament
Mechanical: pregnancy, obesity, fatigue, scoliosis
Degenerative: osteoarthritis
Infections: osteomyelitis, subarachnoid or spinal abscess, tuberculosis, meningitis, basilar pneumonia
Metabolic: osteoporosis, osteomalacia
Vascular: leaking aortic aneurysm, subarachnoid or spinal hemorrhage/infarction
Neoplastic: myeloma, Hodgkin's disease, carcinoma of pancreas; metastatic neoplasm from breast, prostate, lung
GI: penetrating ulcer, pancreatitis, cholelithiasis, IBD
Renal: hydronephrosis, calculus, neoplasm, renal infarction, pyelonephritis
Hematologic: sickle cell crisis, acute hemolysis
Gynecologic: neoplasm of uterus or ovary, dysmenorrhea, salpingitis, uterine prolapse
Inflammatory: ankylosing spondylitis, psoriatic arthritis, Reiter's syndrome
Lumbosacral strain
Psychogenic: malingering, hysteria, anxiety
Endocrine: adrenal hemorrhage or infarction
Blood transfusion reaction

10 BREAST MASS

Fibrocystic breasts
Benign tumors (fibroadenoma, papilloma)
Mastitis (acute bacterial mastitis, chronic mastitis)
Malignant neoplasm
Fat necrosis
Hematoma
Duct ectasia
Mammary adenosis

11 BREATH ODOR

Sweet, fruity: DKA, starvation ketosis
Fishy, stale: uremia (trimethylamines)
Ammonia-like: uremia (ammonia)
Musty fish, clover: fetor hepaticus (hepatic failure)
Foul, feculent: intestinal obstruction/diverticulum
Foul, putrid: nasal/sinus pathology (infection, foreign body, cancer), respiratory infections (empyema, lung abscess, bronchiectasis)
Achalasia
Halitosis: tonsillitis, gingivitis, respiratory infections, Vincent's angina, gastroesophageal reflux
Cinnamon: pulmonary tuberculosis

12 BULLOUS DISEASES

Bullous pemphigoid
Pemphigus vulgaris
Pemphigus foliaceus
Paraneoplastic pemphigus
Cicatricial pemphigoid
Erythema multiforme
Dermatitis herpetiformis
Herpes gestationis
Impetigo
Erosive lichen planus
Linear IgA bullous dermatosis
Epidermolysis bullosa acquisita

13 CHEST PAIN (NONPLEURITIC)

Cardiac: myocardial ischemia/infarction, myocarditis
Esophageal: spasm, esophagitis, ulceration, neoplasm, achalasia, diverticula, foreign body
Referred pain from subdiaphragmatic GI structures:
Gastric and duodenal: hiatal hernia, neoplasm, PUD
Gallbladder and biliary: cholecystitis, cholelithiasis, impacted stone, neoplasm
Pancreatic: pancreatitis, neoplasm
Dissecting aortic aneurysm
Pain originating from skin, breasts, and musculoskeletal structures: herpes zoster, mastitis, chest wall phlebitis, cervical spondylosis
Mediastinal tumors: lymphoma, thymoma
Pulmonary: neoplasm, pneumonia, pulmonary embolism/infarction
Psychoneurosis
Chest pain associated w/MVP

14 CHEST PAIN (PLEURITIC)

Cardiac: pericarditis, postpericardiotomy/Dressler's syndrome
Pulmonary: pneumothorax, hemothorax, embolism/infarction, pneumonia, empyema, neoplasm, bronchiectasis, pneumomediastinum, tuberculosis, carcinomatous effusion
GI: liver abscess, pancreatitis, esophageal rupture, Whipple's disease w/associated pericarditis or pleuritis
Subdiaphragmatic abscess
Pain originating from skin and musculoskeletal tissues: costochondritis, chest wall trauma, fractured rib, interstitial fibrositis, myositis, strain of pectoralis muscle, herpes zoster, soft tissue and bone tumors
Collagen-vascular diseases w/pleuritis
Psychoneurosis
Familial Mediterranean fever

15 CLUBBING

Pulmonary neoplasm (lung, pleura)
Other neoplasm (GI, liver, Hodgkin's, thymus, osteogenic sarcoma)
Pulmonary infectious process (empyema, abscess, bronchiectasis, tuberculosis, chronic pneumonitis)
Extrapulmonary infectious process (subacute bacterial endocarditis, intestinal tuberculosis, bacterial or amebic dysentery, arterial graft sepsis)
Pneumoconiosis
Cystic fibrosis
Sarcoidosis
Cyanotic CHD
Endocrine (Graves' disease, hyperparathyroidism)
IBD
Celiac disease
Chronic liver disease, cirrhosis (particularly biliary and juvenile)
Pulmonary arteriovenous malformations
Idiopathic
Thyroid acropachy
Hereditary (pachydermoperiostosis)
Chronic trauma (e.g., in jackhammer operators, machine workers)

16 COLOR CHANGES, CUTANEOUS

Brown
Generalized: pituitary, adrenal, or liver disease; ACTH-producing tumor (e.g., oat cell lung carcinoma)
Localized: nevi, neurofibromatosis
White
Generalized: albinism, anemia
Localized: vitiligo, Raynaud's syndrome
Red (Erythema)
Generalized: fever, polycythemia, urticaria, viral exanthems
Localized: inflammation, infection, Raynaud's syndrome
Yellow
Generalized: liver disease, chronic renal disease, anemia
Generalized (except sclera): hypothyroidism, ↑ intake of vegetables containing carotene
Localized: resolving hematoma, infection, peripheral vascular insufficiency
Blue
Lips, mouth, nail beds: CV and pulmonary diseases, Raynaud's syndrome

17 COMA, NORMAL COMPUTED TOMOGRAPHY

Meningeal Disorders
Bacterial meningitis
Encephalitis

Exogenous Toxins

Sedative drugs and barbiturates
Anesthetics and γ-hydroxybutyrate[*]
Alcohols
Stimulants
Phencyclidine[†]
Cocaine and amphetamine[‡]
Psychotropic drugs
Tricyclic antidepressants
Phenothiazines
Lithium
Anticonvulsants
Opioids
Clonidine[§]
PCNs
Salicylates
Anticholinergics
CO, cyanide, and methemoglobinemia

18 COUGH

Infectious process (viral, bacterial)
Postinfection status
"Smoker's cough"
Rhinitis (allergic, vasomotor, postinfectious)
Asthma
Exposure to irritants (noxious fumes, smoke, cold air)
Drug induced (especially ACEIs, β-blockers)
GERD
ILD
Lung neoplasms
Lymphomas, mediastinal neoplasms
Bronchiectasis
Cardiac (CHF, pulmonary edema, mitral stenosis, pericardial inflammation)
Recurrent aspiration
Inflammation of larynx, pleura, diaphragm, mediastinum
Cystic fibrosis
Anxiety
Other: PE, foreign body inhalation, aortic aneurysm, Zenker's diverticulum, osteophytes, substernal thyroid, thyroiditis

19 CYANOSIS

CHD w/right-to-left shunt
PE
Hypoxia

Pulmonary edema
Pulmonary disease (O_2 diffusion and alveolar ventilation abnlities)
Hemoglobinopathies
↓ CO
Vasospasm
Arterial obstruction
Pulmonary arteriovenous fistulas
↑ hemidiaphragm
Neoplasm (bronchogenic carcinoma, mediastinal neoplasm, intrahepatic lesion)
Substernal thyroid
Infectious process (pneumonia, empyema, tuberculosis, subphrenic abscess, hepatic abscess)
Atelectasis
Idiopathic
Eventration of diaphragm
Phrenic nerve dysfunction (myelitis, myotonia, herpes zoster)
Trauma to phrenic nerve or diaphragm (e.g., surgery)
Thoracic aortic aneurysm
Intra-abdominal mass
Pulmonary infarction
Pleurisy
Radiation Rx
Rib fracture
Superior vena cava syndrome

20 DIPLOPIA, BINOCULAR

Cranial nerve palsy (third, fourth, sixth]
Thyroid eye disease
Myasthenia gravis
Decompensated strabismus
Orbital trauma w/blow-out fracture
Orbital pseudotumor
Cavernous sinus thrombosis

21 DYSPNEA

Upper airway obstruction: trauma, neoplasm, epiglottitis, laryngeal edema, tongue retraction, laryngospasm, abductor paralysis of vocal cords, aspiration of foreign body
Lower airway obstruction: neoplasm, COPD, asthma, aspiration of foreign body
Pulmonary infection: pneumonia, abscess, empyema, tuberculosis, bronchiectasis
Pulmonary HTN
Pulmonary embolism/infarction
Parenchymal lung disease
Pulmonary vascular congestion
Cardiac disease: atherosclerotic heart disease, valvular lesions, cardiac dysrhythmias, cardiomyopathy, pericardial effusion, cardiac shunts
Space-occupying lesions: neoplasm, large hiatal hernia, pleural effusions

---

[*]General anesthetic, similar to γ-aminobutyric acid; recreational drug and body building aid. Rapid onset, rapid recovery often with myoclonic jerking and confusion. Deep coma (2-3 hr; Glasgow Coma Scale = 3) with maintenance of vital signs.
[†]Coma associated with cholinergic signs: lacrimation, salivation, bronchorrhea, and hyperthermia.
[‡]Coma after seizures or status (i.e., a prolonged postictal state).
[§]An antihypertensive agent active through the opiate receptor system; frequent overdose when used to treat narcotic withdrawal.

Disease of chest wall: severe kyphoscoliosis, fractured ribs, sternal compression, morbid obesity

Neurologic dysfunction: GBS, botulism, polio, spinal cord injury

Interstitial pulmonary disease: sarcoidosis, collagen-vascular diseases, desquamative interstitial pneumonitis, Hamman-Rich pneumonitis, others

Pneumoconioses: silicosis, berylliosis, others

Mesothelioma

Pneumothorax, hemothorax, pleural effusion

Inhalation of toxins

Cholinergic drug intoxication

Carcinoid syndrome

Hematologic: anemia, polycythemia, hemoglobinopathies

Thyrotoxicosis, myxedema

Diaphragmatic compression caused by abdominal distention, subphrenic abscess, ascites

Lung resection

Metabolic abnlities: uremia, hepatic coma, DKA

Sepsis

Atelectasis

Psychoneurosis

Diaphragmatic paralysis

Pregnancy

22 DYSURIA

UTI

Estrogen deficiency (in postmenopausal woman)

Vaginitis

Genital infection (e.g., herpes, condyloma)

Interstitial cystitis

Chemical irritation (e.g., deodorant aerosols, douches)

Meatal stenosis or stricture

Reiter's syndrome

Bladder neoplasm

GI origin (diverticulitis, Crohn's disease)

Impaired bladder or sphincter action

Urethral carbuncle

Chronic fibrosis post trauma

Radiation Rx

Prostatitis

Urethritis (gonococcal, chlamydial)

Behçet's syndrome

Stevens-Johnson syndrome

23 EDEMA, GENERALIZED

CHF

Cirrhosis

Nephrotic syndrome

Pregnancy

Idiopathic

Acute nephritic syndrome

Myxedema

Medications (NSAIDs, estrogens, vasodilators), CCBs, glitazones

24 EDEMA, LEG, UNILATERAL

With Pain

DVT

Postphlebitic syndrome

Popliteal cyst rupture

Gastrocnemius rupture

Cellulitis

Psoas or other abscess

Without Pain

DVT

Postphlebitic syndrome

Other venous insufficiency (after saphenous vein harvest, varicosities)

Lymphatic obstruction/lymphedema (carcinoma, lymphoma, sarcoidosis, filariasis, retroperitoneal fibrosis)

25 EDEMA OF LOWER EXTREMITIES

CHF (right sided)

Hepatic cirrhosis

Nephrosis

Myxedema

Lymphedema

Pregnancy

Abdominal mass: neoplasm, cyst

Venous compression from abdominal aneurysm

Varicose veins

Bilateral cellulitis

Bilateral thrombophlebitis

Vena cava thrombosis, venous thrombosis

Retroperitoneal fibrosis

26 ELEVATED HEMIDIAPHRAGM

Neoplasm (bronchogenic carcinoma, mediastinal neoplasm, intrahepatic lesion)

Infectious process (pneumonia, empyema, tuberculosis, subphrenic abscess, hepatic abscess)

Atelectasis

Idiopathic

Eventration

Phrenic nerve dysfunction (myelitis, myotonia, herpes zoster, malignant neoplasm)

Trauma to phrenic nerve or diaphragm (e.g., surgery)

Aortic aneurysm

Intra-abdominal mass

Pulmonary infarction

Pleurisy

Radiation Rx

Rib fracture

27 EMBOLI, ARTERIAL

MI w/mural thrombi

AF

Cardiomyopathies

Prosthetic heart valves

CHF

Endocarditis

Left ventricular aneurysm
Left ventricular apical akinesis
Left atrial myxoma
SSS
Paradoxical embolus from venous thrombosis
Aneurysms of large blood vessels
Atheromatous ulcers of large blood vessels

28 ENCEPHALOPATHY, METABOLIC

Substrate deficiency: hypoxia/ischemia, CO poisoning, hypoglycemia
Cofactor deficiency: thiamine, vitamin B_{12}, pyridoxine (isoniazid administration)
Electrolyte disorders: hyponatremia, hypercalcemia, carbon dioxide narcosis, dialysis, hypermagnesemia, disequilibrium syndrome
Endocrinopathies: DKA, hyperosmolar coma, hypothyroidism, hyperadrenocorticism, hyperparathyroidism
Endogenous toxins: liver disease, uremia, porphyria
Exogenous toxins: drug OD (sedative-hypnotics, ethanol, narcotics, salicylates, tricyclic antidepressants), drug withdrawal, toxicity of therapeutic medications, industrial toxins (e.g., organophosphates, heavy metals), sepsis
Heat stroke
Epilepsy (postictal)
ICU encephalopathy (multifactorial)

29 FEVER AND JAUNDICE

Cholecystitis
Hepatic abscess (pyogenic, amebic)
Ascending cholangitis
Pancreatitis
Malaria
Neoplasm (hepatic, pancreatic, biliary tract, metastatic)
Mononucleosis
Viral hepatitis
Sepsis
Babesiosis
HIV infection (*Cryptosporidium*)
Biliary ascariasis
Toxic shock syndrome
Hemolytic anemia
Yersinia infection, leptospirosis, yellow fever, dengue fever, relapsing fever

30 FEVER AND RASH

Drug hypersensitivity: PCN, sulfonamides, thiazides, anticonvulsants, allopurinol
Viral infection: measles, rubella, varicella, erythema infectiosum, roseola, enterovirus infection, viral hepatitis, infectious mononucleosis, acute HIV infection
Other infections: meningococcemia, staphylococcemia, scarlet fever, typhoid fever, *Pseudomonas* bacteremia, RMSF, Lyme disease, secondary syphilis, bacterial endocarditis, babesiosis, brucellosis, listeriosis
Serum sickness
Erythema multiforme
Erythema marginatum
Erythema nodosum
SLE
Dermatomyositis
Allergic vasculitis
Pityriasis rosea
Herpes zoster
Sweet's syndrome

31 FLANK PAIN

Urolithiasis
Radicular/muscular
Pyelonephritis
Herpes zoster
Renal abscess
Renal vein thrombosis
Renal infarction
AAA
Retroperitoneal hematoma

32 FLUSHING

Physiologic flushing: menopause, ingestion of MSG, ingestion of hot drinks
Drugs: alcohol (w/ or w/o disulfiram, metronidazole, or chlorpropamide), nicotinic acid, diltiazem, nifedipine, levodopa, bromocriptine, vancomycin, amyl nitrate
Neoplastic disorders: carcinoid syndrome, VIPoma syndrome, medullary carcinoma of thyroid, systemic mastocytosis, basophilic CML, renal cell carcinoma
Anxiety disorders
Metabolic abnlities

33 GENITAL DISCHARGE

Physiologic discharge: cervical mucus, vaginal transudation, bacteria, squamous epithelial cells
Individual variation
Pregnancy
Sexual response
Menstrual cycle variation
Infection
Foreign body: tampon, cervical cap, other
Neoplasm
Fistula
Intrauterine device
Cervical ectropion
Spermicide
Nongenital causes: urinary incontinence, urinary tract fistula, Crohn's disease, rectovaginal fistula

34 GENITAL SORES

Herpes genitalis
Syphilis
Chancroid
Lymphogranuloma venereum
Granuloma inguinale
Condyloma acuminatum
Neoplastic lesion
Trauma

35 GYNECOMASTIA

Physiologic (puberty, newborns, aging)
Drugs (estrogen and estrogen precursors, digitalis, testosterone and exogenous androgens, clomiphene, cimetidine, spironolactone, ketoconazole, amiodarone, ACEIs, isoniazid, phenytoin, methyldopa, metoclopramide, phenothiazine)
↑ Prolactin level (prolactinoma)
Liver disease
Adrenal disease
Thyrotoxicosis
↑ Estrogen production (human chorionic gonadotropin–producing tumor, testicular tumor, bronchogenic carcinoma)
Secondary hypogonadism
Primary gonadal failure (trauma, castration, viral orchitis, granulomatous disease)
Defects in androgen synthesis
Testosterone deficiency
Klinefelter's syndrome

36 HALITOSIS

Tobacco use
Alcohol use
Dry mouth (mouth breathing, inadequate fluid intake)
Foods (onion, garlic, meats, nuts)
Disease of mouth or nose (infections, cancer, inflammation)
Medications (antihistamines, antidepressants)
Systemic disorders (diabetes, uremia, cirrhosis)
GI disorders (esophageal diverticula, hiatal hernia, GERD, achalasia)
Sinusitis
Tonsillitis
Pulmonary disorders (bronchiectasis, pneumonia, neoplasms, tuberculosis)

37 HEARING LOSS, ACUTE

Infectious: mumps, measles, influenza, herpes simplex, herpes zoster, CMV, mononucleosis, syphilis
Vascular: macroglobulinemia, sickle cell disease, Berger's disease, leukemia, polycythemia, fat emboli, hypercoagulable states
Metabolic: diabetes, pregnancy, hyperlipoproteinemia
Conductive: cerumen impaction, foreign bodies, otitis media, otitis externa, barotrauma, trauma
Medications: AGs, loop diuretics, antineoplastics, salicylates, vancomycin
Neoplasm: acoustic neuroma, metastatic neoplasm
Meniere's disease

38 HEMARTHROSIS

Trauma
Anticoagulant Rx
Thrombocytopenia, thrombocytosis
Coagulation disorders (e.g., vWD, hemophilias)
Charcot's joint
Idiopathic
Other: pigmented villonodular synovitis, hemangioma, synovioma, arteriovenous fistula, ruptured aneurysm

39 HEMATURIA

Use the mnemonic **TICS**:

T

Trauma: blow to kidney, insertion of Foley catheter or foreign body in urethra, prolonged and severe exercise, very rapid emptying of overdistended bladder
Tumor: hypernephroma, Wilms' tumor, papillary carcinoma of the bladder, prostatic and urethral neoplasms
Toxins: turpentine, phenols, sulfonamides and other abx, cyclophosphamide, NSAIDs

I

Infections: GN, tuberculosis, cystitis, prostatitis, urethritis, *Schistosoma haematobium* infection, yellow fever, blackwater fever
Inflammatory processes: Goodpasture's syndrome, periarteritis, postirradiation status

C

Calculi: renal, ureteral, bladder, urethra
Cysts: simple cysts, polycystic disease
Congenital anomalies: hemangiomas, aneurysms, AV malformation

S

Surgery: invasive procedures, prostatic resection, cystoscopy
Sickle cell disease and other hematologic disturbances: hemophilia, thrombocytopenia, anticoagulants
Somewhere else: bleeding genitals, factitious (e.g., in drug addicts)

40 HEMIPARESIS/ HEMIPLEGIA

CVA
TIA
Cerebral neoplasm
MS or other demyelinating disorder

CNS infection
Migraine
Hypoglycemia
Subdural hematoma
Vasculitis
Todd's paralysis
Epidural hematoma
Metabolic (hyperosmolar state, electrolyte imbalance)
Psychiatric disorders
Congenital disorders
Leukodystrophies

41 HEMOLYSIS AND HEMOGLOBINURIA

Erythrocyte trauma (prosthetic cardiac valves, marching and severe trauma, extensive burns)
Infections (malaria, *Bartonella*, *Clostridium welchii*)
Brown recluse spider bite
Incompatible blood transfusions
AIHAs
Hemolytic-uremic syndrome
TTP
PNH
Drugs (PCNs, quinidine, methyldopa, sulfonamides, nitrofurantoin)
Erythrocyte enzyme deficiencies (e.g., exposure to fava beans in pts w/ G6PD deficiency)

42 HEMOPTYSIS

Cardiovascular
Pulmonary embolism/infarction
Left ventricular failure
Mitral stenosis
Arteriovenous fistula
Severe HTN
Erosion of aortic aneurysm

Pulmonary
Neoplasm (primary or metastatic)
Infection:
  Pneumonia: *Streptococcus pneumoniae*, *Klebsiella pneumoniae*, *Staphylococcus aureus*, *Legionella pneumophila*
  Bronchiectasis
  Abscess
  Tuberculosis
  Bronchitis
  Fungal infections (aspergillosis, coccidioidomycosis)
  Parasitic infections (amebiasis, ascariasis, paragonimiasis)
Vasculitis: Wegener's granulomatosis, Churg-Strauss syndrome, Henoch-Schönlein purpura
Goodpasture's syndrome
Trauma (needle Bx, foreign body, right-sided heart catheterization, prolonged and severe cough)
Cystic fibrosis, bullous emphysema
Pulmonary sequestration
Pulmonary arteriovenous fistula

SLE
Idiopathic pulmonary hemosiderosis
Drugs: ASA, anticoagulants, penicillamine
Pulmonary HTN
Mediastinal fibrosis

Other
Epistaxis, trauma
Laryngeal bleeding (laryngitis, laryngeal neoplasm)
Hematologic disorders (clotting abnlities, disseminated intravascular coagulation, thrombocytopenia)

43 HEPATOMEGALY

Frequent Jaundice
Infectious hepatitis
Toxic hepatitis
Carcinoma: liver, pancreas, bile ducts, metastatic neoplasm to liver
Cirrhosis
Obstruction of CBD
Alcoholic hepatitis
Biliary cirrhosis
Cholangitis
Hemochromatosis w/cirrhosis

Infrequent Jaundice
CHF
Amyloidosis
Liver abscess
Sarcoidosis
Infectious mononucleosis
Alcoholic fatty infiltration
Nonalcoholic steatohepatitis
Lymphoma
Leukemia
Budd-Chiari syndrome
Myelofibrosis w/myeloid metaplasia
Familial hyperlipoproteinemia type I
Other: amebiasis, hydatid disease of liver, schistosomiasis, kala-azar (*Leishmania donovani* infection), Hurler's syndrome, Gaucher's disease, kwashiorkor

44 HIRSUTISM

Idiopathic: familial, possibly ↑ sensitivity to androgens
Menopause
Polycystic ovarian syndrome
Drugs: androgens, anabolic steroids, methyltestosterone, minoxidil, diazoxide, phenytoin, glucocorticoids, cyclosporine
Congenital adrenal hyperplasia
Adrenal virilizing tumor
Ovarian virilizing tumor: arrhenoblastoma, hilus cell tumor
Pituitary adenoma
Cushing's syndrome
Hypothyroidism (congenital and juvenile)
Acromegaly
Testicular feminization
Obesity

45 HOARSENESS

Allergic rhinitis
Infections (laryngitis, epiglottitis, tracheitis, croup, tuberculosis)
Vocal cord polyps
Voice strain
Irritants (tobacco smoke)
Vocal cord trauma (intubation, surgery)
Neoplastic involvement of vocal cord (primary or metastatic)
Neurologic abnlities (MS, amyotrophic lateral sclerosis, parkinsonism)
Endocrine abnlities (puberty, menopause, hypothyroidism)
Other (laryngeal webs or cysts, psychogenic, muscle tension abnlities)

46 HYDROCEPHALUS

Head trauma
Brain neoplasm (primary or metastatic)
Spinal cord tumor
Cerebellar infarction
Exudative or granulomatous meningitis
Cerebellar hemorrhage
Subarachnoid hemorrhage
Aqueductal stenosis
Third ventricle colloid cyst
Hindbrain malformation
Viral encephalitis
Mets to leptomeninges
NPH

47 HYDRONEPHROSIS

Urinary stones
Neoplastic disease
Prostatic hypertrophy
Neurologic disease
Urinary reflux
UTI
Medication effects
Trauma
Congenital abnlity of urinary tract
Foley catheter dysfunction
Retroperitoneal fibrosis

48 HYPERPIGMENTATION

Pregnancy
Drug induced (i.e., antimalarials, melanotropic hormone injection, cytotoxic agents)
PUVA Rx (psoralen administration) for psoriasis and vitiligo
Addison's disease
ACTH- or MSH-producing tumors (e.g., oat cell carcinoma of the lung)
Hemochromatosis ("bronze" diabetes)
Malabsorption syndrome (Whipple's disease and celiac sprue)
Melanoma
Pheochromocytoma
Porphyrias (porphyria cutanea tarda and variegate porphyria)
Progressive systemic sclerosis and related conditions
Arsenic ingestion

49 HYPERTROPHIC OSTEOARTHROPATHY

Paget's disease
Reiter's syndrome
Psoriasis
Osteoarthritis
RA
Osteomyelitis

50 HYPOGONADISM

Hypergonadotropic Hypogonadism
Hormone resistance (androgen, luteinizing hormone insensitivity)
Gonadal defects (e.g., Klinefelter's syndrome, myotonic dystrophy)
Drug induced (e.g., spironolactone, cytotoxins)
Alcoholism or radiation induced
Mumps orchitis
Anatomic defects, castration

Hypogonadotropic Hypogonadism
Pituitary lesions (neoplasms, granulomas, infarction, hemochromatosis, vasculitis)
Drug induced (e.g., glucocorticoids)
Hyperprolactinemia
Genetic disorders (Laurence-Moon-Biedl syndrome, Prader-Willi syndrome)
Delayed puberty
Other: chronic disease, nutritional deficiency, Kallmann's syndrome, idiopathic isolated luteinizing hormone or FSH deficiency

51 HYPOPIGMENTATION

Vitiligo
Tinea versicolor
Atopic dermatitis
Chemical leukoderma
Idiopathic hypomelanosis
Sarcoidosis
SLE
Scleroderma
Oculocutaneous albinism
Phenylketonuria
Nevoid hypopigmentation

52 HYPOTENSION, POSTURAL

Antihypertensive medications (especially α-blockers, diuretics, ACEIs)
Volume depletion (hemorrhage, dehydration)
Impaired CO (constrictive pericarditis, AS, cardiac tamponade)
Peripheral autonomic dysfunction (DM, GBS)
Idiopathic orthostatic hypotension
Central autonomic dysfunction (Shy-Drager syndrome)
Peripheral venous disease
Adrenal insufficiency

53 JAUNDICE

Predominance of Direct (Conjugated) Bilirubin

Extrahepatic obstruction:
    Common duct abnlities: calculi,
        neoplasm, stricture, cyst, sclerosing
        cholangitis
    Metastatic carcinoma
    Pancreatic carcinoma, pseudocyst
    Ampullary carcinoma

Hepatocellular disease: hepatitis,
    cirrhosis

Drugs: estrogens, phenothiazines,
    captopril, methyltestosterone,
    labetalol

Cholestatic jaundice of pregnancy

Hereditary disorders: Dubin-Johnson
    syndrome, Rotor's syndrome

Recurrent benign intrahepatic
    cholestasis

Predominance of Indirect (Unconjugated) Bilirubin

Hemolysis: hereditary and acquired
    hemolytic anemias

Inefficient marrow production

Impaired hepatic conjugation:
    chloramphenicol

Neonatal jaundice

Hereditary disorders: Gilbert's
    syndrome, Crigler-Najjar syndrome

54 JOINT SWELLING

Trauma
Osteoarthritis
Gout
Pyogenic arthritis or infectious arthritis
Pseudogout
RA
Viral syndrome

55 JUGULAR VENOUS DISTENTION

Right-sided heart failure
Cardiac tamponade
Constrictive pericarditis
Goiter
Tension pneumothorax
Pulmonary HTN
Cardiomyopathy (restrictive)
Superior vena cava syndrome
Valsalva maneuver
Right atrial myxoma
COPD

56 LEG CRAMPS, NOCTURNAL

Diabetic neuropathy
Medications
Electrolyte abnlities (hypokalemia,
    hyponatremia, hypocalcemia,
    hyperkalemia, hypophosphatemia)
Respiratory alkalosis
Uremia
Hemodialysis
Peripheral nerve injury

Amyotrophic lateral sclerosis
Alcohol use
Heat cramps
Vitamin B_{12} deficiency
Hyperthyroidism
Contractures
DVT
Hypoglycemia
Peripheral vascular insufficiency
Baker's cyst

57 LEG ULCERS

Vascular

Arterial: arteriosclerosis,
    thromboangiitis obliterans,
    arteriovenous malformation,
    cholesterol emboli

Venous: superficial varicosities,
    incompetent perforators, deep venous
    thrombosis, lymphatic abnlities

Vasculitis, Hematologic

Sickle cell anemia, thalassemia, PV,
    leukemia, cold agglutinin disease

Macroglobulinemia, protein
    C and protein S deficiency,
    cryoglobulinemia, lupus anticoagulant,
    antiphospholipid syndrome

Infectious

Fungus: blastomycosis,
    coccidioidomycosis, histoplasmosis,
    sporotrichosis

Bacteria: furuncle, ecthyma, septic
    emboli

Protozoal: leishmaniasis

Metabolic

Necrobiosis lipoidica diabeticorum
Localized bullous pemphigoid
Gout, calcinosis cutis, Gaucher's disease

Tumors

Basal cell carcinoma, squamous cell
    carcinoma, melanoma

Mycosis fungoides, Kaposi's sarcoma,
    metastatic neoplasms

Trauma

Burns, cold injury, radiation dermatitis
Insect bites
Factitial, excessive pressure

Neuropathic

Diabetic trophic ulcers
Tabes dorsalis, syringomyelia

Drugs

Warfarin, IV colchicine extravasation,
    methotrexate, halogens, ergotism,
    hydroxyurea

Panniculitis

Weber-Christian disease
Pancreatic fat necrosis, alpha$_1$-
    antitrypsin deficiency

58 LEUKOCORIA

Cataract
Retinal detachment
Retinoblastoma

Retinal telangiectasia
Retrolentricular vascularized membrane
Familial exudative vitreoretinopathy
Toxocariasis, retinal telangiectasia,
retinopathy of prematurity

59 LIVEDO RETICULARIS
Emboli (subacute bacterial endocarditis,
left atrial myxoma, cholesterol
emboli)
Thrombocythemia or polycythemia
Antiphospholipid Ab syndrome
Cryoglobulinemia, cryofibrinogenemia
Leukocytoclastic vasculitis
SLE, RA, dermatomyositis
Pancreatitis
Drugs (quinine, quinidine, amantadine,
catecholamines)
Physiologic (cutis marmorata)
Congenital

60 LYMPHADENOPATHY
Generalized
AIDS
Lymphoma: Hodgkin's disease, non-
Hodgkin's lymphoma
Leukemias, reticuloendotheliosis
Infectious mononucleosis, CMV, and
other viral infections
Diffuse skin infection: generalized
furunculosis, multiple tick bites
Parasitic infections: toxoplasmosis,
filariasis, leishmaniasis, Chagas'
disease
Serum sickness
Collagen-vascular diseases (RA, SLE)
Dengue (arbovirus infection)
Sarcoidosis and other granulomatous
diseases
Drugs: isoniazid, hydantoin derivatives,
antithyroid and antileprosy drugs
Secondary syphilis
Hyperthyroidism, lipid storage diseases

Localized
Cervical nodes
  Infections of the head, neck, ears,
    sinuses, scalp, pharynx
  Mononucleosis
  Lymphoma
  Tuberculosis
  Malignant neoplasm of head and neck
  Rubella
Scalene/supraclavicular nodes
  Lymphoma
  Lung neoplasm
  Bacterial or fungal infection of thorax
    or retroperitoneum
  GI malignant neoplasm
Axillary nodes
  Infections of hands and arms
  Cat-scratch disease
  Neoplasm (lymphoma, melanoma,
    breast carcinoma)
  Brucellosis
Epitrochlear nodes

Infections of the hand
Lymphoma
Tularemia
Sarcoidosis, secondary syphilis
  (usually bilateral)
Inguinal nodes
  Infections of leg or foot, folliculitis
    (pubic hair)
  Lymphogranuloma venereum, syphilis
  Lymphoma
  Pelvic malignant neoplasm
  Pasteurella pestis infection
Hilar nodes
  Sarcoidosis
  Tuberculosis
  Lung carcinoma
  Fungal infections, systemic
Mediastinal nodes
  Sarcoidosis
  Lymphoma
  Lung neoplasm
  Tuberculosis
  Mononucleosis
  Histoplasmosis
Abdominal/retroperitoneal nodes
  Lymphoma
  Tuberculosis
  Neoplasm (ovary, testes, prostate,
    colon, and other malignant
    neoplasms)

61 MIOSIS
Medications (e.g., morphine,
  pilocarpine)
Neurosyphilis
Congenital
Iritis
CNS pontine lesion
CNS infections
Cavernous sinus thrombosis
Inflammation/irritation of cornea or
  conjunctiva

62 MUSCLE WEAKNESS
Physical deconditioning
Impaired CO (e.g., mitral stenosis,
  MR, CHF)
Uremia, liver failure
Electrolyte abnlities (hypokalemia,
  hyperkalemia, hypophosphatemia,
  hypercalcemia), hypoglycemia
Drug induced (e.g., statin myopathy)
Muscular dystrophies
Steroid myopathy
Alcoholic myopathy
Myasthenia gravis, Lambert-Eaton
  syndrome
Infections (polio, botulism, HIV
  infection, hepatitis, diphtheria, tick
  paralysis, neurosyphilis, brucellosis,
  tuberculosis, trichinosis)
Pernicious anemia, other anemias,
  beriberi
Psychiatric illness (depression,
  somatization syndrome)
Organophosphate or arsenic poisoning

Inflammatory myopathies (e.g., collagen-vascular disease, RA, sarcoidosis)
Endocrinopathies (e.g., adrenal insufficiency, hypothyroidism, diabetic neuropathy
Other: motor neuron disease, mitochondrial myopathy, L-tryptophan (eosinophilia-myalgia), rhabdomyolysis, glycogen storage disease, lipid storage disease, muscle phosphorylase deficiency

63 MYDRIASIS

Coma
Medications (cocaine, atropine, epinephrine, others)
Glaucoma
Cerebral aneurysm
Ocular trauma
Head trauma
Optic atrophy
Cerebral neoplasm
Iridocyclitis

64 MYELOPATHY AND MYELITIS

Inflammatory
Infectious: spirochetal, tuberculosis, herpes zoster, rabies, HIV infection, polio, rickettsial, fungal, parasitic
Noninfectious: idiopathic transverse myelitis, MS

Toxic/Metabolic
DM, pernicious anemia, chronic liver disease, pellagra, arsenic

Trauma, Compression
Spinal neoplasm, cervical spondylosis, epidural abscess, epidural hematoma

Vascular
Arteriovenous malformation, SLE, PAN, dissecting aortic aneurysm

Physical Agents
Electrical injury, irradiation

Neoplastic
Spinal cord tumors, paraneoplastic myelopathy

65 MYOTONIA

Myotonia congenita (Thomsen's disease)
  May be autosomal dominant or recessive (two distinct varieties)
  The disease is limited to muscles and causes hypertrophy and stiffness after rest. Muscle function nlizes w/exercise. There is no weakness. Sx are exacerbated by exposure to cold.
Paramyotonia congenita
  Autosomal dominant disease
  Weakness and stiffness of facial muscles and distal upper extremities, especially or exclusively on cold exposure
Muscular dystrophies
Inflammatory myopathies (polymyositis)
Metabolic muscle diseases
Myasthenic syndromes
Motor neuron disease

66 NAIL CLUBBING

COPD
Pulmonary malignant neoplasm
Cirrhosis
IBD
Chronic bronchitis
CHD
Endocarditis
AV malformations
Asbestosis
Trauma
Idiopathic

67 NECK MASS

Congenital Anomalies
Thyroglossal duct cyst
Bronchial apparatus anomalies
Teratomas
Ranula
Dermoid cysts
Hemangioma
Laryngoceles
Cystic hygroma

Non-Neoplastic Inflammatory Etiologies
Folliculitis
Adenopathy secondary to peritonsillar abscess
Retropharyngeal or parapharyngeal abscess
Salivary gland infections
Viral infections (mononucleosis, HIV, CMV)
Tuberculosis
Cat-scratch disease
Toxoplasmosis
Actinomycosis
Atypical mycobacterial infection
Jugular vein thrombus
Neoplasm (primary or metastatic)
Lipoma

68 NYSTAGMUS

Medications (meperidine, barbiturates, phenytoin, phenothiazines, others)
MS
Congenital
Neoplasm (cerebellar, brainstem, cerebral)
Labyrinthine or vestibular lesions (otoliths)
CNS infections
Optic atrophy
Other: Arnold-Chiari malformation, syringobulbia, chorioretinitis, meningeal cysts

69 OPHTHALMOPLEGIA

Bilateral
Botulism
Myasthenia gravis

Wernicke's encephalopathy
Acute cranial polyneuropathy
Brainstem stroke

Unilateral

Carotid, posterior (third cranial nerve, pupil involved, communicating aneurysm)
Diabetic, idiopathic (third or sixth cranial nerve, pupil spared)
Myasthenia gravis
Brainstem stroke

70 PALPITATIONS

Anxiety
Electrolyte abnlities (hypokalemia, hypomagnesemia)
Exercise
Hyperthyroidism
Ischemic heart disease
Ingestion of stimulant drugs (cocaine, amphetamines, caffeine)
Medications (digoxin, β-blockers, Ca channel antagonists, hydralazines, diuretics, minoxidil)
Hypoglycemia
MVP
WPW syndrome
SSS
AF

71 PAPILLEDEMA

CNS infections (viral, bacterial, fungal)
Medications (lithium, cisplatin, corticosteroids, tetracycline, others)
Head trauma
CNS neoplasm (primary or metastatic)
Pseudotumor cerebri
Cavernous sinus thrombosis
SLE
Sarcoidosis
Subarachnoid hemorrhage
Carbon dioxide retention
Arnold-Chiari malformation and other developmental or congenital malformations
Orbital lesions
Central retinal vein occlusion
Hypertensive encephalopathy
Metabolic abnlities

72 PARAPLEGIA

Trauma: penetrating wounds to motor cortex, fracture-dislocation of vertebral column w/compression of spinal cord or cauda equina, prolapsed disk, electrical injuries
Neoplasm: parasagittal region, vertebrae, meninges, spinal cord, cauda equina, Hodgkin's disease, non-Hodgkin's lymphoma, leukemic deposits, pelvic neoplasms
MS and other demyelinating disorders
Mechanical compression of spinal cord, cauda equina, or lumbosacral plexus: Paget's disease, kyphoscoliosis, herniation of intervertebral disk, spondylosis, ankylosing spondylitis, RA, aortic aneurysm
Infections: spinal abscess, syphilis, tuberculosis, poliomyelitis, leprosy
Thrombosis of superior sagittal sinus
Polyneuritis: GBS, diabetes, alcohol, beriberi, heavy metals
Heredofamilial muscular dystrophies
Amyotrophic lateral sclerosis
Congenital and familial conditions: syringomyelia, myelomeningocele, myelodysplasia
Hysteria

73 PARESTHESIAS

MS
Nutritional deficiencies (thiamine, vitamin B_{12}, folic acid)
Compression of spinal cord or peripheral nerves
Medications (e.g., isoniazid, lithium, nitrofurantoin, gold, cisplatin, hydralazine, amitriptyline, sulfonamides, amiodarone, metronidazole, dapsone, disulfiram, chloramphenicol)
Toxic chemicals (e.g., lead, arsenic, cyanide, mercury, organophosphates)
DM
Myxedema
Alcohol
Sarcoidosis
Neoplasms
Infections (HIV, Lyme disease, herpes zoster, leprosy, diphtheria)
Charcot-Marie-Tooth syndrome and other hereditary neuropathies
Guillain-Barré neuropathy

74 PELVIC MASS

Hemorrhagic ovarian cyst
Simple ovarian cyst (follicle or corpus luteum)
Ovarian carcinoma, carcinoma of fallopian tube, colorectal carcinoma, metastatic carcinoma, prostate carcinoma, bladder carcinoma, lymphoma, Hodgkin's disease
Cystadenoma, teratoma, endometrioma
Leiomyoma
Leiomyosarcoma
Diverticulitis, diverticular abscess
Appendiceal abscess, tubo-ovarian abscess
Ectopic pregnancy, intrauterine pregnancy
Paraovarian cyst
Hydrosalpinx

75 PNEUMONIA, RECURRENT

Mechanical obstruction from neoplasm
Chronic aspiration (tube feeding, alcoholism, CVA, neuromuscular disorders, seizure disorder, inability to cough)

Bronchiectasis
Kyphoscoliosis
COPD, CHF, asthma, silicosis, pulmonary fibrosis, cystic fibrosis
Pulmonary tuberculosis, chronic sinusitis
Immunosuppression (HIV infection, corticosteroids, leukemia, chemoRx, splenectomy)

76 POLYURIA
DM
Diabetes insipidus
Primary polydipsia (compulsive water drinking)
Hypercalcemia
Hypokalemia
Postobstructive uropathy
Diuretic phase of ARF (specifically ATN)
Drugs: diuretics, caffeine, alcohol, lithium
Sickle cell trait or disease, chronic pyelonephritis (failure to concentrate urine)
Anxiety, cold weather

77 POPLITEAL SWELLING
Phlebitis (superficial)
Lymphadenitis
Trauma: fractured tibia or fibula, contusion, traumatic neuroma
DVT
Ruptured varicose vein
Baker's cyst
Popliteal abscess
Osteomyelitis
Ruptured tendon
Aneurysm of popliteal artery
Neoplasm: lipoma, osteogenic sarcoma, neurofibroma, fibrosarcoma

78 POSTMENOPAUSAL BLEEDING
Hormone replacement Rx
Neoplasm (uterine, ovarian, cervical, vaginal, vulvar)
Atrophic vaginitis
Vaginal infection
Polyp
Extragenital (GI, urinary)
Tamoxifen
Trauma

79 PROPTOSIS
Thyrotoxicosis
Orbital pseudotumor
Optic nerve tumor
Cavernous sinus arteriovenous fistula, cavernous sinus thrombosis
Cellulitis
Metastatic tumor to orbit

80 PROTEINURIA
Nephrotic syndrome as a result of primary renal diseases
Malignant HTN

Malignant diseases: MM, leukemias, Hodgkin's disease
CHF
DM
SLE, RA
Sickle cell disease
Goodpasture's syndrome
Malaria
Amyloidosis, sarcoidosis
Tubular lesions: cystinosis
Functional (after heavy exercise)
Pyelonephritis
Pregnancy
Constrictive pericarditis
Renal vein thrombosis
Toxic nephropathies: heavy metals, drugs
Radiation nephritis
Orthostatic (postural) proteinuria
Benign proteinuria: fever, heat, or cold exposure

81 PRURITUS
Dry skin
Drug-induced eruption, fiberglass exposure
Scabies
Skin diseases
Myeloproliferative disorders: mycosis fungoides, Hodgkin's lymphoma, MM, PV
Cholestatic liver disease
Endocrine disorders: DM, thyroid disease, carcinoid, pregnancy
Carcinoma: breast, lung, gastric
Chronic renal failure
Iron deficiency
AIDS
Neurosis
Sjögren's syndrome

82 PRURITUS ANI
Fecal irritation:
  Poor hygiene
  Anorectal conditions (fissure, fistula, hemorrhoids, skin tags, perianal clefts)
  Spicy foods, citrus foods, caffeine, colchicine, quinidine
Contact dermatitis: anesthetic agents, topical corticosteroids, perfumed soap
Dermatologic disorders: psoriasis, seborrhea, lichen simplex or sclerosus
Systemic disorders: chronic renal failure, myxedema, DM, thyrotoxicosis, PV, Hodgkin's disease
STDs: syphilis, HSV, HPV
Other infectious agents: pinworms, scabies
Bacterial infection, viral infection

83 PTOSIS
Third nerve palsy
Myasthenia gravis
Horner's syndrome
Senile ptosis

84 PURPURA

Trauma
Septic emboli, atheromatous (cholesterol) emboli
Disseminated intravascular coagulation
Thrombocytopenia
Meningococcemia
RMSF
Hemolytic-uremic syndrome
Viral infection: echovirus, coxsackievirus
Scurvy
Other: left atrial myxoma, cryoglobulinemia, vasculitis, hyperglobulinemic purpura, leukemia, bacterial endocarditis

85 RED EYE

Infectious conjunctivitis (bacterial, viral)
Allergic conjunctivitis
Acute glaucoma
Keratitis (bacterial, viral)
Iritis
Trauma
Foreign body

86 SEIZURES

Syncope
Alcohol abuse/withdrawal
TIA
Hemiparetic migraine
Psychiatric disorders
Carotid sinus hypersensitivity
Hyperventilation, prolonged breath holding
Hypoglycemia
Narcolepsy
Movement disorders (tics, hemiballismus)
Hyponatremia
Brain tumor (primary or metastatic)
Tetanus
Strychnine, phencyclidine poisoning
Epilepsy
Cerebral anoxia from any cause

87 SPASTIC PARAPLEGIAS

Cervical spondylosis
Friedreich's ataxia
MS
Spinal cord tumor
HIV infection
Tertiary syphilis
Vitamin B_{12} deficiency
Spinocerebellar ataxias
Syringomyelia
Spinal cord AV malformations
Adrenoleukodystrophy

88 SPLENOMEGALY

Hepatic cirrhosis
Neoplastic involvement: chronic myelogenous leukemia, CLL, lymphoma, MM
Bacterial infections: tuberculosis, infectious endocarditis, typhoid fever, splenic abscess
Viral infections: infectious mononucleosis, viral hepatitis, HIV infection
Gaucher's disease and other lipid storage diseases
Sarcoidosis
Parasitic infections (malaria, kala-azar, histoplasmosis)
Hereditary and acquired hemolytic anemias
Idiopathic thrombocytopenic purpura
Collagen-vascular disorders: SLE, RA (Felty's syndrome), polyarteritis nodosa
Serum sickness, drug hypersensitivity reaction
Splenic cysts and benign tumors: hemangioma, lymphangioma
Thrombosis of splenic or portal vein
PV, myeloid metaplasia

89 TASTE AND SMELL LOSS

Taste
Local: radiation Rx
Systemic: cancer, renal failure, hepatic failure, nutritional deficiency (vitamin B_{12}, zinc), Cushing's syndrome, hypothyroidism, DM, infection (influenza), drugs (antirheumatic and antiproliferative)
Neurologic: Bell's palsy, familial dysautonomia, MS

Smell
Local: allergic rhinitis, sinusitis, nasal polyposis, bronchial asthma
Systemic: renal failure, hepatic failure, nutritional deficiency (vitamin B_{12}), Cushing's syndrome, hypothyroidism, DM, infection (viral hepatitis, influenza), drugs (nasal sprays, abx)
Neurologic: head trauma, MS, Parkinson's disease, frontal brain tumor

90 URINARY RETENTION, ACUTE

Mechanical obstruction: urethral stone, foreign body, urethral stricture, benign prostatic hypertrophy, prostate carcinoma, prostatitis, trauma w/hematoma formation or obstructive clots
Neurogenic bladder
Neurologic disease (MS, parkinsonism, tabes dorsalis, CVA)
Spinal cord injury
CNS neoplasm (primary or metastatic)
Spinal anesthesia
Lower urinary tract instrumentation
Medications (antihistamines, antidepressants, narcotics, anticholinergics)
Abdominal or pelvic surgery
Alcohol toxicity
Pregnancy

Anxiety
Encephalitis
Postoperative pain
Spina bifida occulta

91 VERTIGO

Peripheral
Otitis media
Acute labyrinthitis
Vestibular neuronitis
Benign positional vertigo
Meniere's disease
Ototoxic drugs: streptomycin, gentamicin
Lesions of the eighth nerve: acoustic neuroma, meningioma, mononeuropathy, metastatic carcinoma
Mastoiditis

Central Nervous System or Systemic
Vertebrobasilar artery insufficiency
Posterior fossa tumor or other brain tumors
Infarction/hemorrhage of cerebral cortex, cerebellum, or brainstem
Basilar migraine
Metabolic: drugs, hypoxia, anemia, fever
Hypotension/severe HTN
MS
CNS infections: viral, bacterial
Temporal lobe epilepsy
Arnold-Chiari malformation, syringobulbia
Psychogenic: ventilation, hysteria

92 VISION LOSS, ACUTE, PAINFUL

Acute angle-closure glaucoma
Corneal ulcer
Uveitis
Endophthalmitis
Factitious
Somatization syndrome
Trauma
Giant cell arteritis

93 VISION LOSS, ACUTE, PAINLESS

Retinal artery occlusion
Optic neuritis
Retinal vein occlusion
Vitreous hemorrhage
Retinal detachment
Exudative macular degeneration
CVA
Ischemic optic neuropathy
Factitious
Somatization syndrome, anxiety reaction
Giant cell arteritis

94 VISION LOSS, CHRONIC, PROGRESSIVE

Cataract
Macular degeneration
Cerebral neoplasm

Refractive error
Open-angle glaucoma

95 VISUAL FIELD DEFECTS
See Figure 2-1.

96 VOCAL CORD PARALYSIS

Neoplasm: primary or metastatic (e.g., lung, thyroid, parathyroid, mediastinum)
Neck surgery (parathyroid, thyroid, carotid endarterectomy, cervical spine)
Idiopathic
Viral, bacterial, tuberculous, or fungal infection
Trauma (intubation, penetrating neck injury)
Cardiac surgery
RA
MS
Parkinsonism
Toxic neuropathy
CVA
CNS abnlities: hydrocephalus, Arnold-Chiari malformation, meningomyelocele

97 WEAKNESS, ACUTE, EMERGENT

Demyelinating disorders (GBS, chronic inflammatory demyelinating polyneuropathy)
Myasthenia gravis
Infectious (poliomyelitis, diphtheria)
Toxic (botulism, tick paralysis, paralytic shellfish toxin, puffer fish, newts)
Metabolic (acquired or familial hypokalemia, hypophosphatemia, hypermagnesemia)
Metals poisoning (arsenic, thallium)
Porphyria
CVA

98 WEIGHT GAIN

Sedentary lifestyle
Fluid overload
Discontinuation of tobacco abuse
Endocrine disorders (hypothyroidism, hyperinsulinism associated w/ maturity-onset DM, Cushing's syndrome, hypogonadism, insulinoma, hyperprolactinemia, acromegaly)
Medications (nutritional supplements, oral contraceptives, glucocorticoids, others)
Anxiety disorders w/compulsive eating
Laurence-Moon-Biedl syndrome, Prader-Willi syndrome, other congenital diseases
Hypothalamic injury (rare; <100 cases reported in medical literature)

99 WEIGHT LOSS

Malignant disease
Psychiatric disorders (depression, anorexia nervosa)

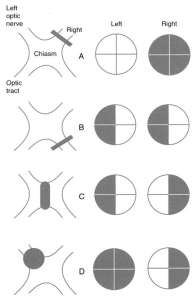

FIGURE 2-1. Visual field defects. **A,** Transection of right optic nerve: ipsilateral monocular blindness. **B,** Lesion of right optic tract: left homonymous hemianopia. **C,** Chiasmal lesion: bitemporal hemianopia. **D,** Lesion of left optic nerve and chiasm: ipsilateral blindness and right temporal deficit. *(From Noble J [ed]: Textbook of Primary Care Medicine, 2nd ed. St. Louis, Mosby, 1996.)*

New-onset DM
Malabsorption
COPD
AIDS
Uremia, liver disease
Thyrotoxicosis, pheochromocytoma, carcinoid syndrome
Addison's disease
Intestinal parasites
PUD
IBD
Food faddism
Postgastrectomy syndrome

ILD
Infections (pneumonia, bronchitis, bronchiolitis, epiglottitis)
Cardiac asthma
GERD w/aspiration
Foreign body aspiration
PE
Anaphylaxis
Obstruction airway (neoplasm, goiter, edema or hemorrhage from trauma, aneurysm, congenital abnlities, strictures, spasm)
Carcinoid syndrome

100 WHEEZING

Asthma
COPD

Cardiovascular Disease 3

A. DIAGNOSTIC AIDS IN CARDIOLOGY

1 CARDIOVASCULAR FORMULAS
See Box 3-1.

2 THE CARDIAC CYCLE
See Figure 3-1.

3 ECG: INTERPRETATION
Proper positioning of precordial leads is shown in Figure 3-2. Figure 3-3 illustrates the axis of electrical activation.

a. Determine the **HR.** Nl HR is 50 to 100 beats/min (bpm). If the heart rhythm is regular, the HR can be determined by dividing 300 by the number of boxes in the R-R interval (e.g., if R-R interval contains 4 large boxes, the HR is 75 bpm [HR = 300/4]). The HR can also be calculated by use of the following formula: each large square = 0.2 sec; 5 large squares/sec. For specific rate, measure large squares between R waves as follows:
   i. 1 = 300 bpm
   ii. 2 = 150 bpm

Box 3-1 • Cardiovascular Formulas

Output of left ventricle

$$= \frac{O_2 \text{consumption (mL/min)}}{[CaO_2 - C\bar{v}O_2]}$$

$$= \frac{250 \text{ mL/min}}{190 \text{ mL/L arterial blood}} - 140 \text{ mL/L venous blood in pulmonary artery}$$

$$= \frac{250 \text{ mL/min}}{50 \text{ mL/L}} = 5 \text{ L/min}$$

CI = Cardiac output/Body surface area
  Normal = 3.0-3.4 L/min/m²

$$EF = \frac{(\text{End-diastolic volume}) - (\text{end-systolic volume})}{(\text{End-diastolic volume})} = \%$$

Mean arterial (or pulmonary) pressure = DBP + ⅓(SBP – DBP)
Mean pulmonary arterial pressure = DPP + ⅓(SPAP – DPAP)
Pulmonary vascular resistance index (PVRI) = 79.92 (mean PAP – PAOP)/CI
  Normal = 255-285 dyne-sec/cm⁻⁵
Shunt % = (Qs/Qt)

$$Qs/Qt \ (\%) = \frac{Cco_2 - Cao_2}{Cco_2 - C\bar{v}o_2}$$

Cco_2 = Hgh in g × 1.34 + (alveolar PO_2 × 0.003)
  Normal = <10%
  Considerable disease = 20%-29%
  Life-threatening = >30%
SV = (end-diastolic volume) – (end-systolic volume)
Systemic vascular resistance index (SVRI) = 79.92 (MAP – CVP/CI)

Venous blood O_2 content ($C\bar{v}o_2$) = $P\bar{v}o_2$ × 0.003 +
  (1.34 × Hgh in g × venous blood Hgh O_2 sat %)

Normal = 13-16 mL/dL

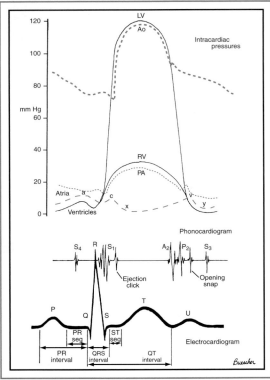

FIGURE 3-1. The cardiac cycle. *(From Tschudy MM, Arcara KM: The Harriet Lane Handbook, 19th ed. Philadelphia, Mosby, 2012.)*

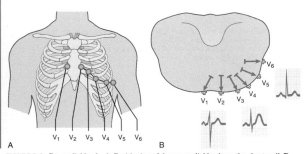

FIGURE 3-2. Precordial leads. **A,** Positioning of the precordial leads on the chest wall. **B,** Normal cardiac activation as manifested in the precordial leads. Note the small r wave and deep S wave in lead V_1, the transition at around V_3 or V_4, and the "septal" q wave and large R wave in lead V_6. *(From Goldman L, Schafer AI [eds]: Goldman's Cecil Medicine, 24th ed. Philadelphia, Saunders, 2012.)*

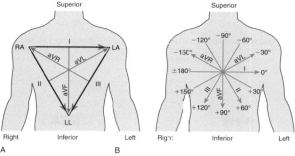

FIGURE 3-3. Axis of electrical activation. **A,** Vectors for the limb leads (LL) in the frontal plane. **B,** Hexaxial reference for determining the frontal plane axis. Note that the vectors for the leads I, II, and III are in the same direction as in **A.** But now, like the augmented limb leads, these standard limb lead vectors have been moved so that they emanate from the center of the figure. *(From Goldman L, Schafer AI [eds]: Goldman's Cecil Medicine, 24th ed. Philadelphia, Saunders, 2012.)*

  iii. 3 = 100 bpm
  iv. 4 = 75 bpm
  v. 5 = 60 bpm
  vi. 6 = 50 bpm
b. Determine the **heart rhythm.**
  i. Is the rhythm regular?
  ii. Are there P waves (Fig. 3-4)?
  iii. Is the P wave related to the QRS (i.e., are P waves "married" to the QRS)?
  iv. The P wave should always be upright in lead I if there is sinus rhythm (unless there is reversal of leads or dextrocardia). Normal P wave duration is <0.12 sec (120 msec). If the rhythm is irregular, the P wave can help w/ the dx (e.g., w/sinus arrhythmia, the P waves will be identical; w/wandering pacemaker, the P waves will have different shapes; w/AF, the P waves are not discernible).

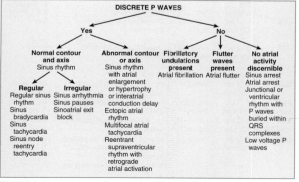

FIGURE 3-4. An approach to the interpretation of the ECG. *(From Goldman L, Ausiello D [eds]: Cecil Textbook of Medicine, 22nd ed. Philadelphia, Saunders, 2004.)*

c. Evaluate the **intervals.**
   i. **PR interval:** NI is 0.09 (90 msec) to 0.20 sec (200 msec) [for practical purposes, the PR interval is nl if it does not exceed a large box]. The PR interval becomes shorter as the rate ↑.
   ii. **QRS interval** (Fig. 3-5): NI QRS duration is 0.075 (75 msec) to 0.11 sec (110 msec). For practical purposes, the QRS interval should not be > half a large box. If the QRS is wide, evaluate for BBB (Table 3-1).

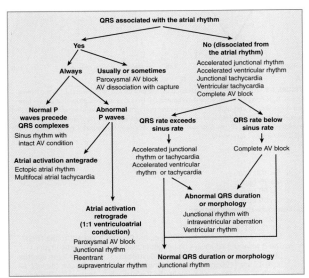

FIGURE 3-5. The QRS rhythm. *(From Goldman L, Ausiello D [eds]: Cecil Textbook of Medicine, 22nd ed. Philadelphia, Saunders, 2004.)*

TABLE 3-1 ■ Fascicular and Bundle Branch Blocks

	QRS Duration	Axis	QRS Morphology	ST Segments and T Waves
LAFB	<0.12 sec (120 msec)	−45 to −90 degrees	Delayed transition across the precordium qR aVL	Normal
LPFB	<0.12 sec (120 msec)	+90 to +180 degrees	Delayed transition across the precordium rS in I, aVL qR in III, aVF	Normal
RBBB	≥0.12 sec (120 msec)	Normal	rsr', rsR', rSR' in V_1 (and usually V_2); wide S in V_6 and I	Discordant in V_1 and V_2
RBBB with LAFB	≥0.12 sec (120 msec)	−45 to 90 degrees	rsr', rsR', rSR' in V_1 (and usually V_2); wide S in V_6 and I	Discordant in V_1 and V_2
RBBB with LPFB	≥0.12 sec (120 msec)	+ 90 to +180 degrees	rsr', rsR', rSR' in V_1 (and usually V_2); wide S in V_6 and I	Discordant in V_1 and V_2
LBBB	≥0.12 sec (120 msec)	Variable	rS or QS in V_1 (S wide and notched); wide notched R without q in V_5, V_6, and I Wide notched R with or without small q in aVL	Discordant in V_1 to V_6

From Goldman L, Schafer AI (eds): Goldman's Cecil Medicine, 24th ed. Philadelphia, Saunders, 2012.
LAD, left axis deviation.

- **LBBB:** The following may be seen:
  - Wide slurred R in V_{5-6}.
  - QRS prolonged ≥0.12 sec, lengthened VAT or intrinsicoid deflection.
  - AVL similar to V_{5-6}, lead I similar to aVL and V_{5-6} (w/depression of the ST segments and inversion of the T waves).
- **RBBB:**
  - QRS ≥0.12 sec.
  - Wide slurred S waves in V_{5-6}, rsR′ complexes in V_3R and V_{1-2}, w/absent Q waves.
  - VAT prolonged in V_3R and V_{1-2}; a wide S wave in lead I.

iii. **QT interval:** The nl QT interval should be < half the R-R interval (if the HR is <100 bpm). Nl QTc interval is 0.45 sec (450 msec) males, 0.46 sec (460 msec) females.

d. Determine the **axis deviation:** QRS axis is −30 to + 90 degrees. Look at the net QRS deflection in leads I and aVF. Table 3-2 summarizes QRS complex axis determination. An algorithm for the detection and dx of interventricular conduction abnormality is described in Figure 3-6.

TABLE 3-2 ■ Rapid QRS Complex Axis Determination

	Lead I	Lead II	Lead III
Normal	Positive QRS	Positive QRS	Positive QRS
Left axis deviation	Positive QRS	Negative QRS	Negative QRS
Right axis deviation	Negative QRS	Varied QRS	Positive QRS
Indeterminate	Negative QRS	Negative QRS	Negative QRS

From Garcia D, Mattu A, Holstege P, Brady WJ: Intraventricular conduction abnormality: An electrocardiographic algorithm for rapid detection and diagnosis. Am J Emerg Med 27:492-502, 2009.

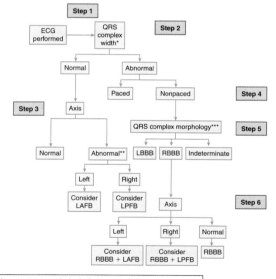

FIGURE 3-6. Electrocardiographic algorithm for the detection and diagnosis of intraventricular conduction abnormality. *(From Garcia D, Mattu A, Holstege P, Brady WJ: Intraventricular conduction abnormality: An electrocardiographic algorithm for rapid detection and diagnosis. Am J Emerg Med 27:492-502, 2009.)*

Figures 3-7 to 3-12 illustrate the criteria for fascicular and bundle branch blocks.

e. **Hypertrophy:** Look for signs of enlargement of the four chambers.

    i. **LVH:** The sum of the deepest S in V_1 or V_2 and the tallest R in V_5 or V_6 is >35 mm (in pts ≥35 years of age); R in lead aVL ≥12 mm; "strain" pattern.

    ii. **Left atrial hypertrophy (P mitrale):** The P waves are notched (M shaped) in the mitral leads (I, II, or aVL), or there is a deep terminal (–) component to the P in lead V_1.

CRITERIA FOR RBBB – A UNIFASCICULAR BLOCK

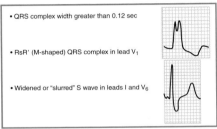

- QRS complex width greater than 0.12 sec

- RsR′ (M-shaped) QRS complex in lead V_1

- Widened or "slurred" S wave in leads I and V_6

FIGURE 3-7. Criteria for RBBB: a unifascicular block. *(From Garcia D, Mattu A, Holstege P, Brady WJ: Intraventricular conduction abnormality: An electrocardiographic algorithm for rapid detection and diagnosis. Am J Emerg Med 27:492-502, 2009.)*

CRITERIA FOR RBBB WITH LAFB – A BIFASCICULAR BLOCK

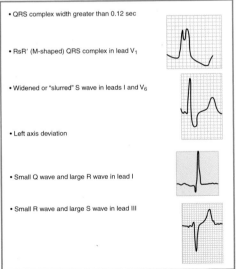

- QRS complex width greater than 0.12 sec

- RsR′ (M-shaped) QRS complex in lead V_1

- Widened or "slurred" S wave in leads I and V_6

- Left axis deviation

- Small Q wave and large R wave in lead I

- Small R wave and large S wave in lead III

FIGURE 3-8. Criteria for RBBB with LAFB: a bifascicular block. *(From Garcia D, Mattu A, Holstege P, Brady WJ: Intraventricular conduction abnormality: An electrocardiographic algorithm for rapid detection and diagnosis. Am J Emerg Med 27:492-502, 2009.)*

iii. Right atrial hypertrophy (**P pulmonale**): The P waves are prominent (≥2.5 mm tall) and peaked in the pulmonary leads (II, III, and aVF).

iv. RVH: Findings suggestive of RVH in adults are right atrial enlargement, RAD, incomplete RBBB, low voltage, tall R wave in V₁, persistent precordial S waves, right ventricular strain.

f. **Infarct:** Look at all leads (except aVR) for:

i. Q waves: Small (nl septal Q waves) are commonly seen in lateral leads (I, aVL, V₄, V₅, and V₆); moderate- or large-sized Q waves may be nl (as an isolated finding) in leads III, aVF, aVL, and V₁.

CRITERIA FOR RBBB WITH LPFB – A BIFASCICULAR BLOCK

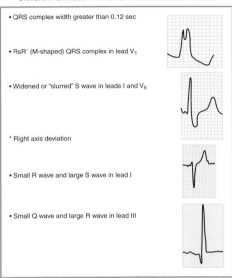

- QRS complex width greater than 0.12 sec

- RsR′ (M-shaped) QRS complex in lead V₁

- Widened or "slurred" S wave in leads I and V₆

* Right axis deviation

- Small R wave and large S wave in lead I

- Small Q wave and large R wave in lead III

FIGURE 3-9. Criteria for RBBB with LPFB: a bifascicular block. *(From Garcia D, Mattu A, Holstege P, Brady WJ: Intraventricular conduction abnormality: An electrocardiographic algorithm for rapid detection and diagnosis. Am J Emerg Med 27:492-502, 2009.)*

CRITERIA FOR LBBB – A BIFASCICULAR BLOCK

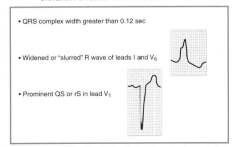

- QRS complex width greater than 0.12 sec

- Widened or "slurred" R wave of leads I and V₆

- Prominent QS or rS in lead V₁

FIGURE 3-10. Criteria for LBBB: a bifascicular block. *(From Garcia D, Mattu A, Holstege P, Brady WJ: Intraventricular conduction abnormality: An electrocardiographic algorithm for rapid detection and diagnosis. Am J Emerg Med 27:492-502, 2009.)*

CRITERIA FOR ISOLATED LAFB – A UNIFASCICULAR BLOCK

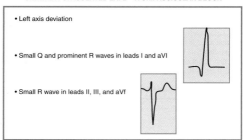

- Left axis deviation

- Small Q and prominent R waves in leads I and aVl

- Small R wave in leads II, III, and aVf

FIGURE 3-11. Criteria for isolated LAFB: a unifascicular block. *(From Garcia D, Mattu A, Holstege P, Brady WJ: Intraventricular conduction abnormality: An electrocardiographic algorithm for rapid detection and diagnosis. Am J Emerg Med 27:492-502, 2009.)*

CRITERIA FOR ISOLATED LPFB – A UNIFASCICULAR BLOCK

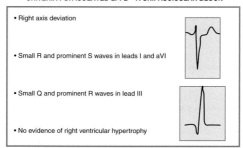

- Right axis deviation

- Small R and prominent S waves in leads I and aVl

- Small Q and prominent R waves in lead III

- No evidence of right ventricular hypertrophy

FIGURE 3-12. Criteria for isolated LPFB: a unifascicular block. *(From Garcia D, Mattu A, Holstege P, Brady WJ: Intraventricular conduction abnormality: An electrocardiographic algorithm for rapid detection and diagnosis. Am J Emerg Med 27:492-502, 2009.)*

  ii. R wave progression: Transition should occur between V_2 and V_4.
  iii. ST segments: Concentrate more on shape (i.e., "smiley" or "frowny") than on the amount of ST segment deviation. Figure 3-13 illustrates ST-T wave changes in nl and abnl conditions.
  iv. T waves: They may normally be inverted in leads III, aVF, aVL, and V_1. T wave changes in nl and abnl conditions are described in Figure 3-14.

4 CARDIAC STRESS TESTING

Stress testing is indicated to r/o CAD. Exercise duration is one of the strongest independent prognostic indicators in ETT and correlates well with outcome. Adequate workload during ETT goal = 85% of max predicted HR [220 – pt's age]. ETT is contraindicated in recent MI (<30 days), severe AS, decompensated acute HF, acute PE, aortic dissection, myopericarditis, uncontrolled arrhythmias. Table 3-3 describes advantages and limitations of various testing modalities in cardiology.

5 ECHOCARDIOGRAM

TTE: useful for evaluation of valve disease, cardiomyopathy, pericardial disease, HF, aortic disease, pulmonary HTN, and congenital heart disorder. Figure 3-15 illustrates 2D echo.

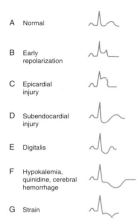

ST-T changes

A Normal

B Early
   repolarization

C Epicardial
   injury

D Subendocardial
   injury

E Digitalis

F Hypokalemia,
   quinidine, cerebral
   hemorrhage

G Strain

FIGURE 3-13. ST-T changes. ST-T wave changes in normal and abnormal conditions. *(From Gazes PC: Clinical Cardiology: A Bedside Approach, 2nd ed. Chicago, Year Book, 1983.)*

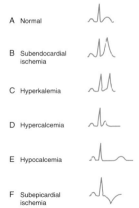

T wave changes

A Normal

B Subendocardial
   ischemia

C Hyperkalemia

D Hypercalcemia

E Hypocalcemia

F Subepicardial
   ischemia

FIGURE 3-14. T wave changes. T wave changes in normal and abnormal conditions. *(From Gazes PC: Clinical Cardiology: A Bedside Approach, 2nd ed. Chicago, Year Book, 1983.)*

Doppler echo: used to assess direction and velocity of blood flow

TEE: requires esophageal intubation and is used for endocarditis evaluation, evaluation of prosthetic valves, suspected lt atrial thrombus, and eval of aortic disease

3D echo: improved imaging, often used during cardiac procedures for device placement, good imaging of mitral valve disease

TABLE 3-3 ■ Diagnostic Testing for CAD

Test	Indication	Pros	Cons	Comments
ETT	Suspected CAD, evaluation of exercise tolerance	Evaluates exercise capacity, HR, BP, provoked symptoms	Cannot be used with baseline ECG abnormalities (LBBB, > 1 mm ST-segment depression, LVH, WPW syndrome, paced rhythm)	Low cost Low sensitivity (65%), specificity (75%) for CAD
Stress echo	Baseline ECG abnormality, localization of ischemia	Evaluates wall motion abnormalities (reversible defect = ischemia, fixed defect = infarct), valve function, pulmonary pressures	Operator dependent Suboptimal image quality in some patients Baseline wall motion abnormalities may affect image interpretation	Lower cost than nuclear imaging No radiation exposure Fast results (<1 hr) Sensitivity 75%, specificity 90% for CAD
Nuclear SPECT perfusion	Baseline ECG abnormality, localization of ischemia	Localizes ischemia (reversible defect = ischemia, fixed defect = infarct), evaluates LV function	Higher cost Radiation exposure Diaphragm interference or breast tissue can result in attenuation artifacts Obesity may result in false + image artifacts	Sensitivity 90%, specificity 75% Technetium has better tissue penetration and superior images but takes longer than thallium
Dobutamine echo	Suspected CAD in patients that cannot exercise	Evaluates wall motion abnormalities, valve function, pulmonary pressures in pts unable to exercise	Dobutamine cannot be used with severe baseline hypertension and arrhythmias (may precipitate tachyarrhythmias) Echo image quality suboptimal in some pts	Continuous acquisition of images allows rapid stoppage of test when ischemia is detected Hold β-blockers before the test
Dobutamine nuclear perfusion	Baseline ECG abnormality, localization of ischemia in pts who cannot exercise	Localizes ischemia and evaluates LV function with sensitivity and specificity equivalent to echo	Radiation Higher cost Dobutamine cannot be used with severe baseline hypertension and arrhythmias (may precipitate tachyarrhythmias)	Hold β-blockers before the test
Adenosine, dipyridamole, regadenoson (vasodilator) nuclear perfusion	Baseline ECG abnormality, localization of ischemia in pts who cannot exercise and have contraindication to dobutamine	Localizes ischemia in pts who cannot exercise and have contraindication to dobutamine	May precipitate bronchospasm and bradycardia	Caffeine (adenosine receptor antagonist) should be withheld for ≥24 hr before administration of adenosine Vasodilators with demonstrate CAD but will not accurately dx ischemia
Coronary angiography	To define the location and extent of CAD	Allows angioplasty and stent placement	Radiation Potential adverse reaction to radiocontrast dye	Invasive
CT and MR coronary imaging	Identification of CAD in selected patients with intermediate risk for CAD	Can identify anomalous coronary arteries MR accurate in proximal and middle segments	CT does not provide detailed images of distal anatomy MR contraindicated in pts with pacemaker, ICD, other implanted devices	Noninvasive Best images in pts with sinus rhythm and slower heart rates MR not useful in claustrophobic pts CT angiography requires a high-resolution CT scanner
Coronary artery calcium (CAC) score	Detects and quantitates coronary calcium Useful in selected pts with intermediate risk	Moderate/good predictor of CAD risk CAC score: <100 = low risk, >300 = high risk	Radiation Sensitive but not specific for CAD Expensive, limited insurance coverage	Not recommended for use in asymptomatic patients at either high or low risk of coronary event

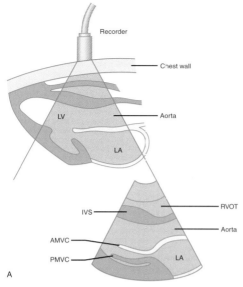

A

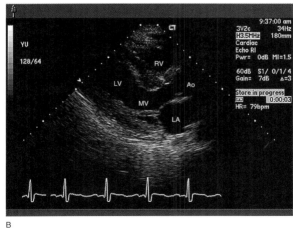

B

FIGURE 3-15. Echocardiogram: an example of a two-dimensional long-axis view. **A,** Diagram showing the anatomy of the area scanned and a diagrammatic representation of the echocardiogram. **B,** Two-dimensional long-axis view. *AMVC,* anterior mitral valve cusp; *IVS,* interventricular septum; *PMVC,* posterior mitral valve cusp; *RVOT,* right ventricular outflow tract. (*From Ballinger A: Kumar & Clark's Essentials of Clinical Medicine, 6th ed. Edinburgh, Saunders, 2012.*)

6 RADIAL ARTERY CANNULATION (A-LINE)

Indications

- Monitoring of BP during use of potent vasoactive agents (e.g., nitroprusside, dopamine)
- Monitoring of BP in critically ill hypotensive pts (e.g., shock) or during major surgery (e.g., CV)
- Frequent ABG analysis or other blood tests in pts w/limited vascular access

Procedure

1. Evaluate patency of the ulnar artery w/the ***Allen test.*** Simultaneously compressing the radial and ulnar arteries, have the pt clench and elevate the fist to let blood drain from the hand; keep pressure on both arteries until the hand blanches; then have the pt open the hand while pressure is maintained on both arteries. Release the ulnar artery and observe the hand for blushing. The presence of blushing and return of nl color to the hand indicate patency of the ulnar artery and adequate blood supply if radial occlusion occurs w/the catheter.
2. Hyperextend the hand over a wrist roll, and immobilize it and the lower arm.
3. Sterile drape and clean the area w/povidone-iodine solution.
4. Anesthetize the skin and then insert the angiocatheter through the skin at a 30- to 45-degree angle, advancing it parallel to the artery; gently cannulate the artery (as evidenced by the blush of blood within the catheter). Advance the catheter over the needle until it locks into place. It should easily advance over the needle. If it does not easily advance, the artery is probably no longer cannulated.
5. Detach the syringe and connect the catheter to the pressure tubing and functioning irrigation system; an arterial pressure tracing indicates intra-arterial positioning.
6. Secure the catheter line to the skin w/silk ligature; apply sterile dressing and adhesive tape to prevent accidental disconnection.
7. Remove the wrist from its hyperextended position, and splint the dorsal aspect to prevent accidental disconnection.

7 CENTRAL VENOUS ACCESS (CVP LINE)

Indications

- Inadequate peripheral venous access
- TPN, use of vasopressor agents that cannot be given through peripheral lines
- Chemotherapeutic administration
- Central venous and PA pressure monitoring
- Frequent blood draws w/difficult IV access

Anatomy for Central Venous Catheter Placement

- **External jugular vein:** formed at the angle of the mandible by the posterior facial veins and the posterior auricular vein. It passes caudally over the SCM muscle to enter the subclavian vein lateral to the anterior scalene muscle.
- **Internal jugular vein:** arises from the base of the skull in the carotid sheath posterior to the internal carotid artery and terminates in the subclavian vein anterior and *lateral* to the common carotid artery. It runs medial to the SCM in its upper part, posterior in triangle between two heads of the SCM and behind the clavicular head in its lower part.
- **Subclavian vein:** continuation of axillary vein at the lateral border of the first rib; passes over the first rib anterior to the anterior scalene muscle, continues behind the medial third of the clavicle, where it is fixed to the rib and clavicle; joins the internal jugular to form the innominate vein behind the sternocostoclavicular joint. The subclavian artery and apical pleura lie behind the vein at the medial third of the clavicle.
- **Femoral vein:** used as a last resort because of the ↑ frequency of thrombosis, embolism, and infection. The vein is located *medial* to the femoral artery in the femoral sheath below the inguinal ligament. The artery may be found at the midpoint of a line connecting the anterior superior iliac spine and the pubic symphysis; the vein is one fingerbreadth medial. A useful mnemonic is NAVEL (Nerve, Artery, Vein, Empty space, Lymphatics).

Principles of Internal Jugular and Subclavian Vein Catheterization

1. Check the INR, APTT, and Plt count before puncture attempts to r/o coagulopathy.
2. Equipment needed: prepackaged sterile kit that contains apparatus for catheterization by the Seldinger technique. The use of bedside U/S to verify the internal jugular location is increasing and is standard of care in many hospitals.

3. Place a rolled towel vertically between the shoulder blades; put the pt in the Trendelenburg position w/the neck extended. If the pt is anxious and hemodynamically stable, consider sedation.
4. Wear gown, mask, and sterile gloves; prepare and drape the pt.
5. Infiltrate local anesthesia at the puncture site w/25-gauge needle, then a 20-gauge needle; infiltrate track toward the vein, aspirating before instilling anesthetic. It is especially important in subclavian venipuncture to anesthetize the clavicle edge.
6. Flush the catheter w/sterile fluid; estimate the length to the sternomanubrial junction to place in the SVC.
7. Mount an 18-gauge thin-walled needle on the syringe.
8. Insert slowly, while aspirating, until blood returns; advance a few millimeters farther until blood return ↑. Bright red blood usually means arterial puncture; remove needle and apply pressure for 10 minutes.
9. If no blood returns, withdraw needle slowly under (−) pressure; blood may still return into syringe. If still no blood returns, reattempt.
10. After blood returns, stabilize needle, carefully unscrew syringe, and prevent air embolism by occluding the needle w/a finger.
11. Place a guide wire through the needle gently; it should advance easily. Withdraw the needle, holding the wire in position.
12. Nick the skin w/the #11 blade, slide the dilator over the wire to enlarge the skin site and track, remove the dilator, then advance the catheter over the wire into the desired position.
13. Remove the wire, check blood return on each port and flush it w/NS, and attach IV tubing or caps.
14. Suture at skin and place sterile occlusive dressing.

Specific Sites

Internal Jugular: Central Approach
1. Locate the triangle formed by the two heads of the SCM and the clavicle.
2. Insert a 22-gauge localizing needle at the apex of the triangle formed by the two heads of the SCM.
3. Aim the needle parallel to the clavicular head toward the ipsilateral nipple at a 45- to 60-degree angle until the vein is entered. Keep a finger of the nondominant hand on the pulse of the carotid artery to be cognizant of its location.
4. If the needle is inserted 3 cm w/o blood return, attempt a new puncture in a slightly more lateral position.
5. Do not proceed medially because the carotid artery may be punctured.

Internal Jugular: Posterior Approach
1. Insert the needle under the SCM three fingerbreadths above the clavicle, and aim anteriorly to the suprasternal notch at a 45-degree angle to the sagittal and horizontal planes.
2. The vein should be entered within 5 to 7 cm of needle penetration.

Subclavian Vein Catheterization (Infraclavicular)
1. Insert the needle 1 to 2 cm below the junction of the medial and middle thirds of clavicle.
2. Advance the needle parallel to the frontal plane until the clavicle is located.
3. March the needle down the clavicle until it just passes below it, aiming just above the suprasternal notch and keeping the needle parallel to the frontal plane.
4. When the vein is entered, carefully rotate the needle 90 degrees to aim the bevel caudally so that the wire will pass into the innominate vein.

Contraindications

- Thrombosis of central veins
- Coagulopathy: a relative contraindication. Many coagulopathies can be temporarily overcome w/transfusion of FFP, cryoprecipitate, or Plt, followed by immediate venipuncture. It is preferable to place deep lines in areas that are compressible in the event of bleeding (i.e., femoral, brachial, internal jugular). Also consider cutdown of antecubital veins.
- Bullous emphysema: Avoid subclavian approach.

Complications

- Catheter misplacement: poor blood return, cardiac irritability, pain in neck or ear. Corrective options include the following:
  - Reposition under fluoroscopy.
  - Reattempt entire procedure.
- Arterial puncture (subclavian, carotid, femoral)
- Hemorrhage: venous or arterial

- Pneumothorax: Always check CXR after placement and after failed attempts and before reattempting central venipuncture on the contralateral side.
- Thoracic duct injury with or w/o chylothorax
- Extravasation of fluid, hyperalimentation, and so forth
- Neural injury (brachial plexus)
- Air embolism
- Catheter or wire embolization
- Hydrothorax
  - Primary: placement of the catheter into pleural or mediastinal spaces
  - Secondary: erosion of the catheter through SVC after successful placement
- Infection
  - Cellulitis at puncture site
  - Bacteremia from catheter colonization (catheter sepsis)
  - ↑ incidence w/use of multilumen catheters
- Thrombosis (central venous): Clinical signs include unilateral upper extremity edema, upper extremity and neck venous distention, and neck pain. Rx: similar to that of iliofemoral DVT. Remove the catheter, heparinize, and follow w/long-term warfarin administration because there is a well-described incidence of PE after subclavian vein thrombosis.

8 PULMONARY ARTERY (PA) CATHETERIZATION (SWAN-GANZ)

Useful in dx cause of hemodynamic shock, locating intracardiac shunts, obtaining cardiac data on hemodynamically unstable pts. Figure 3-16 illustrates typical waveforms and pressures. Table 3-4 summarizes hemodynamic measurements and their clinical significance. Box 3-2 shows hemodynamic measurements in specific disease states. Table 3-5 describes the effects of therapeutic measures on hemodynamic measurements, and Table 3-6 describes the effects of inotropic and mixed agents on cardiac parameters.

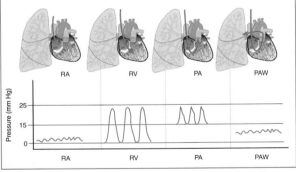

FIGURE 3-16. A Swan-Ganz catheter is introduced into a large vein and advanced in the direction of blood flow. Vena cava pressure and RAP are about 0 to 5 mm Hg. Right ventricular pressure is 25/0 mm Hg; pulmonary artery pressure is 25/15 mm Hg. Inflation of the balloon on the catheter allows recording of the PAWP, about 8 mm Hg, which is a good estimate of pulmonary venous BP. *(From Carroll R: Elsevier's Integrated Physiology. Philadelphia, Mosby, 2007.)*

B. CORONARY ARTERY DISEASE

1 CHRONIC STABLE ANGINA

- **Angina pectoris:** discomfort that occurs when myocardial O_2 demand exceeds supply
- Four classes (Canadian Cardiovascular Society classification system):
  - **Class I:** Ordinary physical activity (e.g., walking, climbing stairs) does not cause angina. Angina occurs w/strenuous, rapid, or prolonged exertion at work or recreation.

TABLE 3-4 ■ Hemodynamic Measurements and Their Clinical Significance

Hemodynamic Measurement	Normal Value	Clinical Significance	Abnormalities
RAP	0-8 mm Hg	Equivalent to CVP	↑: Right ventricular failure, PE, tricuspid valve abnormalities, pericardial tamponade, right ventricular infarction ↓: Hypovolemia
PAP	Systolic: 15-30 mm Hg Diastolic: 5-12 mm Hg Mean: 10-20 mm Hg	PAP is equal to RAP during systole while the pulmonary valve is open If the pulmonary vascular resistance is normal, the PADP is 1-4 mm Hg > PCWP and can be substituted for it in following the patient's hemodynamic measurements	↑: PE, chronic lung disease, VSD, cardiogenic shock, right ventricular infarction If the PADP is 5 mm Hg > PCWP, consider ARDS, pulmonary emboli, or COPD
PCWP	5-12 mm Hg	PCWP is normally equal to left atrial pressure; it is therefore a sensitive indicator of the presence of pulmonary congestion and left-sided CHF PCWP is not equal to LVEDP in the following situations: PCWP > LVEDP: Mitral stenosis Patient receiving PEEP Left atrial myxoma Pulmonary venous obstruction PCWP < LVEDP: "Stiff" left ventricle ↑ LVEDP (>25 mm Hg)	↑: Left ventricular failure w/resultant pulmonary congestion, acute mitral insufficiency, tamponade ↓: Left ventricular compliance (hypertrophy, infarction)
CO	3.5-7 L/min	CO = SV × HR	↓: Cardiac dysrhythmias, ↓ contracting muscle mass (myocardial ischemia, MI), mitral insufficiency, VSD
CI	2.5-4 L/m²	CI relates CO to BSA CI = CO/BSA	↑: High-output failure secondary to fluid overload, hepatocellular failure, renal disease, septic shock ↓: Hypovolemia, cardiogenic shock, PE, hypothyroidism, CHF w/failing ventricle
SVR	900-1300 dyne-sec/cm⁻⁵	Resistance against which the left ventricle must work to eject its SV SVR = (MAP − RAP) × 80/CO	↑: Hypervolemic vasoconstrictive states (HTN, cardiogenic shock, traumatic shock) ↓: Septic shock, acute renal failure, pregnancy
PVR	155-255 dyne-sec/cm⁻⁵	PVR = (PAP − PAWP) × 8C/CO	↑: Cor pulmonale, PE, valvular heart disease, CHF ↓: Hypervolemic states, pregnancy

---

Box 3-2 • Hemodynamic Measurements in Specific Disease States

Septic shock
Early: ↓ PCWP, ↓ SVR, ↑ CO
Late: ↓ PCWP, ↑ SVR, ↓ CO
Neurogenic shock: ↓ PCWP, ↓ SVR, N/↓ CO
Cardiac tamponade: ↑ PCWP, ↑ SVR, ↓ CO, ↓ CI
CVP = PADP = PCWP
Pulmonary embolism: normal PCWP, ↑ PADP, ↓ CI
Cardiogenic shock: ↑ PCWP, ↑ PADP, ↓ CO, ↓ CI, ↑ SVR
Hypovolemic shock: ↓ PCWP, ↓ CO, ↑ SVR, ↓ CI
Right ventricular infarct: RAP/PCWP ≥0.8

N, No effect.

TABLE 3-5 ■ Effects of Therapeutic Measures on Hemodynamic Measurements			
Therapeutic Measure	CO	SVR	PCWP
IV fluids	N/↑	N/↑	↑
Diuretics	N/↓↓	↓/Secondary ↑	↓
Nitrates	N/↓	↓	↓
Nitroprusside	↑	↓↓	N/↓
Catecholamines	N/↑	↑↑↑	N/↑
Dopamine	N/↑	↑↑	N/↑↑
Dobutamine	↑↑	↓	N/↓

N, no effect.

TABLE 3-6 ■ Effects of Inotropic and Mixed Agents on Cardiac Parameters					
Agent	CO	SVR	MAP	HR	CVP
Dobutamine $\beta_1 > \beta_2$ (inotropic)	↑↑	↓	↑	↑	↔
Milrinone PDE inhibitor (inotropic)	↑↑	↓	↓	↑	↔
Norepinephrine α_1, β_1 (mixed)	↑↓	↑↑	↑	↔	↑
Epinephrine α_1, α_2, β_1, β_2 (mixed)	↑↑	↑↑	↑	↔	↑
Dopamine >5 µg/kg/min β (mixed)	↑	↑	↑↑	↑↑	↑
Dopamine >10 µg/kg/min α, β (mixed)	↑	↑↑	↑↑	↑↑	↑

- **Class II:** Slight limitation of ordinary activity. Angina occurs on walking or climbing stairs rapidly; walking uphill; walking or stair climbing pc, in cold, in wind, or under emotional stress; or only during the few hr after awakening. Angina occurs on walking more than two blocks on the level and climbing more than one flight of ordinary stairs at a nl pace and in nl conditions.
- **Class III:** Marked limitations of ordinary physical activity. Angina occurs on walking one to two blocks on the level and climbing one flight of stairs in nl conditions and at a nl pace.
- **Class IV:** Inability to carry on any physical activity w/o discomfort—anginal sx may be present at rest.

Risk Factors
- **Uncontrollable:** Advanced age, male sex, genetic predisposition
- **Modifiable:** Smoking (risk is almost double), HTN, impaired fasting glucose or DM, obesity (weight >30% above ideal), hypothyroidism, LVH, sedentary lifestyle, oral contraceptive use, cocaine use, vasculitis, depression, ↑ hs-CRP, ↑ fibrinogen, ↑ homocysteine, ↑ lipoprotein-associated phospholipase A_2

Diagnosis
H&P
- The most important dx factor is the hx (e.g., chest pain, pressure, jaw pain, lt arm pain).
- PE is little diagnostic help and may be nl in many pts, although the presence of an S_4 gallop suggests ischemic chest pain.

ECG
- During the acute episode may show transient T wave inversion or ST-segment depression or elevation, but some pts may have a nl tracing.

Stress Testing
See Table 3-3.

Imaging
- Echo: indicated in pts w/systolic murmur suggestive of AS, MVP, or hypertrophic cardiomyopathy. Echo combined w/treadmill exercise (stress echo) or pharmacologic stress w/dobutamine can be used to detect regional wall abnlities that occur during myocardial ischemia associated w/CAD.
- Cardiac cath: if + stress test result

Labs
- Cardiac troponins in pts presenting with sx suggestive of myocardial ischemia
- Lipid panel, FBS to evaluate risk factors

TABLE 3-7 ■ Likelihood of Ischemic Etiology and Short-Term Risk

Part I. Chest Pain Patients without ST-Segment Elevation: Likelihood of Ischemic Etiology

	A. High Likelihood	B. Intermediate Likelihood	C. Low Likelihood
	High likelihood that chest pain is of ischemic etiology if patient has *any* of the findings in the column below:	Intermediate likelihood that chest pain is of ischemic etiology if patient has *no findings* in column A and *any* of the findings in the column below	Low likelihood that chest pain is of ischemic etiology if patient has *no* findings in column A or B; patients may have any of the findings in the column below:
History	Chief symptom is chest or left arm pain or discomfort *plus* Current pain reproduces pain of previous documented angina and known CAD, including MI	Chief symptom is chest or left arm pain or discomfort Age >70 yr Male sex Diabetes mellitus	Probably ischemic symptoms Recent cocaine use
Physical exam	Transient mitral regurgitation Hypotension Diaphoresis Pulmonary edema or rales	Extracardiac vascular disease	Chest discomfort reproduced by palpation
ECG	New (or presumed new) transient ST deviation (≥0.5 mm) or T wave inversion (≥2 mm) with symptoms	Fixed Q waves Abnormal ST segments or T waves that are not new	Normal ECG *or* T wave flattening *or* T wave inversion in leads with dominant R waves
Cardiac markers	Elevated troponin I or T Elevated CK-MB	*Any finding in column B above plus* Normal cardiac markers	Normal cardiac markers

Part II. Risk of Death or Nonfatal MI during the Short Term in Patients with Chest Pain with High or Intermediate Likelihood of Ischemia (Columns A and B in Part I)

	High Risk	Intermediate Risk	Low Risk
	Risk is high if patient has *any* of the following findings:	Risk is intermediate if patient has *any* of the following findings:	Risk is low if patient has *no* high- or intermediate-risk features; may have any of the following:
History	Accelerating tempo of ischemic symptoms during previous 48 hr	Prior MI *or* Peripheral artery disease *or* Cerebrovascular disease *or* CABG, previous aspirin use	
Character of Pain	Prolonged, continuing (>20 min) rest pain	Prolonged (>20 min) rest angina is now resolved (moderate to high likelihood of CAD) Rest angina (<20 min) or relieved by rest or sublingual nitrates	New-onset functional angina (class III or IV) in past 2 wk without rest pain (but with moderate or high likelihood of CAD)

Reprinted with permission from 2005 American Heart Association Guidelines for cardiopulmonary resuscitation and emergency cardiovascular care, part 8: Stabilization of the patient with acute coronary syndromes. Circulation 112(Suppl IV), 2005.

TABLE 3-8 ■ Likelihood of Ischemic Etiology and Short-Term Risk

	Low Risk	High Risk	Intermediate Risk
Physical exam	Pulmonary edema secondary to ischemia New or worse mitral regurgitation murmur Hypotension, bradycardia, tachycardia S₃ gallop or new or worsening rales Age >75 yr	Age > 70 yr	
ECG	Transient ST deviation (≥0.5 mm) with rest angina New or presumably new BBB Sustained VT	T wave inversion ≥2 mm Pathologic Q waves or T waves that are not new	Normal or unchanged ECG during an episode of chest discomfort
Cardiac markers	Elevated cardiac troponin I or T Elevated CK-MB	Any of the above findings plus Normal cardiac markers	Normal cardiac markers

Risk stratification

Tables 3-7 and 3-8 describe the likelihood of ischemic etiology and short-term risk.

Treatment

Medical

- Major classes of antianginal agents are nitrates, β-blockers, CCB, and ASA; can be used alone or in combination.
- Ranolazine (selective inhibitor of the late Na^+ channel) can be added in pts with persistent symptoms.
- Add ACEI in pts with DM, ↓ EF, or HTN.
- Add statins to keep LDL chol <100 mg/dL (optimal goal is <70 mg/dL).
- Correct possible aggravating factors (e.g., anemia, HTN, DM, hyperlipidemia, thyrotoxicosis, hypothyroidism).

Coronary Revascularization

- Reserved for pts who remain symptomatic despite optimal medical Rx
- *PCI* (angioplasty and coronary stents): for pts w/one- or two-vessel disease that usually does not involve the main left coronary artery and ventricular function is nl or nearly nl. Some noncomplex lesions of the left main coronary involving the ostium and proximal and midvessel may be amenable to PCI. PCI improves symptoms but does not improve survival or ↓ future cardiovascular events. Following PCI, continue ASA (81 mg/day) indefinitely, clopidogrel for 1 yr when using drug-eluting stent, or 1 month when using bare-metal stent.
- *CABG surgery:* for pts w/left main coronary disease, for those w/symptomatic 3-vessel disease, and for those w/left ventricular EF <40% and critical (>70% stenosis) in all 3 major coronary arteries. Surgical Rx improves prognosis, particularly in diabetic pts w/multivessel disease.

Secondary Prevention

- Smoking cessation
- BP control (<140/90 mm Hg, <130/80 mm Hg in diabetes or renal disease)
- Lipid management (LDL <70 mg/dL)
- Exercise (30 min at least 5 days/wk); weight loss if overweight (keep BMI 18.5-24.9); waist circumference <40 inches in men, <35 inches in women
- Antiplatelet Rx: ASA 75-162 mg
- β-Blockers (unless contraindicated)

Clinical Pearl

- Within 12 mo of initial dx, 10% to 20% of pts w/dx of stable angina progress to MI or unstable angina.

2 CORONARY ARTERY SYNDROMES (ACS)

- **ACS** are manifestations of ischemic heart disease and represent a broad clinical spectrum that includes non–ST-segment elevation ACS (collectively UA/**NSTEMI**) and **STEMI**. Pts presenting with STEMI usually have complete occlusion of the coronary artery, whereas those with UA/NSTEMI have partial occlusion
- **STEMI:** defined as ST-segment elevation >0.1 mV in ≥2 contiguous precordial or adjacent limb leads, a new LBBB, or a true posterior MI.
- According to the European Society of Cardiology/ACC, either one of the following criteria for acute evolving or recent MI satisfies the dx:
  - Typical and gradual fall (troponin) or more rapid and fall (CK-MB) of biochemical markers of myocardial necrosis w/at least one of the following:
    - Ischemic sx
    - Development of pathologic Q waves on ECG
    - ECG changes indicative of ischemia (ST-segment elevation or depression)
    - Coronary artery intervention (e.g., coronary angioplasty)
  - Pathologic findings of acute MI: ST elevation MI (area of ischemic necrosis that penetrates the entire thickness of the ventricular wall and results in ST-segment elevation)
- **NSTEMI:** coronary arterial plaque rupture w/fragmentation and distal arterial embolization resulting in myocardial necrosis. It usually occurs w/o ST elevation and is thus termed NSTEMI.

Etiology

- Coronary atherosclerosis
- Coronary artery spasm
- Coronary embolism (caused by infective endocarditis, rheumatic heart disease, intracavitary thrombus)
- Periarteritis and other coronary artery inflammatory diseases

- Dissection into coronary arteries (aneurysmal or iatrogenic)
- Congenital abnlities of coronary circulation
- **MINC syndrome:** more frequent in younger pts and cocaine addicts. The risk of acute MI is by a factor of 24 during the 60 min after the use of cocaine in persons who are otherwise at relatively low risk. Most pts w/cocaine-related MI are young, nonwhite, male cigarette smokers w/o other risk factors for arteriosclerotic heart disease who have a h/o repeated cocaine use. Blood and urine toxicology screen for cocaine is recommended in all young pts who present w/acute MI.
- Hypercoagulable states, blood viscosity (polycythemia vera)

Diagnosis

H&P

- Crushing substernal chest pain or pressure usually >20 min
  - Unrelieved by rest or sublingual NTG or is rapidly recurring
  - Radiates to the left or right arm, neck, jaw, back, shoulders, or abd and is not pleuritic in character
  - May be associated w/dyspnea, diaphoresis, N/V
  - Pain in 20% of infarctions (usually in diabetic or elderly pts)
- Diaphoresis, w/pallor (because of ↓ O₂)
- Rales possibly present at the bases of lungs (indicative of CHF)
- Cardiac auscultation may reveal an apical systolic murmur caused by MR secondary to papillary muscle dysfunction. S_3 or S_4 may also be present.

Labs

- See Figure 3-17.
- Cardiac troponin levels: cTnT and cTnI after muscle damage (3-12 hr), peak within 24 hr, and may be present up to 7 days for cTnI and up to 10-14 days for cTnT. cTnT can be falsely + in pts w/renal failure.

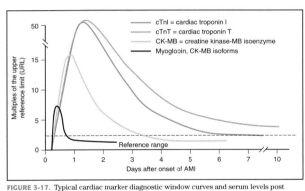

FIGURE 3-17. Typical cardiac marker diagnostic window curves and serum levels post acute MI. *(From Lehman CA [ed]: Saunders Manual of Clinical Laboratory Science. Philadelphia, Saunders, 1998.)*

Imaging

- CX
- ECG (Fig. 3-18 and Table 3-9)
- STEMI
  - Inverted T waves (area of ischemia)
  - ↑ ST segment (area of injury): leads V_1-V_6 = anterior or anterolateral MI; leads I and aVL = lateral MI; leads II, III, or aVF = inferior wall MI
  - Q waves (area of infarction, usually develop during 12-36 hr)
- NSTEMI
  - Hx and enzyme elevations are compatible w/MI.
  - ECG shows no ST-segment elevation and sometimes shows a small depression of the ST segment, T wave inversion.
- UIA
  - enzymes normal
  - ECG may show changes similar to NSTEMI

A ST-segment elevation (⇒ *injury*)

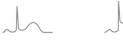

Early ("hyperacute")
stage

Coved ("frowny") ST-segment
elevation (= ***acute injury pattern***)

B T wave inversion (⇒ *ischemia*)

Early T wave
inversion

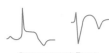

Deeper, symmetric T wave
inversion (= ***ischemia***)

C Development of Q waves

Early Q wave
development

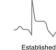

Established
Q wave stage

QS complex

D Reciprocal ST-segment depression

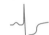

Mirror-image
ST depression

Subtler reciprocal
ST-segment depression

FIGURE 3-18. Principal ECG indicators of acute infarction. *(From Goldman L, Ausiello D [eds]: Cecil Textbook of Medicine, 22nd ed. Philadelphia, Saunders, 2004.)*

TABLE 3-9 ■ Electrocardiographic Location of ST-Elevation MI

Area of Infarction	ECG Abnormality	Artery Involved
Anterior wall	Q waves in V_1-V_4	LAD
Anteroseptal	Q waves in V_1-V_2	Proximal LAD
Anteroapical	Q waves in V_2-V_3	LAD or branches of LAD
Anterolateral	Q waves in V_4-V_6, I, aVL	Mid-LAD or CFX
Lateral wall	Q waves in I, aVL	CFX
Inferior wall	Q waves in II, III, aVF	RCA
Posterior wall	R > S in V_1	PDA
	Q wave in V_6	

CFX, Left circumflex artery; *LAD*, left anterior descending; *PDA*, posterior descending artery; *RCA*, right coronary artery.

Risk Stratification
■ The TIMI risk store: Estimation of short-term risk for death/non-fatal MI for pts presenting with UA and NSTEMI is described in Table 3-10.

Treatment
UA/NSTEMI
■ Low TIMI (0-2): ASA, β-blockers, nitrates, statin, clopidogrel or prasugrel; predischarge or outpt stress test
■ Intermediate TIMI (3-4) or high TIMI (5-7): ASA, β-blocker, nitrates, anticoagulation (UFH, enoxaparin, or bivalirudin), thienopyridine (clopidogrel or prasugrel), statin. Consider glycoprotein (GP) IIb/IIIa inhibitor in pts with ongoing angina, HF, dynamic ECG changes, DM. Consider early coronary angiography and PCI or surgical revascularization depending on angiography results. In pts on clopidogrel, CABG should be delayed by ≥5 days after stopping clopidogrel.

TABLE 3-10 ■ TIMI Risk Score for Patients with Unstable Angina and Non–ST-Segment Elevation MI: Predictor Variables

Predictor Variable	Point Value of Variable	Definition
Age ≥65 years	1	
≥3 risk factors for CAD	1	Risk factors: Family history of CAD Hypertension Hypercholesterolemia Diabetes Current smoker
Aspirin use in last 7 days	1	
Recent, severe symptoms of angina	1	≥2 anginal events in the last 24 hr
Elevated cardiac markers	1	CK-MB or cardiac-specific troponin level
ST deviation ≥0.5 mm	1	S⁻ depression ≥0.5 mm is significant; transient ST elevation >0.5 mm for <20 min is treated as ST-segment depression and is high risk; ST elevation ≥1 mm for >20 min places these patients in the STEMI treatment category
Prior coronary artery stenosis ≥50%	1	Risk predictor remains valid even if this information is unknown
Calculated TIMI Risk Score	**Risk of ≥1 Primary Endpoint* in ≤14 days**	**Risk Status**
0 or 1	5%	Low
2	8%	
3	13%	Intermediate
4	20%	
5	26%	High
6 or 7	41%	

Reprinted with permission from 2005 American Heart Association guidelines for cardiopulmonary resuscitation and emergency cardiovascular care, part 8: Stabilization of the patient with acute coronary syndromes. Circulation 112(Suppl IV), 2005.

*Primary endpoints: new or recurrent MI or need for urgent revascularization.

STEMI

- On arrival →ASA (325 mg chewed), antithrombotics (UHF or enoxaparin), antiplatelets (clopidogrel or prasugrel), O_2, MSO_4 IV for pain, nitrates (except in IWMI, RV infarction), β-blockers (metoprolol, esmolol but avoid β-blockers in HF, BP systolic <90, HR, 50/min). Within 24 hr →statin, ACEI
- Pts w/STEMI who present <12 hr of sx onset and have no contraindications should receive immediate reperfusion Rx (fibrinolysis [streptokinase, alteplase, reteplase, or tenecteplase] or PCI).
- Figure 3-19 describes an Rx algorithm for STEMI.
- Figure 3-20 illustrates coronary anatomy.
- Rescue PCI is reasonable in those w/<50% resolution of ST-segment elevation 90 min after initiation of fibrinolytic Rx and a moderately large area of myocardium at risk.
- Hemodynamic categories in acute MI are described in Table 3-11.
- Post-STEMI complications:
  - **Papillary muscle rupture:** seen with IWMI, or IW-PWMI, holosystolic murmur @ LSB & apex, pulm edema. Dx with echo (severe MR, flail mitral valve leaflet with papillary muscle head), PA cath (large v waves in wedge pressure tracing). Rx IABP, afterload reduction (diuretics, nitroprusside), surgery
  - **RV infarct:** >1 mm ST-segment elevation in V_3R and V_4R, JVD but clear lung fields, ↓↓ BP, echo shows ↓ systolic function, dilated RV, PA cath shows ↑ RA and RV pressures, ↓ PWP. Rx with aggressive IV fluids, inotropic support, revascularization
  - **VSD:** Holosystolic murmur @ LSB, PA cath shows step-up O_2 sat from RA to RV, echo shows fast lt → rt systolic jet within ventricular septum. Rx with IABP, vasopressors, urgent surgical repair
  - **LV thrombus** (10%-20% of pts): dx with echo, Rx with warfarin for 3 to 6 mo

Secondary Prevention Post STEMI

- Smoking cessation

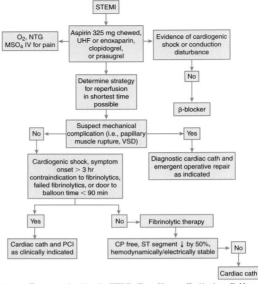

FIGURE 3-19. Treatment algorithm for STEMI. *(From Vincent JL, Abraham E, Moore FA, et al [eds]: Textbook of Critical Care, 6th ed. Philadelphia, Saunders, 2011.)*

- BP control (<140/90 mm Hg, <130/80 mm Hg in diabetes or renal disease)
- Lipid management (LDL <70 mg/dL)
- Exercise (30 min at least 5 days/wk); weight loss if overweight (keep BMI 18.5-24.9); waist circumference <40 inches in men, <35 inches in women
- Antiplatelet Rx: ASA 75-162 mg or prasugrel 10 mg qd, clopidogrel 75 mg qd (if stent placed)
- β-Blockers (unless contraindicated)
- ACEIs reduce left ventricular dysfunction and dilation and slow the progression of CHF. Use ARBs in pts intolerant to ACEIs.

C. HEART FAILURE (HF)

Definition
HF is a pathophysiologic state characterized by congestion in the pulmonary or systemic circulation resulting from the heart's inability to pump sufficient oxygenated blood to meet the metabolic needs of the tissues. **Systolic dysfunction** refers to loss of contractile strength of myocardium in the setting of ventricular dilatation. **Diastolic dysfunction** occurs when filling of one or both ventricles is impaired in the setting of nl emptying capacity.

Classification
ACC and AHA: Four Stages
A. At high risk for heart failure but w/o structural heart disease or sx of heart failure (e.g., CAD, HTN)
B. Structural heart disease but w/o sx of heart failure
C. Structural heart disease w/prior or current sx of heart failure
D. Refractory heart failure requiring specialized interventions

The NYHA Four Functional Classes
I. Asymptomatic (no limitations of physical activity)
II. Slight limitation of physical activity (symptomatic w/moderate exertion)

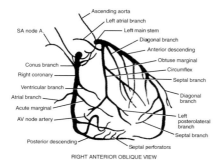

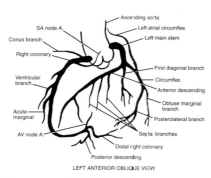

RIGHT ANTERIOR OBLIQUE VIEW

LEFT ANTERIOR OBLIQUE VIEW

FIGURE 3-20. The coronary vessels in the right and left anterior oblique views are shown. The major arteries are the left main, left anterior descending, circumflex, and right coronary arteries. *(From the Pulmonary Disease Section, University of Oklahoma Health Sciences Center, Oklahoma City, Oklahoma, as reprinted in Williamson JO: Acid-base disorders: classification and management strategies. Am Fam Physician 52:584-590, 1995.)*

III. Marked limitation of physical activity
    IIIA. Symptoms with < then ordinary exertion
    IIIB. Symptomatic w/minimal exertion
IV. Symptomatic at rest (unable to carry on any physical activity w/o symptoms)

Diagnosis

H&P

- The findings on PE in pts w/HF vary according to the severity and whether the failure is right sided or left sided.
- Common clinical manifestations are:
  - Dyspnea on exertion initially, then w/progressively less strenuous activity, and eventually manifesting when pt is at rest; caused by pulmonary congestion
  - Orthopnea caused by venous return in the recumbent position (↑ pillows to sleep)
  - PND resulting from multiple factors (venous return in the recumbent position, ↓ Pao₂, ↓ adrenergic stimulation of myocardial function)
  - Nocturnal angina resulting from cardiac work (secondary to venous return)
  - *Cheyne-Stokes respiration:* alternating phases of apnea and hyperventilation caused by prolonged circulation time from lungs to brain
  - Fatigue, lethargy resulting from low CO
- **Left-sided HF:** pulmonary rales, tachypnea, S₃ gallop, cardiac murmurs (AS, AR, MR), paradoxical splitting of S₂

TABLE 3-11 ■ Hemodynamic Categories in Acute MI				
Condition	CI (L/min/m²)	PCWP (mm Hg)	Systolic BP (mm Hg)	Treatment
NI in acute MI	>2.5	≤18	>100	
Hypovolemia	<2.5	<15	<100	Successive boluses of 100 mL NS If inferior MI in evolution and RAP >10, consider RV infarction
Volume overload	>2.5	>18	>100	Diuretic (e.g., furosemide 10-20 mg IV) NTG, topical paste or IV
LV failure	<2.5	>18	>100	Diuretic (e.g., furosemide 10-20 mg IV) IV NTG, or if markedly HTN, use IV sodium nitroprusside
Severe LV failure	<2.5	>18	<100	If BP ≥90, IV dobutamine ± IV NTG or sodium nitroprusside If BP <90, IV dopamine If accompanied by pulmonary edema, attempt diuresis w/IV furosemide; may be limited by hypotension May require intra-aortic balloon pump
Cardiogenic shock	<1.8	>18	<90 w/ oliguria and confusion	IV dopamine Intra-aortic balloon pump Emergency coronary angioplasty or CABG may be lifesaving

From Noble J (ed): Textbook of Primary Care Medicine, 2nd ed. St. Louis, Mosby, 1996.

- **Right-sided HF:** JVD, peripheral edema, perioral and peripheral cyanosis, congestive hepatomegaly, ascites, HJR
- Acute precipitants of CHF exacerbations are noncompliance w/salt restriction, pulmonary infections, arrhythmias, medications (e.g., CCBs, antiarrhythmic agents), and inappropriate reductions in CHF Rx.

Labs
- CBC (to r/o anemia, infections), BUN, Cr, lytes, liver enzymes, TSH
- ↑ BNP

ECG
- May reveal: prior MI, arrhythmias, low voltage (hypothyroidism)

Imaging
- CXR: pulmonary venous congestion, cardiomegaly w/dilation of the involved heart chamber, pleural effusions
- 2D echo: useful to assess global and regional LV function and to estimate EF
- CMR: useful for dx cardiomyopathies

Etiology

Left Ventricular Failure
- HTN
- Valvular heart disease (AS, AR, MR)
- Cardiomyopathy, myocarditis
- Bacterial endocarditis
- MI
- HCM
- Left ventricular failure is traditionally differentiated according to systolic dysfunction (↓ EF), now known as **"Heart failure with reduced ejection fraction"** (**HFREF**), and diastolic dysfunction, known as **"Heart failure with preserved ejection fraction"** (**HFPEF**).
- Common causes of HFREF are previous MI, cardiomyopathy, myocarditis.
- Causes of HFPEF are hypertensive CVD, valvular heart disease (AS, AR, MR, HCM), restrictive cardiomyopathy.

Right Ventricular Failure
- Valvular heart disease (mitral stenosis)
- Pulmonary HTN
- Bacterial endocarditis (right sided)
- Right ventricular infarction

Biventricular Failure
- Left ventricular failure
- Cardiomyopathy
- Myocarditis
- Arrhythmias

- Anemia
- Thyrotoxicosis
- AV fistula
- Paget's disease
- Beriberi

Treatment
- Determine whether HF is secondary to HFREF or HFPEF and Rx accordingly.
- Identify and correct precipitating factors (i.e., anemia, thyrotoxicosis, infections, Na$^+$ load, medical noncompliance).
- ↓ Cardiac workload in pts w/systolic dysfunction: Restrict pt's activity only during periods of acute decompensation.
- ↓ Na intake to <2 g/day
- ↓ Fluid intake to <2 L in pts w/hyponatremia

Treatment HF Secondary to HFREF
- ACEIs
- β-Blockers (carvedilol, bisoprolol, or metoprolol)
- ARBs in pts unable to tolerate ACEIs. Avoid combination ACE/ARB.
- Loop diuretics (furosemide)
- Aldosterone antagonists: Low-dose spironolactone or eplerenone Rx should be considered in pts w/NYHA class III or IV who remain symptomatic despite Rx w/ ACEIs and β-blockers.
- Direct vasodilating drugs (hydralazine and isosorbide): in pts who are intolerant of both ACEIs and ARBs. These drugs should also be considered in African American pts as an add-on to standard Rx w/ACE and ARBs in symptomatic heart failure NIHA class II/IV.
- Digitalis is of limited value in pts w/mild CHF and nl sinus rhythm. When used, it should be reserved for pts w/symptomatic NYHA class II-IV CHF. Digoxin has a narrow therapeutic window. Its beneficial effects are found w/a low dose that results in a serum concentration of approximately 0.7 ng/mL. Higher doses may be detrimental.

Treatment HF Secondary to HFPEF
- The initial treatment of HFPEF should be directed at ↓ the congestive state w/the use of diuretics, with care taken to avoid excessive diuresis. Long-term goal is to control HTN, tachycardia, congestion, and ischemia. Rx options are determined by the cause.
- HTN: CCBs, ACEIs, β-blockers, diuretics, ARBs
- AS: aortic valve replacement in pts w/critical stenosis, diuretics
- AI, MR: ACEs, surgery
- HCM: β-blockers or verapamil; restoration of intravascular volume w/IV saline solution if necessary in acute pulmonary edema. DDD pacing is useful in selected pts.

Device Rx Indications
- **ICD:** NYHA class II, or III *and* an overall life expectancy >12 mo *and*
  - Hx cardiac arrest or hemodynamically significant ventricular arrhythmia *or*
  - Nonischemic cardiomyopathy with EF ≤35 % or ischemic cardiomyopathy ≥40 days post MI
- **Biventricular pacemaker (cardiac resynchronization Rx):** NYHA class III or IV, EF ≤35%, ventricular dyssynchrony (QRS interval ≥120 msec) despite max medical Rx

D. VALVULAR HEART DISEASE

1 CARDIAC MURMURS
a. Grading of cardiac murmurs (Table 3-12)
b. Response of selected murmurs to physiologic intervention (Table 3-13)

TABLE 3-12 ■ Grading Cardiac Murmurs	
Grade	Description
1	Faintest audible; can be heard only w/special effort
2	Faint but easily audible
3	Moderately loud
4	Loud; associated with a thrill
5	Very loud; associated with a thrill; may be heard w/stethoscope off chest
6	Maximum loudness; associated with a thrill; heard w/o stethoscope

TABLE 3-13 ■ Response of Selected Murmurs to Physiologic Intervention

Cardiac Murmur	Accentuation	Decrease
Systolic		
Aortic stenosis	Valsalva release Sudden squatting Passive leg raising	Handgrip Valsalva Standing
Hypertrophic obstructive cardiomyopathy	Valsalva strain Standing	Handgrip Squatting Leg elevation
Mitral regurgitation	Sudden squatting Isometric handgrip	Valsalva Standing
Pulmonic stenosis	Valsalva release	Expiration
Tricuspid regurgitation	Inspiration Passive leg raising	Expiration
Diastolic		
Aortic insufficiency	Sudden squatting Isometric handgrip	
Mitral stenosis	Exercise Left lateral position Isometric handgrip Coughing	
Tricuspid stenosis	Inspiration Passive leg raising	Expiration

TABLE 3-14 ■ Mitral Valve

Condition	Valve Area (cm²)	LA Pressure (mm Hg)
Normal	4-6	<10
Symptomatic during exercise	1-4	>20
Symptomatic at rest	<1	>35

2 MITRAL STENOSIS (MS)

- Narrowing of the mitral valve orifice
- Table 3-14 describes valve areas and pressures.

Etiology
- Progressive fibrosis, scarring, and calcification of the valve
- Rheumatic fever (still a common cause in underdeveloped countries); heart valves most frequently affected in rheumatic heart disease (in descending order of occurrence): mitral, aortic, tricuspid, and pulmonary
- Congenital defect (parachute valve)
- Rare causes: endomyocardial fibroelastosis, malignant carcinoid syndrome, SLE

Pathophysiology
- MS results in ↑ pressures in LA, pulmonary vein and pulmonary artery (Fig. 3-21) → dyspnea, AF (with ↑ risk of thromboembolism).

Severity Grade
See Table 3-15.

Diagnosis
H&P
- Prominent jugular A waves
- A murmur that becomes audible when the valve orifice becomes <2 cm²
- Opening snap in early diastole. Short (<0.07 second) A_2 to opening snap interval indicates severe mitral stenosis.
- Apical mid-diastolic or presystolic rumble that does not radiate
- Accentuated S_1 (because of delayed and forceful closure of the valve)
- If pulmonary HTN is present, there may be an accentuated P_2 or a soft, early diastolic decrescendo murmur (**Graham Steell murmur**) secondary to pulmonary regurgitation (best heard along LSB, may be confused w/AI).
- Palpable right ventricular heave at LSB
- Sx of left-sided HF: dyspnea on exertion, PND, orthopnea
- RV dysfunction (in late stages): peripheral edema, enlarged and pulsatile liver, ascites

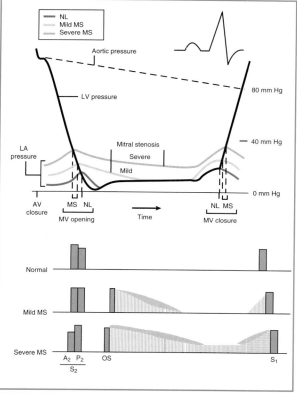

FIGURE 3-21. Schematic representation of LV, aortic, and LA pressures, showing nl (NL) relationships and alterations with mild and severe mitral stenosis (MS). Corresponding classic auscultatory signs of MS are shown at the bottom. Compared with mild MS, with severe MS the higher left atrial v wave causes earlier pressure crossover and earlier MV opening, thus leading to a shorter time interval between aortic valve (AV) closure and the opening snap (OS). The higher left atrial end-diastolic pressure with severe MS also results in later closure of the mitral valve. With severe MS, the diastolic rumble becomes longer and there is accentuation of the pulmonic component (P_2) of the second heart sound (S_2) in relation to the aortic component (A_2). *(From Zipes DP, Libby, P, Bonow RO, Braunwald E: Braunwald's Heart Disease, 7th ed. Philadelphia, Saunders, 2005.)*

TABLE 3-15 ▪ Mitral Stenosis Severity Gradient and Recommended Echocardiography Monitoring

Stage	Mitral Valve Area (MVA) (cm²)	Mean Pressure Gradient (MPG) (mm Hg)	Pulmonary Artery Systolic Pressure (PASP) (mm Hg)	ECHO F/up
Mild	>1.5	<5	<30	Every 3 yr
Moderate	1.0-1.5	5-10	30-50	Every 2 yr
Severe	<1.0	>10	>50	Every yr

Imaging
- Echo (Fig. 3-22): markedly diminished E to F slope of the anterior mitral valve leaflet during diastole, fusion of the commissures, resulting in anterior movement of the posterior mitral valve leaflet during diastole (calcification in the valve may also be noted)
- TEE: to r/o lt atrial appendage clot and estimate MR severity in all pts being considered for percutaneous balloon valvotomy

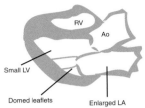

FIGURE 3-22. Features of mitral stenosis. *(From Weissleder R, Wittenberg J, Harisinghani MG, Chen JW: Primer of Diagnostic Imaging, 5th ed. St. Louis, Mosby, 2011.)*

Treatment
Surgical
- *Percutaneous mitral (balloon) valvotomy (PMV):* symptomatic pts with less than moderate MR and no LA thrombus
- *Valve replacement:* when PA systolic pressure ≥50 mm Hg at rest or ≥60 mm Hg during exercise. Consider valve commissurotomy if valve is noncalcified and if there is pure mitral stenosis w/o significant subvalvular disease.

Medical
- Symptomatic pts: β-blockers (carvedilol) → allow ↑ diastolic filling time of LV = improved symptoms
- AF: anticoagulation with warfarin, IV diltiazem or esmolol when a rapid ↓ in HR is required
- HF: diuretics, Na restriction

3 MITRAL REGURGITATION (MR)
- Retrograde blood flow through the left atrium secondary to an incompetent mitral valve
- Table 3-16 describes severity gradients in MR.

TABLE 3-16 ■ Mitral Regurgitation Severity Gradient				
Stage	Vena Contracta (VC) Width (cm)	Regurgitant Orifice Area (ROA) (cm²)	Regurgitant Fraction (RF) (%)	Regurgitant Volume (RV) (mL/beat)
Mild	<0.3	<0.20	<30	<30
Moderate	0.3-0.69	0.20-0.39	30-49	30-59
Severe	≥0.7	≥0.4	>50	≥60

Etiology
- Papillary muscle dysfunction (as a result of ischemic heart disease)
- Ruptured chordae tendineae
- Infective endocarditis
- Calcified mitral valve annulus
- Left ventricular dilation
- Rheumatic valvulitis
- Primary or secondary MVP
- Hypertrophic cardiomyopathy
- Idiopathic myxomatous degeneration of the mitral valve
- Myxoma
- SLE
- Fenfluramine, dexfenfluramine

Diagnosis

H&P
- Hyperdynamic apex, often w/palpable left ventricular lift and apical thrill
- Holosystolic murmur at apex w/radiation to base or to left axilla; poor correlation between the intensity of the systolic murmur and the degree of regurgitation
- Apical early to mid-diastolic rumble (rare)

Imaging
- Echo: Enlarged left atrium, hyperdynamic LV (erratic motion of the leaflet is seen in pts w/ruptured chordae tendineae); Doppler echo will show evidence of MR.

Treatment

Surgery
- Early intervention in symptomatic pts despite optimal medical Rx
- Mitral valve replacement indications:
  - Pulmonary HTN (PA systolic pressure ≥50 mm Hg at rest or ≥60 mm Hg during exercise)
  - LVEEF <60%
  - LV end-diastolic diameter >40 mm
  - New-onset AF
- Mitral valve repair: option in selected pts with favorable anatomy (annular dilatation, mitral leaflet prolapse, or myxomatous changes without calcification or stenosis)

Medical
- Medical Rx is primarily directed toward treatment of the source or its complications (e.g., AF, HF, ischemic heart disease, infective endocarditis).
- The utility of afterload reduction (to ↓ the regurgitant fraction and to ↑ CO) depends on the etiology of MR and the administration of afterload reducers. In acute MR, IV nitroprusside has shown some utility. Long-term use of oral afterload reducers (e.g., ACEIs or ARBs) has shown mixed results but may be given if another indication for their use exists (HTN, LV dysfunction, DM).

4 MITRAL VALVE PROLAPSE (MVP)
- Posterior bulging of interior and posterior leaflets in systole
- MVP syndrome refers to a constellation of MVP and associated sx (e.g., autonomic dysfunction, palpitations) or other physical abilities (e.g., pectus excavatum).

Etiology
- Myxomatous degeneration of connective tissue of mitral valve
- Congenital deformity of mitral valve and supportive structures
- Secondary to other disorders (e.g., Ehlers-Danlos, pseudoxanthoma elasticum)

Diagnosis

H&P
- Usually young female pt w/narrow AP chest diameter, low BW, low BP
- Mid to late click, heard best at the apex
- Crescendo mid to late diastolic murmur
- Findings accentuated in the standing position
- Most pts asymptomatic; sx (if present): chest pain, palpitations
- Neuro abnormalities (e.g., TIA or stroke) rare

Imaging
- Echo: anterior and posterior leaflets bulging posteriorly in systole

Treatment
- β-Blockers (↓ HR = ↓ stretch on prolapsing valve leaflets); useful in symptomatic pts (e.g., palpitations, chest pain)
- Valve replacement or valve repair in severe MR secondary to MVP

5 AORTIC STENOSIS (AS)
- Obstruction to systolic left ventricular outflow across the aortic valve. Valve area measurements are described in Table 3-17.

TABLE 3-17 ▪ Aortic Valve	
Condition	Valve Area
Normal	2.0-4.0 cm²
Symptomatic at exercise	<1.0 cm²
Symptomatic at rest	<0.75 cm²

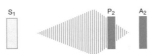

FIGURE 3-23. Graphic representation of an aortic stenosis murmur. *(From Lehman CA [ed]: Saunders Manual of Clinical Laboratory Science. Philadelphia, Saunders, 1998.)*

Etiology
- Rheumatic inflammation of aortic valve
- Progressive stenosis of congenital bicuspid valve (found in 1%-2% of population)
- Idiopathic calcification of the aortic valve
- Congenital (major cause of AS in pts <30 yr)

Diagnosis
H&P
- Rough, loud, systolic diamond-shaped murmur (Fig. 3-23), best heard at base of heart and transmitted into neck vessels; often associated w/a thrill or ejection click; may also be heard well at the apex
- Absence or ↓ intensity of sound of aortic valve closure (in severe AS)
- Late, slow-rising carotid upstroke w/↓ amplitude
- Strong apical pulse
- Narrowing of pulse pressure in later stages of AS
- Medical hx should focus on sx and potential complications: angina, syncope (particularly w/exertion), HF, GI bleeding (in pts w/associated hemorrhagic telangiectasia [AVM]).

Imaging
- Echo: thickening of LV wall, LVH (Fig. 3-24). If the pt has valvular calcifications, multiple echoes may be seen from within the aortic root, and there is poor separation of the aortic cusps during systole. Gradient across the valve can be estimated but is less precise than w/cardiac cath.
- ECG:
  - LVH (found in >80% of pts)
  - ST-T wave changes
  - AF: frequent
- Severity gradient (Table 3-18)

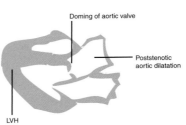

FIGURE 3-24. Features of aortic stenosis. *(From Weissleder R, Wittenberg J, Harisinghani MG, et al: Primer of Diagnostic Imaging, 4th ed. St. Louis, Mosby, 2007.)*

TABLE 3-18 ■ **Aortic Stenosis Gradient and Recommended Echocardiography Monitoring**

Stage	Mean Gradient (mm Hg)	Aortic Valve Area (AVA) (cm²)	Maximum Aortic Jet Velocity (Vmax) (m/sec)	Echo F/up
Mild	<25	>1.5	<3	3-5 yr
Moderate	25-40	1.0-1.5	3-4	1-2 yr
Severe	>40	<1.0	>4	Every yr

Treatment
Surgical
- Valve replacement indications:
  - Symptomatic pts
  - Rapidly progressive stenosis
  - LVEF <50 %
  - Abn BP response with exercise (↓ BP)
  - Moderate stenosis and need for other cardiac surgery
- Balloon valvuloplasty: useful in infants and children or poor surgical candidates who do not have calcified valve apparatus. It can be done as an intermediate procedure to stabilize high-risk pts before surgery.

Medical
- Diuretics and Na⁺ restriction if CHF is present. ACEIs are relatively contraindicated.
- CCB verapamil is useful to control rate of AF if present.

6 AORTIC REGURGITATION (AR), AORTIC INSUFFICIENCY (AI)
Retrograde blood flow into the LV from the aorta secondary to incompetent aortic valve

Etiology
- Infective endocarditis
- Rheumatic fibrosis
- Trauma w/valvular rupture
- Congenital bicuspid aortic valve
- Myxomatous degeneration
- Syphilitic aortitis
- Rheumatic spondylitis
- SLE
- Aortic dissection
- Fenfluramine, dexfenfluramine
- Takayasu's arteritis, granulomatous arteritis

Diagnosis
H&P
- Clinical presentation varies according to whether AI is acute or chronic.
  - Chronic AI is well tolerated (except when secondary to infective endocarditis), and pts remain asymptomatic for years. Common manifestations after significant deterioration of LV function are dyspnea on exertion, syncope, chest pain, and HF.
  - Acute AI manifests primarily w/hypotension in response to a sudden fall in CO. A rapid rise in left ventricular diastolic pressure results in a further ↓ in coronary blood flow.
- Physical findings in chronic AI:
  - Widened pulse pressure (markedly ↑ SBP, ↓ DBP)
  - Bounding pulses, head "bobbing" w/each systole (*de Musset's sign*) are present. "Water-hammer" or collapsing pulse (*Corrigan's pulse*) can be palpated at the wrist or on the femoral arteries ("pistol shot" femorals) and is caused by rapid rise and sudden collapse of the arterial pressure during late systole; capillary pulsations (*Quincke's pulse*) may occur at the base of the nail beds.
  - A to-and-fro *double Duroziez murmur* may be heard over femoral arteries w/ slight compression.
  - Popliteal systolic pressure is ↑ >20 mm Hg over brachial systolic pressure (*Hill's sign*) with a 40 to 60 mm difference in moderate AR and >60 mm difference in severe AR.
- Cardiac auscultation:
  - Displacement of cardiac impulse downward and to the pt's left
  - S₃ heard over the apex
  - Decrescendo, blowing diastolic murmur heard along LSB
  - Low-pitched apical diastolic rumble (*Austin-Flint murmur*) caused by contrast of the aortic regurgitant jet w/the left ventricular wall
  - Early systolic apical ejection murmur
  - In pts w/acute AI, both the wide pulse pressure and the large SV are absent. A short blowing diastolic murmur may be the only finding on PE.

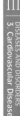

Stage	Vena Contracta (VC) Width (cm)	Regurgitant Orifice Area (ROA) (cm²)	Regurgitant Fraction (RF) (%)	Regurgitant Volume (RV) (mL/beat)
Mild	<0.3	<0.10	Normal EF	<30
Moderate	0.3-0.6	0.10-0.29	30-49	30-59
Severe	>0.6	≥0.3	>50	≥60

TABLE 3-19 ■ Aortic Regurgitation Severity Gradient

Imaging
- Echo: coarse diastolic fluttering of the anterior mitral leaflet; LVH in pts w/chronic AI
- Cardiac catheterization: assesses degree of left ventricular dysfunction, confirms the presence of a wide pulse pressure, assesses surgical risk, and determines if there is coexistent CAD
- CXR:
  - LVH (chronic AI)
  - Aortic dilation
  - Nl cardiac silhouette w/pulmonary edema: possible in pts w/acute AI
- ECG: LVH
- Severity gradient (Table 3-19)

Treatment
Surgical
- Valve replacement with ascending aorta graft replacement if enlarged
- Indications:
  - Symptomatic pts w/chronic AI despite optimal medical Rx
  - LVEF <50%
  - LV dilatation (end-systolic dimension >55 mm or end-diastolic dimension >75 mm)
  - Pts w/acute AI (i.e., infective endocarditis) producing LVH

Medical
- Diuretics, ACEIs, and Na⁺ restriction for HF; IV afterload reduction (nitroprusside) and inotropic support (dobutamine) in pts w/acute AI
- Long-term vasodilator Rx w/vasodilators (ACEIs, hydralazine, nifedipine) for reducing or delaying the need for aortic valve replacement in asymptomatic pts w/ severe aortic regurgitation and nl LV function

7 INFECTIVE ENDOCARDITIS
- Infection of the endocardial surface of the heart that most commonly involves heart valves. Staphylococcal infection is the leading cause of native valve, prosthetic valve, and cardiac device infections.
- Lesions (vegetations) are composed of microorganisms, inflammatory cells, fibrin, and plts.
- It is classified as acute or subacute on the basis of the temporal profile and severity of the clinical presentation and progression.

Etiology
- Acute endocarditis: usually caused by *S. aureus, Streptococcus pyogenes, Streptococcus pneumoniae,* and *Neisseria* organisms; classic clinical presentation of high fever, + blood cultures, vascular and immunologic phenomena
- Subacute endocarditis: usually caused by viridans streptococci in the presence of valvular disease; less toxic, often indolent presentation w/lower fevers, night sweats, fatigue
- Endocarditis in IV drug users: *S. aureus* or *Pseudomonas aeruginosa* w/variation that may be geographically influenced; tricuspid or multiple valvular involvement; mortality rate of 50% to 60%
- Prosthetic valve endocarditis (early): usually caused by *S. aureus* (leading cause) within 2 mo of valve replacement; other organisms include *Staphylococcus epidermidis,* gram(–) bacilli, diphtheroids, *Candida* organisms
- Prosthetic valve endocarditis (late): typically develops >60 days after valvular replacement; involved organisms similar to early prosthetic valve endocarditis, including viridans streptococci, enterococci, and group D streptococci
- Nosocomial endocarditis: secondary to IV catheters, TPN lines, pacemakers; coagulase(–) staphylococci, *S. aureus,* and streptococci most common
- Non-HACEK gram(–) bacillus endocarditis is not primarily a disease of injection drug users. More than half of all cases are associated w/health care contact.
- *Streptococcus bovis* suggests bowel pathology (new name: *Streptococcus gallolyticus*).

TABLE 3-20 ■ Diagnostic Criteria for Endocarditis
Major Criteria
Positive Blood Cultures for Infective Endocarditis
Typical microorganism for infective endocarditis from two separate blood cultures in the absence of a primary focus: *Streptococcus viridans, Streptococcus bovis*
HACEK group: *Haemophilus* species, *Actinobacillus actinomycetemcomitans, Cardobacterium hominis, Eikenella corrodens,* and *Kingella kingae*
Community-acquired *Staphylococcus aureus* or enterococci
Persistently positive blood cultures, defined as recovery of a microorganism consistent with infective endocarditis from blood cultures drawn more than 12 hours apart or all of three or the majority of four or more separate blood cultures, with first and last drawn at least 1 hr apart
Single positive blood culture for *Coxiella burnetii* or antiphase IgG antibody titer > 1:800
Evidence for Endocardial Involvement
TTE (TEE in prosthetic valve) showing oscillating intracardiac mass on a valve or supporting structures, in the path of regurgitant jet or on implanted material, in the absence of an alternative anatomic explanation, or
Abscess, or
New partial dehiscence of prosthetic valve
Minor Criteria
Predisposition (e.g. prosthetic valve, intravenous drug use)
Fever > 38°C
Vascular phenomena
Immunologic phenomena
Microbiologic evidence: positive blood culture but not meeting major criteria

From Ballinger A: Kumar & Clark's Essentials of Clinical Medicine, 5th ed. Ecinburgh, Saunders, 2012.

Diagnosis

- Requires 2 major criteria *or* 1 major criteria and 3 minor criteria *or* 5 minor criteria (Table 3-20). Pathologic criteria (organisms demonstrated by culture or histologic exam of a vegetation) is also definite criteria for endocarditis.

H&P

- Heart murmur: usually present in subacute bacterial endocarditis but may be absent in acute bacterial endocarditis and right-sided endocarditis
- Fever: generally present; may be absent in elderly or immunocompromised pts
- Flame-shaped retinal hemorrhages w/pale centers (***Roth's spots***)
- Painless erythematous papules and macules on the palms of the hands and soles of the feet (***Janeway's lesions***), have an embolic or immunologic cause
- Painful erythematous SC papules (***Osler's nodes***) generally found in the fleshy pads of fingers or toes and caused by local vasculitis
- Petechiae (microemboli)
- Subungual splinter hemorrhages (microemboli)
- Splenomegaly (splenic sequestration), hepatomegaly (passive congestion)
- Other: headaches, backache, arthralgias, confusion

Labs

- Blood cultures: + in 85% to 95% of pts
- CBC: ↓ Hgb/Hct secondary to ↓ RBC production caused by inflammatory state; WBC, usually w/shift to left

Imaging

- Echo: useful to demonstrate valvular vegetations and to evaluate valvular damage, perivalvular abscess and left ventricular function. However, a nl echo does not r/o endocarditis; if nl, should be repeated in 1 wk.
- 2D echo is preferred to M mode because of sensitivity (can detect 80%-85% of vegetations); TEE further enhances sensitivity and is preferred to TTE.

Treatment

Initial IV abx Rx (before culture results) is aimed at the most likely organism:

- **Native valve (no hx IV drugs) empiric Rx awaiting cultures:** pen G 20 million U IV q24h continuous or div q4h or ampicillin 12g IV q24h continuous or div q4h + (nafcillin or oxacillin 2 g IV q4h) + gentamicin 1 mg/kg IM or IV q8h or vancomycin 15 mg/kg (assuming CrCl ≥80 mL/min) IV q12h + gentamicin 1 mg/kg IM or IV q8h
- **Native valve (IV drug use ± evidence rt-sided endocarditis) empiric Rx:** vancomycin 30 to 60 mg/kg/day in 2 to 3 divided doses for trough 15 to 20 mcg/mL or daptomycin 6 mg/kg IV q24h

- **Native valve [culture (+)]:** pen G 12 to 18 million U/day IV, divided q4h × 2 wk + (gentamicin IV 1 mg/kg q8h IV ×2 wk [target level peak 3 mcg/mL, trough <1 mcg/mL] or ceftriaxone 2 g IV q24h ×4 wk)
- **Staphylococcal endocarditis (aortic &/or mitral valve)**
  - **MSSA:** nafcillin (or oxacillin) 2 g IV q4h × 4 to 6 wk or cefazolin 2 g IV q8h × 4 to 6 wk or vancomycin 15 mg/kg IV q12h (check level if >2g/day) × 4 to 6wk
  - **MRSA:** vancomycin 30 to 60 mg/kg/day 2 to 3 div doses w/ trough conc 15 to 20 mcg/mL
- **Pts w/prosthetic valves or native valves who are allergic to PCN:** vancomycin (1 g IV q12h × 4 wk) + rifampin 600 mg PO qd and gentamicin (1 mg/kg IV q8h × 2 wk), assuming nl renal function in adult pts
- Abx Rx after identification of the organism should be guided by susceptibility testing, preferably by formal testing by MIC (minimum inhibitory concentration).
- **Endocarditis prophylaxis** (Table 3-21):
  - Indications: previous bacterial endocarditis, prosthetic heart valves, unrepaired cyanotic heart disease
  - Procedures: dental procedures only. Prophylaxis is no longer recommended for GI and GU procedures.

TABLE 3-21 ■ Prophylactic Regimens for Dental Procedures

Situation	Agent	Regimen*
Standard general prophylaxis	Amoxicillin	Adults: 2 g; children: 50 mg/kg PO 1 hr before procedure
Unable to take oral medications	Ampicillin	Adults: 2 g IM or IV; children: 50 mg/kg IM or IV within 30 min before procedure
Allergic to penicillin	Clindamycin *or*	Adults: 600 mg; children: 20 mg/kg PO 1 hr before procedure
	Cephalexin† *or* cefadroxil†	Adults: 2 g; children: 50 mg/kg PO 1 hr before procedure
	Azithromycin *or* clarithromycin	Adults: 500 mg; children: 15 mg/kg PO 1 hr before procedure
Allergic to penicillin and unable to take oral medications	Clindamycin *or*	Adults: 600 mg; children: 20 mg/kg IV within 30 min before procedure
	Cefazolin†	Adults: 1 g; children: 25 mg/kg IM or IV within 30 min before procedure

Reprinted with permission from Dajani AS, Taubert KA, Wilson W, et al: Prevention of bacterial endocarditis: Recommendations by the American Heart Association. JAMA 277:1794-1801, 1997.

*Total children's dose should not exceed adult dose.

†Cephalosporins should not be used in individuals with immediate-type hypersensitivity reaction (urticaria, angioedema, or anaphylaxis) to penicillins.

8 PROSTHETIC VALVES

Artificial valves can be mechanical or biologic.
- **Mechanical prosthetic valves:** Preferred valve substitutes in adult pts who are already taking anticoagulants (e.g., for AF). The most important risk linked to these valves is valvular thrombosis requiring lifelong anticoagulation (60 μ INR 2.5 – 3.5).
  - *Ball-cage prosthesis:* Constructed as a ball in a metallic cage (e.g., Starr-Edwards valve). The ball prosthesis partially obstructs blood flow, and flow through the prosthesis is turbulent. Benefit: low cost. Disadvantage: trauma to RBCs can result in hemolytic anemia. Prosthesis is also very bulky.
  - *Tilting disk prosthesis:* The mobile element of these valves is a tilting disk held in place by two welded struts. Older models consisted of the Bjork-Shiley valve; a newer model is the Medtronic Hall Omnicarbon prosthesis.
  - *Bileaflet prostheses:* Made of two semicircular pivoting disks constructed from pyrolytic carbons, a material considered to be less thrombogenic. Introduced in 1977, the prototype is the St. Jude valve, the most commonly implanted prosthetic valve. Newer models include the CarboMedics prosthesis.
- **Biologic valves:** These valves are divided into three groups based on the origin of the biologic material: heterografts (animal origin), homografts (human donor), and autografts (tissues originating from the pt).
  - *Bioprostheses (heterografts):* Porcine bioprosthetic valves such as the Carpentier-Perimount are derived from pig aortic leaflets mounted on metal-coated stents.

A major concern in these valves is degradation over time, usually manifested as a valvular leak caused by a torn and prolapsed cusp or by commissural detachment. As a rule, most pts >75 years of age are offered a bioprosthesis.

- **Homograft valves:** Valves harvested from human donors. They have an excellent hemodynamic profile and are particularly useful in the management of infectious endocarditis because of the absence of prosthetic material.
- **Autograft valves:** The main use of autograft valves is the transfer of the pulmonary valve to the aortic position (Ross procedure) w/the subsequent implantation of a pulmonary homograft into the prior position of the pulmonary valve. The Ross procedure is the operation of choice for aortic valve replacement.

E. PERICARDIAL DISEASE

1 PERICARDITIS

- Inflammation (or infiltration) of the pericardium.
- *Myopericarditis:* myocardial injury associated with pericarditis. Occurs in 15% of pts with pericarditis. Dx: ↑ troponins, ST-segment elevation, new segmental or global LV dysfunction

Etiology

- Idiopathic (possibly postviral). In 90%, cause is either viral or unknown (idiopathic).
- Infectious (viral, bacterial [1%-2%], tuberculous [4%], fungal, amebic, toxoplasmosis)
- Collagen-vascular disease (SLE, RA, scleroderma, vasculitis, dermatomyositis): 3% to 5% of cases
- Drug-induced lupus syndrome: procainamide, hydralazine, phenytoin, isoniazid, rifampin, doxorubicin, mesalamine
- Acute MI
- Traumatic or post-traumatic
- Post MI (Dressler's syndrome)
- Post pericardiotomy
- Post mediastinal irradiation (e.g., pts w/Hodgkin's disease)
- Uremia

TABLE 3-22 ■ Diagnostic Pathway and Sequence of Performance in Acute Pericarditis	
Diagnostic Measure	**Characteristic Findings**
Obligatory	
Auscultation	Pericardial rub (monophasic, biphasic, or triphasic)
ECG	Stage I: anterior and inferior concave ST-segment elevation; PR segment deviations opposite to P wave polarity
	Early stage II: all ST junctions return to the baseline; PR segments deviated.
	Late stage II: T waves progressively flatten and invert
	Stage III: generalized T wave inversions in most or all leads
	Stage IV: ECG returns to prepericarditis state
Echocardiography	Effusion types B to D (Horowitz)
	Signs of tamponade
Blood analyses	Erythrocyte sedimentation rate, C-reactive protein, lactate dehydrogenase, leukocytes (inflammation markers)
	Troponin I, CK-MB (markers of myocardial involvement)
Chest radiograph	Ranging from normal to "water bottle" shape of the heart shadow
	Performed primarily to reveal pulmonary or mediastinal pathology
Mandatory in Tamponade, Optional in Large/Recurrent Effusions or If Previous Tests Inconclusive in Small Effusions	
Pericardiocentesis/drainage	Polymerase chain reaction and histochemistry for etiopathogenetic classification of infection or neoplasia
Optional or If Previous Tests Inconclusive	
CT	Effusions, pericardium, and epicardium
MRI	Effusions, pericardium, and epicardium
Pericardioscopy, pericardial/epicardial biopsy	Establishing the specific etiology

From Vincent JL, Abraham E, Moore FA, et al (eds): Textbook of Critical Care, 6th ed. Philadelphia, Saunders, 2011.

- Sarcoidosis
- Neoplasm (primary or metastatic [breast, lung, leukemia, lymphoma]): 7% of cases
- Leakage of aortic aneurysm in pericardial sac
- Familial Mediterranean fever
- RF
- Other: anticoagulants, amyloidosis, ITP

Diagnosis
See Table 3-22.

H&P
- Severe, constant pain that localizes over the anterior chest and may radiate to arms and back. It can be differentiated from myocardial ischemia because the pain intensifies w/inspiration and is relieved by sitting up and leaning forward (the pain of myocardial ischemia is not pleuritic).
- Pericardial friction rub: best heard w/pt upright and leaning forward and by pressing the stethoscope firmly against the chest; it consists of 3 short, scratchy sounds:
  • Systolic component
  • Diastolic component
  • Late diastolic component (associated w/atrial contraction)
- Cardiac tamponade may be occurring if the following are observed:
  • Tachycardia
  • BP and pulse pressure
  • Distended neck veins
  • Paradoxical pulse

Imaging
- Echo: to detect and to determine amount of pericardial effusion; absence of effusion does not r/o dx of pericarditis. Divergence of right and left ventricular systolic pressures is present in cardiac tamponade and constrictive pericarditis.
- CXR: cardiac silhouette appears enlarged if >250 mL of fluid has accumulated. Calcifications around the heart may be seen w/constrictive pericarditis.
- ECG varies w/the evolutionary stage of pericarditis (see Table 3-22).

Treatment
- NSAIDs (ibuprofen 800 mg tid or ASA 650 mg q 4-6 h) for 3 to 4 wks
- Colchicine 0.6 mg bid × 3 months: alternative in pts intolerant of NSAIDs or added to NSAIDs
- Prednisone 60 mg qd, tapered over several months: third-line agent for refractory cases (before use of prednisone, tuberculous pericarditis must be excluded)
- Close observation of pts for signs of cardiac tamponade
- Avoidance of anticoagulants (risk of hemopericardium)
- Treat underlying cause of pericarditis.

2 PERICARDIAL EFFUSION

Etiology
- Pericarditis (viral, tuberculous, bacterial, idiopathic)
- Uremia
- Myxedema
- Neoplasm (leukemia, lymphoma, metastatic)
- Hemorrhage (trauma, leakage of thoracic aneurysm)
- SLE, rheumatoid disease
- MI and post cardiac surgery
- Dressler's syndrome

Diagnosis
- Hx: may be asymptomatic if small effusion
- Echo, CXR, labs (CBC, Cr, TSH, ANA), PPD
- Consider pericardiocentesis (following CMR) in suspected malignancy, TB, bacterial infection, persistent effusion (>3 months). Test fluid for culture, cytology, adenosine deaminase activity. Consider pericardial bx.

Treatment
- Infection: IV antibiotics, drainage
- Malignancy: catheter drainage, surgical decompression, pericardial sclerosis, percutaneous balloon pericardiotomy
- Idiopathic chronic pericardial effusion: pericardiotomy

3 CARDIAC TAMPONADE

Pericardial effusion significantly impairs diastolic filling of the heart.

Diagnosis

H&P

- Dyspnea, orthopnea
- Interscapular pain
- **_Beck's triad:_** distended neck veins, distant heart sounds, hypotension. (Note: JVD may be absent with severe hypovolemia.)
- ↓ Apical impulse
- Diaphoresis, tachypnea
- Tachycardia (compensatory to maintain CO)
- **_Ewart's sign:_** an area of dullness at the angle of the left scapula, caused by compression of the lung by the pericardial effusion
- **_Pulsus paradoxus_** (↓ in systolic BP >10 mm Hg during inspiration)
- Hypotension
- Narrowed pulse pressure

Imaging

- CXR: cardiomegaly (water bottle configuration of the cardiac silhouette) w/clear lung fields. CXR may be nl when acute tamponade occurs rapidly in absence of prior pericardial effusion.
- ECG: ↓ amplitude of the QRS complex, variation of the R wave amplitude from beat to beat (**_electrical alternans_**). This results from the heart oscillating in the pericardial sac from beat to beat. It is more common w/ neoplastic effusions.
- Echo: detects effusions as small as 30 mL (they are seen as an echo-free space). Paradoxical wall motion can also be seen.
  - Two-dimensional echo may reveal prolonged diastolic collapse or inversion of right atrial free wall.
  - Early diastolic collapse of right ventricular wall also suggests cardiac tamponade.
  - Paradoxical movement of the septum
  - Echo may miss localized effusions laterally adjacent to right atrium.
- Cardiac catheterization
  - Equalization of pressures within chambers of the heart
  - Elevation of RAP w/a prominent x but no significant y descent.
- MRI

Treatment

- Volume resuscitation & vasopressors if hypotensive. IABP in refractory cases
- Immediate pericardiocentesis (under echo, fluoroscopy, or CT) or surgical drainage (preferred when tamponade results from aortic dissection, malignant effusions)

4 CONSTRICTIVE PERICARDITIS

Diagnosis

- PE: JVD, **Kussmaul's sign** (↑ in JVD during inspiration as a result of ↑ venous pressure), **pericardial knock** (early diastolic filling sound heard 0.06 to 0.1 sec after S₂), clear lungs, tender hepatomegaly, pedal edema, ascites, scrotal edema, and possible anasarca
- CXR: clear lung fields, normal or slightly enlarged heart, pericardial calcification
- ECG: low-voltage QRS complex
- Echo: respiratory inflow variation over the mitral and tricuspid valves (from variations in the diastolic ventricular pressure gradients with respiration), pericardial thickening
- Cardiac cath: ↑ right-sided filling pressures, ↑ and equalized diastolic LV and RV pressures (within 5 mm Hg), prominent y descent in the RA tracing, a "dip and plateau" tracing of the RV pressure and discordance of RV and LV systolic pressures during respiration

Treatment

Surgical stripping or removal of both layers of the constricting pericardium

Effusive-Constrictive Pericarditis

- Syndrome characterized by concomitant tamponade caused by tense pericardial effusion and constriction caused by the visceral pericardium
- Rx: Idiopathic cases may resolve spontaneously.
- Extensive epicardiectomy in symptomatic/persistent cases

III

DISEASES AND DISORDERS
3. Cardiovascular Disease

F. ADULT CONGENITAL HEART DISEASE

1 PATENT FORAMEN OVALE (PFO)

Etiology
- Vestige of the fetal circulation (failure of the primum and secundum septa to fuse postnatally)
- Persistence of the one-way flap valve overlying this foramen ovale allows right-to-left blood flow when RAP exceeds that of the left.

Diagnosis
H&P
- Most pts with isolated PFO are asymptomatic.
- PFO cannot be detected on clinical examination.
- ↑ risk of cryptogenic stroke (paradoxical embolization, in situ thrombosis within the canal of the PFO, associated atrial arrhythmia and concomitant hypercoagulable state)
- TEE, especially when performed with contrast injected during a cough or Valsalva maneuver, is the most sensitive and preferred test for diagnosing PFO.

Treatment
- Most pts with a PFO as an isolated finding: no Rx
- PFO is associated with an otherwise unexplained neurologic event → Rx with ASA alone in low-risk pts, combined with warfarin in high-risk pts
- Percutaneous method of closure indications: recurrent cryptogenic stroke resulting from presumed paradoxical embolism through PFO while on adequate medical Rx with antiplatelets or anticoagulants
- Surgical closure (open thoracotomy) indications: PFO >25 mm in size, inadequate rim of tissue around the defect, percutaneous device failure in the presence of other indication for open heart surgery

2 ATRIAL SEPTAL DEFECT (ASD)

Abnl opening in the atrial septum that allows blood flow between the atria
- Ostium primum: defect low in the septum
- Ostium secundum: occurs mainly in the region of the fossa ovalis
- Sinus venosus defect: less common form, involves the upper part of the septum

Diagnosis
H&P
- Exertional dyspnea may be present; small defects are generally asymptomatic.
- Pansystolic murmur best heard at apex secondary to MR (ostium primum defect), widely split S_2, visible and palpable pulmonary artery pulsations, ejection systolic flow murmur, prominent RV impulse, cyanosis, and clubbing (severe cases)

Imaging
- TTE w/saline bubble contrast and Doppler flow studies may demonstrate the defect and the presence of shunting. TEE is more sensitive than TTE.
- Cardiac cath confirms the dx in pts who are candidates for surgery. It calculates pulmonary-to-systemic blood flow ratio (Qp/Qs).
- ECG
  - Ostium primum defect: LAD, RBBB, prolongation of PR interval
  - Sinus venosus defect: leftward deviation of P axis
  - Ostium secundum defect: RAD, RBBB

Treatment
- Closure is indicated in symptomatic pts and Qp/Qs ratio >1.5:2.
- Surgery should be avoided in pts w/pulmonary HTN w/reversed shunting (Eisenmenger's syndrome) because of risk of right-sided HF.
- Transcatheter closure in children is performed when feasible.

3 VENTRICULAR SEPTAL DEFECT (VSD)

VSDs are the most common congenital heart abnormalities (30% of all congenital cardiac defects).

Diagnosis
H&P
- Clinical presentation depends on the direction and volume of the VSD shunt.
  - Defects of ≤25% of the aortic annulus diameter: small shunt lt → rt, no LV volume overload, and no PAH
  - Defects that are 25% to 75% of aortic annulus diameter: shunt lt → rt, mild to moderate LV volume overload, mild or no PAH

- Defects of ≥75% of the aortic annulus diameter: LV volume overload and PAH, CHF
- In adults with VSD, shunt is lt → rt in the absence of pulmonary stenosis and pulmonary HTN; left-sided HF results from left ventricular volume overload (e.g., shortness of breath, orthopnea, dyspnea on exertion).
- PE: machine-like holosystolic murmur that is heard best along the LSB, systolic thrill, mid-diastolic rumble heard at the apex, S_3 heart sound

Imaging
- Echocardiography: imaging modality of choice for the Dx of VSD

Treatment

Closure is indicated in adults with a Qp/Qs of ≥2 and clinical evidence of left ventricular volume overload or a hx of endocarditis.

4 PATENT DUCTUS ARTERIOUS (PDA)

Etiology
- Maternal rubella and neonatal prematurity predispose fetus to persistence of ductus arteriosus after birth.
- PDA may be isolated abnl or assoc with other congenital cardiac defects (VSD, ASD).

Clinical Findings
- PDA produces AV fistula with continuous "machinery" murmur enveloping S_2 best heard beneath the left clavicle.
- Sx heart failure, bounding pulses, and wide pulse pressure
- Ddx: any AV fistula, ruptured sinus of Valsalva aneurysm, VSD with AI

Diagnosis
- Transthoracic echocardiography with color flow Doppler
- Severe pulmonary arterial HTN (PDA difficult to visualize)
- CT and CMR imaging possibly useful for ancillary information
- ECG: LA enlargement, LV hypertrophy with PAH: RV hypertrophy
- CXR: cardiomegaly, ↑ pulmonary vascular markings, occasional calcification of PDA, prominent central pulmonary arteries, reduced peripheral pulmonary vascular markings
- Cardiac catheterization reserved for moderate-sized PDA with ↑ pulmonary artery pressure or severe pulmonary arterial HTN to determine reversibility
- Angiography (confirms size and shape of PDA)

Treatment
- Closure of PDA is indicated for LA or LV enlargement in the absence of PAH or in the presence of net left-to-right shunting.

5 TETRALOGY OF FALLOT

Four Features
1. VSD
2. Infundibular stenosis that leads to the obstruction of the RV outflow tract or pulmonary valve stenosis
3. An aorta that overrides the VSD by <50% of its diameter
4. Concentric RV hypertrophy

Diagnosis
H&P
- Cyanosis of the nail beds and lips, dyspnea on exertion, digital clubbing, squatting position after exercise to ↑ systemic vascular resistance, thereby decreasing right-to-left shunting
- Systolic thrill along the left sternal border, single second heart sound comprised of aortic component only
- A grade 3 to 5 crescendo/decrescendo murmur is heard along the LSB with posterior radiation.

Imaging
- CXR: boot-shaped heart (*coeur en sabot*)
- Echo
- Cardiac catheterization and angiography
- CMR
- Multislice spiral CT

Treatment
- Palliative or complete surgical repair before adulthood

G. CARDIOMYOPATHIES

1 DILATED (CONGESTIVE) CARDIOMYOPATHY

Etiology
- Idiopathic
- Alcoholism (15%-40% of all cases in Western countries)
- Collagen-vascular disease (SLE, RA, polyarteritis, dermatomyositis)
- Post myocarditis
- Peripartum (last trimester of pregnancy or 6 mo post partum)
- Heredofamilial neuromuscular disease
- Toxins (cobalt, lead, phosphorus, CO, mercury, doxorubicin, daunorubicin)
- Nutritional (beriberi, selenium deficiency, carnitine deficiency, thiamine deficiency)
- Cocaine, heroin, organic solvents ("glue sniffer's heart")
- Irradiation
- Acromegaly, osteogenesis imperfecta, myxedema, thyrotoxicosis, diabetes
- Hypocalcemia
- Antiretroviral agents (zidovudine, didanosine, zalcitabine)
- Phenothiazines
- Infections (viral [HIV], rickettsial, mycobacterial, toxoplasmosis, trichinosis, Chagas' disease)
- Hematologic (e.g., sickle cell anemia)

Diagnosis
H&P
- Pulmonary rales, hepatomegaly, peripheral edema
- JVP
- ↓ Pulse pressure
- S_3, S_4
- MR, TR (less common)

Imaging
- CXR: cardiac enlargement, possible interstitial pulmonary edema
- Echo: ↓ EF w/global akinesia
- ECG: LVH w/ST-T wave changes, RBBB or LBBB, arrhythmias (AF, PVC, PAC, VT)

Treatment
- Treat HF (cause of death in 70% of pts) w/ Na^+ restriction, diuretics, ACEIs, β-blockers, spironolactone, and digitalis.
- Vasodilators (combined w/nitrates and ACEIs) in symptomatic pts w/LV dysfunction
- Oral anticoagulants in pts w/AF and in pts w/moderate or severe failure
- Low-dose β-blockade w/carvedilol or other β-blockers may improve ventricular function by interrupting the cycle of reflex sympathetic activity and controlling tachycardia.
- Diltiazem and ACEIs in idiopathic dilated cardiomyopathy
  - ICD in pts w/severe LV dysfunction or symptomatic and sustained VT
  - Surgical revascularization in pts w/dilated cardiomyopathy (LVEF <25%) and associated coronary atherosclerosis (angina, ECG changes, reversible defects on thallium scan)
- Heart transplantation for young pts (<60 yr old) who are no longer responsive to medical Rx (dilated cardiomyopathy accounts for 45% of heart transplants)

2 RESTRICTIVE CARDIOMYOPATHY

Restrictive cardiomyopathies are characterized by ↓ ventricular compliance, usually secondary to infiltration of the myocardium.

Etiology
- Infiltrative and storage disorders (glycogen storage disease, amyloidosis, sarcoidosis, hemochromatosis)
- Scleroderma
- Radiation
- Endocardial fibroelastosis
- Endomyocardial fibrosis
- Idiopathic
- Anthracycline
- Carcinoid heart disease, metastatic cancers
- Diabetic cardiomyopathy
- Eosinophilic cardiomyopathy (Löffler's endocarditis)

Diagnosis
H&P
- PE: edema, ascites, hepatomegaly, distended neck veins, regurgitant murmur, prominent apical impulse, Kussmaul's sign
- Fatigue and weakness (secondary to ↓ output)

Imaging
- Echo: wall thickness and thickened cardiac valves (especially in pts w/amyloidosis)
- Cardiac cath can be used to distinguish restrictive cardiomyopathy from constrictive pericarditis (see constrictive pericarditis). MRI may also be useful to distinguish restrictive cardiomyopathy from constrictive pericarditis (thickness of the pericardium >5 mm in the latter).
- CXR: moderate cardiomegaly, CHF (pulmonary vascular congestion, pleural effusion)
- ECG: ↓ voltage w/ST-T wave changes. Arrhythmias, LAD, and AF may also be present.

Treatment
- Volume overload: cautious use of diuretics. B-blockers, verapamil, diltiazem may improve diastolic filling.
- Hemochromatosis: repeated phlebotomies to ↓ iron deposition in the heart
- Sarcoidosis: corticosteroids
- Eosinophilic cardiomyopathy: corticosteroid and cytotoxic drugs
- There is no effective Rx for other causes of restrictive cardiomyopathy.

3 HYPERTROPHIC CARDIOMYOPATHY (HCM)

Primary myocardial disease manifesting with diffuse or focal LVH in absence of disorders that ↑ afterload

Etiology
- Autosomal dominant trait w/variable penetrance caused by mutations in any of 1 to 10 genes, each encoding proteins of cardiac sarcomere
- Sporadic occurrence

Diagnosis
H&P
- Dyspnea
- Syncope (usually seen w/exercise)
- Angina (↓ angina in recumbent position)
- Palpitations
- PE: harsh, systolic, diamond-shaped murmur at the LSB or apex that ↑ w/Valsalva maneuver (decreased preload) and ↓ w/squatting or leg elevation (increased venous return)

Imaging
- Two-dimensional echo: LV wall thickness >15 mm, ratio of septum thickness to left ventricular wall thickness >1.3:1; 30 % of pts will manifest systolic anterior motion of the anterior leaflet of the mitral valve, causing obstruction of the LVOT. Stress echo can unmask outflow obstruction.
- MRI useful in identifying segmental LVH undetectable by echo
- CXR: nl or cardiomegaly
- ECG (abnl in 75%-95% pts): LVH, abnl Q waves in anterolateral and inferior leads
- 24-hr Holter monitor to screen for potential lethal arrhythmias (principal cause of syncope or sudden death in HCM)

Major Risk Factors for Sudden Death
- Spontaneous VT
- VF, cardiac arrest
- + Family hx of sudden death
- Unexplained syncope
- HF & dilated cardiomyopathy with EF ≤35%, NYHA class II or III symptoms
- ↓ in systolic BP with exercise or blunted ↑ (<20 mm Hg)
- LV diastolic wall thickness ≥30 mm

Treatment
- Asymptomatic pts with no major risk factors: no Rx or β-blockers, avoidance of vigorous exercise in pts with phenotypic features of HCM
- Symptomatic pts with HF and preserved systolic function:
  - β-Blockers [↓ HR = prolongation of diastole = passive ventricular filling]
  - DDD pacing for hemodynamic and symptomatic benefit
  - ICD for pts with major risk factors (see earlier)
  - Heart transplant for HCM with advanced HF

- Long-term warfarin anticoagulation in pts with CHADS2 ≥2
■ Surgical Rx (septal myectomy) is reserved for pts who have both a large outflow gradient (≥50 mm Hg) and severe sx of HF that are unresponsive to medical Rx. The risk of sudden death from arrhythmias is not altered by surgery. Alcohol septal ablation is an alternative Rx for pts with high surgical risk.

4 ARRHYTHMOGENIC RIGHT VENTRICULAR DYSPLASIA (ARVD)

■ Disorder characterized by replacement of the nl myocardium by fibrofatty tissue, RV myocyte loss, and RV wall thinning, and represents a kind of cardiomyopathy. It is defined clinically by life-threatening ventricular arrhythmias in otherwise healthy young people.
■ Autosomal dominant with variable penetrance and polymorphic phenotypic expression

Diagnosis
■ Suspect when young male pts present with syncope, sudden cardiac arrest, ventricular tachycardia, PVCs originating from the right ventricle
■ Resting ECG: T wave inversions in anterior precordial leads V_1-V_6, *epsilon waves,* and VT with LBBB pattern
■ Endomyocardial biopsy with immunohistochemical analysis: preferred method for Dx of ARVD (specificity >90%)
■ EPS: to identify delayed potentials that can lead to tachycardiac events
■ CMR: most sensitive method to detect ARVD, but ↑ false + rates: thinning and aneurysmal dilation of the RV anterior wall and outflow tract
■ Echo: RV dilatation with regional wall motion abnlities

Treatment
■ Avoidance of activity that may trigger tachycardia
■ Right ventriculotomy
■ Cardiac transplantation
■ Antiarrhythmic Rx with sotalol, amiodarone, propafenone, β-blocker alone or in combination can be used
■ Radiofrequency ablation is used in cases of refractory VT, frequent tachycardia after defibrillator placement, or localized arrhythmia sites.
■ Implantable cardioverted defibrillators hold promise

5 TAKOTSUBO CARDIOMYOPATHY (STRESS CARDIOMYOPATHY, SC)

The term *takotsubo* is the Japanese name for an octopus trap (*takotsubo*), which has a similar shape of the LV in systole during a left ventriculogram.

Diagnosis
Mayo Clinic criteria (2008): All 4 criteria are required to make Dx.
1. Transient hypokinesis, akinesis, or dyskinesis of the left ventricular mid segments with or without apical involvement. The RWMA typically extend beyond a single epicardial coronary distribution. A stressful trigger is often but not always present.
2. Absence of obstructive CAD or angiographic evidence of acute plaque rupture
3. New ECG abnormalities: either ST-segment ↑ and/or T wave inversion or modest ↑ in cardiac troponin
4. Absence of pheochromocytoma or myocarditis

Imaging
■ Echo: may show apical ballooning
■ Cardiovascular MRI
■ Cardiac cath: The lt ventriculogram is diagnostic.

Treatment
■ β-blockers, ACEIs, and diuretics for systolic dysfunction
■ Pts in shock without significant LVOT: Rx with IABP
■ Repeat Echo (in 4 to 6 wk) to ensure nlization of systolic function (most pts nlize by this time)
■ Duration of medical Rx is debatable.

H. MYOCARDITIS

Inflammatory disorder of the myocardium

Etiology
■ Infection, drugs, collagen-vascular disorders, radiation, post partum

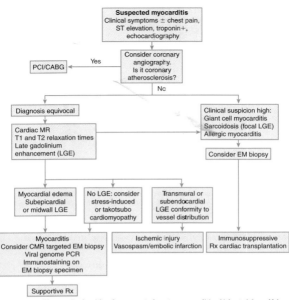

FIGURE 3-25. Diagnostic algorithm for suspected acute myocarditis. (*Adapted from Nelson KH, Li T, Afonso L. Diagnostic approach and role of the assessment of acute myocarditis. Cardiol Rev 17:24-30, 2009.*)

Diagnosis

H&P

- Persistent tachycardia out of proportion to fever
- Faint S_1, S_4 sound on auscultation
- Murmur of MR
- Pericardial friction rub if associated w/pericarditis
- Signs of biventricular failure (hypotension, hepatomegaly, peripheral edema, distention of neck veins, S_3)
- H/o recent influenza-like syndrome (fever, arthralgias, malaise), dyspnea (72%), chest pain (32%), arrhythmias (18%)
- **W/up** (Fig. 3-25)

Treatment

- Rx of underlying cause, supportive care, Rx of systolic HF (if present)

I. DISEASES OF THE AORTA

1 THORACIC AORTIC ANEURYSM

Risk Factors

- Heritable
  - Marfan's (lens dislocation, arm span > height, tall, scoliosis, arachnodactyly, MVP, pectus carinatum, thumb and wrist signs)
  - Ehlers-Danlos (joint hypermobility, thin translucent skin)
  - Loeys-Dietz (craniosynostosis, cleft palate, hypertelorism)
  - Familial TAAD
- Degenerative: HTN, smoking, atherosclerosis
- Other: Takayasu's arteritis, untreated syphilis

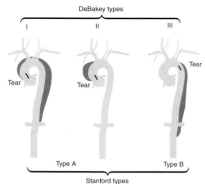

DeBakey types

I   II   III

Type A   Type B

Stanford types

FIGURE 3-26. Classification of aortic dissection. (*From Weissleder R, Wittenberg J, Harisinghani MG, Chen JW: Primer of Diagnostic Imaging, 5th ed. St. Louis, Mosby, 2011.*)

Diagnosis
- Most detected incidentally; compressive sx (hoarseness, stridor, dysphagia)
- If phenotypic expression of genetic disease recognized, aortic imaging warranted

Imaging
- Echo: good for aortic root/proximal aorta, poor for aortic arch
- MRI: good for entire aorta
- CT: good for entire aorta but radiation and contrast dye exposure

Treatment
- BP control (β-blockers, ACEIs, particularly useful in Marfan's)
- Stop smoking
- CT or MRI annually
- Repair if ≥5.5 cm for degenerative disease, ≥5 cm for Marfan's, >4.5 cm for other heritable causes. **However, rapid expansion (>0.5 cm/yr) may be an indication for repair regardless of absolute diameter.**

2 ACUTE AORTIC SYNDROMES (AORTIC DISSECTION, INTRAMURAL HEMATOMA, PENETRATING ATHEROSCLEROTIC ULCER)
- **Dissection:** Intimal tear allows blood to dissect between medial layers of the aorta.
- **Intramural hematoma:** secondary to microtears in intima or rupture of vasa vasorum
- **Penetrating atherosclerotic ulcer:** HTN + atherosclerosis = plaque rupture and pseudoaneurysm

Classification
Based on the location of dissection (Fig. 3-26)
- DeBakey: type I, ascending and descending aorta; II, ascending aorta; III, descending aorta
- Stanford: type A, ascending aorta (proximal); type B, descending aorta (distal)

Diagnosis
H&P
- Sudden onset of severe chest pain often described as sharp, tearing, or ripping. Pain can be anterior w/ascending aortic dissection or back pain w/descending aortic dissection.
- Pulse and BP differentials common (38%), caused by partial compression of subclavian arteries
- Most pts present w/severe HTN. Hypotension (25%) can indicate bleeding, cardiac tamponade, or severe AI.

Imaging
- TEE: study of choice in unstable pts. Sensitivity is 97% to 100%.
- MRI: gold standard and gives best information to surgeons. Sensitivity is 90% to 100%, but length of test and difficult access are not suitable for stable intubated pts.
- CXR: may show widened mediastinum (62%)

Treatment
- Target SBP <120, HR <70 bpm to ↓ aortic wall stress
- IV β-blockers: metoprolol 5 mg IV q5min, esmolol 500 mcg/kg/min IV × 1 min followed by 30 to 50 mcg/kg/min for 5 min or labetalol 20 mg IV, then 20 to 80 mg q10min, followed by IV nitroprusside 1 to 8 mcg/kg/min IV
- Nitroprusside should not be used w/o β-blockade because vasodilation can induce reflex sympathetic stimulation and aortic sheer stress.
- Type A dissection: emergency surgery (open surgical revascularization) to prevent rupture or pericardial effusion
- Type B dissection: most treated medically unless distal organ involvement (visceral or limb ischemia, impending rupture [penetrating ulcer ≥20 mm diameter, >10 mm depth, or associated intramural hematoma] or progressive dilatation despite med Rx)
- Evolving role for endovascular repair as less invasive

3 ABDOMINAL AORTIC ANEURYSM

Diagnosis
Imaging
- Abd U/S: preferred initial imaging modality; estimates size within 0.4 cm; not very good in estimating proximal extension to renal arteries or involvement of iliac arteries
- CT scan and angiography: more accurate, used preoperatively

Causes
- Atherosclerotic (degenerative or nonspecific): risk factors are older age, smoking, male sex, white race, FHx AAA, occlusive atherosclerotic disease
- Genetic (e.g., Ehlers-Danlos syndrome)
- Trauma
- Cystic medial necrosis (Marfan's syndrome)
- Arteritis, inflammatory
- Mycotic, syphilitic

Treatment
- Monitoring by U/S or CT q 6 mo for AA measuring >4.5 cm. In pts w/AAA 3.5 to 4.4 cm, monitor yearly; 3.0 to 3.4 cm q 3 yr; and <3 cm, q 5 years is reasonable.
- Vascular surgical referral should be made in asymptomatic pts w/AAA ≥4.0 cm or in rapidly expanding aneurysms of 0.6 to 0.8 cm/yr, especially if sx are present.
- Surgical repair: open repair or EVAR. EVAR is a better choice for high-risk pts (↓ hospital stay, lower hospital morbidity, but no difference in total mortality).

Clinical Pearls
- Mortality rate for elective repair of nonruptured aneurysms is 4%.
- Mortality after rupture is >80%.
  - 70% of AAAs are asymptomatic. U/S of AA to screen for AAA. Consider in all male smokers 65 to 75 y.o.

J. ARRHYTHMIAS

1 AV CONDUCTION DEFECTS

a. First-degree heart block
- PR interval >200 msec
- Delay in impulse conduction in AV node
- No Rx needed
- Asymptomatic but small ↑ risk of AF and need for pacer over long term

b. Second-degree heart block
Types of second-degree AV block:
- **Mobitz type I (Wenckebach)** (Fig. 3-27)
  - Progressive prolongation of the PR interval before an impulse is completely blocked. The cycle repeats periodically.
  - Cycle w/dropped beat is <2 times the previous cycle.
  - Site of block is usually AV node (proximal to the bundle of His).
- **Mobitz type II** (Fig. 3-28)
  - Sudden interruption of AV conduction occurs w/o prior prolongation of the PR interval.
  - Site of block is infranodal.

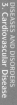

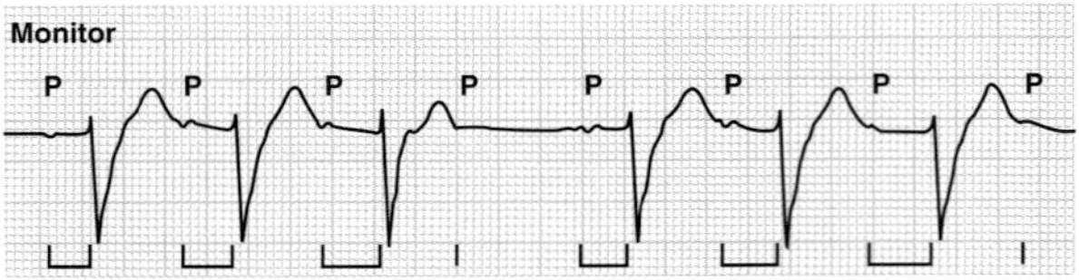

Monitor

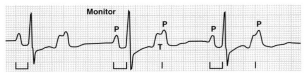

FIGURE 3-27. Mobitz I second-degree atrioventricular block (Wenckebach). *(From Goldberger AL, Goldberger E: Clinical Electrocardiography: A Simplified Approach, 5th ed. St. Louis, Mosby, 1994.)*

Monitor

FIGURE 3-28. Mobitz II second-degree atrioventricular block. Note that every alternate P wave is blocked. *(From Goldberger E: Treatment of Cardiac Emergencies, 5th ed. St. Louis, Mosby, 1990.)*

Etiology
Mobitz Type I
- Vagal stimulation
- Degenerative changes in the AV conduction system
- Ischemia at the AV nodes (particularly in inferior wall MI)
- Drugs (digitalis, quinidine, procainamide, adenosine, CCBs, β-blockers)
- Cardiomyopathies
- AI
- Lyme carditis
Mobitz Type II
- Degenerative changes in the His-Purkinje system
- Acute anterior wall MI
- Calcific AS

Treatment
Mobitz Type I
- Rx generally is not necessary (block is usually transient).
- If symptomatic (e.g., dizziness): atropine 1 mg (may repeat once after 5 min). If no response, insert temporary pacemaker.
- If block is secondary to drugs (e.g., digitalis), discontinue the drug.
- If associated w/anterior wall MI and wide QRS escape rhythm, consider insertion of temporary pacemaker.
Mobitz Type II
- Pacemaker insertion

c. Third-degree heart block
Diagnosis
H&P
- Pts may present w/dizziness, palpitations, Stokes-Adams syncopal attacks, CHF, angina.
- ECG (Fig. 3-29)
- P waves constantly change their relationship to the QRS complexes.
- Ventricular rate is usually <50 bpm (may be higher in congenital forms).
- Ventricular rate is generally lower than the atrial rate.
- QRS complex is wide.
Causes
- Degenerative changes in His-Purkinje system
- Acute anterior wall MI
- Calcific AS
- Cardiomyopathy
- Trauma

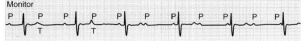

A

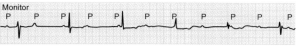

B

FIGURE 3-29. Third-degree atrioventricular block. Strips **A** and **B** were taken several hours apart. **A,** Atrial rate of 75 bpm. Ventricles are beating independently at a slow rate of approximately 40 bpm. **B,** A few hours later, same patient, with variations in shape of QRS complex from beat to beat. *(From Goldberger E: Treatment of Cardiac Emergencies, 5th ed. St. Louis, Mosby, 1990.)*

TABLE 3-23 ■ Commonly Programmed Modes of Pacemaker Function	
AAI	Demand atrial pacing; output inhibited by sensed atrial signals
AAIR	Demand atrial pacing; output inhibited by sensed atrial signals
	Atrial pacing rates ↓ and in response to sensor input up to the programmed sensor-based upper rate
VVI	Demand ventricular pacing; output inhibited by sensed ventricular signals
VVIR	Demand ventricular pacing; output inhibited by sensed ventricular signals
	Ventricular paced rates ↓ and in response to sensor input up to the programmed sensor-based upper rate
VDD	Paces ventricle, senses in both atrium and ventricle
	Synchronizes w/atrial activity and paces ventricle after a preset atrioventricular interval up to the programmed upper rate
VDDR	Paces ventricle, senses in both atrium and ventricle
	Synchronizes w/atrial activity and paces ventricle after a preset atrioventricular interval up to the programmed upper rate; in absence of spontaneous atrial activity, functions as VVIR
DDD	Paces and senses in both atrium and ventricle
	Paces ventricle in response to sensed atrial activity up to programmed upper rate
DDDR	Atrial and ventricular paced rates can both and ↓ in response to sensor input up to the programmed sensor-based upper rate

From Goldman L, Braunwald E (eds): Primary Cardiology. Philadelphia, Saunders, 1998.
A, Atrium; *D,* dual (both atrium and ventricle); *I,* inhibition and triggering (pacing in response to another event); *R,* rate adaptation available; *V,* ventricle.

- CV surgery
- Congenital

Treatment

- Pacemaker insertion (unless the pt has congenital third-degree AV block and is completely asymptomatic)

2 PACEMAKERS

- Table 3-23 describes commonly programmed modes of pacemaker function.
- Indications for permanent pacing
  - 3rd-degree heart block or advanced 2nd-degree heart block
  - Symptomatic 2nd-degree heart block
  - Symptomatic HR <40/min or sinus pauses
  - Alternating BBB
  - AF with pauses ≥5 sec
- Pacemaker indications in acute MI are described in Table 3-24.

3 APPROACH TO THE PATIENT WITH TACHYCARDIA

- Evaluate QRS interval: Nl QRS duration is 0.075 (75 msec) to 0.11 sec (110 msec).
- Subdivide tachycardia in narrow QRS vs broad QRS complex.
- Figure 3-30 describes the ddx for narrow QRS complex tachycardia. A testing guideline for narrow QRS complex tachycardia is shown in Figure 3-31.

TABLE 3-24 ■ Guidelines of the ACC and the AHA for Temporary or Permanent Implantation of Pacemakers in Patients with Acute MI		
Class*	Indications for Temporary Pacing	Indications for Permanent Pacing
I	Asystole Symptomatic bradycardia (including sinus brady-cardia or Mobitz type I block with hypotension) Bilateral BBB (alternating BBB or RBBB alternat-ing with LAFB or LPFB) Bifascicular block that is new or of indeterminate age (RBBB with LAFB or LPFB or LBBB) with a prolonged PR interval Mobitz type II second-degree AV block	Persistent second-degree AV block in the His-Purkinje system, with bilateral BBB or third-degree AV block within or below the His-Purkinje system after MI Transient advanced (second- or third-degree) infranodal AV block and associated BBB† Persistent and symptomatic second-or third-degree AV block
IIa	RBBB and LAFB or LPFB that is new or of indeterminate age RBBB with a prolonged PR interval LBBB that is new or of indeterminate age Recurring sinus pauses not responsive to atropine	None
IIb	Bifascicular block of indeterminate age Isolated RBBB that is new or of indeterminate age	Persistent second- or third-degree AV block at the level of the AV node
III	Prolonged PR interval Type I second-degree AV block with normal hemodynamics Accelerated idioventricular rhythm BBB or fascicular block known to exist before acute MI	Transient AV conduction disturbances in the absence of intraventricular conduction defects Transient, isolated AV block in the presence of isolated LAFB Acquired LAFB in the absence of AV block Persistent first-degree AV block in the presence of BBB that is old or of indeterminate age

Adapted with permission from Ryan TJ, Antman EM, Brooks NH, et al: 1999 update: ACC/AHA guidelines for the management of patients with acute myocardial infarction—executive summary and recommendations. A report of the American College of Cardiology/American Heart Association Task Force on Practical Guidelines (Committee on Man-agement of Acute Myocardial Infarction). Circulation 100:1016-1030, 1999; and Gregoratos G, Abrams J, Epstein AE, et al: ACC/AHA/NASPE 2002 guideline update for implantation of cardiac pacemakers and antiarrhythmia devices. Summary article: A report of the American College of Cardiology/American Heart Association Task Force on Practical Guidelines (ACC/AHA/NASPE). Circulation 106:2145, 2002.

LAFB, Left anterior fascicular block; LPFB, left posterior fascicular block.

*Class designations refer to the level of evidence supporting the effectiveness of the procedure or treatment, where class I indicates that the evidence is very strong and class III that it is absent or that the procedure is not useful and may be harmful.

†An electrophysiologic study may be useful to determine the site of the block.

- The ddx and testing algorithms for wide QRS complex tachycardia are shown in Figures 3-32 and 3-33.
- Antiarrhythmic meds can be classified using the Vaughn-Williams classification (Table 3-25).

4 ATRIAL FIBRILLATION AND ATRIAL FLUTTER

a. Atrial Fibrillation

Totally chaotic atrial activity caused by simultaneous d/c of multiple atrial foci. Subdivided in 4 types:
- *Lone AF:* no clinical or echo evidence of cardiac disease, including HTN in pt < 60 y.o.
- *Paroxysmal AF:* self-terminating
- *Persistent AF:* sustained AF >7 days' duration
- *Permanent AF:* >1 yr's duration

Etiology
- CAD
- MS, MR, AS, AR
- Thyrotoxicosis
- PE, COPD
- Pericarditis
- Myocarditis, cardiomyopathy
- Tachy-brady syndrome
- Alcohol abuse
- MI
- WPW syndrome

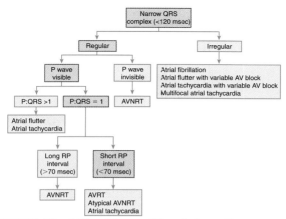

FIGURE 3-30. Differential diagnosis for narrow QRS complex (presumably supraventricular) tachycardias. Note that ventricular tachycardia may manifest with narrow QRS complexes (e.g., fascicular tachycardia). *(From Vincent JL, Abraham E, Moore FA, et al [eds]: Textbook of Critical Care, 6th ed. Philadelphia, Saunders, 2011.)*

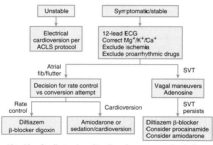

FIGURE 3-31. Algorithm for diagnosis and testing of narrow-complex tachycardia. *fib,* fibrillation. *(From Vincent JL, Abraham E, Moore FA, et al [eds]: Textbook of Critical Care, 6th ed. Philadelphia, Saunders, 2011.)*

- Obesity
- ↑ Pulse pressure (SBP-DBP)
- Others: LA myxoma, ASD, CO poisoning, pheochromocytoma, idiopathic, hypoxia, hypokalemia, sepsis, pneumonia; medications: zoledronic acid, alendronate, amphetamines, antihistamines

Diagnosis

H&P
- Most common complaint: palpitations
- Cardiac auscultation revealing irregularly irregular rhythm

Labs
- TSH, free T_4
- Serum electrolytes

Imaging
- ECG (Fig. 3-34)
  - Irregular, nonperiodic waveforms (best seen in V_1) reflecting continuous atrial reentry

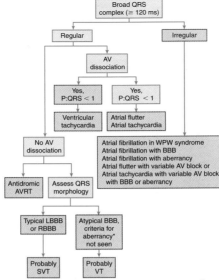

FIGURE 3-32. Differential diagnosis for wide QRS complex tachycardias. *Criteria for aberrancy: rate dependency, triphasic QRS complexes, rSR in V_1, with R >, QRS width <140 msec, QRS deflections are discordant in precordial leads, absence of fusion and capture beats. *(From Vincent JL, Abraham E, Moore FA, et al [eds]: Textbook of Critical Care, 6th ed. Philadelphia, Saunders, 2011.)*

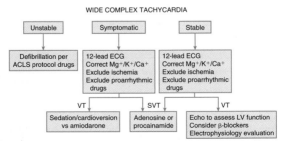

WIDE COMPLEX TACHYCARDIA

FIGURE 3-33. Algorithm for diagnosis and testing of wide-complex tachycardia. *(From Vincent JL, Abraham E, Moore FA, et al [eds]: Textbook of Critical Care, 6th ed. Philadelphia, Saunders, 2011.)*

- Absence of P waves
- Conducted QRS complexes showing no periodicity
■ Echo: to evaluate left atrial size and detect valvular disorders

Treatment

■ New-onset AF: 2 options
  • Pt hemodynamically unstable, angina, preexcited AF → immediate cardioversion
  • Pt hemodynamically stable: rate control → anticoagulation → cardioversion

TABLE 3-25 ■ Antiarrhythmic Meds Classification

Class	Meds	Mechanism/Effect	Rx
IA*	Procainamide, quinidine, disopyramide	Na+ and K+ channel blockade = ↓ conduction, ↑ repolarization	Ventricular arrhythmias, preexcited AF, SVT
IB*	Lidocaine, mexiletine, phenytoin	Na+ channel blockade = ↓ repolarization, ↓ conduction in diseased tissues	Ventricular arrhythmias
IC*	Flecainide, propafenone	Na+ channel blockade = ↓↓ conduction, ↑ repolarization	AF/flutter, SVT, ventricular arrhythmias
II*	Propranolol, atenolol, metoprolol	β-Blockade = ↓ automaticity, ↓ AV node conduction	Rate control (SVT, atrial arrhythmias), ventricular arrhythmias
III*	Amiodarone, sotalol, dofetilide, dronedarone	K+ channel blockade = ↑ action potential duration	AF/flutter, ventricular arrhythmias
IV*	Diltiazem, verapamil	Ca2+ channel blockade = ↓ SA node automaticity, ↓ AV node conduction	Rate control (SVT, atrial arrhythmias)
A1 receptor agonist	Adenosine	↓ block SA and AV node conduction	SVT termination
Vagal activity stimulant	Digoxin	↓ AV node conduction	Rate control atrial

*Vaughn/Williams classification.

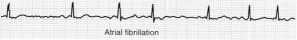

Atrial fibrillation

FIGURE 3-34. Atrial fibrillation with slow ventricular response. *(From Goldberger E: Treatment of Cardiac Emergencies, 5th ed. St. Louis, Mosby, 1990.)*

■ **Rate control**: usually with β-blockers or CCB (Table 3-26)
■ **Anticoagulation**
  • Determine whether AF duration is >48 hr.
    • If AF duration <48 acute anticoagulation (IV UFH or SC LMWH) may not be necessary hr (>50% spontaneous conversion in 24 hr).
    • If AF duration >48 hr, 3 options:
    • Warfarin × 3 wk → cardioversion followed by warfarin × 4 wk
    • TEE → (–) thrombus → immediate cardioversion – warfarin × 4 wk
    • TEE → (+) thrombus → anticoagulate for 3 wk → cardioversion + warfarin × 4 wk
  • Long-term anticoagulation is indicated for AF indicated in all pts w/AF and associated CVD (see CHADS2 score later in this section), including the following:
    • Rheumatic valvular disease (MS, MR, AI)
    • AS
    • Mechanical heart valves
    • H/o previous embolism
    • Persistent atrial thrombus on TEE
    • CHF
    • Cardiomyopathy w/poor LV function
    • Nonrheumatic heart disease (e.g., hypertensive CVD, CAD, ASD)
  • Use CHADS2 score (Table 3-27) to evaluate risk of stroke in nonvalvular AF. CHADS2 score:
    • = 0 → ASA* or no anticoagulation
    • =1 → ASA*, warfarin, dabigatran†, rivaroxaban‡, or apixaban‡
    • ≥2 → warfarin, dabigatran, or rivaroxaban
  • Interruption of anticoagulation for procedures → bridge with heparin if interruption >1 week, mechanical valve, recent stroke, CHADS2 ≥3, rheumatic mitral valve.

---

*Adding clopidogrel to ASA = ↓ stroke risk but ↑ major bleeding
†Direct thrombin inhibitor, approved only for nonvalvular AF, ↓ stroke risk but ↑ risk GI bleeding
‡Factor Xa inhibitors, approved only for nonvalvular AF, ↓ intracranial hemorrhage but ↑ risk of thrombosis × 4 wks after stopping; requires overlapping with another anticoagulant × 4 wks when stopping it

TABLE 3-26 ■ Acute Pharmacologic Rate Control in Atrial Tachyarrhythmia*

Drug	Route of Administration	Dose	Onset	Potential Adverse Effects
Verapamil	Intravenous	5-10 mg (0.075-0.15 mg/kg) over 2 min; if no response, additional 5-10 mg after 15-30 min; 3-10 mg every 4-6 hr for rate control	3-5 min	Hypotension, bradycardia, heart block, possible deterioration of ventricular function in the presence of organic heart disease
Diltiazem	Intravenous	0.25 mg/kg over 2 min; if no response, additional 0.35 mg/kg after 15-30 min; followed by 5-15 mg/hr infusion for rate control	2-7 min	
Esmolol	Intravenous	0.5 mg/kg over 1 min, followed by 0.05-0.2 mg/kg/min for 4 min; if no response after 5 min, 0.5 mg/kg for 1 min, followed by 0.1 mg/kg for 4 min; infusion 0.05-0.2 mg/kg/min for rate control	2-3 min	Hypotension, bradycardia, heart block, possible deterioration of ventricular function in the presence of organic heart disease
Metoprolol	Intravenous	2.5-5 mg over 2 min followed by repeat doses if necessary (total 10-15 mg)	5 min	
Atenolol	Intravenous	2.5 mg over 2 min, followed by repeat doses if necessary (total 10 mg) or infusion 0.15 mg/kg for 20 min	5-10 min	
Propranolol	Intravenous	1 mg over 1 min (total 10-12 mg; 0.15 mg/kg)	5 min	
Digoxin	Intravenous	0.5-1 mg, followed by 0.25 mg every 2-4 h (maximum, 1.5 mg)	30-60 min	Bradycardia, atrioventricular block, atrial arrhythmias, ventricular tachycardia

From Vincent JL, Abraham E, Moore FA, et al (eds): Textbook of Critical Care, 6th ed. Philadelphia, Saunders, 2011.
*Intravenous amiodarone can also be effective in rate control, especially in patients with poor left ventricular function, but there is insufficient evidence to support this recommendation. The rate-slowing effect of amiodarone is usually delayed by 1-2 hours.

TABLE 3-27 ■ CHADS2 Score

Disease/Disorder	Points
CHF	1
HTN	1
Age ≥75 yr	1
DM	1
Prior TIA/stroke	2

Interpretation: 0 = low risk, 1 to 2 = moderate risk, ≥3 = high risk.

■ Rhythm control
  • Restoration of sinus rhythm does not confer any ↓ mortality or stroke risk. Asymptomatic pts with HR <110/min and EF >40 % do not need rhythm control.
  • Attempts at medical (pharmacologic) intervention should be considered in symptomatic pts only after proper anticoagulation because cardioversion can lead to systemic emboli. After successful cardioversion, anticoagulation should be continued based on CHADS2 score because of persistent systemic embolism risk from potential episodic AF.
  • Useful agents for pharmacologic conversion are described in Table 3-28. Consider "pill-in-pocket" approach in symptomatic pts with paroxysmal AF but no BBB, long QT, sinus or AV block or structural heart disease → Pt takes short-acting CCB or β-blocker and 30 min later takes class 1C drug (flecainide, propafenone).

TABLE 3-28 ■ Antiarrhythmic Drugs for Pharmacologic Conversion of Atrial Tachyarrhythmias

Drug	Route of Administration	Dose	Potential Adverse Effects
Flecainide	Oral or intravenous	Loading oral dose 200-300 mg or slow injection 1.5-2 mg/kg over 10-20 min; if no response, infusion 1.5 mg/kg for 1 hr, then 0.1-0.25 mg/kg over 24 hr	Rapidly conducted atrial flutter, possible deterioration of ventricular function in the presence of organic heart disease, monomorphic ventricular tachycardia
Propafenone	Oral or intravenous	Loading oral dose 450-600 mg or 1.5-2 mg/kg over 10-20 min, followed by infusion 5-10 mg/kg if needed	
Ibutilide	Intravenous	1 mg over 10 min; if no response, additional 1 mg	QT prolongation, torsades de pointes, hypotension
Amiodarone	Intravenous (preferable central line)	5-7 mg/kg over 30-60 min, followed by infusion 20 mg/kg for 25 hr (total 1,200-1,800 mg)	Hypotension, bradycardia, QT prolongation, torsades de pointes (?), gastrointestinal upset, constipation, phlebitis

From Vincent JL, Abraham E, Moore FA, et al (eds): Textbook of Critical Care, 6th ed. Philadelphia, Saunders, 2011.

- • Factors associated w/maintenance of sinus rhythm after cardioversion:
  - • Left atrium diameter <60 mm
  - • Absence of mitral valve disease
  - • Short duration of AF
- ■ Surgical Rx of AF
  - • *Maze procedure* → preservation of sinus rhythm in >95% of pts w/o the use of long-term antiarrhythmic medication post procedure
  - • Reserved for pts w/rapid HR refractory to pharmacologic Rx or who cannot tolerate pharmacologic Rx
  - • Catheter-based radiofrequency ablation procedures designed to eliminate AF represent newer approaches to AF
  - • Pulmonary vein ablation for chronic AF → sinus rhythm maintained long term in the majority of pts w/chronic AF by means of circumferential pulmonary vein ablation
  - • Implantable pacemakers and defibrillators that combine pacing and cardioversion

b. Atrial flutter
Rapid atrial rate of 250-350 bpm w/varying degrees of intraventricular block.

Etiology
- ■ CAD
- ■ MI
- ■ Thyrotoxicosis
- ■ PE
- ■ Mitral valve disease
- ■ Cardiac surgery
- ■ COPD

Diagnosis
H&P
- ■ Fast pulse rate (approximately 150 bpm)
- ■ Dyspnea, lightheadedness, chest pain

Labs
- ■ TSH, free T_4, serum electrolytes
- ■ ECG (Fig. 3-35)
- ■ Regular, sawtooth, or F wave pattern, best seen in II, III, and aVF and secondary to atrial depolarization; AV conduction block (2:1, 3:1, or varying)

Treatment
- ■ Management is similar to AF (including thromboprophylaxis).
- ■ Valsalva maneuver or carotid sinus massage usually slows the ventricular rate (grade of AV block) and may make flutter waves more evident.
- ■ DC cardioversion: Rx of choice for acute management of atrial flutter. Electrical cardioversion is given at low energy levels (20-25 J). Sedation of a conscious pt is highly recommended before cardioversion is performed.

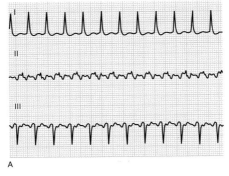

A

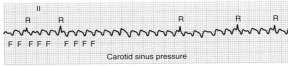

Carotid sinus pressure

B

FIGURE 3-35. Atrial flutter waves (F). **A,** The flutter waves are not apparent in lead I but are obvious in leads II and III. **B,** Carotid sinus pressure slowed the ventricular rate but did not change the atrial flutter rate. *(From Goldberger E: Treatment of Cardiac Emergencies, 5th ed. St. Louis, Mosby, 1990.)*

- Radiofrequency ablation (ablation in isthmus between inferior vena cava and tricuspid valve) → effective for pts w/chronic or recurring atrial flutter and is generally considered first-line Rx in those w/recurrent episodes of atrial flutter.

5 SUPRAVENTRICULAR TACHYCARDIAS (SVT)

a. Paroxysmal atrial tachycardia (PAT, Paroxysmal supraventricular tachycardia [PSVT])

SVT includes all forms of tachycardia that either arise above the bifurcation of the bundle of His or that have mechanisms dependent on the bundle of His.
- **AVNRT:** common type (60%) of SVT involves a slow and a fast pathway within the AV node
- **xAVRT:** involves an AV reentry circuit mediated by an accessory pathway (*Kent bundles* [a short muscle bundle directly connecting the atria and ventricles])
- **Atrial tachycardia:** resulting from ectopic areas of micro-reentry that fire faster than sinus rate

Etiology
- Young pts w/o evidence of cardiac disease (and, thus, the etiology is really just a reentrant tract)
- Preexcitation syndromes (e.g., WPW syndrome)
- ASD
- Acute MI
- When evaluating pts, it is important to assess for triggers (e.g., intake of alcohol, caffeine, and other drugs) and presentation (in contrast to sinus tachycardia, which accelerates and decelerates gradually, SVTs have sudden onset and termination).

Diagnosis
- ECG (Fig. 3-36):
  • Absolutely regular rhythm at rate of 150-220 bpm is present.
  • P waves may or may not be seen (the presence of P waves depends on the relationship of atrial to ventricular depolarization). In *short-RP tachycardias* (AVNRT, AVRT), the P wave is closer to the preceding QRS complex; in

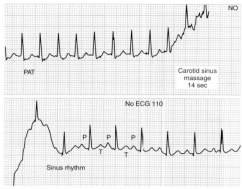

FIGURE 3-36. Supraventricular tachycardia (PAT). The *upper* and *lower rows* are part of one continuous strip. In the *upper row*, no definite P waves are visible. The diagnosis of this ECG is therefore supraventricular tachyarrhythmia. The ventricular rate is approximately 185/min. In the *lower strip*, taken at the end of the carotid sinus massage, sinus rhythm has appeared. However, the heart rate is still rapid (approximately 135/min). *(From Goldberger E: Treatment of Cardiac Emergencies, 5th ed. St. Louis, Mosby, 1990.)*

long-RP tachycardias (junctional reciprocating tachycardia, atypical AVNRT, atrial tachycardia, sinus tachycardia), the P wave is closer to the following QRS complex.
- AVRT with wide QRS complex (>0.12 sec) w/initial slurring (*delta wave;* see Fig. 3-37) during sinus rhythm and short PR (≤0.12 sec) are characteristic of WPW pattern (see later).

Treatment
- Valsalva maneuver in the supine position → most effective way to terminate SVT; carotid sinus massage (after excluding occlusive carotid disease [absence of carotid bruit and no hx suggestive of carotid artery disease]) or application of an ice pack to the face in children is also commonly used to elicit vagal efferent impulses.
- Synchronized DC shock if pt shows signs of cardiogenic shock, angina, or CHF
- Adenosine: for Rx of PSVT that is unresponsive to vagal maneuvers; the dose is 6 mg given as a rapid IV bolus under ECG monitoring; tachycardia is usually terminated within a few seconds in 60% to 80% of pts; if necessary, the drug can be given again w/12-mg IV bolus (effective in terminating PSVT in >90% of pts). Contraindications are second- or third-degree AV block, SSS, AF, and VT. Adenosine is also contraindicated in heart transplant pts and should be used w/caution in COPD pts. It may also cause bronchospasm in asthmatic pts.
- If adenosine is not effective, verapamil 2.5 to 5 mg IV q5min to a max of 15 mg is generally effective.
- Verapamil should be used cautiously in pts w/SVT and h/o hypotension. If the pt is truly hypotensive w/SVT, immediate synchronized cardioversion is indicated.
- Slow injection of Ca chloride (10 mL of a 10% solution) given during 5 to 8 min before verapamil administration may ↓ the hypotensive effect w/o compromising its antiarrhythmic effect.
- Repeat carotid massage after IV verapamil if SVT persists.
- β-Blockers (metoprolol [5 mg IV q2min up to 15 mg] or esmolol [500 mg/kg IV bolus, then 50 mg/kg/min]) or IV diltiazem, IV procainamide, IV propafenone, IV flecainide, or IV ibutilide may also be effective in the treatment of SVT; however, these agents generally have little role in acute management of PSVT. Digoxin should also be avoided in pts w/WPW syndrome and narrow QRS tachycardia (risk of AF during AV reentrant tachycardia).

b. Wolff-Parkinson-White Syndrome (WPW)
- Accessory pathways (Kent bundles) → earlier than nl ventricular depolarization following the atrial impulse → tachyarrhythmias

WPW preexcitation

- Short PR
- Wide QRS
- Delta wave (arrow)

FIGURE 3-37. Preexcitation through the bypass tract in WPW syndrome is associated with the triad of findings shown here. (*From Goldberger AL, Goldberger E: Clinical Electrocardiography: A Simplified Approach, 5th ed. St. Louis, Mosby, 1994.*)

Diagnosis

- ECG (Fig. 3-37)
  - PR interval <120 msec
  - QRS complex >120 msec w/a slurred, slowly rising onset of QRS in some leads (delta wave)
  - Secondary ST-T wave changes directed in opposite direction to major delta and QRS vectors

Treatment

- No Rx in the absence of tachyarrhythmias
- Acute tachyarrhythmia: adenosine, verapamil, or diltiazem
- Cardioversion if hemodynamic impairment present

c. Atrial Tachycardia, Multifocal Atrial Tachycardia (MAT)

- Atrial tachycardias result from ectopic areas of micro-reentry that fire faster than sinus rate. MAT is chaotic, irregular atrial activity at rates of 100-180 bpm.

Etiology

- COPD
- Metabolic disturbances (hypoxemia, hypokalemia, hypomagnesemia)
- Sepsis
- Theophylline toxicity
- CHF
- Acute MI

Diagnosis

- ECG (Fig. 3-38):
  - Variable P-P intervals
  - Morphology of the P wave varies from beat to beat, w/min. of 3 different forms of P wave besides those from the sinus node.
  - Each QRS complex is preceded by a P wave.

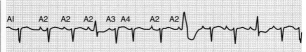

FIGURE 3-38. Multifocal atrial tachycardia. Letter designations A1, A2, A3, and A4 show premature contractions from varying foci. Notice that the fourth, eighth, and eleventh QRS complexes are aberrant. (*From Ferri FF: Ferri's Best Test: A Practical Guide to Clinical Laboratory Medicine and Diagnostic Imaging, 2nd ed. Philadelphia, Mosby, 2010.*)

Treatment

- Treat underlying cause (e.g., improve oxygenation, correct electrolyte abnormalities).
- Verapamil 5 mg IV at a rate of up to 1 mg/min (may repeat after 20 min). Gluca gluconate, 1 g IV given 5 min before treatment w/verapamil, may ↓ drug-induced hypotension w/o affecting the antiarrhythmic effect.
- Metoprolol or esmolol used in absence of COPD, CHF, or bronchospasm
- Amiodarone useful in refractory cases

d. Sick Sinus Syndrome (SSS, Tachy-Brady Syndrome, Brady-Tachy Syndrome)

- Group of cardiac rhythm disturbances characterized by abnormalities of the sinus node, including:
  - Sinus bradycardia
  - Sinus arrest or exit block

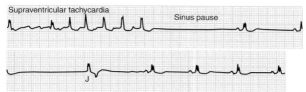

Supraventricular tachycardia — Sinus pause

FIGURE 3-39. Brady-tachy (sick sinus) syndrome. This rhythm strip shows a narrow-complex tachycardia (probably atrial flutter) followed by a sinus pause, an AV junctional escape beat (J), and then sinus rhythm. *(From Goldberger AL, Goldberger E: Clinical Electrocardiography: A Simplified Approach, 5th ed. St. Louis, Mosby, 1994.)*

- Combinations of sinoatrial or AV conduction defects
- Supraventricular tachyarrhythmias.
- These abnormalities may coexist in a single pt so that a pt may have episodes of bradycardia and episodes of tachycardia.

Etiology
- Fibrosis or fatty infiltration involves the sinus node, the AV node, or the His bundle or its branches.
- In addition, inflammatory or degenerative changes of the nerves and ganglia surrounding the sinus nodes and other sclerodegenerative changes may be found.

Diagnosis
H&P
- Clinical presentation: lightheadedness, dizziness, syncope, palpitation
Imaging
- ECG (Fig. 3-39)
- Ambulatory cardiac rhythm monitoring
- 24-hr ambulatory ECG (Holter)
- Event recorder

Treatment
- Permanent pacemaker placement if sx are present
- Drug Rx of the tachycardia (β-blockers, CCB) may worsen or bring out the bradycardia and become the reason for pacemaker requirement.

6 VENTRICULAR ARRHYTHMIAS

a. Long QT Syndrome (LQTS)
- Corrected QT interval >0.44 sec associated w/ ↑ risk of life-threatening ventricular arrhythmias, most common channelopathy (1:5,000)

Etiology
- Cardiac repolarization abnormality
- Congenital cause (chromosome 3 or chromosome 7 abnormality)
- Acquired causes:
  - Drugs (dofetilide, ibutilide, bepridil, quinidine procainamide, sotalol, amiodarone, ranolazine, disopyramide, phenothiazines anc antiemetic agents [droperidol, domperidone], tricyclic antidepressants, quinolones, azithromycin, methadone, astemizole or cisapride given w/ketoconazole or erythromycin, clarithromycin, and antimalarials), particularly among pts w/asthma or those using hypokalemic meds
  - Hypokalemia, hypomagnesemia, hypocalcemia
  - Liquid protein diet
  - CNS lesions
  - MVP
  - Hypothyroidism

Diagnosis
H&P
- Palpitations, presyncope
- Syncope caused by VT
- Sudden death
- Familial (associated w/deafness): autosomal recessive
- Familial associated w/nl hearing: autosomal dominant (incidence unknown)
- Although inheritance of LQTS is autosomal dominant, female predominance has often been observed and has been attributed to a susceptibility to cardiac arrhythmias in women.

TABLE 3-29 ■ ECG Criteria for Congenital Long QT Syndrome	
Corrected QT >480 msec	3 points
Corrected QT 460-480 msec	2 points
Corrected QT 450-460 msec (men)	1 point
Torsades de pointes	2 points
T wave alternans	1 point
Notched T wave in 3 leads	1 point
Bradycardia	0.5 point
History	
Syncope w/stress	2 points
Syncope w/o stress	1 point
Congenital deafness	0.5 point
Definite FHx of long QT	1 point
Unexplained cardiac death in first-degree relative age <30 yr	0.5 point

Total score = 4: definite long QT syndrome.

Total score 2 to 3: intermediate probability.

Total score = 1: low probability.

ECG
- QT interval usually >460 msec, torsades de pointes. Diagnostic criteria for the congenital LQTS are given in Table 3-29.

Treatment
- Asymptomatic sporadic forms w/no complex ventricular arrhythmias: no Rx
- Risk stratification
  - High risk (>50% of cardiac event): QTc >500 msec and LQT1 and LQT2 or male pt w/LQT3
  - Moderate risk (30%-50%): QTc >500 msec in female pt w/LQT3 or QTc <500 msec in male pt w/LQT2 or in female pt w/LQT2 or 3
  - Low risk (<30%): QTc <500 msec and LQT1 or male pt w/LQT2
- General recommendations:
  - Avoid competitive sports.
  - β-Blocker is taken at the max tolerated dose.
  - Cardiology referral is recommended for all cases.
  - Pacemaker and implantable defibrillator are recommended for survivors of cardiac arrest, for pts w/syncope while receiving β-blockers, and for primary prevention in pts w/characteristics that suggest risk (these include LQT2, LQT3, and QTc interval >500 msec).

b. Short QT Syndrome
- Dx: QT interval <350 msec
  - ECG: may show AF, VT, VF
- Hx: syncope, cardiac arrest
- Rx: ICD, quinidine

c. Brugada Syndrome
- Repolarization disorder (autosomal dominant, mutation of *SCN5A* gene → loss of Na^+ channel function) characterized by:
  - ST-segment elevation in rt anterior precordial leads (V_1 to V_3)
  - Incomplete RBBB
  - Susceptibility to ventricular tachyarrhythmias

Diagnosis
- The syndrome manifests usually in third to fourth decade w/cardiac events (syncope, cardiac arrest), often occurring during sleep or at rest.
- Male-to-female ratio is 8:1.
- Role of PES to identify pts at higher risk of cardiac arrest is controversial.

Treatment
- ICD

Clinical Pearl
Concealed forms may be unmasked only by provocative drug testing w/selected class IC drugs (flecainide, procainamide).

d. Ventricular Tachycardia (VT)
- Three consecutive beats of ventricular origin (wide QRS) at a rate between 100 and 200 bpm (Fig. 3-40)

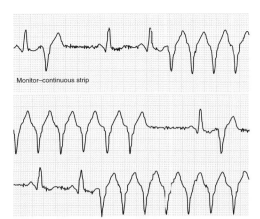

Monitor–continuous strip

FIGURE 3-40. Ventricular tachycardia. *(From Goldberger E: Treatment of Cardiac Emergencies, 5th ed. St. Louis, Mosby, 1990.)*

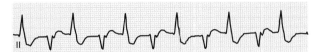

FIGURE 3-41. This digoxin toxic arrhythmia is a special type of ventricular tachycardia (bidirectional tachycardia) with QRS complexes that alternate in direction from beat to beat. No P waves are present. *(From Goldberger AL, Goldberger E: Clinical Electrocardiography: A Simplified Approach, 5th ed. St. Louis, Mosby, 1994.)*

Diagnosis
- ECG:
  - *Monomorphic VT:* QRS complexes of the VT are of the same shape and amplitude.
  - *Polymorphic VT:* QRS complexes vary in shape and amplitude.
  - *Bidirectional VT:* QRS alternate in direction from beat to beat (Fig. 3-41).
  - *Torsades de pointes (see next section):* Polymorphic VT occurring in the presence of a long QT
- Differentiation between ventricular beats and SVT w/aberrant ventricular conduction may be very difficult; because most wide-complex tachycardias are VT, wide-QRS tachycardia in the conscious adult should be considered VT until proved otherwise, especially in the presence of underlying heart disease. Table 3-30 describes ECG criteria favoring VT.

Treatment
- Refer to the ACLS algorithm.

e. Torsades de Pointes
VT manifested by episodes of alternating electrical polarity, w/the amplitude of the QRS complex twisting around an isoelectric baseline resembling a spindle (Fig. 3-42). The rhythm usually starts w/a PVC and is preceded by widening of the QT interval.

Etiology
- Torsades may be caused by electrolyte disturbances (hypokalemia, hypomagnesemia, hypocalcemia), antiarrhythmic drugs that prolong the QT interval (procainamide, quinidine, disopyramide), N-acetylprocainamide, droperidol, amiodarone, phenothiazines, haloperidol, tricyclic antidepressants, terfenadine, astemizole, ketoconazole, erythromycin, TMP-SMZ, high-dose methadone, or cocaine. Torsades de pointes is also associated w/hereditary long QT interval syndromes.

TABLE 3-30 ■ ECG Criteria Favoring Ventricular Tachycardia
AV Relationship
Dissociated P waves
Fusion beats
Capture beats
A/V ratio <1
QRS Duration
>160 msec with LBBB pattern
>140 msec with RBBB pattern
QRS during WCT is narrower than in NSR
Onset QRS to peak (+ or −) in lead II >50 msec
QRS Axis
Axis shift of >40 degrees between NSR and WCT
Right superior (northwest) axis
Left axis deviation with RBBB morphology
Right axis deviation with LBBB morphology
Precordial QRS Concordance
Positive concordance
Negative concordance
QRS Morphology in RBBB Pattern WCT
Monophasic R, biphasic qR complex, or broad R (>40 msec) in lead V_1
Rabbit ear sign: double-peaked R wave in lead V_1 with the left peak taller than the right peak
rS complex in lead V_6
Contralateral BBB in WCT and NSR
QRS Morphology in LBBB Pattern WCT
Broad initial R wave of ≥40 msec in lead V_1 or V_2
R wave in lead V_1 during WCT taller than the R wave during NSR
Slow descent to the nadir of the S, notching in the downstroke of the S wave in lead V_1
RS interval >70 msec in lead V_1 or V_2
Q or QS wave in lead V_6

From Issa Z, Miller JM, Zipes DP: Clinical Arrhythmology and Electrophysiology, 2nd ed. Philadelphia, Saunders, 2012.

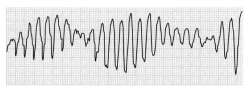

FIGURE 3-42. Torsades de pointes. *(From Cerra FB: Manual of Critical Care. St. Louis, Mosby, 1998.)*

Treatment
- Electrical termination of the tachycardia w/cardioversion when the ventricular tachyarrhythmia is sustained
- ICD

K. PERIPHERAL ARTERIAL DISEASE (PAD)

Stenotic, occlusive, and aneurysmal diseases of the aorta and its branch arteries, exclusive of the coronary arteries. The primary cause of PAD is atherosclerosis.

Diagnosis
- Based on the presence of limb sx or a low ankle-brachial index (ABI) ≤0.90
- The ABI is calculated by dividing the highest ankle systolic pressure in either the dorsalis pedis or posterior tibial artery by the highest systolic pressure from either arm.
- The severity of PAD is based on the ABI at rest and during treadmill exercise (1-2 mph, 5 min, or sx limited):
  - Mild: ABI at rest 0.71 to 0.90 or ABI during exercise 0.50 to 0.90
  - Moderate: ABI at rest 0.41 to 0.70 or ABI during exercise 0.20 to 0.50
  - Severe: ABI at rest <0.40 or ABI during exercise <0.20

- >50% of the pts w/PAD are asymptomatic.
- 33% present w/intermittent claudication (aching or cramping leg pain brought on by exertion and relieved w/rest).
- Other manifestations:
  - Painful cramping in buttocks, hip, or leg that occurs while walking but goes away while resting
  - Diminished pedal pulses
  - Bruits heard over the distal aorta, iliac, or femoral arteries
  - Changes in skin color, especially on feet (rubor w/prolonged capillary refill on dependency or delayed pallor)
  - Cool skin temperature
  - Trophic changes of hair loss and muscle atrophy
  - Nonhealing ulcers, necrotic tissue, and gangrene
  - Weakness, numbness, or a feeling of heaviness in legs
  - Aching or burning in toes and feet during rest and especially while lying flat

Labs
- Lipid profile, FBS

Imaging
- CTA or MRA to localize and quantify arterial stenosis
- Catheter-based digital-subtraction angiography (DSA): gold standard for visualizing the arterial anatomy before revascularization

Treatment

Medical
- Smoking cessation
- HTN control w/goal <140/90 or <130/80 mm Hg if the pt has DM or CKD
- Tight glycemic control: HbA_{1c} <7 % in DM
- Control dyslipidemia: goal for LDL <70 mg/dL in very high-risk pts
- Antiplatelet Rx: ASA 81 mg qd. Clopidogrel 75 mg qd in pts who cannot tolerate ASA
- Cilostazol 100 mg bid: effective for intermittent claudication.

Surgical
- Revascularization (surgery or percutaneous transluminal angioplasty) in pts w/claudication that limits their lifestyle and is unresponsive to exercise and pharmacologic Rx
- Endarterectomy (with possible surgical patch repair) for revascularization of common femoral artery
- Endovascular Rx preferred in pts ≤50 y.o. because they have a higher risk of graft failure after surgical Rx than do older pts.

L. CARDIAC RISK ASSESSMENT FOR NONCARDIAC SURGERY

Risk of Major Perioperative Cardiovascular Event by Type of Surgery
- High risk (death or MI >4%): thoracic, vascular
- Intermediate risk (2%-4%): abd, head and neck
- Low risk (<1%): breast, eye, gyn, skin, urologic

Clinical Risk Stratification: Risk of MI
- High (4.1%): CAD almost certain (MI by hx/ECG; typical angina; prior angiography or revascularization)
- Intermediate (0.8%): PVD, prior stroke/TIA, atypical chest pain but no evidence of CAD
- Low (<0.8%): risk factors for CAD but no obvious disease, age >75 yr, ECG abnl

Simplified Approach
- No h/o sx of CAD, fully active → no additional recommended tests
- High likelihood of CAD, stable CAD functional class I, II → cardiac stress testing
- Unstable CAD functional class III or IV → cardiac catheterization

M. HYPOTENSION

- Figure 3-43 describes the suggested approach to pts with low systemic arterial pressure.

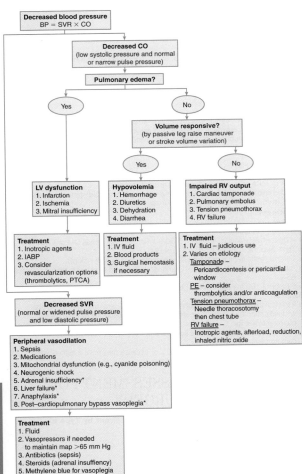

FIGURE 3-43. Initial approach to a patient with low systemic arterial blood pressure. *Adrenal insufficiency, liver failure, post–cardiopulmonary bypass vasoplegia, and anaphylaxis are commonly listed as vasodilatory shock; however, data are inconclusive, and components of other types of shock (hypovolemic, cardiogenic) may also be present. (*From Vincent JL, Abraham E, Moore FA, et al [eds]: Textbook of Critical Care, 6th ed. Philadelphia, Saunders, 2011.*)

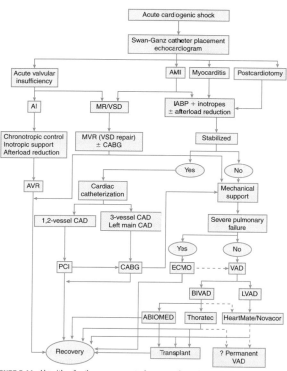

FIGURE 3-44. Algorithm for the management of acute cardiogenic shock. *(From Vincent JL, Abraham E, Moore FA, et al [eds]: Textbook of Critical Care, 6th ed. Philadelphia, Saunders, 2011.)*

N. ACUTE CARDIOGENIC SHOCK

- Figure 3-44 describes an algorithm for the management of acute cardiogenic shock.

O. DYSLIPIDEMIA

- *Primary hyperlipoproteinemia* = group of genetic disorders of the lipid transport proteins in the blood, manifested as abnl levels of cholesterol, TGs, or both in the serum of affected pts.
- *Hypercholesterolemia* = blood cholesterol measurement >200 mg/dL.

Etiology

Primary
- Genetics
- Obesity
- Dietary intake

Secondary
- Hypothyroidism
- Diabetes mellitus
- Nephrotic syndrome
- Obstructive liver disease: hepatoma, extrahepatic biliary obstruction, primary biliary cirrhosis

- Alcohol or tobacco use
- Drugs: oral contraceptives, progesterone, corticosteroids, thiazide diuretics, β-blockers, androgenic steroids, retinoic acid derivatives

Labs
- TC, LDL, HDL, TG chol/HDL ratio
- If TG <400, LDL = TC−HDL − (TG/5)

PE
May include:
- Tendon xanthomas (on elbows, hands, Achilles) → LDL >300
- Xanthelasma (yellow streaks on eyelids) → TG >600
- Arcus corneae in young pt
- Arterial bruits

Treatment
- First line of Rx: dietary Rx (use of NCEP-ATP III Therapeutic Lifestyle Change TLC Diet can result in 5% to 15% ↓ in LDL cholesterol level)
- Composition of the TLC diet:
  - Total fat: 25% to 30% of total calories
  - Polyunsaturated fat: up to 10% of total calories
  - Monounsaturated fat: up to 20% of total calories
  - Saturated fats: <7% of total calories
  - Carbohydrate: 50% to 60% of total calories
  - Protein: 15% of total calories
  - No more than 200 mg/day of cholesterol
  - Fiber: 20 to 30 g/day
- ↑ Physical activity: Encourage 20 to 30 min of aerobic exercise 3 to 4 ×/wk.
- Weight reduction
- Smoking cessation
- Counseling on CAD risk factors
- ↑ LDL cholesterol is the primary target of cholesterol-lowering Rx.
- Risk assessment should be made based on the presence of risk factors:
  - Cigarette smoking
  - HTN (BP ≤140/90 mm Hg or on meds)
  - Low HDL (<40 mg/dL); HDL >60 mg/dL counts as (−) risk factor.
  - Family hx premature CHD (<55 yr in first-degree male relative, <65 yr in female)
  - Age (men >45 yr, women >55 yr)
- Evaluate the presence of CHD equivalents: DM, AAA, PAD, symptomatic carotid artery disease (stroke, TIA), 10-yr risk for CAD >20% with Framingham risk calculator.
- Determine Framingham risk:
  - High risk: CHD or CHD equivalents or ≥2 risk factors & >20% 10-yr risk
  - Mod high risk: ≥2 risk factors & 10% to 20% 10-yr risk
  - Mod risk: ≥2 risk factors & <10% 10-yr risk
  - Lower risk: 0 to 1 risk factor
- Drug Rx in pts with:
  - LDL >190 and 0 to 1 risk factor
  - LDL >160 and ≥2 risk factors and <10% 10-yr risk
  - LDL >130 and ≥2 risk factors and 10% to 20% 10-yr risk
  - LDL >100 with CHD, CHD risk equivalents, and >20% 10-yr risk
- Optional goal is LDL <70 mg/dL for "very high-risk" pts, which includes the presence of established CVD + multiple major risk factor (especially DM), severe and poorly controlled risk factors (especially continued cigarette smoking), multiple risk factors of the metabolic syndrome, and in pts with ACS.
- Non–HDL cholesterol should be secondary target of Rx in pts with ↑ triglycerides (>200 mg/dL). The non–HDL cholesterol goal is 30 mg/dL > LDL goal.
- Optimal fasting triglyceride level is <100 mg/dL.
- Medications that can be used:
  1. HMG-CoA reductase inhibitors (statins)
  2. Niacin
  3. Bile acid sequestrants (rarely used due to side effects)
  4. Fibric acids
  5. Ezetimibe
  6. Omega-3 fatty acids

- Statin use = 30% reduction in coronary events and a 12% ↓ in total mortality.
- Fenofibrates have not been shown to reduce morbidity and mortality in pts.
- No cardiovascular benefit exists from taking ER niacin.

P. METABOLIC SYNDROME

Any 3 of the following criteria:
- Abdominal waist circumference >94 cm (37 in) in men and >80 cm (31 in) in women
- Serum hypertriglyceridemia ≥150 mg/dL (1.7 mmol/L) or drug Rx for ↑ triglycerides
- HDL <40 mg/dL (1 mmol/L) in men and <50 mg/dL (1.3 mmol/L) in women or drug Rx for ↓ HDL-C
- BP ≥130/85 mm Hg or drug Rx for ↑ BP
- Fasting glucose ≥100 mg/dL (5.6 mmol/L) or drug Rx for ↑ blood glucose

Treatment
- Lifestyle modification (weight loss, physical activity, smoking cessation)
- Treat HTN: systolic BP >130/80 mm Hg. Consider ACEIs/ARBs.
- Treat hyperlipidemia: goal LDL <80. Consider statin.
- Treat diabetes: goal fasting blood glucose <100 mg/dL. Consider metformin.

Q. SYNCOPE

- Temporary loss of consciousness results from an acute global reduction in cerebral blood flow.

Diagnosis

Hx
- Can provide clues to cause of syncope
- Sudden loss of consciousness: Consider cardiac arrhythmias, vertebrobasilar TIA.
- Gradual loss of consciousness: Consider orthostatic hypotension, vasodepressor syncope, hypoglycemia.
- Pt's activity at the time of syncope:
  • Micturition, coughing, defecation: syncope caused by ↓ venous return
  • Turning the head while shaving: carotid sinus syndrome
  • Physical exertion in pt w/murmur: AS
  • Arm exercise: subclavian steal syndrome
  • Assuming an upright position: orthostatic hypotension
- Associated events:
  • Chest pain: MI, PE
  • Palpitations: dysrhythmias
  • H/o aura, incontinence during episode, and transient confusion after "syncope": seizure disorder
  • Psychic stress: consider vasovagal syncope
  • Current meds, particularly anti-HTN drugs: hypotension induced by meds

PE
- BP: If low, consider orthostatic hypotension. If unequal in both arms (difference >20 mm Hg), consider subclavian steal or dissecting aneurysm. BP and HR should be recorded in the supine, sitting, and standing positions.
- Pulse: If pt has tachycardia, bradycardia, or irregular rhythm, consider dysrhythmia.
- Mental status: If pt is confused after the syncopal episode, consider postictal state.
- Heart: If murmurs are present, suggestive of AS or HOCM, consider syncope secondary to LV outflow obstruction; if JVD and distant heart sounds are present, consider cardiac tamponade.
- Carotid sinus pressure can be dx if it reproduces sx and other causes are excluded. A pause ≥3 sec or a systolic BP drop >50 mm Hg w/o sx or <30 mm Hg w/sx when sinus pressure is applied separately on each side for ≤5 sec is considered abnl; this test should be avoided in pts w/carotid bruits or cerebrovascular disease. ECG monitoring, IV access, and bedside atropine should be available when carotid sinus pressure is applied.

Initial Diagnostic Tests
- See Figure 3-45.
- Routine blood tests rarely yield diagnostically useful information and should be done only when they are specifically suggested by the results of H&P. The following tests should be considered:
  • CBC: R/o anemia, infection.

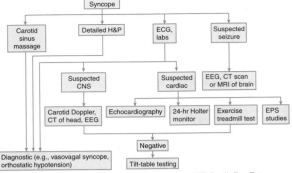

FIGURE 3-45. Diagnostic algorithm for syncope. *(From Ferri FF: Ferri's Best Test: A Practical Guide to Clinical Laboratory Medicine and Diagnostic Imaging, 2nd ed. Philadelphia, Mosby, 2010.)*

- Electrolytes, BUN, Cr, Mg, and Ca: R/o electrolyte abnlities, hypomagnesemia, and hypocalcemia; evaluate fluid status.
- ECG: R/o arrhythmias; may be diagnostic in 5% to 10% of pts.
- CXR: Evaluate cardiac size, lung fields.
- ABGs: R/o PE, hyperventilation.
- Pregnancy test in women of childbearing age
■ Tilt table testing
  - Useful to support the dx of neurocardiogenic syncope and to identify pts w/ prominent bradycardic response who may benefit from a permanent pacemaker
  - Indicated in pts w/recurrent episodes of unexplained syncope. Pts >50 yr should have stress testing before undergoing tilt table testing.
■ Additional diagnostic tests may be indicated, depending on H&P.
  - If arrhythmias are suspected, 24-hr Holter monitor and admission to a telemetry unit are appropriate; in general, Holter monitoring is rarely useful, revealing a cause of syncope in <3% of cases. Loop recorders that can be activated after a syncopal event and retrieve information about the cardiac rhythm during the preceding 4 min have added considerable diagnostic yield in pts w/unexplained syncope.
  - Echo: indicated in pts w/heart murmur to r/o AS, HCM, or atrial myxoma
  - CT of brain and EEG: when seizure disorder is suspected
  - CT of chest: when PE is suspected
  - Cardiac isoenzymes or troponin in pt w/h/o chest pain before syncopal episode
  - Blood and urine toxicology when toxicity or drug abuse is suspected

Treatment
■ Varies w/etiology of syncope

Prognosis
■ Varies w/the age of the pt and the cause of the syncope
■ Benign prognosis (low 1-year morbidity and mortality) in pts:
  - Aged ≤30 yr and having noncardiac syncope
  - Aged ≤70 yr and having vasovagal or psychogenic syncope
■ Poor prognosis (high morbidity and mortality) in pts w/cardiac syncope. Pts w/ syncope of unknown cause are also at risk for death from any cause.
■ Pts w/≥3 of the following risk factors have a >30% 1-yr mortality risk: abnl ECG, h/o ventricular arrhythmias, h/o CHF, age >45 yr.

R. HYPERTENSION

■ JNC 7: nl BP in adults: systolic BP <120 mm Hg and diastolic <80 mm Hg
■ *Prehypertension:* systolic BP 120 to 139 mm Hg or diastolic BP 80 to 89 mm Hg
■ *Stage 1 HTN:* systolic BP 140 to 159 mm Hg or diastolic BP 90 to 99 mm Hg
■ *Stage 2 HTN:* systolic BP ≥160 mm Hg or diastolic BP ≥100 mm Hg

Diagnosis

■ ECG: LVH with strain pattern

Treatment

Lifestyle modifications:

■ Lose weight if overweight (target BMI <25).
■ Limit alcohol intake to 1 oz of ethanol per day (<2 drinks/day) in men or 0.5 oz (<1 drink/day) in women.
■ Perform regular aerobic exercise (at least 30 min/day on most days).
■ Reduce Na^+ intake to <100 mmol/day (<1.5 g of Na^+/day).
■ Maintain adequate dietary K^+ (>3500 mg/day) intake in pts with nl kidney function.
■ Stop smoking.

According to the JNC 7:

■ For pts with pre-HTN and no other complications, recommend lifestyle modifications to prevent progression to sustained HTN.
■ For pts with pre-HTN and DM or CKD, aggressive pharmacologic Rx should be undertaken to reduce BP to <130/80 mm Hg.
■ Antihypertensive drug Rx should be initiated in pts with stage 1 HTN. Thiazide diuretics are preferred for initial Rx unless there are compelling indications to use other agents for initial Rx.
■ Compelling indications for individual drug classes:
  • CHF resulting from systolic dysfunction: ACEIs, ARBs, β-blockers, diuretics, aldosterone antagonists
  • Post MI: β-blockers, ACEIs, aldosterone antagonists
  • High cardiovascular risk: β-blockers, ACEIs, CCBs, diuretics
  • Diabetes: ACEIs, ARBs, CCBs, β-blockers, diuretics
  • Chronic kidney disease: ACEIs, ARBs
  • Recurrent stroke prevention: ACEIs, diuretics
■ A two-drug combination is necessary for most pts with stage 2 HTN. The combination of a diuretic with another agent is preferred unless there is a compelling indication to use other agents.

1 HYPERTENSIVE CRISES

Definition

■ *Malignant HTN:* life-threatening situation secondary to BP. The rate of BP is a critical factor. Clinical manifestations are grade IV hypertensive retinopathy (exudates, hemorrhages, and papilledema), CV or renal compromise, and encephalopathy. It requires immediate BP ↓ (not necessarily to nl ranges) to prevent or to limit target organ disease.
■ *Hypertensive emergencies:* situations that require rapid (within 1 hr) ↓ of BP to avoid end-organ damage
■ *Hypertensive urgencies:* significant BP ↑ that should be corrected within 24 hr of presentation. These situations are not associated w/target organ damage; however, the risk of such damage is high.

Etiology

■ Abrupt ↑ in BP in pts w/chronic HTN
■ Withdrawal from antihypertensive agents (most commonly centrally acting agents and β-agonists)
■ Use of sympathomimetic agents (e.g., cocaine, phencyclidine, amphetamines)
■ Other: renovascular HTN, eclampsia, pheochromocytoma, coarctation of aorta, vasculitis, collagen-vascular disease, acute pyelonephritis, autonomic hyperactivity (e.g., spinal cord syndromes, GBS)

Treatment

■ Choice of therapeutic agent varies w/the cause and manifestation of the hypertensive crisis. Table 3-31 lists medications commonly used in hypertensive emergencies.
■ The initial goal of antihypertensive Rx is not to achieve a *nl* BP but rather to *gradually reduce* the BP. W/exception of pts w/aortic dissection, the initial goal in hypertensive emergencies is to ↓ the MAP by 25% within 2 hr and DBP to <100 mm Hg within 2 to 6 hr.

2 RENAL ARTERY STENOSIS (RAS)

■ Acute RAS (via emboli/in situ thrombosis):
  • Flank or abdominal pain with hematuria (microscopic/gross)
  • Fever, nausea/vomiting
  • ↑ WBC, ↑ AST, ↑ LDH (up to 4× nl), and alk phos

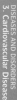

TABLE 3-31 ■ Parenteral Drugs for Treatment of Hypertensive Emergencies

Drug	Dose	Onset of Action	Duration of Action	Adverse Effects*	Special Indications
Vasodilators					
Sodium nitroprusside	0.25-10 μg/kg/min as IV infusion† (max dose for 10 min only)	Immediate	1-2 min	N/V, muscle twitching, sweating, thiocyanate and cyanide intoxication	Most hypertensive emergencies; caution w/high ICP or azotemia
Nicardipine hydrochloride	5-15 mg/hr IV	5-10 min	1-4 hr	Tachycardia, headache, flushing, local phlebitis	Most hypertensive emergencies except acute heart failure; caution w/coronary ischemia
Fenoldopam mesylate	0.1-0.3 μg/kg/min IV infusion	<5 min	30 min	Tachycardia, headache, nausea, flushing	Most hypertensive emergencies; caution w/ glaucoma
Nitroglycerin	5-100 μg/min as IV infusion†	2-5 min	3-5 min	Headache, vomiting, methemoglobinemia, tolerance w/ prolonged use	Coronary ischemia
Enalaprilat	1.25-5 mg q6h IV	15-30 min	6 hr	Precipitous fall in pressure in high-renin states; response variable	Acute left ventricular failure; avoid in acute MI
Hydralazine hydrochloride	10-20 mg IV / 10-50 mg IM	10-20 min / 20-30 min	3-8 hr	Tachycardia, flushing, headache, vomiting, aggravation of angina	Eclampsia
Diazoxide	50-100 mg IV bolus repeated, or 15-30 mg/min infusion	2-4 min	6-12 hr	Nausea, flushing, tachycardia, chest pain	Now obsolete; when no intensive monitoring is available
Adrenergic Inhibitors					
Labetalol hydrochloride	20-80 mg IV bolus q10min, 0.5-2.0 mg/min IV infusion	5-10 min	3-6 hr	Vomiting, scalp tingling, burning in throat, dizziness, nausea, heart block, orthostatic hypotension	Most hypertensive emergencies except acute heart failure
Esmolol hydrochloride	250-500 μg/kg/min for 1 min, then 50-100 μg/kg/min for 4 min; may repeat sequence	1-2 min	10-20 min	Hypotension, nausea	Aortic dissection; perioperative
Phentolamine	5-15 mg IV	1-2 min	3-10 min	Tachycardia, flushing, headache	Catecholamine excess

Modified with permission from Joint National Committee on Prevention, Detection, Evaluation, and Treatment of High Blood Pressure and the National High Blood Pressure Education Program Coordinating Committee: The sixth report of the Joint National Committee on Prevention, Detection, Evaluation, and Treatment of High Blood Pressure. JAMA 289:2560-2572, 2003.

*Hypotension may occur with all agents.
†Requires special delivery system.

- Chronic RAS:
  - Fibromuscular dysplasia: new onset HTN at age <30 yr
  - Atherosclerotic renal artery disease: new-onset HTN at age >55 yr, with risk factors for or evidence of atherosclerotic disease
  - Uncontrolled HTN refractory to ≥3 meds
  - Abdominal bruit (40% of cases)

Diagnosis
- Onset/refractory/accelerated HTN age <30 yr or severe HTN age >55 yr or HTN with end-organ damage (acute renal failure, acute decompensated HF, new visual or neurologic disturbance, and/or retinopathy)
- New AKI or ARF after ACEI/ARB

Labs/Imaging
- CBC, BMP, GFR, UA
- ECG (r/o AF/MI)
- Hypercoagulable w/up in setting of thrombosis or embolic disease
- Duplex U/S, CT angiography, MRA

Treatment
- Acute renal artery thrombosis:
  - Thrombolytics
  - Anticoagulation with BP control
  - Revascularization (endovascular stenting/angioplasty).
- Renal artery thrombosis/emboli: If atrial fibrillation with therapeutic INR, consider INR 2.5 to 3.5.
- Cholesterol emboli: supportive care
- Renal artery stenosis:
  - ACEI/ARBs Rx renovascular HTN
  - β-Blockers Rx HTN in all etiologies of RAS
  - Angioplasty/stent or surgical revascularization reserved for ptw/difficult BP control

3 ECLAMPSIA

Definition
Seizures/coma in setting of preeclampsia

Risks
Multifetal gestation (3.6% in twin gestation), molar pregnancy, nonimmune hydrops fetalis, uncontrolled HTN, preexisting HTN, renal disease

Diagnosis
H&P
- Facial twitching → generalized tonic-clonic state → respiratory cessation → postictal amnesia, agitation, and confusion
- Generalized edema with rapid ↑ wt (>2 lb/wk) may be early sign
- Persistent occipital headache and hyperreflexia with clonus (80% pts)

Labs
- Proteinuria: severe (49%), mild to moderate (29%), absent (22%)
- ↑ Hct, ↓ platelets, ↑ BUN/Cr
- Hyperuricemia: >6.9 mg/dL (70%)
- ABG: maternal acidemia and hypoxia

Treatment
- Fetal resuscitation/HR monitoring, maternal oxygenation with left lateral positioning
- Mg^{2+} sulfate 6 g IV load over 20 min, then 3 g/hr maintenance, for recurrent seizure prophylaxis. If repeated convulsions, may give an additional 2 g IV over 3 to 5 min. Check Mg^{2+} level 1 hr after loading dose, then q6h (therapeutic range 4 to 6 mg/dL). Antidote for toxicity is Ca^{2+} gluconate 10 mL of 10% solution.
- Na^+ amobarbital 250 mg IV over 3 min for persistent seizures.
- Treat BP if >160 mm Hg/110 mm Hg with labetalol 20- to 40-mg IV bolus, hydralazine 10 mg IV, or nifedipine 10 to 20 mg sublingual q20min.
- Phenytoin has been used as an alternative in pts in whom Mg^{2+} sulfate is contraindicated (renal insufficiency, heart block, myasthenia gravis, hypoparathyroidism).

III

DISEASES AND DISORDERS
3. Cardiovascular Disease

4 Dermatology

A. HERPES ZOSTER (SHINGLES)

Diagnosis
- Pain localized to the dermatome that will be affected by the skin lesions → precedes skin manifestation by 3-5 days.
- Rash: erythematous maculopapules affecting one dermatome → maculopapules evolve into vesicles and pustules of various sizes (a distinguishing characteristic from HSV, in which the vesicles are of uniform size) by the 4th day → vesicles subsequently become umbilicated and then form crusts that generally fall off within 3 wk.
- *Ramsay Hunt syndrome:* involvement the trigeminal nerve → painful ear, w/vesicles on the pinna and external auditory canal, facial palsy.

Treatment
- PO antivirals can ↓ acute pain, inflammation, and vesicle formation when Rx is begun within 72 hr of onset of rash. Rx options are (adjust dose for renal failure):
  - Valacyclovir 1000 mg × 7 days
  - Famciclovir 500 mg tid × 7 days
  - Acyclovir 800 mg 5× qd × 7-10 days
- Immunocompromised pts: IV acyclovir 10 mg/kg q8h (infusion over 1 hr) for 7-14 days
- Consider adding prednisone in pts >50 yr old within 72 hr of clinical presentation or if new lesions are still appearing. Initial dose is prednisone 40 mg/day ↓ by 5 mg/day until finished. Corticosteroids ↓ in the use of analgesics and time to resumption of usual activities, but there is no effect on the incidence and duration of postherpetic neuralgia.
- Postherpetic neuralgia Rx:
  - Gabapentin 100-600 mg tid
  - Lidocaine patch 5% applied to intact skin to cover the most painful area for up to 12 hr within a 24-hr period

Vaccination
- Immunocompetent adults ≥50 yr old: single dose of varicella-zoster vaccine (VZV, Zostavax)
- Adults who are VZV sero(–) (never had varicella): immunize w/2 doses of varicella vaccine (Varivax).

B. PRESSURE ULCERS

- **Stage I:** Nonblanchable erythema of intact skin and/or boggy, mushy texture.
- **Stage II:** Partial-thickness skin loss involving the epidermis and/or dermis. May also manifest as an intact or ruptured serum-filled blister.
- **Stage III:** Full-thickness loss/damage or necrosis of subcutaneous tissue that may extend down to underlying fascia/muscle. Possible undermining/tunneling.
- **Stage IV:** Full-thickness skin loss with exposed muscle, bone, or joint capsule. Sloughing or eschar may be present, often with undermining/tunneling.
- **Deep tissue injury:** Purple/maroon localized area of discolored, intact skin or blood-filled blister resulting from damage of underlying tissue from pressure and/or shear.
- **Unstageable:** Full-thickness tissue loss with the base of the ulcer covered by slough or eschar in wound bed.

Treatment
- ↓ Prolonged skin exposure to moisture, urine, or stool. Rx dry, cracking skin.
- Use repositioning and pressure-reducing devices for support while in bed or chair.
- Clean at each dressing change; necrotic tissue should be débrided quickly because it delays wound healing (except for heel ulcers).
- Wound irrigation should not exceed 15 psi; best done with an 18-gauge angiocatheter.

- ↓ Pressure by using foam mattress, dynamic support surface (e.g., low-air loss bed), and frequent repositioning (e.g., q2h or, in cases of poor perfusion, more frequently).
- (–) Pressure devices (Vac devices) help in wounds that have significant drainage.
- Correct poor nutrition through improved diet.

C. PSORIASIS

- Primary psoriatic lesion: erythematous papule topped by a loosely adherent scale. Scraping the scale results in several bleeding points (***Auspitz's sign***).
- Chronic plaque psoriasis (80% cases): symmetric, sharply demarcated, erythematous, silver-scaled patches affect primarily the intergluteal folds, elbows, scalp, fingernails, toenails, and knees.
- Guttate psoriasis: multiple droplike lesions on the extremities and the trunk are usually preceded by strep pharyngitis.
- Psoriasis at the site of any physical trauma (sunburn, scratching) is known as ***Koebner's phenomenon.***
- Joint involvement → sacroiliitis, spondylitis.

Treatment
- Limited disease (<20% of the body):
  - Topical steroids
  - Calcipotriene (vitamin D analogue)
  - Tar products (Estar, LCD, PsoriGel) + UVB light (Goeckerman's regimen)
  - Anthralin + UVB
  - Retinoids (tazarotene 0.05%, 0.1% cream or gel)
  - Others: tape or occlusive dressing, UVB and lubricating agents, and interlesional steroids
- Generalized disease (affecting >20% of the body)
  - UVB light exposure 3x/wk
  - Oral PUVA administered 2-3x/wk
- Systemic Rxs: methotrexate 25 mg/wk, etretinate, cyclosporine, alefacept, etanercept, efalizumab, adalimumab, ustekinumab, briakinumab

5 Endocrinology

A. DIABETES MELLITUS (DM)

Definition
- The American Diabetes Association (ADA) defines DM as follows:
  - FPG ≥126 mg/dL, which should be confirmed with repeat testing on a different day. Fasting is defined as no caloric intake for at least 8 hr.
  - Sx of hyperglycemia and a casual (random) plasma glucose ≥200 mg/dL. Classic sx of hyperglycemia include polyuria, polydipsia, and unexplained weight loss.
  - An OGTT with a plasma glucose ≥200 mg/dL 2 hr after a 75-g (100 g for pregnant women) glucose load
  - HBA_{1c} ≥6.5%
- **Prediabetes:** glucose levels > nl but not high enough to meet the criteria for dx DM
  - Impaired fasting glucose: FBS 100 to 125 mg/dL
  - Impaired glucose tolerance: after OGTT, a 2-hr plasma glucose 140 to 199 mg/dL
  - HBA_{1c} value 5.7% to 6.4%
- Table 5-1 describes diagnostic categories for diabetes mellitus and at-risk states.

PE

Diabetic Retinopathy
- a. Nonproliferative (background diabetic retinopathy)
  - i. Initially: microaneurysms, capillary dilation, waxy or hard exudates, dot and flame hemorrhages, atrioventricular shunts
  - ii. Advanced stage: microinfarcts with cotton wool exudates, macular edema
- b. Proliferative retinopathy: formation of new vessels, vitreous hemorrhages, fibrous scarring, and retinal detachment

Diabetic Neuropathy
- a. Distal sensorimotor polyneuropathy
  - i. Sx: paresthesia, hyperesthesia, or burning pain involving bilateral distal extremities, in a "stocking-glove" distribution. It can progress to motor weakness and ataxia.
  - ii. PE: ↓ pinprick sensation, sensation to light touch, vibration sense, and loss of proprioception. ↓ DTRs and atrophy of interossei muscles can also be seen.
- b. Autonomic neuropathy
  - i. GI: esophageal motility abnlities, gastroparesis, diarrhea (usually nocturnal)
  - ii. GU: neurogenic bladder (hesitancy, weak stream, and dribbling), impotence
  - iii. Orthostatic hypotension: postural syncope, dizziness, lightheadedness
- c. Polyradiculopathy: painful weakness and atrophy in the distribution of ≥1 contiguous nerve roots
- d. Mononeuropathy involving cranial nerves III, IV, or VI or peripheral nerves

Diabetic Nephropathy
Pts have pedal edema, pallor, weakness, uremic appearance.

Foot Ulcers
They occur in 15% of individuals with DM (incidence rate, 2%/yr) → leading causes of hospitalization and amputation in U.S. They result from combination of PVD, repeated trauma (unrecognized because of sensory loss), and superimposed infection.
- a. Sx: less than would be expected from clinical findings, resulting from loss of sensation related to peripheral neuropathy
- b. Dx: assessment of pedal pulses, sensation (using a 10-g monofilament)
- c. Prevention: strict glucose control, pt education, prescription footwear, podiatric care, evaluation for surgical interventions

Neuropathic Arthropathy (Charcot's Joints)
Bone or joint deformities result from repeated trauma (secondary to peripheral neuropathy).

Necrobiosis Lipoidica Diabeticorum
Plaquelike reddened areas with a central area that fades to white yellow are found on the anterior surfaces of the legs.

TABLE 5-1 ■ General Comparison of the Two Types of Diabetes Mellitus

	Type 1	Type 2
Previous terminology	Insulin-dependent diabetes mellitus (IDDM), type I, juvenile-onset diabetes	Non–insulin-dependent diabetes mellitus, type II, adult-onset diabetes
Age at onset	Usually <30 yr, particularly childhood and adolescence, but any age	Usually >40 yr, but any age
Genetic predisposition	Moderate; environmental factors required for expression; 35%-50% concordance in monozygotic twins; several candidate genes proposed	Strong; 6%-90% concordance in monozygotic twins; many candidate genes proposed; some genes identified in maturity-onset diabetes of the young
Human leukocyte antigen associations	Linkage to DQA and DQB, influenced by DRB (3 and 4) (DR2 protective)	None known
Other associations	Autoimmune; Graves' disease, Hashimoto's thyroiditis, vitiligo, Addison's disease, pernicious anemia	Heterogeneous group, ongoing subclassification based on identification of specific pathogenic processes and genetic defects
Precipitating and risk factors	Largely unknown; microbial, chemical, dietary, other	Age, obesity (central), sedentary lifestyle, previous gestational diabetes
Findings at diagnosis	85%-90% of patients have one and usually more autoantibodies to ICA512/Ia-2/IA-2β, GAD65, insulin (IAA)	Possibly complications (microvascular or macrovascular) caused by significant preceding asymptomatic period
Endogenous insulin levels	Low or absent	Usually present (relative deficiency), early hyperinsulinemia
Insulin resistance	Only with hyperglycemia	Mostly present
Prolonged fast	Hyperglycemia, ketoacidosis	Euglycemia
Stress, withdrawal of insulin	Ketoacidosis	Nonketotic hyperglycemia, occasionally ketoacidosis

From Andreoli TE (ed): Cecil Essentials of Medicine, 6th ed. Philadelphia, Saunders, 2005.

GAD, glutamic acid decarboxylase; IA-2/IA-2β, tyrosine phosphatases; IAA, insulin autoantibodies; ICA, islet cell antibody; ICA512, islet cell autoantigen 512 (fragment of IA-2).

DETECTION AND DX OF GESTATIONAL DM (GDM)
■ OGTT
■ Women with GDM should be screened for diabetes 6 to 12 wk post partum.

Lab Screening in Diabetics
■ Screening for diabetic retinopathy: Alb/Cr ratio (microalb) in a random spot urine collection or by 24-hr urine collection for alb, CrCl
■ Dx of microalbuminuria (30-299 mg/24 hr) should be based on 2 to 3 ↑ levels within a 3- to 6-mo period because of marked variability in day-to-day alb excretion
■ Labs in DM: HBA₁c, urine microalbumin, fasting lipid panel, serum Cr, and electrolytes; TSH, vitamin B₁₂ level, IgA TTG Ab (for celiac disease screen) in type 1 DM
■ Daily monitoring with glucose test strips: type 1 DM and pregnant women on insulin ≥3 ×/day. T2 DM not on insulin, 1-2×/day

Treatment
ADA and European Association for the Study of Diabetes recommend: "Intervention at the time of Dx with metformin in combination with life style changes (diet and exercise) and continuing timely augmentation of Rx with additional agents (including early initiation of insulin Rx) as a means of achieving adequate glycemic control
1. *Diet*
   a. Calories
      i. Start with 15 calories/lb of ideal body weight; ↑ 20 calories/lb for an active person and 25 calories/lb if the pt does heavy physical labor.
      ii. The calories are distributed as 45% to 65% carbohydrates; <30% fat, with saturated fat limited to <7% of total calories; and 10% to 30% protein; daily cholesterol <300 mg.
      iii. The emphasis should be on complex carbohydrates rather than simple and refined starches and on polyunsaturated instead of saturated fats in a ratio of 2:1.

iv. The **glycemic index** compares the ↑ in blood sugar after the ingestion of simple sugars and complex carbohydrates with the ↑ that occurs after the absorption of.
2. *Exercise:* Exercise program must be individualized and built up slowly. Consider beginning with 15 min of low-impact aerobic exercise 3 ×/wk and increasing the frequency and duration to 30 to 45 min of moderate aerobic activity (50% to 70% of maximum age predicted heart rate) to 3 to 5 days/wk. In the absence of contraindications, resistance training 3 ×/wk should be encouraged.
3. *Weight loss:* to ideal body weight if the pt is overweight
   - Maintain HbA$_{1c}$ <7%. HbA$_{1c}$ 7.5 or higher may be reasonable in elderly pts with limited life expectancy and ↑ risk of hypoglycemia.
   - When the previous measures fail, oral hypoglycemic agents (Table 5-2) should be added to the regimen in type 2 DM. If renal function is not significantly impaired (creat < 1.3), metformin is the preferred initial hypoglycemic agent. GLP-1 agonists and dipeptidyl peptidase-4 inhibitions are preferred as additional oral hypoglycemics but cost is a limiting factor, especially in elderly patients.
   - Insulin: indicated for all pts with type 1 DM and for pts with type 2 DM whose condition cannot be adequately controlled with diet and oral agents. Insulin Rx may be started with oral agents at 0.3 unit/kg, or as replacement, starting at 0.6 to 1 unit/kg. Table 5-3 describes commonly used types of insulin.
     a. The risks of insulin Rx include weight gain, hypoglycemia, and in rare cases, allergic or cutaneous reactions.
     b. Replacement insulin Rx should mimic nl release patterns.
       i. 50% to 60% of daily insulin can be given as a long-acting insulin (NPH, ultralente, glargine, detemir) injected qd or bid.
       ii. 40% to 50% can be short-acting (regular) or rapid-acting (lispro, aspart, glulisine) to cover mealtime carbohydrates and correct ↑ current glucose levels.
   - Continuous subcutaneous insulin infusion (CSII, or insulin pump) provides better glycemic control than does conventional Rx. It should be considered for DM in childhood or adolescence and during pregnancy.
   - The Diabetes Control and Complications Trial (DCCT) showed that intensive Rx for glucose control ↓ the development and progression of complications of type 1 DM. In this trial, the risks for retinopathy, nephropathy, and neuropathy were ↓ by 70%, 54%, and 64%, respectively.
   - Low-dose aspirin (ASA; 81 mg/day): for primary prevention in diabetic pts with one additional CV risk factor, including age >40 yr, cigarette smoking, HTN, obesity, albuminuria, hyperlipidemia, and family hx of CAD
   - Statins: DM >40 yr with ≥1 risk factor for CAD; LDL goal <100 mg/dL, <70 mg/dL if overt CAD
   - BP control: SBP <130 DBP <80 mm Hg. Use ACEI to ↓ albuminuria and prevent CKD regardless of presence of HTN.
   - Bariatric surgery: consider in adults with BMI >35 kg/m^2 and type 2 diabetes
   - Hypoglycemia Rx: conscious person → glucose tab or gel 15 to 20 g; unconscious → IM glucagon
   - Neuropathy Rx: duloxetine, pregabalin, gabapentin
   - Diabetic gastroparesis Rx: endoscopic injection of botulinum toxin into the pylorus and gastric electrical stimulation (using f electrodes placed laparoscopically in the muscle wall of the stomach antrum and connected to a neurostimulator)
   - Nephropathy: ACEIs or ARBs (if intolerant to ACEIs)
   - Glycemic control in hospitalized pts: Avoid intensive insulin Rx. The ACP recommends a target blood glucose level of 140 to 200 mg/dL if insulin Rx is used. Table 5-4 describes an insulin sliding scale.

1 DIABETIC KETOACIDOSIS

Metabolic decompensation in diabetic pts usually precipitated by an infectious process (≤40% of cases). Poor compliance w/insulin Rx and severe medical illness (e.g., CVA, MI) are other common causes. Consider cocaine abuse in middle age DM w/multiple DKA admissions.

Diagnosis
PE

- Evidence of dehydration (tachycardia, hypotension, dry mucous membranes, sunken eyeballs, poor skin turgor)
- Clouding of mental status
- Tachypnea w/air hunger (Kussmaul's respiration)
- Fruity breath odor (caused by acetone)

TABLE 5-2 ■ Oral Antidiabetic Agents and Monotherapy

	Sulfonylureas	Biguanides	α-Glucosidase Inhibitors	Incretin Mimetics	Megitinides	Dipeptidyl Peptidase-4 Inhibitor
Generic name	Glimepiride, glyburide, glipizide, chlorpropamide, tolbutamide	Metformin	Acarbose, miglitol	Exanatide, liraglutide	Repaglinide, nateglinide	Sitagliptin, inagliptin, saxagliptin
Mode of action	↑↑ Pancreatic insulin secretion chronically	↓↓HGP, ↓ peripheral IR, ↓ intestinal glucose absorption	Delays PP digestion of carbohydrates and absorption of glucose	↑ Insulin secretion	↑↑ Pancreatic insulin secretion acutely	Potentiates insulin synthesis and release
Preferred patient type	Diagnosis age >30 yr, lean, diabetes <5 yr, insulinopenic	Overweight, IR, fasting hyper-glycemia, dyslipidemia	PP hyperglycemia	Type 2 DM	PP hyperglycemia, insulinopenic	
Therapeutic effects						
↓ HBA1c * (%)	1-2	1-2	0.5-1	↓HBA1c by 0.7 -0.9	1-2	↓ HBA1c by 0.5%
↓ FPC* (mg/dL)	50-70	50-80	15-30		40-80	
↓ PPC* (mg/dL)	≈90	80	40-50		30	
Insulin levels	↑	—	—		↑	
Weight	↑	↓↓	—		↑	
Lipids	—	↓ LDL ↓↑TG	—		—	
Side effects	Hypoglycemia	Diarrhea, lactic acidosis	Abdominal pain, flatulence, diarrhea	Nausea, headache, diarrhea	Hypoglycemia (low risk)	
Dose(s)/day	1-3	2-3	1-3	Variable from daily to weekly	1-4+	1
Maximum daily dose (mg)	Depends on agent	2550	150 (<60-kg BW) 300 (>60-kg BW)		16 (repaglinide) 360 (nateglinide)	100
Range/dose (mg)	Depends on agent	500-1000	25-50 (<60-kg BW) 25-100 (>60-kg BW)		0.5-4 (repaglinide) 60, 120 (nateglinide)	50-100
Optimal administration time	≈30 min premeal (some with food, others on empty stomach)	With meal	With first bite of meal		Preferably <15 (0-30 min) before meals (omit if no meal)	
Main site of metabolism/excretion	Hepatic/renal, fecal	Not metabolized/renal	Only 2% absorbed/fecal	Renal	Hepatic/fecal	

From Andreoli TE (ed): Cecil Essentials of Medicine, 6th ed. Philadelphia, Saunders, 2005.

HGP, Hepatic glucose production; *IR*, insulin resistance; *PP*, postprandial; *PPC*, postprandial plasma glucose.

*Values combined from numerous studies; values are also dose dependent.

TABLE 5-3 ■ Types of Insulin

Preparation	Brand	Onset (hr)	Peak (hr)	Duration (hr)	Route
Insulin aspart	NovoLog[†]	<0.25	1-3	3-5	SC
Insulin aspart prot-amine/insulin aspart	NovoLog Mix 70/30[†]	<0.25	1-4	24	SC
Insulin detemir	Levemir[‡]	1	None	24	SC
Insulin glargine	Lantus[†]	1.1	None	≥24	SC
Insulin glulisine	Apidra[†]	≤0.25	1	2-4	SC, IV[§]
Insulin lispro	Humalog[†]	<0.25	1	3.5-4.5	SC
Insulin lispro prot-amine/insulin lispro	Humalog Mix 75/25[†]	≤0.25	0.5-1.5	24	SC
	Humalog Mix 50/50[†]	≤0.25	1	16	SC
Insulin injection regular (R)	Humulin R[*]	0.5	2-4	6-8	SC, IM, IV
	Novolin R[‡]	0.5	2.5-5	8	SC, IM, IV
Insulin isophane suspension (NPH)/regular insulin (R)	Humulin 70/30[*]	0.5	2-12	24	SC
	Humulin 50/50[*]	0.5	3-5	24	SC
	Novolin 70/30[‡]	0.5	2-12	24	SC
Insulin isophane suspension (NPH)	Humulin N[*]	1-2	6-12	18-24	SC
	Novolin N[‡]	1.5	4-12	24	SC

From Ferri FF: Ferri's Clinical Advisor 2010. Philadelphia, Mosby, 2010.

Injectable insulins listed are available in a concentration of 100 units/mL; Humulin R, in a concentration of 500 unit/mL for SC injection only, is available by prescription from Lilly for insulin-resistant patients who are hospitalized or under close medical supervision.

[*]Recombinant (using *E. coli*).
[†]Recombinant human insulin analogue (using *E. coli*).
[‡]Recombinant (using *S. cerevisiae*).
[§]IV to be used in a clinical setting under proper medical supervision.

TABLE 5-4 ■ Regular Insulin (SC) Sliding Scale

Finger Stick Blood Glucose	Mild Scale	Moderate Scale	Aggressive Scale
<60	1 amp (25 g) D50 or orange juice, call MD	1 amp D50 or orange juice, call MD	1 amp D50 or orange juice, call MD
60-150	No insulin	No insulin	No insulin
151-200	No insulin	3 units	4 units
201-250	2 units	5 units	6 units
251-300	4 units	7 units	10 units
301-350	6 units	9 units	12 units
351-400	8 units	11 units	15 units
>400	10 units, call physician	13 units, call physician	18 units, call physician

From Nguyen TC, Abilez OJ (eds): Practical Guide to the Care of the Surgical Patient: The Pocket Scalpel. Philadelphia, Mosby, 2009.

- Lipemia retinalis in some pts
- Possible evidence of precipitating factors (infected wound, pneumonia)
- Abd tenderness in some pts

Labs

- Glucose level is generally >250 mg/dL; urine and serum ketones (+) (usually 7-10 mmol/L).
- ABGs reveal acidosis: arterial pH usually <7.30 w/Pco_2 >40 mm Hg.
- Serum electrolytes:
  - Serum bicarbonate is usually <18 mEq/L.
  - Serum K^+: may be ↓, nl, or ↑. There is always significant total body K^+ depletion regardless of the K^+ level.
  - Serum Na^+: usually ↓ (pseudohyponatremia) as a result of ↑↑ glucose, dehydration, and lipemia. Assume 1.6 mEq/L ↓ in extracellular Na^+ for each 100 mg/dL↑ in glucose.
  - Calculate the AG: AG = $Na^+ - (Cl^- + HCO_3^-)$.
  - In DKA, the AG is ↑ (generally >15); hyperchloremic metabolic acidosis may be present in unusual circumstances when both the GFR and the plasma volume are well maintained.

Adult patient with DKA or HHS

Complete initial evaluation, including (but not limited to):
Medical history and physical examination
Complete blood count with differential
Fingerstick blood glucose
Serum chemistries ("Chem-10" plus serum ketones)
Urine for urinalysis and ketones
Cultures as indicated (wound, blood, urine, etc.)
Chest ± abdominal x-ray
12-lead ECG

Concurrently, begin empirical fluid resuscitation with 0.9% NaCl at 1000 mL/hr
Consider volume expanders if hypovolemic shock is present
Continue fluid resuscitation until volume status and cardiovascular parameters (pulse, BP) have been restored

IV Fluids
Based on corrected serum sodium*
If high/normal, use 0.45% NaCl
If low/normal, use 0.9% NaCl
Continue IV fluids at 250–1000 mL/hr, depending on volume status, cardiovascular history, and cardiovascular status (pulse, BP)

Insulin Therapy
Regular insulin bolus, 0.15 U/kg
IV infusion, 0.10 U/kg/hr
Check serum glucose hourly—should fall by 50–80 mg/dL/hr

If serum glucose falling too rapidly, back off on insulin infusion
If serum glucose rising or falling too slowly, increase insulin infusion rate by 50–100%

Continuing Management:
Follow and replete serum electrolytes (including divalent cations) q2–4h until stable
After resolution of hyperglycemic state, follow blood glucose q4h and initiate sliding scale regular insulin coverage
Convert IV insulin to subcutaneous injections (or resumption of prior therapy), ensuring adequate overlap
Begin clear liquid diet and advance as tolerated. Encourage resumption of ambulation and activity
Review and update diabetes education, with special attention to prevention of further hyperglycemic crises

When serum glucose reaches 250–300 mg/dL:
For DKA, add dextrose to IV fluids and reduce insulin infusion, adjusted to maintain serum glucose ~200 mg/dL until anion gap has closed
For HHS, continue IV fluids but may reduce insulin infusion until plasma osmolality drops below 310 mOsm/kg
Begin more exhaustive search for precipitant of metabolic decompensation

Potassium (K$^+$) Repletion
Obtain baseline serum potassium; Obtain 12-lead ECG

[K$^+$] ≥5.5 mEq/L
↓
Hold K$^+$ therapy
↓
Treat hyperkalemia if ECG changes present
↓
Recheck [K$^+$] in 2 hr

[K$^+$] <5.5 mEq/L and adequate urine output
Add K$^+$ to IV fluids (use KCl and/or KPhos)
[K$^+$] = 4.5 – 5.4: add 20 mEq/L IV fluids
[K$^+$] = 3.5 – 4.4: add 30 mEq/L IV fluids
[K$^+$] <3.5: add 40 mEq/L IV fluids

Follow serum [K$^+$] every 2–4 hours until stable: anticipate rapid drop of serum [K$^+$] during therapy, due to dilution and intracellular shifting
Ensure adequate urine output to avoid over-repletion and hyperkalemia
Continue K$^+$ repletion until serum [K$^+$] is stable at 4–5 mEq/L
If refractory hypokalemia, ensure concurrent magnesium repletion
Repletion may need to be continued for several days, as total body losses may reach up to 500 mEq

Bicarbonate Therapy   Obtain ABG; Obtain baseline serum bicarbonate

pH <6.9	6.9≤pH <7.0	pH ≥7.0
100 mEq (2 amps) NaHCO$_3$ over 2 hr	50 mEq (1 amp) NaHCO$_3$ over 1 hr	Bicarbonate therapy usually not necessary

Repeat ABG after bicarbonate administration
Repeat NaHCO$_3$ therapy until pH ≥7.0, then discontinue therapy
Follow serum bicarbonate q4h until stable

*Sodium correction: Serum sodium should be corrected for hyperglycemia. For every 100 mg/dL of glucose elevation above 100 mg/dL, add 1.6 mEq/L to the measured sodium value; this will yield the corrected serum sodium concentration.

FIGURE 5-1. Management of DKA and HHS. (From Goldman L, Schafer AI [eds]: Goldman's Cecil Medicine, 24th ed. Philadelphia, Saunders, 2012.)

- CBC w/diff, U/A, urine and blood cultures to r/o infectious precipitating factor
- Serum Ca^{2+}, Mg^{2+}, and PO_4^{-3}; plasma PO_4^{-3} and Mg^{2+} levels may be significantly depressed and should be rechecked within 24 hr because they may ↓ further w/correction of DKA.
- ↑ BUN and Cr secondary to significant dehydration
- Amylase, LFTs should be checked in pts w/abd pain.

Imaging
CXR is helpful to r/o infectious process. The initial CXR may be nl if the pt has significant dehydration. Repeat CXR after 24 hr if pulmonary infection is strongly suspected.

Treatment
- Fluid replacement (the usual deficit is 6-8 L), insulin Rx, electrolyte replacement
- Consider bicarbonate Rx (Fig. 5-1).

2 HYPEROSMOLAR NON-KETOTIC COMA, HONK

Definition
This is a state of extreme hyperglycemia, marked dehydration, serum hyperosmolarity, mental status changes, and absence of ketoacidosis.

Etiology
- Infections, 20% to 25% (e.g., pneumonia, UTI, sepsis)
- New or previously unrecognized diabetes (30%-50%)
- Reduction or omission of diabetic medication
- Stress (MI, CVA)
- Drugs: diuretics (dehydration), phenytoin, diazoxide (impaired insulin secretion)

Diagnosis
H&P
- Evidence of extreme dehydration (poor skin turgor, sunken eyeballs, dry mucous membranes)
- Neurologic defects (reversible hemiplegia, focal seizures)
- Orthostatic hypotension, tachycardia
- Evidence of precipitating factors (pneumonia, infected skin ulcer)
- Coma (25% of pts), delirium

Labs
- Hyperglycemia: serum glucose usually >600 mg/dL
- Hyperosmolarity: serum osmolarity usually >340 mOsm/L
- Serum Na^+: may be ↓, nl, or ↑; if nl or ↑, the pt is severely dehydrated because glucose draws fluid from intracellular space = ↓ serum Na^+; the corrected Na^+ can be obtained by the serum Na^+ concentration by ↑ 1.6 mEq/dL for every 100 mg/dL ↓ in the serum glucose level above nl.
- Serum K^+: may be ↓, nl, or ↑; regardless of the initial serum level, the total body deficit is approximately 5 to 15 mEq/kg.
- Serum bicarbonate: usually >12 mEq/L
- Arterial pH: usually >7.2 (average is 7.26). Both serum bicarbonate and arterial pH may be lower if lactic acidosis is present.
- ↑ BUN: Azotemia (prerenal) is usually present (BUN generally ranges from 60-90 mg/dL).
- ↓ PO_4^{-3}: hypophosphatemia (average deficit is 70-140 mM)
- ↓ Ca^{2+}: hypocalcemia (average deficit is 50-100 mEq)
- ↓ Mg^{2+}: hypomagnesemia (average deficit is 50-100 mEq)
- CBC w/diff, U/A, blood and urine cultures should be performed to r/o infectious etiology.

Treatment
- Vigorous IV fluid replacement, electrolyte replacement, insulin Rx (see Fig. 5-1)

B. HYPOGLYCEMIA

Definition
Hypoglycemia can be arbitrarily defined as a plasma glucose level <50 mg/dL. To establish the dx, the following 3 criteria are necessary:
- Presence of sx
  - Adrenergic: sweating, anxiety, tremors, tachycardia, palpitations
  - Neuroglycopenic: seizures, fatigue, syncope, headache, behavior changes, visual disturbances, hemiplegia
- ↓ Plasma glucose level in symptomatic pt
- Relief of sx after ingestion of carbohydrates

Etiology

- Reactive hypoglycemia
  - Hypoglycemia usually occurs 2 to 4 hr after a meal rich in carbohydrates.
  - These pts never have sx in the fasting state and rarely experience loss of consciousness secondary to their hypoglycemia.
  - Pts who have had subtotal gastrectomy rapidly absorb carbohydrates. This causes an early plasma glucose level followed by a late insulin surge that reaches its peak when most of the glucose has been absorbed and that results in hypoglycemia.
  - Pts with type 2 (non–insulin-dependent) diabetes can experience hypoglycemia 3 to 4 hr postprandially secondary to a delayed and prolonged second phase of insulin secretion.
  - Congenital deficiencies of enzymes necessary for carbohydrate metabolism and functional (idiopathic) hypoglycemia are additional causes of reactive hypoglycemia.
- Fasting hypoglycemia
  - Sx usually appear in the absence of food intake (at night or during early morning).
  - Etiology: insulinoma, mesenchymal tumors that synthesize insulin-like hormones, adrenal failure, glycogen storage disorders, severe liver disease or renal disease
- Iatrogenic or drug-induced: hypoglycemic drugs, excessive insulin replacement, factitious, ethanol-induced hypoglycemia

Diagnosis

- When the plasma glucose level is ↓ (e.g., fasting state), the plasma insulin level should also be ↓. Any pt presenting w/fasting hypoglycemia of unexplained cause should have the following tests drawn during the hypoglycemic episode (Table 5-5):
  - Plasma glucose
  - Plasma insulin level
  - Plasma C-peptide
  - Plasma and urine metabolites of sulfonylurea levels and meglitinides
- Factitious hypoglycemia should be considered, especially if the pt has ready access to insulin or oral hypoglycemic agents (e.g., medical or paramedical personnel, family members who are diabetic or in the medical profession).
- Pancreatic islet cell neoplasms (insulinomas) are usually small (<3 cm), single, insulin-producing adenomas. Measurement of inappropriately serum insulin levels despite ↓ plasma glucose level after prolonged fasting (24-72 ↑ hr) is pathognomonic of these neoplasms.

TABLE 5-5 ■ Hypoglycemia in Nondiabetic Pt. Laboratory Differentiation of Factitious Hypoglycemia and Insulinoma

Lab	Insulinoma	Exogenous Insulin	Oral Hypoglycemic Agents (Sulfonylurea/Meglitinides)
Plasma glucose	↓	↓	↓
Serum insulin	↑	↑↑	↑
Plasma and urine sulfonylureas/meglitinides	Absent	Absent	Present
C-peptide	↑	N/↓	↑

Treatment

- Variable, depending on etiology of hypoglycemia

C. ANTERIOR PITUITARY DISORDERS

1 HYPOPITUITARISM

Partial or complete loss of secretion of one or more pituitary hormones results from diseases of the hypothalamus or pituitary gland.

Etiology

Hypopituitarism is the result of destruction of pituitary cells caused by

- Pituitary tumors
  - Macroadenomas >10 mm
  - Microadenomas ≤10 mm
- Pituitary apoplexy caused by hemorrhage or infarct on of the pituitary gland
- Pituitary radiation Rx
- Pituitary surgery

- **Empty sella syndrome** w/enlargement of the sella turcica and flattening of the pituitary gland (from extension of the subarachnoid space and filling of CSF into the sella turcica)
- Infiltrative disease including sarcoidosis, hemochromatosis, histiocytosis X, Wegener's granulomatosis, and lymphocytic hypophysitis
- Infection (TB, mycosis, and syphilis)
- Head trauma
- Internal carotid artery aneurysm

Diagnosis

H&P

Sx are related to the lack of one or more hormones or mass effect.
- Mass effect → headaches, visual field disturbances
- Corticotropin deficiency
  - Fatigue and weakness
  - Hypotension, hair loss
- Thyrotropin deficiency
  - Fatigue and weakness, weight gain, cold intolerance, constipation
  - Bradycardia, ↓ DTR, pretibial edema, hair loss
- Gonadotropin deficiency
  - Loss of libido, erectile dysfunction, amenorrhea, hot flashes, dyspareunia, infertility
  - Gynecomastia w/lack of hair growth and ↓ muscle mass
- GH deficiency
  - Growth retardation in children
  - Fatigue, hypoglycemia
  - ↓ Muscle mass, obesity
- Hyperprolactinemia
  - Galactorrhea
  - Hypogonadism
- Vasopressin deficiency
  - Polyuria, polydipsia
  - Hypotension, dehydration

Baseline Labs
- Corticotropin deficiency:
  - ↓ Serum AM cortisol level (<3 g/dL)
- Thyrotropin deficiency:
  - TSH and free T_4 measurements
  - Primary hypothyroidism: ↑ TSH, ↓ free T_4
  - Secondary hypothyroidism: nl/↑ TSH, ↓ free T_4
- Gonadotropin deficiency:
  - FSH, LH, estrogen, and testosterone measurements
  - In men ↓ testosterone levels, nl/↓ FSH and LH levels
  - In premenopausal women w/amenorrhea, ↓ estrogen w/nl/↓ FSH and LH levels
- GH deficiency:
  - ↓ Serum IGF-1

Provocative testing for pituitary insufficiency is summarized in Table 5-6.

Imaging
- MRI of pituitary

Treatment

- Hormone replacement Rx and surgery, irradiation, or medications in pts w/ pituitary tumors
- Acute situations such as adrenal crisis and myxedema coma are discussed separately.
- Long-term Rx: lifelong and requires the following hormone replacement Rx:
  - ACTH deficiency: hydrocortisone 20 mg PO q AM and 10 mg PO q PM or prednisone 5 mg PO q AM and 2.5 mg PO q PM. Dexamethasone or prednisone is often preferred because of longer duration of action.
  - LH and FSH deficiency:
    - In men, testosterone replacement
    - In women who are not interested in fertility, conjugated estrogen 0.3 to 1.25 mg/day and held the last 5 to 7 days of each month w/the addition of medroxyprogesterone 10 mg/day given during days 15 to 25 of the nl menstrual cycle. In those who have secondary hypogonadism and wish to become pregnant, pulsatile GnRH may be of benefit.

TABLE 5-6 ■ Tests of Pituitary Insufficiency

Hormone	Test	Interpretation
Growth hormone (GH)	Insulin tolerance test: Regular insulin (0.05-0.15 U/kg) is given IV and blood drawn at −30, 0, 30, 45, 60, and 90 min for measurement of glucose and GH.	If hypoglycemia occurs (glucose <40 mg/dL), GH should increase to >5 μg/L.
	Arginine-GHRH test: GHRH 1 μg/kg IV bolus followed by 30-min infusion of l-arginine (30 g)	Normal response is GH > 4.1 μg/L.
	Glucagon test: 1 mg IM with GH measurements at 0, 60, 90, 120, 150 and 180 min	Normal response is GH >3 μg/L.
Adrenocorticotropic hormone (ACTH)	Insulin tolerance test: Regular insulin (0.05-0.15 U/kg) is given IV and blood is drawn at −30, 0, 30, 45, 60, and 90 min for measurement of glucose and cortisol.	If hypoglycemia occurs (glucose <40 mg/dL), cortisol should increase by >7 μg/dL or to >20 μg/dL.
	CRH test: 1 μg/kg ovine CRH IV at 8 am with blood samples drawn at 0, 15, 30, 60, 90, 120 min for measurement of ACTH and cortisol	In most normal individuals, the basal ACTH increases twofold to fourfold and reaches a peak (20-100 pg/mL). ACTH responses may be delayed in cases of hypothalamic dysfunction. Cortisol levels usually reach 20-25 μg/dL.
	Metyrapone test: Metyrapone (30 mg/kg to max 2 g) at midnight with measurements of plasma 11-deoxycortisol and cortisol at 8 am. ACTH can also be measured. A 3-day test is also available. Basal cortisol should be >5-6 μg/dL before test.	A normal response is 11-deoxycortisol >7.5 μg/dL or ACTH >75 pg/mL. Plasma cortisol should fall below 4 μg/dL to ensure an adequate response.
	ACTH stimulation test: ACTH 1-24 (cosyntropin), 0.25 mg IM or IV. Cortisol is measured at 0, 30, and 60 min.	A normal response is cortisol >18 μg/dL. In suspected hypothalamic-pituitary deficiency, a low-dose (1-μg) test may be more sensitive.
Thyroid-stimulating hormone (TSH)	Basal thyroid function tests: free T4, free T3, TSH	Low free thyroid hormone levels in the setting of TSH levels that are not appropriately increased.
Luteinizing hormone (LH), follicle-stimulating hormone (FSH)	Basal levels of LH, FSH, testosterone, estrogen	Basal LH and FSH should be increased in postmenopausal women. Low testosterone levels in conjunction with low or low-normal LH and FSH are consistent with gonadotropin deficiency.
	GnRH test: GnRH (100 μg) IV with measurements of serum LH and FSH at 0, 30, and 60 min	In most normal persons, LH should increase by 10 IU/L and FSH by 2 IU/L. Normal responses are variable, and repeated stimulation may be required.
	Clomiphene test: Clomiphene citrate (100 mg) is given orally for 5 days. Serum LH and FSH are measured on days 0, 5, 7, 10, and 13.	A 50% increase should occur in LH and FSH, usually by day 5.
Multiple hormones	Combined anterior pituitary test: GHRH (1 μg/kg), CRH (1 μg/kg), GnRH (100 μg) are given sequentially IV. Blood samples are drawn at −30, 15, 30, 60, 90, and 120 min for measurements of GH, ACTH, LH, and FSH.	Combined or individual releasing hormone responses must be evaluated in the context of basal hormone values and may not be diagnostic (see text).

From Goldman L, Schafer AI (eds): Goldman's Cecil Medicine, 24th ed. Philadelphia, Saunders, 2012.

*Values are with polyclonal assays.

- TSH deficiency: levothyroxine 0.05 to 0.15 mg/day
- GH deficiency: GH is generally not used in adults; however, it can be given at 0.04 to 0.08 mg/kg/day SC in children.
- ADH deficiency: Desmopressin (DDAVP) 10 to 20 μg by intranasal spray or 0.05 to 0.1 mg PO bid is used in pts w/DI.

- Pituitary adenomas are classified by their size (macroadenomas ≥10 mm) and function
  - GH→ acromegaly
  - PRL→ prolactinoma
  - ACTH→ Cushing's disease

H&P

Prolactinomas

- Females: galactorrhea, amenorrhea, oligomenorrhea with anovulation, infertility
- Estrogen deficiency leading to hirsutism, ↓ vaginal lubrication, osteopenia
- Males: ↓ libido or hypogonadism

GH-Secreting Pituitary Adenoma: Acromegaly

- Coarse facial features, oily skin, prognathism, carpal tunnel syndrome
- Osteoarthritis, hx of ↑ hat, glove, or shoe size, visual field deficits

Corticotropin-Secreting Pituitary Adenoma: Cushing's Disease

- Truncal obesity, round facies (moon face)
- Dorsocervical fat accumulation (buffalo hump), hirsutism, acne, menstrual disorders
- HTN, striae, bruising, thin skin, hyperglycemia

Thyrotropin-Secreting Pituitary Adenoma

- Sx: thyrotoxicosis, goiter, visual impairment

Diagnosis

Prolactinoma

- ↑ PRL levels are correlated with tumor size.
- Level >200 ng/mL is diagnostic, with levels of 100 to 200 ng/mL being equivocal.

Acromegaly

- First screening tests are the measurement of serum IGF-1 ↑, postprandial serum GH, and TRH stimulation test.
- Follow with an OGTT.
- Failure to suppress serum GH to <2 ng/mL with an oral load of 100 g glucose is considered conclusive.
- A GH-releasing hormone level >300 ng/mL is indicative of an ectopic source of GH.

Cushing's Disease

- Nl or slightly ↑ corticotropin levels ranging from 20 to 200 pg/mL
- Level <10 pg/mL usually indicates an autonomously secreting adrenal tumor.
- Level >200 pg/mL suggests an ectopic corticotropin-secreting neoplasm.
- Cushing's disease can be assessed by absence of cortisol suppression with the low-dose dexamethasone test but with the presence of cortisol suppression after the high-dose test.
- 24-hr urine collection should demonstrate an ↑ level of cortisol excretion.

Thyrotropin-Secreting Pituitary Adenoma

- Highly sensitive thyrotropin assays, which evaluate the presence of thyrotoxicosis, are among the ways to detect a thyrotropin-secreting tumor.
- Free α subunit is secreted by >80% of tumors, with the ratio of the α subunit to thyrotropin <1.
- With central resistance to thyroid hormone, the ratio is <1.
- ↑ serum levels of both T_3 and T_4

Imaging

- MRI of the pituitary and hypothalamus
- CT scan only when MRI is unavailable or is otherwise contraindicated

Treatment

Surgery

- Selective transsphenoidal resection of the adenoma is used for acromegaly, Cushing's disease, and thyrotropin-secreting pituitary adenomas.
- RadioRx is reserved for pts who have not responded to surgical Rx and who still have sx of the adenoma.
- Bilateral adrenalectomy is performed in pts with Cushing's disease after failure of other therapies; complications requiring lifelong hormone replacement or Nelson's syndrome may occur.

RadioRx

- Generally reserved for pts who have not responded to surgical Rx
- Used with varying degrees of success in all the different pituitary adenomas

Medical

Prolactinoma

- Bromocriptine or cabergoline

Acromegaly
- Octreotide

Cushing's Disease
- Ketoconazole, which inhibits the cytochrome P-450 enzymes involved in steroid biosynthesis, is effective in managing mild to moderate disease in daily oral doses of 600 to 1200 mg.
- Metyrapone and aminoglutethimide can be used to control hypersecretion of cortisol but are generally used when preparing a pt for surgery or while waiting for a response to radioRx.

Thyrotropin-Secreting Pituitary Adenoma
- Ablative Rx with either radioactive iodide or surgery
- Octreotide

D. FLUID HEMOSTASIS DISORDERS

1 DIABETES INSIPIDUS (DI)

Definition
This polyuric disorder results from insufficient production of ADH (pituitary [central, neurogenic] DI) or unresponsiveness of the renal tubules to ADH (nephrogenic DI).

Etiology
Central (Neurogenic) DI
- Idiopathic
- Neoplasms of brain or pituitary fossa (craniopharyngiomas, metastatic neoplasms from breast or lung)
- Post-therapeutic neurosurgical procedures (e.g., hypophysectomy)
- Head trauma (e.g., basal skull fx)
- Granulomatous disorders (sarcoidosis or TB)
- Histiocytosis (Hand-Schüller-Christian disease eosinophilic granuloma)
- Familial (autosomal dominant)
- Other: interventricular hemorrhage, aneurysms, meningitis, postencephalitis, MS

Nephrogenic DI
- Drugs: lithium, amphotericin B, demeclocycline, methoxyflurane anesthesia
- Familial: X-linked
- Metabolic: hypercalcemia or hypokalemia
- Other: sarcoidosis, amyloidosis, pyelonephritis, polycystic disease, sickle cell disease, postobstructive condition

Diagnosis
H&P
- Polyuria: urinary volumes ranging from 2.5 to 6 L/day
- Polydipsia (predilection for cold or iced drinks)
- Neurologic manifestations (seizures, headaches, visual field defects)
- Evidence of volume contractions

Labs
- ↓ Urine specific gravity (≤1.005)
- ↓ Urine osmolality (usually <200 mOsm/kg) even in the presence of high serum osmolality
- Hypernatremia, plasma osmolarity, hypercalcemia, hypokalemia
- Water deprivation test confirms dx.

Imaging
- MRI of the brain if neurogenic DI is confirmed

Treatment
- Central DI: desmopressin acetate (DDAVP)
- Nephrogenic DI: adequate hydration, low-Na$^+$ diet and chlorothiazide to induce mild Na$^+$ depletion, amiloride 5 mg PO bid initially

2 SYNDROME OF INAPPROPRIATE ANTIDIURETIC HORMONE (SIADH, SIAD) SECRETION

This syndrome is characterized by excessive secretion of ADH in absence of nl osmotic or physiologic stimuli.

Etiology
- Neoplasm: lung, oropharynx, stomach, duodenum, pancreas, brain, thymus, bladder, prostate, endometrium, mesothelioma, lymphoma, Ewing's sarcoma

III

DISEASES AND DISORDERS
5. Endocrinology

- Pulmonary disorders: pneumonia, aspergillosis, pulmonary abscess, TB, bronchiectasis, emphysema, CF, status asthmaticus, respiratory failure associated w/positive-pressure breathing
- Intracranial disease: trauma, neoplasms, infections (meningitis, encephalitis, brain abscess), hemorrhage, hydrocephalus, MS, GBS
- Postoperative period: surgical stress, ventilators w/positive pressure, anesthetic agents
- Drugs: nicotine, chlorpropamide, thiazide diuretics, vasopressin, desmopressin, oxytocin, chemotherapeutic agents (vincristine, vinblastine, cyclophosphamide), carbamazepine, phenothiazines, MAOIs, tricyclic antidepressants, narcotics, nicotine, clofibrate, haloperidol, SSRIs, NSAIDs
- Other: acute intermittent porphyria, myxedema, psychosis, delirium tremens, ACTH deficiency (hypopituitarism), general anesthesia, endurance exercise

Diagnosis
H&P
- Delirium, lethargy, and seizures may be present if the hyponatremia is severe or of rapid onset.
- Manifestations of the underlying disease may be evident (e.g., fever from an infectious process or headaches and visual field defects from an intracranial mass).
- ↓ DTR and extensor plantar responses may occur w/severe hyponatremia.
- The pt is generally normovolemic or slightly hypervolemic; edema is absent.

Labs
- Demonstration through laboratory evaluation of excessive secretion of ADH in absence of appropriate osmotic or physiologic stimuli. Labs reveal
  - Hyponatremia
  - Urinary osmo > serum osmo
  - Urinary Na^+ >30 mEq/L
  - Normal BUN, Cr (indicative of nl renal function and absence of dehydration)
  - ↓ Uric acid
- For diagnostic purposes, pt should have nl thyroid, adrenal, and cardiac function and no recent or concurrent use of diuretics.

Imaging
- CXR: r/o neoplasm, pneumonia

Treatment
- In emergency situations (seizures, coma), SIADH can be treated w/combination of
  - Hypertonic saline solution (slow infusion of 250 mL of 3% NaCl). Infuse 3% saline (513 mmol/L) at a rate of 1 to 2 mL/kg of BW/hr to ↑ serum Na^+ by 1-2 mmol/L/hr.
  - Furosemide, 20 to 40 mg IV: ↑ serum Na^+ concentration by causing diuresis of urine that is more dilute than plasma and prevents extracellular fluid volume expansion.
- The rapidity of correction varies according to the degree of hyponatremia and if the hyponatremia is acute or chronic; in general, the serum Na^+ concentration should be corrected only halfway to nl in the initial 24 hr. A prudent approach is to ↑ serum Na^+ concentration by <0.5 mEq/L/hr and to limit the total ↑ to 8 to 12 mmol/L during the first 24 hr.
- Close monitoring of the rate of correction (every 2-3 hr) is recommended to avoid overcorrection. In pts w/hyponatremia of chronic duration, correction of serum Na^+ level by >12 mmol/L during a period of 24 hr = ↑ risk of osmotic demyelination.
- Conivaptan (20-40 mg/day IV) and tolvaptan (15 mg PO initially) are selective arginine vasopressin (AVP) antagonists useful in selected hospitalized pts w/ moderate to severe hyponatremia. Potential problems associated w/their use are infusion site reactions (50% of pts) and risk of osmotic demyelination if serum Na^+ levels are corrected too rapidly.

Long-term Rx
- Depending on the underlying cause, fluid restriction may be needed indefinitely. Monthly monitoring of electrolytes is recommended in pts w/chronic SIADH.
- Demeclocycline 300 to 600 mg PO bid: useful in pts w/chronic SIADH (e.g., secondary to neoplasm), but use w/caution in pts w/hepatic disease; side effects include nephrogenic DI and photosensitivity. This medication is also very expensive.

Clinical Pearl
- SIAD is the most frequent cause of hyponatremia (50% of hyponatremia cases in hospital setting).

E. THYROID DISORDERS

1 INTERPRETATION OF THYROID FUNCTION STUDIES

See Table 5-7 and Figure 5-2.

TABLE 5-7 ■ Findings in Thyroid Function Tests in Various Clinical Conditions							
Condition	T4	FT4I	T3	FT3I	TSH	TSI	TRH Stimulation
Hyperthyroidism							
Graves' disease	↑	↑	↑	↑	↓	+	↓
Toxic nodular goiter	↑	↑	↑	↑	↓	–	↓
Pituitary TSH-secreting tumors	↑	↑	↑	↑	↑	–	↓
T3 thyrotoxicosis	N	N	↑	↑	↓	+, –	↓
T4 thyrotoxicosis	↑	↑	N	N	↓	+, –	↓
Hypothyroidism							
Primary	↓	↓	↓	↓	↑	+, –	↑
Secondary	↓	↓	↓	↓	↓, N	–	↓
Tertiary	↓	↓	↓	↓	↓, N	–	N
Peripheral unresponsiveness	↑, N	↑, N	↑, N	↑	↑, N	–	N, ↑

From Tilton RC, Barrows A: In Hohnadel DC, Reiss R (eds): Clinical Laboratory Medicine. St. Louis, Mosby, 1992.
-, variable; FT3I, free T3 index; FT4I, free T4 index; TSI, thyroid-stimulating immunoglobulin.

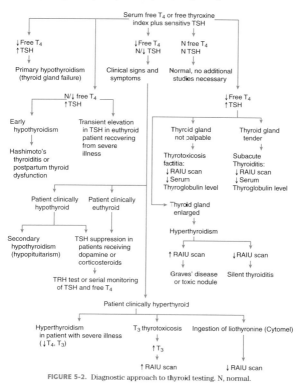

FIGURE 5-2. Diagnostic approach to thyroid testing. N, normal.

2 HYPERTHYROIDISM

Etiology

- Graves' disease (diffuse toxic goiter): 80% to 90% of all cases of hyperthyroidism
- Toxic multinodular goiter (Plummer's disease)
- Toxic adenoma
- Iatrogenic and factitious
- Transient hyperthyroidism (subacute thyroiditis, Hashimoto's thyroiditis)
- Rare causes: hypersecretion of TSH (e.g., pituitary neoplasms), struma ovarii, ingestion of large amount of iodine in a pt w/preexisting thyroid hyperplasia or adenoma (Jod-Basedow phenomenon), hydatidiform mole, carcinoma of thyroid, amiodarone Rx

Diagnosis

H&P

- Tachycardia, tremor, hyperreflexia, anxiety, irritability, emotional lability, panic attacks, heat intolerance, sweating, appetite, diarrhea, weight loss, menstrual dysfunction (oligomenorrhea, amenorrhea). The presentation may be different in elderly pts (see later).
- Pts w/Graves' disease may present w/exophthalmos, lid retraction, lid lag (*Graves' ophthalmopathy*). The following signs and sx of ophthalmopathy may be present: blurring of vision, photophobia, lacrimation, double vision, deep orbital pressure. Clubbing of fingers associated w/periosteal new bone formation in other skeletal areas (*Graves' acropachy*) and pretibial myxedema may also be noted.

Labs (Fig. 5-3)

- ↑ Free T_4
- ↑ Free T_3: generally not necessary for dx
- ↓ TSH (unless hyperthyroidism is a result of the rare hypersecretion of TSH from a pituitary adenoma in which case ↑ TSH)
- Thyroid Abs useful in selected cases to differentiate Graves' disease from toxic multinodular goiter (absent thyroid Abs)

Imaging

- 24-hr RAIU is useful to distinguish hyperthyroidism from iatrogenic thyroid hormone synthesis (thyrotoxicosis factitia) and from thyroiditis.
- An overactive thyroid = ↑ uptake, whereas iatrogenic thyroid ingestion and painless or subacute thyroiditis = nl or ↓ uptake.

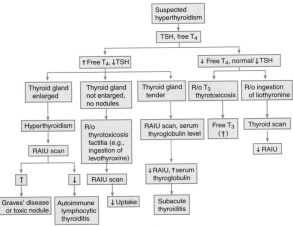

FIGURE 5-3. Diagnostic algorithm for hyperthyroidism.

- The RAIU results also vary w/the etiology of the hyperthyroidism:
  - Graves' disease: diffuse homogeneous uptake
  - Multinodular goiter: heterogeneous uptake
  - Hot nodule: single focus of uptake

Treatment
- Antithyroid drugs (thionamides): methimazole inhibits thyroid hormone synthesis by blocking production of thyroid peroxidase. Adjunctive Rx to alleviate α-adrenergic sx of hyperthyroidism involves propranolol 20 to 40 mg PO q6h; dosage is gradually ↑ until sx are controlled.
- RAI is the Rx of choice for pts >21 yr of age who have not achieved remission after 1 yr of antithyroid drug Rx.
- Subtotal thyroidectomy is indicated in obstructing goiters, in any pt who refuses RAI and cannot be adequately managed w/antithyroid medications (e.g., pts w/ toxic adenoma or toxic multinodular goiter), and in pregnant pts who cannot be adequately managed w/antithyroid medication or develop side effects to them.

Clinical Pearl
- Elderly hyperthyroid pts may have only subtle signs (weight loss, tachycardia, fine skin, brittle nails). This form is known as **apathetic hyperthyroidism** and is manifested by lethargy rather than with hyperkinetic activity. An enlarged thyroid gland may be absent. Coexisting medical disorders (most commonly cardiac disease) may also mask the sx. These pts often have unexplained CHF or new-onset AF.

3 THYROID STORM
Acute life-threatening exacerbation of hyperthyroidism

Diagnosis
- Tremor, tachycardia/tachyarrhythmias, fever (as high as 105.8° F)
- Sweating, diarrhea, vasodilatation
- Lid lag, lid retraction, proptosis, goiter
- Change in mental status (psychosis, coma, seizures)
- Other: precipitating factors (infection, trauma) CHF, hepatosplenomegaly, jaundice

Labs
- ↑ Free T_4, ↓ TSH

Treatment
- Replace fluid deficit aggressively (daily fluid requirement may reach 6 L); use solutions containing glucose and add multivitamins to the hydrating solution.
- Propylthiouracil (PTU) 800 mg initially (PO/NG tube)/PR, then 200 to 300 mg PO/PR q6h (allergy PTU, methimazole 80-100 mg PO/PR followed by 40 mg PO/PR q8h).
- Inhibition of stored thyroid hormone from the gland:
  - Iodide can be administered as Telepaque (iopanoic acid) 1 g PO once daily or Na^+ iodine 250 mg IV q6h, or, saturated solution of K^+ iodide (SSKI), 5 gtt PO q8h, or Lugol's solution, 10 gtt PO q8h. It is important to administer PTU or methimazole 1 hr before the iodide to prevent the oxidation of iodide to iodine and its incorporation in the synthesis of additional thyroid hormone.
  - Corticosteroids: Dexamethasone 1 to 2 mg IV q6h or hydrocortisone 100 mg IV q6h for approximately 48 hr is useful to inhibit thyroid hormone release, impair peripheral conversion of T_3 from T_4, and provide additional adrenocortical hormone to correct deficiency (if present).
- Suppression of peripheral effects of thyroid hormone: β-adrenergic blockers: Administer propranolol 80 to 120 mg PO q4 to 6h. Propranolol may also be given IV 1 mg/min for 2 to 10 min under continuous ECG and blood pressure monitoring. β-Adrenergic blockers must be used with caution in pts with severe CHF or bronchospasm. Cardioselective β-blockers (e.g., esmolol or metoprolol) may be more appropriate for pts with bronchospasm, but these pts must be closely monitored for exacerbation of bronchospasm because these agents lose their cardioselectivity at ↑ doses.
- Control of fever with acetaminophen 325 to 650 mg q4h; avoid aspirin because it displaces thyroid hormone from its binding protein
- Rx of any precipitating factors (e.g., abx if infection is strongly suspected)

4 HYPOTHYROIDISM

Etiology
- Primary hypothyroidism >90% of the cases
  - Hashimoto's thyroiditis: most common cause of hypothyroidism after 8 yr of age
  - Idiopathic myxedema (nongoitrous form of Hashimoto's thyroiditis)
  - Previous Rx of hyperthyroidism (radioiodine Rx, subtotal thyroidectomy)

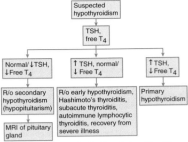

FIGURE 5-4. Diagnostic algorithm for hypothyroidism.

- Subacute thyroiditis
- Radiation Rx to the neck (usually for malignant disease)
- Iodine deficiency or excess
- Drugs (lithium, PAS, sulfonamides, phenylbutazone, amiodarone, thiourea)
- Congenital (approximately 1 case per 4000 live births)
- Prolonged Rx w/iodides
- Secondary hypothyroidism: pituitary dysfunction, postpartum necrosis, neoplasm, infiltrative disease causing deficiency of TSH
- Tertiary hypothyroidism: hypothalamic disease (granuloma, neoplasm, or irradiation causing deficiency of TRH)
- Tissue resistance to thyroid hormone: rare

Diagnosis
H&P
- Skin: dry, coarse, thick, cool, sallow (yellow color caused by carotenemia); nonpitting edema in skin of eyelids and hands (*myxedema*) secondary to infiltration of SC tissues by a hydrophilic mucopolysaccharide substance
- Hair: brittle and coarse; loss of outer third of eyebrows
- Facies: dulled expression, thickened tongue, thick, slow-moving lips
- Thyroid gland: may or may not be palpable (depending on the cause of the hypothyroidism)
- Heart sounds: distant, possible pericardial effusion
- Pulse: bradycardia
- Neurologic: delayed relaxation phase of the DTRs, cerebellar ataxia, hearing impairment, poor memory, peripheral neuropathies w/paresthesia
- Musculoskeletal: carpal tunnel syndrome, muscle stiffness, weakness

Labs (see Table 5-7; Fig. 5-4)
- TSH: ↑ TSH may be nl if pt has secondary or tertiary hypothyroidism, pt is receiving dopamine or corticosteroids, or the level is obtained after severe illness.
- ↓ Free T_4
- Other common laboratory abnlities: hyperlipidemia, hyponatremia, and anemia
- Antimicrosomal and antithyroglobulin Ab titers: useful only when autoimmune thyroiditis is suspected as the cause of the hypothyroidism

Treatment
- Levothyroxine 25 to 100 μg/day, depending on pt's age and severity of the disease. The dose may be ↑ every 6 to 8 wk, depending on the clinical response and serum TSH level. Elderly pts and pts w/CAD should be started w/12.5 to 25 μg/day (higher doses may precipitate angina).

Clinical Pearls
- Periodic monitoring of TSH level is an essential part of Rx. Pts should be evaluated w/office visit and TSH levels every 6 to 8 wk until the pt is clinically euthyroid and the TSH level is normalized.
- For monitoring Rx in pts w/central hypothyroidism, measurement of serum free T_4 level rather than TSH is appropriate; it should be maintained in the upper half of the nl range.
- Pregnant pts also have ↑ requirements. Women w/hypothyroidism should generally ↑ their levothyroxine dose by approximately 30% as soon as pregnancy is confirmed and have frequent testing.

5 SUBCLINICAL HYPOTHYROIDISM

- Frequency: 10% to 15% of elderly
- Labs: ↑ serum TSH and a nl free T_4 level
- Associated with an ↑ risk of CHD events (particularly in those with a TSH concentration of ≥10 mU/L)
- Rx: Levothyroxine if TSH ≥10 mU/L and with presence of goiter or thyroid autoantibodies

6 MYXEDEMA COMA

- This is a life-threatening complication of hypothyroidism.

Etiology

- Decompensation of hypothyroidism secondary to
  - Sepsis
  - Exposure to cold weather
  - CNS depressants (sedatives, narcotics, antidepressants)
  - Trauma, surgery

Diagnosis
H&P

- Profound lethargy or coma
- Hypothermia (rectal temperature <35° C [<95° F]); often missed by using ordinary thermometers graduated only to 34.5° C
- Bradycardia, hypotension (secondary to circulatory collapse)
- Delayed relaxation phase of DTR, areflexia
- Myxedema facies
- Alopecia, macroglossia, ptosis, periorbital edema, nonpitting edema, doughy skin
- Bladder dystonia and distention

Labs

- ↑↑ TSH (if primary hypothyroidism), ↓ free T_4

Treatment

- Levothyroxine 5 to 8 µg/kg (300-500 µg) IV infused over 15 min, then 100 µg IV q24h.
- Glucocorticoids should also be administered until coexistent adrenal insufficiency can be r/o → hydrocortisone hemisuccinate 100 mg IV bolus, followed by 50 mg IV q12h or 25 mg IV q6h until initial plasma cortisol level is confirmed nl.
- IV hydration w/D5NS

7 THYROIDITIS

Classification and Etiology

- Hashimoto's thyroiditis (autoimmune)
- Painful subacute thyroiditis (follows URI): subacute thyroiditis, giant cell thyroiditis, de Quervain's thyroiditis, subacute granulomatous thyroiditis, pseudogranulomatous thyroiditis
- Painless postpartum thyroiditis: subacute lymphocytic thyroiditis
- Suppurative thyroiditis (infectious etiology thus febrile with nuchal rigidity/erythema)
- Riedel's thyroiditis (slowly enlarging hard mass): fibrous thyroiditis

Labs

- TSH, free T_4: may be nl, ↓, ↑
- ↑ WBC with left shift occurs with subacute and suppurative thyroiditis.
- Antimicrosomal Abs (>90%), Hashimoto's thyroiditis, (65%) silent thyroiditis
- Serum thyroglobulin levels ↑ subacute and silent thyroiditis, factitious hyperthyroidism (↓ or absent serum thyroglobulin level)

Imaging

- 24 hr RAIU: Graves' disease (↑ RAIU), thyroiditis (nl cr ↓ RAIU)

Treatment

- If hypothyroid: levothyroxine 25 to 50 µg/day initially and monitor TSH q 6 to 8wk
- Control sx of hyperthyroidism: β-blocker (e.g., propranolol 20-40 mg PO q6h)
- If pain → NSAIDs, if refractory → prednisone 20 to 40 mg qd
- If suppurative thyroiditis → IV abx and drain abscess

8 EVALUATION OF THYROID NODULE

Epidemiology and Risk Factors for Malignancy

- Incidence of thyroid nodules ↑ after age 45 yr, more frequently in women
- ↑ Risk malignancy: nodule ≥2 cm, regional lymphadenopathy, fixation to adjacent tissues, age <40 yr, sx of local invasion (dysphagia, hoarseness, neck pain, male sex, family hx of thyroid cancer or polyposis [Gardner syndrome]), rapid growth during levothyroxine Rx

- FNA biopsy best diagnostic study; accuracy can be >90%
- TSH, T_4, and serum thyroglobulin levels
- Serum calcitonin if suspect medullary carcinoma of the thyroid/family hx
- Thyroid U/S to evaluate size, composition (solid vs. cystic), and dimensions
- Thyroid scan with technetium-99m pertechnetate, iodine-123, or iodine-131 in selected pts (Fig. 5-5)

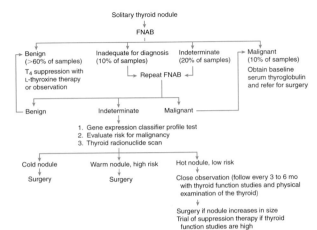

FIGURE 5-5. Diagnostic evaluation of solitary thyroid nodule in euthyroid patient. High risk for malignancy: nodule >2 cm, age <40 years, male sex, regional lymphadenopathy, fixation to adjacent tissues, history of previous head and neck irradiation.

9 THYROID CARCINOMA

Three major types are recognized (Table 5-8).

- Papillary carcinoma
  - Psammoma bodies (calcific bodies present in papillary projections)
  - Spread via lymphatics/local invasion
- Follicular carcinoma
  - Incidence ↑ with age
  - May metastasize hematogenously to bone → pathologic fractures
  - Tends to concentrate iodine (useful for radiation Rx)

TABLE 5-8 ■ Characteristics of Thyroid Cancers

Type of Cancer	Percentage of Thyroid Cancers (%)	Age of Onset (yr)	Treatment	Prognosis
Papillary	80	40-80	Thyroidectomy, followed by radioactive iodine ablation	Good
Follicular	15	45-80	Thyroidectomy, followed by radioactive iodine ablation	Fair to good
Medullary	3	20-50	Thyroidectomy and central compartment lymph node dissection	Fair
Anaplastic	1	50-80	Isthmusectomy followed by palliative x-ray treatment	Poor
Lymphoma	1	25-70	X-ray therapy and/or chemotherapy	Fair

From Andreoli TE, Benjamin IJ, Griggs RC, Wing EJ: Andreoli and Carpenter's Cecil Essentials of Medicine, 8th ed. Philadelphia, Saunders, 2010.

- Anaplastic carcinoma
  - Two very aggressive histologic types: small cell (less aggressive, 5-yr survival 20%) and giant cell (death usually within 6 mo of dx)
- MTC:
  - Unifocal: found sporadically in elderly pts
  - Bilateral: assoc w/MEN-II pheochromocytoma + hyperparathyroidism (↑ plasma calcitonin)

H&P
- Presence of thyroid nodule/painless swelling
- Most common type (50%-60%) is papillary carcinoma.
- Median age at dx: 45 to 50 yr; female 3:1
- Hoarseness and cervical lymphadenopathy

W/up
- FNA biopsy; thyroid function studies are generally nl.
- Thyroid U/S, thyroid scanning with iodine-123 or technetium-99m

Treatment
- Thyroidectomy

F. CALCIUM HOMEOSTASIS DISORDERS

1 CALCIUM FORMULAS
See Box 5-1.

Box 5-1 • Calcium Formulas

The correction of Ca based on the serum albumin and globulin levels is calculated as:

$$\% \; Ca^{2+} \; bound = 8(albumin) + 2(globulin) + 3$$

Another formula to correct C_{Ca} based on total protein is:

$$Corrected \; Ca^{2+} = Measured \; Ca^{2+}/(0.6 + [total \; protein/8.5])$$

A quick bedside formula for calculation of the corrected Ca is:

$$Corrected \; Ca^{2+} = Measured \; Ca^{2+} - albumin + 4$$

---

2 HYPERCALCEMIA

Etiology
- Malignant disease (20%-30% of cancers), 4 types:
  - Humoral hypercalcemia of malignancy (80%): breast cancer, MM, and lymphoma; caused by secretion of PTHrP by the tumors → bone resorption and renal retention of Ca^{2+}
  - Local osteolytic hypercalcemia (<20%): squamous cell cancer (e.g., lung, head and neck, esophagus), renal or ovarian cancer, breast cancer, some lymphomas, and endometrial cancer; caused by osteoclastic bone resorption in areas surrounding the malignant cells within the marrow space
  - Secretion of 1,25(OH)$_2$D by lymphomas (<1%) → osteoclastic bone resorption and intestinal absorption of Ca^{2+}
  - Ectopic hyperparathyroidism (<0.01%); caused by ectopic secretion of PTH
- Hyperparathyroidism bone resorption, GI absorption, and renal absorption from
  - Parathyroid hyperplasia, adenoma
  - Hyperparathyroidism or renal failure w/secondary hyperparathyroidism
- Granulomatous disorders → GI absorption (e.g., sarcoidosis)
- Paget's disease → bone resorption (seen only during periods of immobilization)
- Vitamin D intoxication, milk-alkali syndrome → GI absorption
- Thiazides → renal absorption
- Other causes: familial hypocalciuric hypercalcemia, thyrotoxicosis, adrenal insufficiency, prolonged immobilization, vitamin A intoxication, recovery from acute kidney injury (AKI), lithium administration, pheochromocytoma, SLE

Diagnosis
H&P
- GI: constipation, anorexia, N/V, pancreatitis, ulcers
- CNS: confusion, obtundation, psychosis, lassitude, depression, coma
- GU: nephrolithiasis, renal insufficiency, polyuria, ↓ urine-concentrating ability (nephrogenic DI), nocturia, nephrocalcinosis
- Musculoskeletal: myopathy, weakness, osteoporosis, pseudogout, bone pain

- Other: HTN, metastatic calcifications, band keratopathy, pruritus
- Most pts are asymptomatic at the time of dx.

Hx
- FHx of hypercalcemia such as MEN syndromes or familial hypocalciuric hypercalcemia (the latter is a benign autosomal dominant condition of ↑ serum Ca^{2+}, ↓ urinary Ca^{2+}, ↓ fractional excretion of Ca^{2+} [generally <1%], and a nl PTH → parathyroidectomy not indicated)
- Inquire about intake of milk and antacids (milk-alkali syndrome), intake of thiazides, lithium, large doses of vitamins A or D.
- Inquire whether pt has any bone pain (MM, metastatic disease) or abd pain (pancreatitis, PUD).

PE
- Look for evidence of primary neoplasm (e.g., breast, lung).
- Check eyes for evidence of band keratopathy (found in medial and lateral margin of the cornea).

Labs (Fig. 5-6)
- Initial labs: serum Ca^{2+}, alb, PO_4^{-3}, Mg, alk phos, electrolytes, BUN, Cr, PTH, and 24-hr urine Ca^{2+} collection. In pts w/abnl alb levels, it is important to measure the serum level of ionized Ca^{2+} to correct for the abnl alb. If the ionized Ca^{2+} is not available, the total Ca^{2+} can be corrected for a low alb level by adding 0.8 mg/dL to the total Ca^{2+} level for every 1.0 g/dL of serum alb below the level of 3.5 g/dL.
- If the hx suggests ↓ intake of vitamin D (e.g., in food faddists w/intake of megadoses of fat-soluble vitamins), check serum vitamin D level (1,25-dihydroxyvitamin D).
- The iPTH distinguishes primary hyperparathyroidism from hypercalcemia caused by malignant disease when the serum Ca level is >12 mg/dL.
- ↑↑ Urinary cyclic AMP = primary hyperparathyroidism, although certain nonparathyroid malignant neoplasms also produce levels of urinary cyclic AMP.
- ↑ PTHrP = hypercalcemia-associated malignant neoplasms.

Imaging
- Bone survey may show evidence of subperiosteal bone resorption (suggesting PTH excess).
- Parathyroid localization w/technetium-99m sestamibi: high sensitivity and specificity for single adenomas
- ECG: shortening of the QT interval

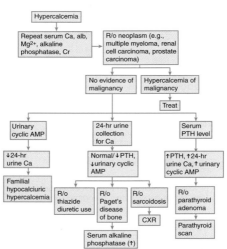

FIGURE 5-6. Diagnostic algorithm for hypercalcemia. *(From Ravel R: Clinical Laboratory Medicine, 6th ed. St. Louis, Mosby, 1995.)*

Treatment

Acute Severe Hypercalcemia (serum Ca ≥13 mg/dL or symptomatic pt)

- Vigorous IV hydration w/NS. Usual administration rate is 200 to 500 mL/hr, depending on the baseline level of dehydration, renal function, and the CV and mental status of the pt.
- NS infusion = inhibition of proximal tubular Na^+ and Ca^{2+} reabsorption → increased delivery of Na^+ and water to distal nephron → ↑ urinary Ca^{2+} excretion
- IV bisphosphonates to inhibit osteoclast bone resorption: zoledronate (4 mg IV over a 15-min period in a solution of 50 mL of NS or D_5W). In pts with impaired kidney function can use denosumab to ↓ osteoclast mediated bone resorption
- PO_4^{-3} repletion: Hypophosphatemia occurs in most pts w/hypercalcemia due to cancer. Serum PO_4^{-3} level should be kept in the range of 2.5 to 3 mg/dL. Serum phosphorus and Cr levels should be closely monitored. PO_4^{-3} replacement should be PO (e.g., 250 mg Neutra-Phos PO qid until serum phosphorus level is >3.0 mg/dL).
- Loop diuretics (e.g., furosemide 20-40 mg IV) can worsen dehydration and should not be administered until full hydration has been achieved. Thiazide diuretics are contraindicated because they will stimulate rather than inhibit renal Ca reabsorption.

3 HYPOCALCEMIA

Etiology

- Renal insufficiency: hypocalcemia caused by
  - ↑ Ca deposits in bone and soft tissue secondary to ↑ serum PO_4^{-3} level
  - ↓ Production of 1,25-dihydroxyvitamin D
  - ↑ Loss of 25-OHD (nephrotic syndrome)
- Hypoalbuminemia: Each ↓ in serum alb (g/L) will ↓ serum Ca by 0.8 mg/dL but will not change free (ionized) Ca.
- Vitamin D deficiency
- Malabsorption (most common cause)
  - Inadequate intake
  - ↓ Production of 1,25-dihydroxyvitamin D (vitamin D–dependent rickets, renal failure)
  - ↓ Production of 25-OHD (parenchymal liver disease)
  - ↑ 25-OHD catabolism (phenytoin, phenobarbital)
  - End-organ resistance to 1,25-dihydroxyvitamin D
- Hypomagnesemia: hypocalcemia caused by
  - ↓ PTH secretion
  - Inhibition of PTH effect on bone
- Pancreatitis, hyperphosphatemia, osteoblastic mets: Hypocalcemia is secondary to Ca deposits (bone, abd).
- **Pseudohypoparathyroidism:** autosomal recessive, short stature, shortening of metacarpal bones, obesity, mental retardation The hypocalcemia is secondary to congenital end-organ resistance to PTH.
- Idiopathic hypoparathyroidism, surgical removal of parathyroids (e.g., neck surgery)
- **Hungry bones syndrome:** rapid transfer of Ca from plasma into bones after removal of a parathyroid tumor
- Sepsis
- Massive blood transfusion (as a result of EDTA and calcium chelation in blood)

Diagnosis

H&P

- Neuromuscular irritability
  - **Chvostek's sign:** facial twitch after a gentle tapping over the facial nerve (can occur in 10%-25% of nl adults)
  - **Trousseau's sign:** carpedal spasm after inflation of BP cuff above the pt's systolic BP for a 2- to 3-min duration
- Tetany, paresthesias, myopathy, seizures, muscle spasm or weakness
- Psychiatric disturbances: psychosis, depression, impaired cognitive function
- Soft tissue calcifications, ocular cataracts
- CV: arrhythmias, CHF, QT interval, hypotension

Labs (Table 5-9 and Fig. 5-7)

- Serum alb: to r/o hypoalbuminemia
- BUN, Cr: to r/o renal failure
- Serum Mg: to r/o severe hypomagnesemia
- Serum PO_4^{-3}, alk phos: to differentiate hypoparathyroidism from vitamin D deficiency

TABLE 5-9 ■ Laboratory Differential Diagnosis of Hypocalcemia

	Plasma Tests					Urine Tests					Comments
Diagnosis	Ca	PO₄	PTH	25(OH)D	1,25(OH)₂D	cAMP	cAMP After PTH	TmP/GFR	TmP/GFR After PTH	Ca	
Hypoparathyroidism	↓	↑	N/↓	N	↓	↓	↑↑	↑	↓↓	N/↓	Deficiency of PTH
Pseudohypoparathyroidism											
Type I	↓	↑	↑↑	N	↓	↓	NC	↑	↑	N/↓	Resistance to PTH; patients may have Albright's hereditary osteodystrophy and resistance to multiple hormones
Type II	↓	N	↑↑	N	↓	↑	↑	↑	↑	N/↓	Renal resistance to cAMP
Vitamin D deficiency	↓	N/↓	↑↑	↓↓	N/↓	↑	↑	↑	↑	↓↓	Deficient supply (e.g., nutrition) or absorption (e.g., pancreatic insufficiency) of vitamin D
Vitamin D-dependent rickets											
Type I	↓	N/↓	↑↑	N	↑	↑		↑		↓↓	Deficient activity of renal 25[OH]D-1α-hydroxylase
Type II	↓	N/↓	↑↑	N	↑↑	↑		↑		↓↓	Resistance to 1,25[OH]₂D

From Moore WT, Eastman RC: Diagnostic Endocrinology, 2nd ed. St. Louis, Mosby, 1996.

(OH)D, hydroxycholecalciferol D; OH₂D, dihydroxycholecalciferol; TmP, renal threshold for phosphorus.

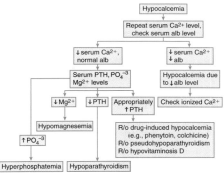

FIGURE 5-7. Diagnostic algorithm for hypocalcemia. *(From Ferri FF: Ferri's Best Test: A Practical Guide to Clinical Laboratory Medicine and Diagnostic Imaging, 2nd ed. Philadelphia, Mosby, 2010.)*

- Serum PTH
  - $\uparrow\uparrow$ PTH: pseudohypoparathyroidism
  - $\uparrow$ PTH: vitamin D deficiency
  - $\downarrow$ PTH: hypoparathyroidism

Treatment

- Acute, severe symptomatic hypocalcemia caused by hypoparathyroidism or vitamin D deficiency: Give a slow IV bolus (over 15 min) of 10 to 30 mL of a 10% Ca gluconate solution followed by an infusion of 4 g Ca gluconate in 500 mL D_5W over 4 hr (1 g Ca gluconate = 10 mL 10% Ca gluconate).
- Hypoalbuminemia
  - Improve nutritional status.
  - Ca replacement is not indicated because the free (ionized) Ca is nl.
- Hypomagnesemia: Correct the Mg deficiency.
  - Severe hypomagnesemia (serum Mg level <0.8 mEq/L): Give 1 g (8 mEq) of a 10% Mg sulfate solution IV slowly (during 15 min).
  - Moderate to severe hypomagnesemia (serum Mg level 0.8-1.3 mEq/L): Give one 2-mL ampule of a 50% Mg solution IM; may repeat q4-6h.
- Chronic hypocalcemia caused by hypoparathyroidism or vitamin D deficiency
  - Ca supplementation: 1 to 4 g/day of elemental Ca (e.g., Ca carbonate, 650 mg PO qid, will provide 1 g of elemental Ca/day)
  - Vitamin D replacement
- Chronic hypocalcemia caused by renal failure
  - Reduction of hyperphosphatemia w/phosphate-binding antacids
  - Vitamin D and oral Ca supplementation (as noted earlier)

G. ADRENAL GLAND DISORDERS

1 CUSHING'S SYNDROME

This clinical disorder is associated w/glucocorticoid excess secondary to exaggerated adrenal cortisol production or chronic glucocorticoid Rx. **Cushing's disease** is Cushing's syndrome caused by pituitary ACTH excess.

Etiology

- Iatrogenic from chronic glucocorticoid Rx (most common) ($\downarrow$ ACTH, $\uparrow$ cortisol)
- Pituitary ACTH excess (Cushing's disease) ($\uparrow$ ACTH, $\uparrow$ cortisol)
- Adrenal neoplasms (30%) ($\downarrow$ ACTH, $\uparrow$ cortisol)
- Ectopic ACTH production (neoplasms of lung, pancreas, kidney, thyroid, thymus; 10%) ($\uparrow\uparrow$ ACTH, $\uparrow\uparrow$ cortisol)

Diagnosis

H&P

- HTN
- Central obesity w/rounding of the facies (**moon facies**); thin extremities

- Hirsutism, menstrual irregularities, hypogonadism
- Skin fragility, ecchymoses, red-purple abd striae, acne, poor wound healing, hair loss, facial plethora, hyperpigmentation (when there is ACTH excess)
- Psychosis, emotional lability, paranoia
- Muscle wasting w/proximal myopathy

Labs
- Initial screening test is the overnight dexamethasone suppression test (Fig. 5-8):
  - Dexamethasone 1 mg PO given at 11 PM
  - Plasma cortisol level measured 9 hr later (8 AM)
  - Plasma cortisol level <2 μg/dL (55 nmol/L) excludes Cushing's syndrome. Levels >5 μg/dL (138 nmol/L) suggest Cushing's syndrome. Levels 2 to 5 μg/dL (55-138 nmol/L) require additional testing with 24-hr urine free cortisol testing (>100 μg/24 hr in Cushing's syndrome) and midnight salivary cortisol measurement (↑ in Cushing's syndrome). Nl diurnal variation leads to a cortisol nadir around midnight; therefore, a cortisol level >7.5 μg/dL is 96% sensitive and 100% specific for the dx of Cushing's syndrome.
  - If necessary, dx of Cushing's syndrome can be confirmed with low-dose 2-day dexamethasone suppression and dexamethasone plus CRH.
  - Other lab tests reveal hypokalemia, hypochloremia, metabolic alkalosis, hyperglycemia, hypercholesterolemia.
  - Plasma ACTH is useful to determine the cause of Cushing's syndrome (see Fig. 5-8).

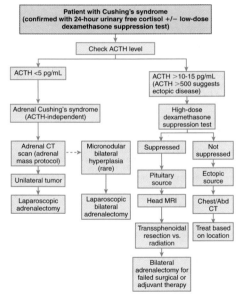

FIGURE 5-8. Clinical diagnosis and management of Cushing's syndrome. *(From Cameron AM: Current Surgical Therapy, 10th ed. Philadelphia, Saunders, 2011.)*

Imaging
- CT scan of adrenal glands: indicated in suspected adrenal Cushing's syndrome
- MRI of pituitary gland w/gadolinium: indicated in suspected pituitary Cushing's syndrome

Treatment
Rx varies w/cause:
- Pituitary adenoma: Transsphenoidal microadenomectomy is the Rx of choice in adults. Pituitary irradiation is reserved for pts not cured by transsphenoidal surgery. In children, pituitary irradiation may be considered initial Rx because

85% of children are cured by radiation. Stereotactic radioRx (photon knife or gamma knife) is effective and exposes the surrounding neuronal tissues to less irradiation than in conventional radioRx. Total bilateral adrenalectomy is reserved for pts not cured by transsphenoidal surgery or pituitary irradiation.

- Adrenal neoplasm: surgical resection of the affected adrenal; glucocorticoid replacement for approximately 9 to 12 mo after the surgery to allow time for the contralateral adrenal to recover from its prolonged suppression
- Bilateral micronodular or macronodular adrenal hyperplasia: bilateral total adrenalectomy
- Ectopic ACTH: surgical resection of the ACTH-secreting neoplasm; control of cortisol excess w/metyrapone, aminoglutethimide, mifepristone, or ketoconazole; control of the mineralocorticoid effects of cortisol and 11-deoxycorticosteroid w/ spironolactone. Bilateral adrenalectomy is a rational approach to pts w/indolent, unresectable tumors.

2 PRIMARY ADRENOCORTICAL INSUFFICIENCY (ADDISON'S DISEASE)

Disorder characterized by inadequate secretion of corticosteroids resulting from partial or complete destruction of all three layers of the adrenal glands.

Etiology
- Autoimmune destruction of the adrenals (80% of cases)
- TB (15% of cases)
- Carcinomatous destruction of the adrenals
- Adrenal hemorrhage (anticoagulants, trauma, coagulopathies, pregnancy, sepsis); adrenal infarction (arteritis, thrombosis)
- AIDS (adrenal insufficiency develops in 30% of pts w/advanced AIDS)
- Other: sarcoidosis, amyloidosis, postoperative, fungal infection, megestrol acetate Rx, etomidate Rx

Diagnosis
H&P
- Hyperpigmentation, hypotension, generalized weakness, amenorrhea, and loss of axillary hair in female pts

Labs (Fig. 5-9)
- Perform rapid ACTH (cosyntropin) test: 250 μg ACTH by IV push; measure cortisol level at 0, 30, 60 min. Cortisol level <18 μg/dL at 30 min or 60 min suggests adrenal insufficiency. Measure plasma ACTH level: ↑ level indicates primary adrenal insufficiency, nl/↓ level indicates secondary adrenal insufficiency.
- ↑ K^+, ↓ Na^+ and Cl^-, ↓ glucose, ↑ BUN/Cr ratio (prerenal azotemia), mild normocytic normochromic anemia, neutropenia, lymphocytosis, eosinophilia (significant dehydration may mask the hyponatremia and anemia), ↓ 24-hr urinary cortisol, 17-OHCS, and 17-KS and ↑ ACTH (if primary adrenocortical insufficiency)

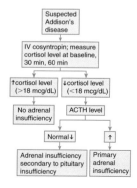

FIGURE 5-9. Diagnostic algorithm for adrenal insufficiency (Addison's disease). *(From Ferri FF: Ferri's Best Test: A Practical Guide to Clinical Laboratory Medicine and Diagnostic Imaging, 2nd ed. Philadelphia, Mosby, 2010.)*

Treatment
Chronic Adrenocortical Insufficiency
- Hydrocortisone, 15 to 20 mg PO q AM and 5 to 10 mg in late afternoon or prednisone 5 mg in AM and 2.5 mg at hs

- Oral fludrocortisone 0.05 to 0.20 mg/day (if the pt has primary adrenocortical insufficiency). The dose is adjusted on the basis of the serum Na^+ level and the presence of postural hypotension or marked orthostasis.
- Monitor serum electrolytes, VS, and BW periodically: Advise liberal Na^+ intake.
- Pts should be instructed to ↑ glucocorticoid replacement in times of stress and to receive parenteral glucocorticoids if diarrhea or vomiting occurs.

Addisonian Crisis
- Acute complications of adrenal insufficiency characterized by circulatory collapse, dehydration, N/V, hypoglycemia, and hyperkalemia
- Draw plasma cortisol level; do not delay Rx until confirming lab results are obtained.
- Administer hydrocortisone 50 to 100 mg IV q6h for 24 hr; if pt shows good clinical response, gradually taper dosage and change to PO maintenance dose (usually prednisone, 7.5 mg/day).
- Provide adequate volume replacement w/D5NS solution until hypotension, dehydration, and hypoglycemia are completely corrected. Large volumes (2-3 L) may be necessary in the first 2 to 3 hr to correct the volume deficit and hypoglycemia and to avoid further hyponatremia.
- Identify and correct any precipitating factor (e.g., sepsis, hemorrhage).

3 DISORDERS OF MINERALOCORTICOID SECRETION

a. Hypoaldosteronism

Etiology
- Hyporeninemic hypoaldosteronism (renin-angiotensin dependent): ↓ aldosterone production as a result of ↓ renin production; pt has renal disease secondary to various factors (e.g., DM, interstitial nephritis, MM).
- Hyperreninemic hypoaldosteronism (renin-angiotensin independent): Renin production by the kidneys is intact; defect is in aldosterone biosynthesis or in the action of angiotensin II. Common causes are meds (ACEIs, heparin), lead poisoning, aldosterone enzyme defects, and severe illness.

H&P
- HTN, muscle weakness, cardiac arrhythmias

Diagnosis
Labs
- ↑ K^+, nl or ↓ Na^+
- Hyperchloremic metabolic acidosis (caused by the absence of hydrogen-secreting action of aldosterone)
- ↑ BUN and Cr (secondary to renal disease)
- Hyperglycemia (DM is common in these pts)

W/up
- Measurement of PRA after 4 hr of upright posture can differentiate hyporeninemic from hyperreninemic causes. Nl/↓ renin levels = renin-angiotensin dependent, ↑ renin levels = renin-angiotensin independent.
- Renin-aldosterone stimulation test
  - Hyporeninemic hypoaldosteronism: ↓ stimulated renin and aldosterone levels
  - End-organ refractoriness to aldosterone action: ↑ stimulated renin and aldosterone levels
  - Adrenal gland abnlity: ↑ stimulated renin and ↓ aldosterone levels

Treatment
- Low-K diet with liberal Na intake (≥4 g of NaCl/day)
- Avoidance of ACEIs and K^+-sparing diuretics
- Judicious use of fludrocortisone (0.05 to 0.1 mg PO every morning) in pts with aldosterone deficiency associated with deficiency of adrenal glucocorticoid hormones
- Furosemide 20 to 40 mg qd to correct hyperkalemia of hyporeninemic hypoaldosteronism

b. Hyperaldosteronism (Conn's syndrome)
Syndrome characterized by hypokalemia, HTN, ↓ PRA, and ↑ aldosterone secretion

Etiology
- Aldosterone-producing adenoma (>60%)
- Idiopathic hyperaldosteronism (>30%)
- Glucocorticoid-suppressible hyperaldosteronism (<1%)
- Aldosterone-producing carcinoma (<1%)

Diagnosis

- 24-hr urine test for aldosterone and K^+ levels (K^+ >40 mEq and aldosterone >15 μg)
- The renin-aldosterone stimulation test (posture test) to differentiate idiopathic hyperaldosteronism (IHA) from aldosterone-producing adenoma (APA). Pts with APA have a ↓ in aldosterone levels at 4 hr, whereas pts with IHA have an ↑ in aldosterone levels.
- As a screening test for primary aldosteronism, an ↑ plasma aldosterone-renin ratio (ARR), drawn randomly from pts taking hypertensive drugs, is predictive of primary aldosteronism. ARR is calculated by dividing plasma aldosterone (mg/dL) by PRA (mg/mL/hr). ARR >100 is considered ↑.
- Bilateral adrenal vein sampling (AVS) may be done to localize APA when adrenal CT scan is equivocal. In APA, ipsilateral/contralateral aldosterone level is >10:1, and ipsilateral venous aldosterone concentration is very high (>1000 ng/dL).

H&P

- If significant hypokalemia: muscle cramping, weakness, paresthesias
- HTN
- Polyuria, polydipsia

Labs

- Routine labs can be suggestive but are not diagnostic of primary aldosteronism. Common abnlities are
  - Spontaneous hypokalemia or moderately severe hypokalemia while receiving conventional doses of diuretics
  - Possible alkalosis and hypernatremia

Imaging

- Adrenal CT scans (with 3-mm cuts) or MRI to localize neoplasm
- Adrenal scanning with iodocholesterol (NP-59) or 6-β-iodomethyl-19-norcholesterol after dexamethasone suppression. The uptake of tracer is ↑ in those with aldosteronoma and absent in those with IHA and adrenal carcinoma.

Treatment

- Low-Na$^+$ diet
- Control of BP and hypokalemia with spironolactone, amiloride, or ACEIs
- Surgery (unilateral adrenalectomy) for APA

H. PHEOCHROMOCYTOMA

Definition

Catecholamine-producing tumors that originate from chromaffin cells of the adrenergic system. Secrete both NE and epi, but NE is predominant amine; 25% of pheos are familial (MEN II, neurofibromatosis, von Hippel–Lindau).

Diagnosis

H&P

- HTN: sustained (55%) or paroxysmal (45%)
- Headache (80%): paroxysmal, described as "pounding" and severe
- Palpitations (70%): w/ or w/o tachycardia
- Hyperhidrosis (60%): most evident during paroxysmal attacks of HTN
- PE may be entirely nl if done in a sx-free interval; during a paroxysm, there is ↑↑ BP, profuse sweating, visual disturbances (caused by hypertensive retinopathy), dilated pupils (secondary to catecholamine excess), paresthesias in the LEs (caused by severe vasoconstriction), tremor, tachycardia.

Labs

- Plasma-free metanephrines show ↑ normetanephrines >2.5 pmol/mL or ↑ metanephrine >1.4 pmol/mL.
- 24-hr urine collection for metanephrines reveals ↑ metanephrines.
- Clonidine suppression test: Used to distinguish between levels of plasma norepinephrine caused by release from sympathetic nerves and those from pheo. A ↓ (<50%) in plasma NE levels after clonidine administration is nl, whereas persistent ↑ = pheochromocytoma.

Imaging

- Abd CT (88% sensitivity): useful in locating pheochromocytomas >0.5 inch in diameter (90%-95% accurate); >90 % of pheos arise in adrenal medulla
- MRI: 100% sensitivity
- Scintigraphy w/^{131}I-MIBG: 100% sensitivity. NE analogue localizes in adrenergic tissue; useful in locating extra-adrenal pheochromocytomas.

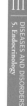

- 6-[^{18}F]Fluorodopamine PET: used when biochemical test results are + but other imaging cannot locate the tumor

Treatment

Laparoscopic removal of the tumor (surgical resection for both benign and malignant disease):

- Preoperative stabilization w/combination of phenoxybenzamine, β-blocker, metyrosine, and liberal fluid and salt intake starting 10 to 14 days before surgery
- HTN crisis preoperatively and intraoperatively controlled w/phentolamine 2 to 5 mg IV q1-2h PRN or nitroprusside used in combination w/β-adrenergic blockers

I. CARCINOID SYNDROME

- Sx complex characterized by paroxysmal vasomotor disturbances, diarrhea, and bronchospasm resulting from amines and peptides (serotonin, bradykinin, histamine) produced by tumors arising from neuroendocrine cells
- Located in appendix (40%), small bowel (20%; 15% in the ileum), rectum (15%), bronchi (12%), esophagus, stomach, colon (10%), ovary, biliary tract, pancreas (3%)

Diagnosis

H&P

- Cutaneous flushing (75%-90%)
- Red-purple flushes starting in the face, then spreading to the neck and upper trunk
- The flushing episodes last from a few minutes to hr (longer lasting flushes may be associated w/bronchial carcinoids).
- Dizziness, tachycardia, and hypotension may be associated w/the cutaneous flushing.
- Diarrhea (>70%): often associated w/abd bloating and audible peristaltic rushes
- Intermittent bronchospasm (25%)
- Facial telangiectasia
- Tricuspid insufficiency, pulmonic stenosis from carcinoid heart lesions

Labs

- ↑ 24-hr urinary 5-hydroxyindoleacetic acid (5-HIAA)
- Biochemical screening can also be done w/plasma chromogranin A.

Imaging

- CXR: to detect bronchial carcinoids
- CT of abd to detect liver mets
- Iodine-123–labeled somatostatin (^{123}I-SS) scintigraphy

Treatment

- Surgical resection
- Octreotide or lanreotide for flushing and diarrhea
- Interferon α may be used as an additive Rx when sx persist.
- Percutaneous embolization and ligation of the hepatic artery can ↓ the bulk of the tumor in the liver and provide palliative Rx of tumors w/hepatic mets.

J. MULTIPLE ENDOCRINE NEOPLASIA

CLASSIFICATION

MEN I (Wermer's Syndrome)

Tumors or hyperplasia of anterior pituitary, enteropancreatic neuroendocrine system (insulinoma, gastrinoma, glucagonoma), parathyroid, and other tissues . MENI is commonly known as the 3P's (pituitary, pancreas, parathyroid tumors)

- Possible associated conditions:
  - Adrenocortical adenoma or hyperplasia
  - Thyroid adenoma or hyperplasia
  - Renal cortical adenoma
  - Carcinoid tumors
  - GI polyps
  - Skin angiofibromas and skin collagenomas
- Clinical manifestations:
  - Peptic ulcer and its complications (gastrinoma)
  - Hypoglycemia (insulinoma)
  - Hypercalcemia or nephrocalcinosis

- Watery diarrhoea (vipoma)
- Headache, visual field defects, secondary amenorrhea
- Multiple SC lipomas
- Other: flushing, acromegaly, Cushing's syndrome, hyperthyroidism

MEN II (Sipple's Syndrome, MEN IIA)

Associated w/MTC, pheochromocytoma, and hyperparathyroidism

- Clinical manifestations:
  - Neck mass (caused by MTC)
  - HTN
  - Headache, palpitations, sweating
  - Hypercalcemia, nephrocalcinosis, osteitis fibrosa cystica
- Relatives of affected persons should be screened to detect medullary carcinoma at an early stage; screening can be accomplished with
  - Pentagastrin test: unreliable because it does not distinguish C-cell hyperplasia from small carcinomas
  - DNA analysis: reliable method for identification of MEN IIA gene carriers

MEN III (Multiple Mucosal Neuroma Syndrome, MEN IIB)

Associated w/MTC, pheochromocytoma, and multiple mucosal neuromas. Possible associated conditions: intestinal ganglioneuromatosis, marfanoid habitus

- Clinical manifestations:
  - Neck mass (caused by MTC)
  - Headache, palpitations, sweating, HTN
  - Mucosal neuromas (initially noted as whitish, yellow-pink nodules involving lips and anterior third of tongue)
  - Marfan-like habitus (w/absence of CV abnlities and lens subluxation)
  - Peripheral neuropathy (caused by neuromatous plaques overlying the posterior columns of the spinal cord, cauda equina, and sciatic nerve)

6 Gastroenterology

A. ACUTE GASTROINTESTINAL BLEEDING

GENERAL APPROACH
- Evaluate the extent (severity) of the bleeding and assess hemodynamic stability.
- Locate the site of the bleeding:
  - Upper GI bleeding (above the ligament of Treitz): PUD (40%–79%), gastritis/duodenitis (5%–30%), esophageal or gastric varices (6%–21%), Mallory-Weiss tears (3%–15%), tumors (2%–3%), AV (<1%) and aortoenteric fistulas (<1%)
  - Lower GI bleeding (below the ligament of Treitz): Acute *massive* lower GI bleeding causes are diverticular disease (17%–40%), angiodysplasia (2%–30% of colonic bleeding, 70%–80% of small bowel bleeding), neoplasm (11%–14%), IBD (9%–21%), ischemic colitis (5%), solitary rectal ulcer (2%–5%), NSAID-induced colonic ulceration (1%), acute infectious colitis (1%), pseudomembranous colitis (1%), postpolypectomy bleeding (2%–5%), radiation colitis (2%–5%), hemorrhoids (1%), and anal fissures (1%).

Hx
- Meds (ASA, steroids, "blood thinners," NSAIDs)
- Prior GI or vascular surgery
- H/o GI dx or bleeding
- Smoking
- Alcohol intake (gastritis, esophageal varices)
- Sx of PUD
- Associated diseases (CAD, diabetes, HTN, hematologic disorders, renal failure)
- Protracted retching and vomiting (consider gastric or gastroesophageal tear [Mallory-Weiss syndrome])
- Weight loss, anorexia (consider carcinoma)
- Color and character of stool (i.e., hematochezia or melena, constipation or diarrhea)
- Presence or absence of hematemesis

PE
- VS: tachycardia, hypotension, postural changes (orthostatic hypotension). A pulse ↑ >20 bpm or a postural ↑ in systolic BP >10 to 15 mm Hg indicates blood loss >1 L.
- Pts taking β-adrenergic blockers may not demonstrate significant tachycardia w/volume depletion.
- Cardiorespiratory exam: murmurs (↑ incidence of angiodysplasia in pts w/AS), pulmonary rales, JVD to determine rapidity of volume replacement
- Abd exam:
  - Observe for masses, tenderness, distention, ascites.
  - Auscultate for bowel sounds or abd bruits.
  - Look for evidence of liver disease (hepatomegaly, splenomegaly, abnl vascular patterns, gynecomastia, spider angiomas, palmar erythema, testicular atrophy).
- DRE: Check for masses, strictures, hemorrhoids; test stool for occult blood and inspect it for abnormalities (tarry, blood streaked, bright red, mahogany color).
- Skin: Check for jaundice (liver disease), ecchymoses (coagulation abnormality), cutaneous telangiectasia (Rendu-Osler-Weber disease), buccal pigmentation (Peutz-Jeghers syndrome), and other mucocutaneous changes (Ehlers-Danlos syndrome).
- Look for evidence of metastatic disease (cachexia, firm nodular liver).
- If the pt is not experiencing hematemesis and endoscopy is not immediately available, an NG tube may be placed for gastric lavage while awaiting endoscopy to determine whether the bleeding is emanating from the UGI tract (presence of bright red blood clots or coffee-ground–like guaiac (+) aspirate); however, the sensitivity and specificity of this process are limited. A (–) aspirate does not r/o upper GI bleeding because it could have subsided or the pt could be bleeding from the duodenal bulb w/o reflux into the stomach. Lavage w/500 mL of NS. Failure to clear blood w/gastric lavage indicates persistent bleeding and the need for more urgent endoscopy.

INITIAL MANAGEMENT

- Stabilize the pt: Insert two large-bore (18-gauge) IV catheters and administer lactated Ringer's solution or NS; the rate of volume replacement is based on the estimated blood loss, clinical condition, and h/o CVD, including CHF.
- Type and crossmatch for 2 to 8 U of PRBCs, depending on the estimated blood loss, and transfuse as necessary. Aim for Hct >30 for elderly pts w/multiple comorbid conditions and ≥20 for young, healthy individuals.
- Initial labs:
  - Hgb/Hct
    - Initial value should be considered erroneous until serum volume is replaced by crystalloid fluid.
    - After bleeding ceases, the Hct may continue to ↓ for up to 6 hr, and full equilibration may require 24 hr. Follow the Hgb/Hct q6-8 hr while active bleeding is present.
    - The Hct generally ↓ by 2 to 3 points and the Hgb falls by 1 point for every 500 mL of blood lost.
  - BUN: In the absence of renal disease, the BUN level may help determine the severity of the bleeding; a simultaneous Cr level may also be of value because the disparity in the BUN/Cr ratio will reveal the extent of the bleeding more accurately; BUN/Cr >36 is suggestive of UGI bleeding. BUN levels can be confusing if the bleeding is insidious and may mark prerenal azotemia secondary to the bleeding.
  - PT, APTT, and Plt count should be calculated to exclude bleeding disorders; other useful initial labs are LFTs, serum electrolytes, and glucose.
- ECG: R/o myocardial ischemia secondary to severe anemia in patients with risk factors.

ENDOSCOPIC EZZVALUATION

- EGD is indicated when blood or guaiac (+) coffee ground–like material is obtained from the NG aspirate or if lower endoscopic findings are (–). It should be performed urgently in hemodynamically unstable pts or those found to still be actively bleeding by NG lavage or in those requiring blood transfusion. Otherwise, it should ideally be performed within 24 hr of the hospital admission. In addition, if a therapeutic procedure (e.g., bipolar heater probe, laser cauterization, injection scleroRx, or band ligation) is considered, endoscopy should be done on an emergency basis.
- Colonoscopy should be performed initially if lower GI bleeding is suspected, generally within 24 hr of hospital admission after adequate bowel preparation.

IMAGING

- Arteriography can identify briskly bleeding sources. Overall diagnostic sensitivity of arteriography is 41%. Mesenteric arteriography is useful to identify bleeding from AV malformations.
- Radionuclide scans may be used before angiography to determine which pts are bleeding sufficiently to make (+) angiographic result more likely. Bleeding at rates as low as 0.1 mL/min can be detected by radionuclide scans. A (+) "immediate blush" is a good indication for urgent angiography, whereas a (–) "delayed blush" is an indication for observation and elective colonoscopy.
- Technetium-99m (^{99m}Tc) pertechnetate scan (Meckel scan) selectively tags acid-secreting cells (gastric mucosa); it is used most often for unexplained bleeding in infants and young adults.
- ^{99m}Tc-sulfur colloid scan is very sensitive in detecting lesions w/low bleeding rates; its major drawbacks are as follows:
  - Short half-life (difficulty in detecting intermittent bleeding)
  - Affinity of the colloid for liver and spleen (colonic bleeding may be missed if it originates in a region superimposed on areas of liver or spleen uptake)
- ^{99m}Tc-labeled RBC scan: Its major advantage over the sulfur colloid scan is its long duration; it is useful for intermittent bleeding because the pt can be monitored for GI bleeding for 24 to 48 hr. Its disadvantage is that it has a high false-localization rate.
- Selective angiography:
  - On occasion, this is the first test ordered in actively bleeding pts, but in most situations, it is reserved for massive, ongoing bleeding, especially when endoscopy is not feasible or when endoscopic evaluation is unrevealing w/recurrent or persistent blood loss.
  - Angiography may also be therapeutic because vasoconstrictors, autologous clots, or Gelfoam emboli can be administered intra-arterially at the time of angiography to occlude the bleeding vessel.

- Major drawbacks are the high rate of bleeding (>0.5 mL/min) necessary for dx and the risk of allergic reaction to the contrast dye.
- Advantages include the fact that no bowel preparation is required and anatomic localization is accurate.
- Enhanced helical CT scanning w/IV contrast material is used in selected cases.

Treatment
- Correct bleeding abnormalities by administering FFP or vitamin K if the pt has a coagulopathy and Plt if the pt is severely thrombocytopenic.
- IV PPIs in cases of probable peptic ulcer or gastritis. After endoscopic Rx of bleeding peptic ulcers, IV PPIs ↓ the risk of recurrent bleeding ↑ pH, ↑ platelet function.
- Octreotide: IV bolus of 50 to 100 μg followed by IV infusion of 25 to 50 μg/hr is useful for acute variceal bleeding. Another useful agent is terlipressin.
- Endoscopy:
  - ScleroRx or endoscopic variceal ligation is used for bleeding varices.
  - Injection Rx (e.g., epinephrine, saline), bipolar electrocoagulation, and heater-probe Rx are equally effective modalities in the Rx of bleeding peptic ulcer.
- Balloon tamponade is indicated for severe bleeding from esophageal varices if octreotide or other endoscopic Rx modalities are ineffective.
- Radiologic modalities include localized infusion of vasopressin, autologous clots, or foreign coagulating substances (e.g., Gelfoam) in the bleeding vessel during or after arteriography.
- Surgery is indicated at the onset of dx of aortoduodenal fistula, but it is not suggested as the initial Rx in cases of other causes of GI bleeding until a definitive dx is made and other noninvasive modalities are tried. Surgical approach may be necessary in the following situations:
  - Rebleeding in a hospitalized pt
  - Bleeding episode that requires transfusion of >4 U of PRBCs in 24 hr or >10 U of PRBCs in total
  - Endoscopic visualization of a "naked" vessel in a peptic ulcer unresponsive to injection or coagulation Rx

B. DISORDERS OF THE ESOPHAGUS

1 DYSPHAGIA

a. Oropharyngeal Dysphagia
- Inability to move food from oropharynx via UES → esophagus
- Drooling, postnasal regurgitation, difficulty initiating swallowing, sialorrhea, sensation of food stuck in the neck, coughing/choking during swallowing, dysphonia, and dysarthria

Diagnosis
- First test = modified barium swallow videofluoroscopy, then fiberoptic flexible nasopharyngeal laryngoscopy

b. Esophageal Dysphagia
- Inability to move food from esophagus → stomach
- Dysphagia to solids suggests mechanical obstruction.
- Neuromuscular causes result in dysphagia to both solids and liquids.
- Sx intermittent in pts with esophageal dysphagia from benign causes of structural obstruction or diffuse esophageal spasm; sx progressive in pts with peptic stricture, esophageal carcinoma, scleroderma, and achalasia
- Luminal diameter >18 to 20 mm (rarely sx); diameter <13 mm (sx)

Diagnosis
- Esophageal dysphagia: first test = barium esophagography, then EGD

Treatment
- Goal is airway protection and nutrition maintenance.
- Consider consultation with ENT, head and neck surgeon, radiologist, speech pathologist, physical therapist, dietitian, gastroenterologist, physical medicine and rehabilitation specialist, dentist, neurologist, etc., because nursing home pts with oropharyngeal dysphagia and hx of aspiration have 45% mortality rate over 1 yr

2 ESOPHAGEAL MOTILITY DISORDERS
- Table 6-1 compares esophageal motor disorders.

TABLE 6-1 ■ Esophageal Motor Disorders			
	Achalasia	Scleroderma	Diffuse Esophageal Spasm
Symptoms	Dysphagia Regurgitation of nonacidic material	Gastroesophageal reflux disease Dysphagia	Substronal chest pain (angina-like) Dysphagia with pain
Radiographic appearance	Dilated, fluid-filled esophagus Distal bird-beak stricture	Aperistaltic esophagus Free reflux Peptic stricture	Simultaneous noncoordinated contractions
Manometric Findings			
Lower esophageal sphincter	High resting pressure Incomplete or abnormal relaxation with swallow	Low resting pressure	Normal pressure
Body	Low-amplitude, simultaneous contractions after swallowing	Low-amplitude peristaltic contractions or no peristalsis	Some peristalsis Diffuse and simultaneous nonperistaltic contractions, occasionally high amplitude

From Andreoli, T E, Benjamin IJ, Griggs RC, Wing EJ: Andreoli and Carpenter's Cecil Essentials of Medicine, 8th ed. Philadelphia, Saunders, 2010.

3 GERD

■ Motility disorder caused by the reflux of gastric contents into the esophagus

Etiology
■ Incompetent LES
■ Medications ↓ LES pressure (CCBs, β-blockers, theophylline, anti-AChs)
■ Foods ↓ LES pressure (chocolate, yellow onions, peppermint)
■ Tobacco abuse, alcohol, coffee
■ Pregnancy
■ Gastric acid hypersecretion
■ Hiatal hernia (present in 70% w/GERD); however, most w/hiatal hernia asx

Diagnosis
H&P
■ Heartburn, dysphagia, sour taste, regurgitation of gastric contents into mouth, chronic cough/bronchospasm, chest pain, laryngitis, early satiety, abd fullness and bloating w/belching, dental erosions in children

Additional Testing
■ EGD = document type/extent tissue damage; r/o potential malignancy (Barrett's esophagus)
■ 24-hr esophageal pH monitoring: generally not done; useful in atypical manifestations of GERD (chest pain and chronic cough)
■ Esophageal manometry: useful in refractory reflux pt w/surgical Rx planned
■ Upper GI series: identify ulcerations/strictures; may miss mucosal abnormalities. Only one third of pts w/GERD have radiographic signs of esophagitis.

Treatment
■ Lifestyle change (wt loss, ↓ fat intake)/avoidance of exacerbating factors: EtOH, tobacco, citrus/tomato–based products, caffeine, β-blockers, CCBs, α-agonists, theophylline
■ ↑ Head of bed 4 to 8 in. Avoid lying supine directly after late/large meals.
■ Avoid wearing clothing that is tight around the waist.
■ PPIs: preferred Rx (H₂ blockers less effective)
■ Antacids: relief of mild sx; ineffective in severe cases
■ Prokinetic agents (metoclopramide): indicated if PPIs not fully effective. May be used in combination Rx; however, side effects limit use.
■ Nissen fundoplication (refractory cases)
■ Endoscopic radiofrequency heating of GE-jxn (*Stretta procedure*): pts unresponsive to traditional Rx

4 BARRETT'S ESOPHAGUS

■ Squamous lining of lower esophagus replaced by intestinalized metaplastic columnar epithelium; predisposing to neoplasia

H&P
■ Sx ranging from heartburn → dysphagia → nl PE

Diagnosis
- EGD with biopsy

Treatment
- Control GERD sx; maintain healed mucosa via PPI

Monitoring
- Relative risk of adenocarcinoma is 11.3 compared with general population.
- Pts should undergo surveillance EGD and systematic four-quadrant biopsy at intervals determined by the presence and grade of dysplasia.
- Pts who have had two consecutive EGDs showing no dysplasia should have follow-up every 3 to 5 yr.
- Pts with low-grade dysplasia should have extensive mucosal sampling within 6 mo and follow-up every 6 to 12 mo.
- Pts with high-grade dysplasia should have expert confirmation and extensive mucosal sampling. High-grade dysplasia with visible mucosal irregularities should be removed by endoscopic mucosal resection.
- Consider intensive surveillance every 3 mo for patients with focal high-grade dysplasia. Patients with multifocal high-grade dysplasia or carcinoma should be considered for resection or ablation if not an operative candidate.

5 ESOPHAGEAL TUMORS
- 15% in proximal third esophagus, 50% in middle third, 35% in lower third
- Risk factors: EtOH, smoking, achalasia (7× > risk), chronic GERD, HPV (types 16, 18), obesity/hiatal hernia/low-vitamin high-fat diet, ingested carcinogens (nitrates, smoked opiates, fungal toxins [pickled vegetables], betel nut chewing, mucosal damage (long-term exposure tea >70° C, lye ingestion), radiation-induced stricture

H&P
- Dysphagia (74%): initially with solid foods; gradually → semisolids/liquids
- Unintentional weight loss; losing >10% of body mass = poor outcome
- Hoarseness (recurrent laryngeal nerve involvement)
- Cervical adenopathy; usually supraclavicular lymph nodes

Diagnosis
- EGD
- Endoscopic U/S: locoregional staging (depth of invasion/lymph assessment)
- Chest/abd CT and/or integrated CT-PET scans (tumor spread for preop staging)
- Staging laparoscopy may alter Rx plans (20%-30% cases) by more accurately staging regional lymph nodes/detecting occult peritoneal mets.

Treatment
- Surgical resection of squamous cell carcinoma and adenocarcinoma of lower esophageal third indicated for local, resectable disease in the absence of widespread mets detected by CT-PET. Gastric pull-through/colonic interposition is typically used to provide luminal continuity.
- Squamous cell carcinoma is more radiosensitive than adenocarcinoma; used as palliative monoRx of obstructive sx in unresectable/advanced cases.
- Palliative radiation Rx for bone mets
- Preoperative chemoradioRx + surgery in late stage I (T2,3N0), stage II or III ↑ tumoricidal effects
- 5-yr survival 13% (37.3% [local], 18.4% [regional], 3.1% [distant] disease)

C. DISORDERS OF STOMACH AND DUODENUM

1 PEPTIC ULCER DISEASE

Etiology/Epidemiology
- *H. pylori* infection (70%-90% duodenal ulcers)
- NSAIDs (40%-50% gastric ulcers)
- Cigarette smoking, EtOH
- Neoplasia: gastrinoma (ZE syndrome), carcinoid, mastocytosis

Diagnosis
- EGD (preferred), UGI barium studies
- *H. pylori* testing by endoscopic biopsy (gold standard), urea breath test (dx active infection >90% sens/spec), stool antigen test (useful for follow-up s/p Rx), or serology (shows hx but not necessarily current infection, false-[+] possible s/p Rx)

Treatment
- Eradicate if (+) *H. pylori* infection (Table 6-2).
- Lifestyle change: d/c smoking/EtOH.
- Add PPI to ↓ acid secretions.

TABLE 6-2 ■ Overview of Antibiotics Used for *Helicobacter Pylori* Eradication

Drug Class	Drug	Triple Therapy* Dose	Quadruple Therapy† Dose	Sequential Therapy‡ Dose
Acid suppression	Proton pump inhibitor	20-40 mg bid§	20-40 mg bid§	20-40 mg bid§
Standard antimicrobials	Bismuth compound‖	2 tablets bid	2 tablets bid	
	Amoxicillin	1 g bid		1 g bid
	Metronidazole¶	500 mg bid	500 mg tid	500 mg bid
	Clarithromycin	500 mg bid		500 mg bid
	Tetracycline		500 mg qid	
Salvage antimicrobials	Levofloxacin	300 mg bid	300 mg bid	
	Rifabutin	150 mg bid		
	Furazolidone	100 mg bid		
	Doxycycline		100 mg bid	
	Nitazoxanide		1 g bid	

*Triple therapy consists of a proton pump inhibitor or bismuth compound, together with two of the listed antibiotics, usually given for 7-14 days.

†Quadruple therapy consists of a proton pump inhibitor plus either the combination of a bismuth compound, metronidazole, and tetracycline given for 4-10 days, or the combination of levofloxacin, doxycycline, and nitazoxanide for 10 days.

‡Sequential therapy consists of 10 days of proton pump inhibitor treatment, plus amoxicillin during days 1-5 and a combination of clarithromycin and an imidazole (when available, tinidazole; otherwise, metronidazole) during days 6-10.

§Proton pump inhibitor dose equivalent to omeprazole 20 mg bid.

‖Bismuth subsalicylate or subcitrate.

¶An alternative is tinidazole 500 mg bid.

From Goldman L, Schafer AI (eds): Goldman's Cecil Medicine, 24th ed. Philadelphia, Saunders, Elsevier, 2012.

2 GASTROPARESIS
- Sx impaired gastric emptying in absence of mechanical obstruction

Differential Diagnosis and Clinical Pearls
- Diabetes mellitus gastroparesis (HBA_{1c}, fasting glucose)
- Gastric surgery
- Pregnancy
- Hypothyroidism (TSH)
- Cannabinoid hyperemesis syndrome (hx of use; hx of relief of N/V with hot baths/showers)
- Rumination syndrome (hx of passive regurgitation of pleasant tasting food w/o nausea)

Management
- Prokinetic agents (e.g., metoclopramide)
- Refractory cases (↑ risk malnutrition), gastroduodenal manometry to distinguish myopathic from neuropathic process

3 GASTRIC CANCER
- Adenocarcinoma; mostly antral (35%)
- Male-to-female ratio 3:2
- Familiar diffuse gastric cancer (autosomal dominant, mutation E-cadherin gene *CDH1* = cancer at young age)

Physical Exam and Labs
- Wt loss (70%-80%), N/V (20%-40%), dysphagia (20%)
- Dyspepsia (unrelieved by antacids, worse w/food), epigastric/abd mass (40%)
- Microcytic anemia, hemoccult (+) stools
- Hypoalbuminemia

Diagnosis
- Upper endoscopy with biopsy (staging via abd CT scan ± lymph node dissection)

Treatment
- If curable: gastrectomy with regional lymphadenectomy

III

DISEASES AND DISORDERS
6. Gastroenterology

- Perioperative epirubicin, cisplatin, and infused fluorouracil (ECF) ↑ survival
- Gastrectomy pts require vitamin B_{12} replacement

D. DISORDERS OF THE PANCREAS

1 ACUTE PANCREATITIS

■ Inflammatory process w/intrapancreatic enzyme activation possibly also involving peripancreatic tissue/remote organ systems

Etiology
■ >90% of cases: biliary tract disease (calculi or sludge) or EtOH
■ Drugs: thiazides, furosemide, corticosteroids, tetracycline, estrogens, valproic acid, metronidazole, azathioprine, methyldopa, pentamidine, ethacrynic acid, procainamide, sulindac, nitrofurantoin, ACEIs, danazol, cimetidine, piroxicam, gold, ranitidine, sulfasalazine, isoniazid, acetaminophen, cisplatin, opiates, erythromycin
■ Abd trauma, surgery, ERCP, viral infections, PUD, pancreas divisum (congenital failure to fuse of dorsal or ventral pancreas), pregnancy, vascular (vasculitis, ischemic), hypolipoproteinemia (types I, IV, and V), hypercalcemia, pancreatic carcinoma (primary/mets), renal failure, hereditary pancreatitis, occupational exposure (methanol, cobalt, zinc, mercuric chloride, creosol, lead, organophosphates, chlorinated naphthalenes)
■ Others: scorpion bite, obstruction at ampulla region (neoplasm, duodenal diverticula, Crohn's disease), hypotensive shock, autoimmune pancreatitis

Scoring System
■ Table 6-3 describes various scoring systems to assess severity of acute pancreatitis.
■ BUN most accurate in predicting severity

TABLE 6-3 ■ Scoring Systems to Assess Severity of Acute Pancreatitis	
System	**Criteria**
Ranson	At admission
	Age >55 yr
	WBC >16,000/μL
	Glucose >200 mg/dL
	LDH >350 IU/L
	AST >250 IU/L
	Within next 48 hr
	Decrease in hematocrit by >10%
	Estimated fluid sequestration of >6 L
	Serum calcium <8.0 mg/dL
	Pao_2 <60 mm Hg
	BUN increase >5 mg/dL after hydration
	Base deficit >4 mmol/L
APACHE-II	Multiple clinical and laboratory factors. Calculator available at www.mdcalc.com/apache-ii-score-for-icu-mortality
BISAP	BUN >25 mg/dL
	Impaired mental status
	Presence of SIRS
	Age >60 yr
	Pleural effusion
CT	A: Normal pancreas
	B: Focal or diffuse enlargement of pancreas
	C: Grade B plus pancreatic and/or peripancreatic inflammation
	D: Grade C plus a single fluid collection
	E: Grade C plus two or more fluid collections or gas in pancreas
CT severity index	CT grade
	A = 0
	B = 1
	C = 2
	D = 3
	E = 4
	Plus necrosis grade
	No necrosis = 0
	<30% necrosis = 2
	30-50% necrosis = 4
	>50% necrosis = 6

APACHE-II, Acute Physiology and Chronic Health Evaluation II; *BISAP*, bedside index of severity in acute pancreatitis. From Goldman L, Schafer AI (eds): Goldman's Cecil Medicine, 24th ed. Philadelphia, Saunders, Elsevier, 2012.

"Severe Acute Pancreatitis"

The presence of any of the following 4 criteria:

1. Organ failure w/one or more of the following: shock (systolic BP <90 mm Hg), pulmonary insufficiency (Pao_2 <60 mm Hg), renal failure (serum Cr >2 mg/dL after rehydration), and GI bleeding (>500 mL/24 hr)
2. Local complications such as necrosis, pseudocyst, or abscess
3. At least 3 of Ranson's criteria
4. At least 8 of the APACHE II criteria

Diagnosis

H&P

- Fever, epigastric tenderness/guarding; sudder severe pain (peak intensity 10-30 min; lasting several hr w/o relief)
- Hypoactive bowel sounds (secondary to ileus)
- Tachycardia, shock (secondary to ↓ intravascular volume)
- Confusion (secondary to metabolic disturbances)
- ↓ Breath sounds (atelectasis, pleural effusions ARDS)
- Jaundice (secondary to obstruction or compression of biliary tract)
- Ascites (secondary to tear in pancreatic duct, leaking pseudocyst)
- Palpable abd mass (pseudocyst, phlegmon, abscess, carcinoma)
- Hypocalcemia (*Chvostek's sign, Trousseau's sign*)
- Intra-abd bleeding (hemorrhagic pancreatitis):
  - Gray-blue discoloration around umbilicus (*Cullen's sign*)
  - Bluish discoloration involving flanks (*Grey Turner's sign*)
- Tender SC nodules (SC fat necrosis)

Labs

- ↑ Serum amylase (initial 3-5 days), ↑ serum lipase, ↑ serum trypsin
- Rapid urinary trypsinogen-2; useful screening test in pts w/abd pain; (−) dipstick r/o acute pancreatitis w/high degree of probability; (+) test result indicates need for further evaluation.
- CBC: leukocytosis; ↑ Hct (secondary to hemoconcentration); ↓ Hct may indicate hemorrhage/hemolysis.
- ↑ BUN (secondary to dehydration)
- ↑ Serum glucose; in previously nl pt correlates w/pancreatic malfunction
- ↑ AST/LDH (tissue necrosis); ↑ bili/alk phos (CBD obstruction); ≥3 ↑ ALT = biliary pancreatitis (95% probability)
- ↓ Serum Ca (saponification, precipitation, and ↓ PTH response)
- ABGs: Pao_2 may be ↓ secondary to ARDS, pleural effusions; pH may be ↓ secondary to lactic acidosis, respiratory acidosis, and renal insufficiency.
- Serum electrolytes: K^+ may be ↑ secondary to acidosis/renal insufficiency; Na^+ may be ↑ secondary to dehydration.

Imaging

- Abd plain film: r/o perforated viscus; may reveal localized ileus (sentinel loop), pancreatic calcifications (chronic pancreatitis), blurring of left psoas shadow, dilation of transverse colon, calcified gallstones
- CXR: elevation of one or both diaphragms, pleural effusions, basilar infiltrates, platelike atelectasis
- Abd U/S: gallstones (sensitivity 60%-70%), pancreatic pseudocysts; limited in presence of distended bowel loops overlying pancreas
- CT abd: superior to U/S in dx extent; also able dx pseudocysts (well-defined area surrounded by high-density capsule); GI fistulation or infection of a pseudocyst (gas within pseudocyst)
- Contrast-enhanced CT (pancreatic necrosis): severity graded by CT scan (see Table 6-3)
- MRCP: useful if surgical procedure not anticipated
- ERCP: avoided during acute stage, unless to remove impacted stone

Treatment

General Measures

- Maintain intravascular volume (vigorous IV hydration).
- NPO until clinically improved, stable, and hungry; enteral feedings preferred to TPN; PN necessary if unable to tolerate enteral/adequate infusion rate cannot be reached within 2 to 4 days.
- NG suction is used to decompress abd in pts w/ileus.
- Control pain with IV morphine or fentanyl.
- Correct metabolic abnormalities (replace Ca, Mg).

III

DISEASES AND DISORDERS
6. Gastroenterology

Specific Measures

- Pancreatic/peripancreatic infection in 40% to 70% pts w/pancreatic necrosis; prophylactic IV abx (5-7 days) justified w/septicemia, pancreatic abscess, or pancreatitis secondary to biliary calculi. Cover *Bacteroides fragilis*/anaerobes (cefotetan, metronidazole, clindamycin, + AG) and enterococcus (ampicillin).
- Surgical Rx indicated: gallstone-induced pancreatitis (cholecystectomy when acute phase subsides), perforated peptic ulcer, excision/drainage necrotic/infected foci w/placement of wide-bore drains for continuous postop irrigation

Complications

- Pseudocyst (dx: CT scan or U/S) Rx: CT scan or U/S-guided percutaneous drainage w/pigtail catheter for continuous drainage (↑ recurrence rate); conservative approach to reevaluate (w/CT scan or U/S) after 6 to 7 wk and surgically drain if no ↓ in size. Pseudocysts <5 cm generally reabsorbed w/o intervention; those >5 cm require surgery after wall maturation.
- Phlegmon (dx: CT scan or U/S) Rx: supportive care
- Pancreatic abscess (dx: CT scan-retroperitoneal bubbles, Gram staining and cultures of fluid from percutaneous biopsy) Rx: surgical/catheter drainage + IV abx (imipenem-cilastatin)
- Pancreatic ascites (dx: paracentesis-amylase/lipase level in fluid, ERCP) Rx: surgery if exudative/does not resolve spontaneously
- GI bleeding: via EtOH gastritis, varices, stress ulcer, or DIC
- Renal failure: via hypovolemia (oliguria or anuria), cortical or tubular necrosis (shock, DIC), or thrombosis of renal artery or vein
- Hypoxia: via ARDS, pleural effusion, or atelectasis

2 CHRONIC PANCREATITIS

- Recurrent/persistent inflammatory process characterized by chronic pain and pancreatic exocrine/endocrine insufficiency

Etiology

- Chronic EtOH, obstruction (ampullary stenosis, tumor, trauma, pancreas divisum, annular pancreas), hereditary pancreatitis, severe malnutrition, untreated hyperparathyroidism (hypercalcemia), mutations of cystic fibrosis transmembrane conductance regulator (*CFTR*) gene (TF genotype)
- *Autoimmune (sclerosing) pancreatitis* (5% cases): manifests w/jaundice (63%) + abd pain (35%). CT = diffusely enlarged pancreas, enhanced peripheral rim of hypoattenuation "halo," and low-attenuation mass in head of pancreas. Labs = ↑ serum IgG4, serum Ig or γ -globulin level, + antilactoferrin Ab, anti–carbonic anhydrase II level, ASMA, or ANA.

Diagnosis

H&P

- Persistent/recurrent epigastric + LUQ pain, may radiate to the back
- Tenderness over the pancreas, muscle guarding
- Significant weight loss, epigastric mass (10%), jaundice (5%-10%)
- Bulky/greasy, foul-smelling stools

Labs

- ↑/NI serum amylase and lipase
- ↑ Glucose, bili, alk phos, glycosuria
- 72-hr fecal fat determination (rarely performed) = excess fecal fat. Fecal elastase test requires 20 g of stool.
- Secretin stimulation test (dx pancreatic exocrine insufficiency)
- Lipid panel: ↑↑ TGs can cause pancreatitis.
- Serum Ca: hyperparathyroidism (rare cause of chronic pancreatitis)
- ↑ Serum IgG4 (sclerosing pancreatitis and autoimmune pancreatitis)
- ↑ Serum Ig or γ-globulin level, antilactoferrin Ab, anti–carbonic anhydrase II level, ASMA, or ANA in autoimmune pancreatitis

Imaging

- Plain abd radiographs: may reveal pancreatic calcifications (95% spec)
- U/S abd: duct dilation, pseudocyst, calcification, presence of ascites
- Contrast-enhanced abd CT scan: calcifications, evaluate ductal dilation, r/o pancreatic cancer
- EUS (97% sens, 60% spec)
- FNAB combined w/EUS = preferred evaluation of modality to r/o malignant cystic/ mass lesions
- MRCP (preferred to ERCP)

■ Steatorrhea Rx w/pancreatic supplements (e.g., pancrease, pancrelipase [Creon] PRN on basis of steatorrhea/weight loss)
■ Glucocorticoids (autoimmune pancreatitis)
■ Surgical intervention if duct obstruction
■ Transduodenal sphincteroplasty/pancreaticojejunostomy if intractable pain

Clinical Pearls
■ 50% of pts die within 10 yr of chronic pancreatitis or malignant neoplasm.

3 PANCREATIC ADENOCARCINOMA

Risk Factors
■ Smoking, chronic EtOH, genetics (5%-10% pts have family hx), dipeptidyl peptidase-4 inhibitors, incretin mimetics

Diagnosis
■ Labs: ↑ alk phos, bili, amylase
H&P
■ Jaundice, abd pain (dull upper abd pain/vague abd discomfort), wt loss
Imaging
■ Multidetector helical CT with IV contrast (imaging procedure of choice)
■ Endoscopic ultrasonography: useful if no identifiable mass on CT + ↑ clinical suspicion

Treatment
Surgery
■ Curative cephalic pancreatoduodenectomy (Whipple's procedure) in 10% to 20% pts whose lesion <5 cm, solitary, and without metastases. Surgical mortality rate is 5%.
■ Palliative surgery (for biliary decompression/diversion)
■ Palliative therapeutic ERCP with stents
■ Celiac plexus block = pain relief in 80% to 90% of cases
ChemoRx
■ Gemcitabine given alone or + platinum agent (erlotinib or fluoropyrimidine)
■ Combination consisting oxaliplatin, irinotecan, fluorouracil, and leucovorin (Folfirinox)
Radiation
■ External-beam radiation for palliation of pain

4 NEUROENDOCRINE PANCREATIC NEOPLASMS

a. Gastrinoma
■ ZE syndrome: hypergastrinemic state via pancreatic/extrapancreatic non–β islet cell tumor (gastrinoma) resulting in peptic ulcer disease
■ 2/3 gastrinomas (sporadic), 60% assoc (MEN-1; AD including hyperparathyroidism, pituitary tumors)
■ 60% gastrinomas = malignant (mets to liver, regional lymph nodes)
■ Neuroendocrine tumors = 1.3% of all cases of pancreatic cancer

Diagnosis
■ Gastric acid secretion: serum gastrin level (fasting) >1000 pg/mL
■ Provocative gastrin level tests:
  • Secretin stimulation
  • Ca²⁺ stimulation
■ Gastrinoma localization via arteriography, abd U/S or CT scan or MRI
  • Selective portal vein branch gastrin level
  • Octreotide scan
H&P
■ 95% sx of peptic ulcer, 60% sx related to GERD, 33% diarrhea, steatorrhea

Treatment
■ Surgical resection; total gastrectomy/vagotomy (palliative in some pts)
■ Medical Rx: PPIs, somatostatin or octreotide, chemo (mets)

b Insulinoma

Diagnosis
H&P
■ Sx typically in ᴀᴍ before meal; fasting hypoglycemia versus reactive hypoglycemia (which is not commonly associated w/insulinoma)
Labs
■ Overnight fasting blood sugar level + simultaneous plasma insulin, proinsulin, and/or C peptide level will establish existence of fasting organic hypoglycemia in 60% of pts.

III

DISEASES AND DISORDERS
6. Gastroenterology

163

- Plasma proinsulin, C-peptide, antibodies to insulin, and plasma sulfonylurea levels to r/o factitious insulin use/hypoglycemic agents/autoantibodies against the insulin receptor or insulin. Refer to Table 5-5 in Chapter 5.

Imaging
- Abdominal CT scan or MRI
- Octreotide scan

Treatment
- Enucleation of single insulinoma
- Partial pancreatectomy for multiple adenomas

E. DISORDERS OF SMALL AND LARGE BOWEL

1 DIARRHEA

- ↑ Frequency (>200 g/24 hr) of stool w/ ↓ consistency compared with baseline; if lasting >3 wk = *chronic diarrhea*

Diagnosis

Hx
- Travel hx (traveler's diarrhea)
- Short duration (1-3 days) assoc w/mild sx usually viral (rotavirus, Norwalk virus); >3 wk probably not bacterial or viral
- Nocturnal diarrhea (common w/diabetic neuropathy)
- Onset within minutes: scombroid poisoning (tuna, mahi-mahi, mackerel) (N/V, flushing, diarrhea)
- Onset within hr: toxins (*Staphylococcus aureus*, toxigenic *Escherichia coli*, *Clostridium perfringens*, *Bacillus cereus*, *Vibrio parahaemolyticus*, [barracuda, grouper, red snapper: ciguatera toxin, causing paresthesia, weakness])
- Diarrhea secondary to *Salmonella, Shigella, Campylobacter, Yersinia* = longer incubation period.
- Stress: "functional" diarrhea, IBS
- Diarrhea alternating w/constipation: IBS
- Foods containing sorbitol/mannitol (osmotic diarrhea), fried rice (*B. cereus*), undercooked hamburger (*E. coli* 157:H7), poultry, eggs (*Campylobacter, Salmonella, S. aureus*), diarrhea after dairy ingestion (lactose intolerance)
- Shellfish ingestion (Norwalk virus, *Vibrio cholerae, Vibrio mimicus, V. parahaemolyticus, Plesiomonas shigelloides*)
- Long-distance runners (bloody diarrhea secondary to bowel ischemia)
- Daycare centers (rotavirus, *Giardia, Salmonella, Shigella, Cryptosporidium, Campylobacter*)
- Medications: (common agents: Mg-containing antacids, misoprostol, PPIs, methylxanthines [caffeine, theophylline], laxatives, lactulose, colchicine, antiarrhythmic agents (quinidine, digitalis, propranolol), metformin, thyroxine. Abx-induced pseudomembranous colitis should be suspected in any pt receiving abx: (+) *Clostridium difficile* toxin w/the stool assay, cytotoxin test.
- Sexual habits: male homosexuals ↑ incidence of (*Giardia, E. histolytica, Cryptosporidium, Salmonella, Neisseria gonorrhoeae, Campylobacter*).
- Relevant medical hx
  - Surgical hx (ileal resection, gastrectomy, cholecystectomy), abd irradiation, DM, hyperthyroidism, watery diarrhea in elderly pts w/chronic constipation via fecal impaction/obstructing carcinoma
  - AIDS: *Cryptosporidium, Salmonella*, CMV, *Mycobacterium avium-intracellulare*, Kaposi's sarcoma involving the gut, AIDS enteropathy, *Cyclospora* spp (cyanobacterium-like bodies)
  - Proteinuria, neuropathy: amyloidosis, DM
  - Organ transplantation, cancer chemoRx, steroid Rx
- Associated sx
  - Tenderness, fever, weight loss (IBD, amebiasis, lymphoma, tuberculosis)
  - Abd pain + weight loss (carcinoma of pancreas/malignant neoplasia)
  - Weight loss despite good appetite (malabsorption, hyperthyroidism)
  - Diarrhea and PUD (ZE-syndrome, gastrinoma, gastrocolic fistula)
  - Flushing and bronchospasm (carcinoid syndrome)
  - LLQ pain, fever and/or bloody diarrhea (diverticulitis)
  - Arthritis (IBD, Whipple's disease)
  - Bloody diarrhea, HUS, thrombocytopenic purpura (*E. coli* O157:H7)

- Characteristics of the stool (from pt's hx)
  - Large, foul smelling (malabsorption)
  - ↑ Mucus (IBS)
  - Watery stools (psychosomal disturbances, fecal impaction, colon carcinoma, IBD or IBS, *Cyclospora* infection, pancreatic cholera [vasoactive intestinal peptide])

PE
- Rectal fistulas, RLQ abd mass (Crohn's disease)
- Arthritis, iritis, uveitis, erythema nodosum (IBD)
- Abd masses (neoplasms of colon, pancreas, or liver; diverticular abscess [LLQ mass], IBD)
- Flushing, bronchospasm (carcinoid syndrome)
- Buccal pigmentation (Peutz-Jeghers syndrome)
- Pigmentation (Addison's disease)
- Ammoniac/urinary breath odor (renal failure)
- Ecchymosis (vitamin K deficiency secondary to malabsorption, fat-soluble vitamins, celiac)
- Fever (IBD, infectious diarrhea, lymphoma)
- Goiter, tremor, tachycardia (hyperthyroidism)
- Lymphadenopathy (neoplasm, lymphoma, tuberculosis, AIDS, Whipple's disease)
- Macroglossia (amyloidosis)
- Kaposi's sarcoma (AIDS)

Initial Evaluation
- Labs (may not be necessary in pts not appearing ill/dehydrated)
  - CBC: ↑↑ WBCs w/left shift (? infection); ↓ Hb/Hct levels (? anemia via blood loss); ↑ Hct (? dehydration)
  - Serum electrolytes: hypokalemia (diarrhea), hypernatremia (dehydration), hyponatremia (ADH compensation)
  - BUN, Cr may be ↑ via dehydration.
  - ELISA stool antigen test if suspect *Giardia*
  - Stool evaluation: most cases self-limited generally not necessary; stool cultures considered if pt febrile + bloody diarrhea or immunocompromised. If obtaining stool sample, consider:
    - Occult blood ([+] IBD, bowel ischemia, some infection)
    - Löffler's alkaline methylene blue stain for fecal leukocytes ([+] inflammatory diarrhea via *Salmonella, Campylobacter, Yersinia, Shigella*, invasive *E. coli*, although low sensitivity)
    - Bacterial cultures if bloody stool w/suspected infection (*Salmonella, Shigella, Campylobacter, Yersinia, E. coli* O157:H7); culture for *N. gonorrhoeae* active male homosexual pts
    - Examine O&P; indirect hemagglutination test (*Entamoeba histolytica*) if suspect amebiasis and stool exam inconclusive.
    - *C. difficile* toxin: r/o pseudomembranous colitis if receiving abx
    - Modified Ziehl-Neelsen stain, acid-fast, or auramine stain in immunocompromised pts w/suspected *Cryptosporidium* infection
- Abd x-rays indicated if abd pain or evidence of obstruction (r/o toxic megacolon, bowel ischemia; pancreatic calcifications = pancreatic insufficiency)

Treatment
- NPO, IV hydration, electrolyte abnl correction, d/c possible causative agents (antacids containing Mg, abx)
- Antiperistaltic agents (diphenoxylate) used w/caution in pts suspected of IBD or infectious diarrhea; loperamide/bismuth subsalicylate helpful in mild cases
- Persistent diarrhea + bacterial/parasitic organism ID, start abx:
  - *Giardia:* metronidazole, 250 mg tid × 7 to 10 days, or tinidazole, quinacrine
  - *E. histolytica:* metronidazole, 750 mg tid × 10 days, + either iodoquinol (650 mg tid × 20 days) or paromomycin
  - *Shigella:* ciprofloxacin (Cipro) 500 mg bid × 3 days, or azithromycin 500 mg qd × 3 days
  - *Campylobacter:* azithromycin 500 mg qd × 3 days or erythromycin 500 mg qid × 3 days
  - *C. difficile:* PO metronidazole or vancomycin
  - *Cyclospora:* TMP-SMX-DS bid × 7 days
  - *Salmonella* (in pts w/sickle cell, HIV, uremia, malignancy, prosthetic device, age <6 mo or >50 yr): Cipro 500 mg bid × 5 to 7 days or TMP-SMX 160 mg/800 mg bid × 5 to 7 days. Mild cases + low-risk pts = no Rx

- *V. cholerae* O1/O39: Cipro 750 mg × 1, or doxycycline 300 mg × 1, or TMP-SMX 160 mg/800 mg bid × 3 days
- *Cryptosporidium:* paromomycin 500 mg tid × 7 days (severe)
- *Yersinia* species: Cipro 500 mg bid × 7 days or TMP-SMX 160 mg/800 mg × 7 days
- *Isospora* species: TMP-SMX 160 mg/800 mg qid × 10 days, then bid × 3 wk
- *Microsporidium* species: albendazole 400 mg bid ×>3 wk
- *Salmonella* HIV pts: amoxicillin 1 g tid × 3 to 14 days, Cipro 500 mg bid× 7 days, or TMP-SMX bid × 14 days
- IBS Rx: psyllium (fiber products) + ↓ caffeine, chocolate, EtOH, stress; antispasmodics (dicyclomine, hyoscyamine) if resistant cases

Evaluation of Pt w/Chronic or Recurrent Diarrhea

Etiology
- Drug induced (including laxative abuse), IBS, lactose intolerance, IBD, malabsorption (mucosal/pancreatic insufficiency, bacterial overgrowth), parasitic infections (giardiasis, amebiasis), functional diarrhea, postsurgical (partial gastrectomy, ileal resection, cholecystectomy)
- Endocrine disturbances: DM (↓ sympathetic input to the gut), hyperthyroidism, Addison's disease, gastrinoma (ZE syndrome), VIPoma (pancreatic cholera), carcinoid tumors (serotonin), medullary thyroid carcinoma (calcitonin)
- Pelvic irradiation, colonic carcinoma (villous adenoma)
- *Collagenous colitis* (middle-aged woman, nl endoscopy, subepithelial acellular collagen band on sigmoid bx or right colon; sx resolution w/sulfasalazine alone or steroid combination)
- *Lymphocytic colitis* (lymphocytic infiltration w/o collagen band)

Diagnosis
- H&P/initial labs same as new-onset diarrhea; additional labs:
  - Sudan III stool stain: presence of fat droplets and meat fibers = malabsorption
  - CBC = macrocytic, obtain vitamin B_{12} + RBC folate levels to r/o megaloblastic anemia secondary to malabsorption
  - Mg-induced diarrhea dx w/quantitative fecal analysis for soluble Mg
  - 24-hr urine for 5-HIAA if suspected carcinoid syndrome; serum gastrin level if suspected ZE syndrome
  - Stool osmolality to evaluate for factitial diarrhea; hypotonic stools (? Munchausen syndrome/malingering because the colon does not excrete free water, hypotonicity indicates addition of water/urine/hypotonic fluid)
- Secretory diarrhea from impaired absorption/excessive secretion of electrolytes via enteric infection, neoplasms of exocrine pancreas (VIP, GIP, secretin, glucagon), bile salt enteropathy, villous adenoma, IBD, carcinoid tumor, celiac, cathartic agent ingestion
- Osmotic diarrhea from impaired water absorption secondary to osmotic effect of nonabsorbable intraluminal molecules such as lactose and other disaccharide excess, pancreatic insufficiency, lactulose/sorbitol/sodium sulfate/antacid induced, postop (gastrojejunostomy, vagotomy, pyloroplasty, intestinal resection)
- Dx *"osmotic gap"* in stool analysis = measured osmolality −2([Na^+] + [K^+])
- Difference between calculated and actual Osm >50 = osmotic diarrhea

2 CONSTIPATION
- DDx: metabolic (hypercalcemia, DM, pregnancy, hypothyroidism), structural (colorectal cancer, strictures, hernias, adhesions, endometriosis, rectocele, diverticular disease, volvulus, intussusception, IBD, hematoma of bowel wall secondary to trauma or anticoagulants), drug induced (opiates, anti-Ach, iron, CCB, antipsychotics, antacids w/aluminum, verapamil), neurologic/psychological (IBS, anorexia, depression, MS), neonatal (Hirschsprung's disease, meconium ileus, atresia), insufficient bulk in diet, travel, old age, spinal cord injury

Treatment
- Fiber (25-30 g/day) and fluid intake essential
- Physiologic testing (DRE, anorectal manometry, rectal balloon expulsion colonic transit) provides insight/possible indication for MR defecography
- Pts >50 yr old or have alarm sx (wt loss, rectal bleeding, change in bowel habits, FHx colon cancer) should undergo colonoscopy

3 MALABSORPTION
- Generalized loss of nutrients, fat, carbohydrates, or protein in digestive tract

Differential Diagnosis

- *Celiac disease* (diarrhea, bloating, wt loss)
  - Rx: gluten-free diet
- *Lactose malabsorption* (osmotic diarrhea, bloating, excess flatus)
  - Dx: hydrogen breath test (>20 pp million)
  - Rx: asx up to 12 g lactose ingestion, dietary diligence
- *Short-bowel syndrome* (<200 cm of small bowel, nl 600 cm) from Crohn's disease, ischemia, volvulus, desmoid tumors, trauma
  - Rx: dietary/electrolyte monitoring, gastric acid control (PPI), hydration
- *Small intestinal bacterial overgrowth:* bacterial overgrowth from change in colonic flora via dysmotility (scleroderma, amyloidosis), altered secretion/anatomy
  - Dx: upper endoscopy with culture $>10^5$ organisms/mL
  - Rx: abx (amoxicillin-clavulanate, fluoroquinolones, tetracyclines, metronidazole)

4 CELIAC DISEASE

- Chronic disease characterized by malabsorption and diarrhea precipitated by ingestion of food products containing gluten. Celiac sprue is considered an autoimmune-type disease, with TTG suggested as a major autoantigen. It results from an inappropriate T-cell–mediated immune response against ingested gluten in genetically predisposed individuals who carry either HLA-DQ2 or HLA-DQ8 genes. There is sensitivity to gliadin, a protein fraction of gluten found in wheat, rye, and barley. In patients with celiac disease, immune responses to gliadin fractions promote an inflammatory reaction, mainly in the upper small intestine, manifested by infiltration of the lamina propria and the epithelium with chronic inflammatory cells and villous atrophy.

Diagnosis

H&P

- Weight loss, pallor (from anemia), dyspepsia, short stature, and failure to thrive in children and infants
- Weight loss, fatigue, pallor, and diarrhea in adults
- Angular cheilitis, aphthous ulcers, atopic dermatitis, and dermatitis herpetiformis frequently associated w/celiac disease

Labs

- IgA TTG antibody by enzyme-linked immunosorbent assay (TTG test) is the best screening serologic test for celiac disease.
- Iron deficiency anemia (microcytic anemia, ↓ ferritin level)
- Folic acid deficiency
- Serum I_fA (small % of patients are I_fA deficient)
- Vitamin B_{12} deficiency, ↓ Mg, ↓ Ca

Treatment

- Gluten-free diet (avoidance of wheat, rye, and barley). Safe grains (gluten free) include rice, corn, oats, buckwheat, millet, amaranth, quinoa.
- Correct nutritional deficiencies w/iron, folic acid, Ca, vitamin B_{12} as needed.
- Prednisone 20-60 mg qd gradually tapered is useful in refractory cases.

Clinical Pearls

- Celiac disease should be considered in pts w/unexplained metabolic bone disease or hypocalcemia, especially because GI sx may be absent or mild. Clinicians should also consider testing children and young adults for celiac disease if unexplained weight loss, abd pain or distention, and chronic diarrhea are present.
- Pts w/celiac disease have an overall risk of cancer that is almost 2× that in the general population: risk of adenocarcinoma of the small intestine and non-Hodgkin's lymphoma, especially of T-cell type and primarily localized in the gut.
- Screening for celiac disease is recommended in first-degree relatives. It should also be considered in type 1 DM and autoimmune disorders such as PBC, primary sclerosing cholangitis, autoimmune hepatitis, IBD, thyroid disease (hypothyroidism occurs in up to 15% of patients with celiac disease), SLE, RA, and Sjögren's syndrome because of the increased risk of celiac disease in these populations. Screening persons with Down's syndrome or Turner's syndrome for celiac disease has also been recommended.

5 INFLAMMATORY BOWEL DISEASE

a. Crohn's Disease

- Inflammatory disease most commonly involving the terminal ileum. Table 6-4 compares Crohn's disease with ulcerative colitis.

TABLE 6-4 ■ Differentiating Features of Ulcerative Colitis and Crohn's Disease

	Ulcerative Colitis	Crohn's Disease
Site of involvement	Involves only colon Rectum almost always involved	Any area of the gastrointestinal tract Rectum usually spared
Pattern of involvement	Continuous	Skip lesions
Diarrhea	Bloody	Usually nonbloody
Severe abdominal pain	Rare	Frequent
Perianal disease	No	In 30% of patients
Fistula	No	Yes
Endoscopic findings	Erythematous and friable Superficial ulceration	Aphthoid and deep ulcers Cobblestoning
Radiologic findings	Tubular appearance resulting from loss of haustral folds	String sign of terminal ileum RLQ mass, fistulas, abscesses
Histologic features	Mucosa only Crypt abscesses	Transmural Crypt abscesses, granulomas (about 30%)
Smoking	Protective	Worsens course
Serology	p-ANCA more common	ASCA more common

From Andreoli, T E, Benjamin IJ, Griggs RC, Wing EJ: Andreoli and Carpenter's Cecil Essentials of Medicine, 8th ed. Philadelphia, Saunders, 2010.

Diagnosis

H&P

- Sx intermittent w/episodic remission:
  - Abd tenderness/mass/distention
  - Chronic or nocturnal diarrhea, wt loss, fever, night sweats
  - Hyperactive bowel sounds (if partial obstruction), bloody diarrhea
  - Delayed growth and failure to thrive in children
  - Perianal and rectal abscesses, mouth ulcers, atrophic glossitis
  - Extraintestinal manifestations: joint swelling and tenderness, hepatosplenomegaly, erythema nodosum, clubbing, SI joint tenderness to palpation

Labs

- ↓ Hgb/Hct (chronic blood loss, bone marrow inflammation, and vitamin B_{12} malabsorption)
- ↓ K, Mg, Ca, alb in pts w/chronic diarrhea
- Vitamin B_{12} and folate deficiency
- ↑ ESR, (+) ASCA, (−) ANCA

Imaging

- Endoscopy: transmural asymmetric/discontinued disease w/deep longitudinal fissures ("**cobblestone**" appearance via submucosal inflammation"), strictures, crypt distortion + inflammation, possible **noncaseating granulomas** + lymphoid aggregates on bx
- Barium imaging (rarely indicated): deep ulcerations (often longitudinal/transverse) and segmental lesions (**skip lesions**), strictures, **fistulas**); "thumbprinting" is common; "string sign" in terminal ileum
- CT abd: helpful in identifying abscesses/complications
- See Table 6-4.

Treatment

- Figure 6-1 describes a treatment algorithm for Crohn's disease.

b. Ulcerative Colitis

Diagnosis

H&P

- Abd distention and tenderness
- Bloody diarrhea, fever, evidence of dehydration
- Extraintestinal manifestations (25% pts): liver disease, sclerosing cholangitis, iritis, uveitis, episcleritis, arthritis, erythema nodosum, pyoderma gangrenosum, aphthous stomatitis

Labs

- Anemia, ↑ ESR
- ↓ K, Mg, Ca, alb
- If persistent diarrhea: Consider stool exam O&P, stool culture, and testing for *C. difficile* toxin.
- (−) ASCA (anti-*Saccharomyces cerevisiae* Ab), (+) p-ANCA (>45% pts; p-ANCA assoc w/relative resistance to medical Rx)

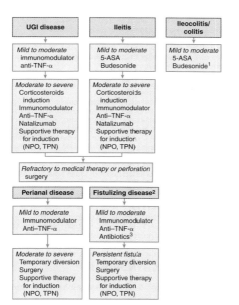

UGI disease	Ileitis	Ileocolitis/colitis
Mild to moderate immunomodulator anti–TNF-α	*Mild to moderate* 5-ASA Budesonide	*Mild to moderate* 5-ASA Budesonide[1]
Moderate to severe Corticosteroids induction Immunomodulator Anti–TNF-α Natalizumab Supportive therapy for induction (NPO, TPN)	*Moderate to severe* Corticosteroids induction Immunomodulator Anti–TNF-α Natalizumab Supportive therapy for induction (NPO, TPN)	

Refractory to medical therapy or perforation
surgery

Perianal disease	Fistulizing disease[2]
Mild to moderate Immunomodulator Anti–TNF-α	*Mild to moderate* Immunomodulator Anti–TNF-α Antibiotics[3]
Moderate to severe Temporary diversion Surgery Supportive therapy for induction (NPO, TPN)	*Persistent fistula* Temporary diversion Surgery Supportive therapy for induction (NPO, TPN)

[1] Proximal colon disease involvement
[2] Abscess should be excluded before initiating medical therapy
[3] Perianal location

FIGURE 6-1. Crohn's disease treatment algorithm. *(From Goldman L, Schafer AI [eds]: Goldman's Cecil Medicine, 24th ed. Philadelphia, Saunders, 2012.)*

Imaging
- Generally not indicated; double-contrast barium enema w/small bowel follow-through used if colonic strictures prevent evaluation, may reveal continuous involvement (including rectum), pseudopolyps, ↓ mucosal pattern, and fine superficial ulcerations.

Treatment
- Rx is based on disease activity. According to Hanauer and Sanborn, disease activity can be defined as follows:
  - *Mild to moderate disease:* The pt is ambulatory and able to take oral alimentation. There is no dehydration, high fever, abdominal tenderness, painful mass, obstruction, or weight loss of >10%.
  - *Moderate to severe disease:* Either the pt has not responded to treatment for mild to moderate disease or has more pronounced symptoms, including fever, significant weight loss, abdominal pain or tenderness, intermittent nausea and vomiting, or significant anemia.
  - *Severe fulminant disease:* Either the pt has persistent symptoms despite outpt steroid Rx or has high fever, persistent vomiting, evidence of intestinal obstruction, rebound tenderness, cachexia, or evidence of an abscess.
- TPN in patients with advanced disease
- Oral salicylates, such as mesalamine (Asacol, Rowasa)
- Corticosteroids have been the mainstay for treating moderate to severe active Crohn's disease. Prednisone 40 to 60 mg/day is useful for acute exacerbation. Steroids are usually tapered over approximately 2 to 3 mo. Some patients require a low dose for a prolonged period of maintenance.
- Steroid analogues are locally active corticosteroids that target specific areas of inflammation in the gastrointestinal tract. Budesonide is available as a

controlled-release formulation and is approved for mild to moderate active Crohn's disease involving the ileum and/or ascending colon.

- Immunosuppressants such as azathioprine 150 mg/day, methotrexate, or cyclosporine can be used for severe, progressive disease. In pts with Crohn's disease who enter remission after treatment with methotrexate, a low dose of methotrexate maintains remission.
- Metronidazole 500 mg qid may be useful for colonic fistulas and treatment of mild to moderate active Crohn's disease. Ciprofloxacin 1 g qd has also been found to be effective in decreasing disease activity.
- TNF inhibitors: Infliximab can induce clinical improvement in 80% of pts with Crohn's disease refractory to other agents. It can be used in combination with other medications such as azathioprine in patients with severe Crohn's disease. Adalimumab and certolizumab are also effective in inducing remissions and may be useful in adult patients with Crohn's disease who cannot tolerate infliximab.
- Natalizumab effective in increasing the rate of remission and response in pts with active Crohn's disease.
- Hydrocortisone enema bid or tid is useful for proctitis.
- Most patients who have anemia associated with Crohn's disease respond to iron supplementation. ESAs are useful in patients with anemia refractory to treatment with iron and vitamins.

6 MICROSCOPIC COLITIS
- Painless, watery diarrhea without bleeding via drugs/idiopathic
- High likelihood (acarbose, ASA, PPIs, ranitidine, sertraline, ticlopidine)
- Intermediate (carbamazepine, lisinopril, simvastatin, paroxetine, flutamide)
  - Dx: colonic biopsy (lymphocytic or collagenous colitis)
  - Rx: drug cessation, antidiarrheal agents, systemic corticosteroids

7 IRRITABLE BOWEL SYNDROME
Rome III dx criteria for IBS:
- Recurrent abd pain/discomfort ≥3 days/month in past 3 mo (with onset >6 mo prior) associated w/2/3 of the following:
  - Pain relived/improved with BM
  - Pain onset assoc with changed frequency of BM
  - Pain onset assoc with changed stool form/appearance
- Risk factors: physical/sexual abuse, infectious gastroenteritis, somatization/psychological traits
- Alarm sx (onset age >50 yr, anemia, nocturnal sx, wt loss, bleeding, FHx colon cancer) should prompt further testing tailored to the clinical scenario.
- Rx: high-fiber diet and PO linaclotide if constipation IBS, SSRIs, loperamide if diarrheal IBS, behavioral + psychoRx

8 APPENDICITIS
Etiology
- Obstruction of appendiceal lumen w/subsequent vascular congestion, inflammation, and edema; common causes of obstruction are
- Fecaliths: 30% to 35% of cases (most common in adults)
- Foreign body: 4% (fruit seeds, pinworms, tapeworms, roundworms, calculi)
- Inflammation: 50% to 60% of cases (submucosal lymphoid hyperplasia [most common in children, teens])
- Neoplasms: 1% (carcinoids, metastatic disease, carcinoma)

Diagnosis
H&P
- Abd pain: initially may be epigastric/periumbilical (50%) → localizing to RLQ within 12 to 18 hr. Pain can be found in back/right flank if retrocecal or malrotated appendix.
- (+) *psoas sign:* pain w/right thigh ext, low-grade fever: Temperature may be >38°C if appendiceal perforation.
- (+) *obturator sign:* pain w/internal rotation of flexed right thigh
- (+) *Rovsing's sign:* RLQ pain on palpation of the LLQ
- PE may reveal right-sided tenderness in pts w/pelvic appendix.
- Point of maximum tenderness = RLQ (*McBurney's point*).
- N/V, tachycardia, cutaneous hyperesthesias at the level of T12

Labs
- CBC w/diff: leukocytosis w/a left shift (>90%). WBC count generally <20,000/mm^3. Higher counts indicative of perforation. ↓ Hgb and Hct in older pt ↑ suspicion of cecal carcinoma.

Imaging
- CT abd/pelvis (sens >90%): distended appendix, periappendiceal inflammation, and thickened appendiceal wall
- U/S (sens 75%-90%): useful in younger/pregnant women if dx unclear. Anl U/S should not deter surgery if H&P suggest appendicitis.

Treatment
- Urgent appendectomy (laparoscopic or open). IV hydration/electrolyte replacement
- IV abx prophylaxis to cover gram(−) bacilli and anaerobes (ampicillin-sulbactam 3 g IV q6h or piperacillin-tazobactam 4.5 g IV q8h in adults)

Clinical Pearl
- Perforation is common (20% adult pts): sx perforation = pain >24 hr, leukocytosis >20,000/mm³, temp >102° F, palpable abd mass, and peritoneal findings

9 DIVERTICULAR DISEASE

Definitions
- *Colonic diverticula:* herniations of mucosa + submucosa through muscularis along the colon's mesenteric border at anatomic weak point (site where vasa recta penetrates the muscle wall)
- *Diverticulosis:* asx presence of multiple colonic diverticula
- *Diverticulitis:* inflammatory process/localized perforation of diverticula

Diagnosis
H&P
- Painful diverticular disease can manifest w/LLC pain, relieved by defecation; location of pain may be anywhere in lower abd due to redundant sigmoid colon.
- Diverticulitis can cause muscle spasm, guarding, and rebound tenderness predominantly affecting the LLQ.
- Diverticular bleed: painless and stops spontaneously in 60% of pts; 70% occurs in right colon

Labs
- WBC w/left shift: diverticulitis
- Microcytic anemia (chronic bleeding); MCV may be ↑ acute bleeding secondary to reticulocytosis.

Imaging
- CT of abd: (sens of 93%-97%, spec ~100%) for diverticulitis. Typical findings = bowel wall thickening, fistulas, and abscess formation. May also reveal (appendicitis, tubo-ovarian abscess, Crohn's disease) accounting for lower abd pain.
- If bleeding suspected:
  - Arteriography if the bleeding >1 mL/min
  - ⁹⁹ᵐTc sulfa colloid
  - ⁹⁹ᵐTc-labeled RBC (detect rates as low as 0.12-5 mL/min)

Treatment
Diverticulosis
- ↑ Fiber intake + regular exercise

Diverticulitis
- Mild: Cipro 500 mg PO bid (aerobic colonic flora) + metronidazole 500 mg q6h (anaerobes) + liquid diet for 7 to 10 days
- Severe: NPO + aggressive IV abx
  - Ampicillin-sulbactam 3 g IV q6h *or* Piperacillin-tazobactam 4.5 g IV q8h *or* Cipro 400 mg IV q12h + metronidazole 500 mg IV q6h *or* (cefoxitin 2 g IV q8h + metronidazole 500 mg IV q6h)
- Life-threatening: imipenem 500 mg IV q6h *or* meropenem 1 g IV q8h
- Surgical: resection of involved area + diverting colostomy w/reanastomosis performed when infection controlled

Diverticular Hemorrhage
- Blood replacement/correction of volume and clotting abnl
- Colonoscopic Rx w/epinephrine injection and/or bipolar coagulation, may prevent recurrent bleeding and ↓ need for surgery.
- Surgical resection if bleeding does not stop spontaneously after administration of 4 to 5 U of pRBCs or recurs w/severity within days; if localization attempts unsuccessful → total abd colectomy w/ileoproctostomy.

III

DISEASES AND DISORDERS
6. Gastroenterology

10 SMALL BOWEL OBSTRUCTION

Etiology
- Adhesions from prior surgery (60%)
- Hernias (25%)
- Malignant tumors (15%)

Diagnosis

H&P
- Colicky abd pain, N/V, abd distention
- Failure to pass gas/feces
- Tachycardia, hypotension, dehydration, fever (if strangulation present)
- Distended abd, tenderness w/ or w/o palpable mass, hyperactive bowel sounds initially followed by ↓ bowel sounds late in obstruction

Labs
- Electrolytes, BUN, Cr, ALT, amylase (generally not helpful)

Imaging
- Plain abd films: dilated loops of small intestine w/o evidence of colonic distention, air-fluid levels
- CT: sensitive for dx complete or high-grade obstruction (less sensitive for partial obstruction); may also ID cause (abscess, neoplasm).
- Barium studies: enteroclysis (PO insertion of a tube into the duodenum and instillation of air and barium) may be useful for low-grade or intermittent obstruction.

Treatment
- IV fluid resuscitation, NG suction to empty stomach
- Prophylactic broad-spectrum abx
- Operative management

11 ADYNAMIC ILEUS
- Abdominal trauma
- Infection (retroperitoneal, pelvic, intrathoracic)
- Laparotomy
- Metabolic disease (hypokalemia)
- Renal colic
- Skeletal injury (rib fracture, vertebral fracture)
- Medications (e.g., narcotics)

12 ISCHEMIC BOWEL DISEASE

a. Mesenteric Ischemia
- Sudden-onset intestinal hypoperfusion via emboli, a/v thrombosis, or vasoconstriction (low-flow states)

Etiology
- Mesenteric arterial embolism: usually LA, LV, or cardiac valves (superior mesenteric artery)
- Mesenteric arterial thrombosis: hx progressive atherosclerotic stenoses, w/superimposed abd trauma or infection
- Mesenteric venous thrombosis: hypercoagulable states, blunt trauma, abd infection, portal HTN, pancreatitis, and portal malignancy
- Nonocclusive mesenteric ischemia: atherosclerotic vascular disease, pt treated w/drugs ↓ intestinal perfusion (recent cardiac surgery/dialysis); cocaine use

Diagnosis

H&P
- Rapid onset of severe periumbilical pain out of proportion to PE findings
- N/V
- Initial abd exam may be nl, w/no rebound or guarding, or show minimal distention or occult blood (+) stool.
- Later in course, may present w/gross distention, absent bowel sounds + peritoneal signs (in elderly change in mental status).

Labs
- Nonspecific (early); later may reveal leukocytosis, acidosis, and ↑ Hct (hemoconcentration).
- Protein C/S, AT III, FV Leiden (? hypercoagulable state)

Imaging
- Mesenteric angiography (gold standard)
- Plain films: nl 25% in early stages; may include ileus, bowel wall thickening, intramural gas.

- Doppler U/S evaluation of intestinal blood flow: often limited by air-filled loops of bowel
- CT scan: nonspecific. Portal venous/intramural gas possible if development of gangrene. CT more useful if mesenteric vein thrombosis causing acute mesenteric ischemia (90% sens).

Treatment
- Rapid blood flow restoration before infarction; correct acidosis, broad-spectrum abx, NG tube decompression
- If peritonitis: laparotomy + infarcted bowel resection
- SMA embolus: embolectomy. Depending on location/degree of occlusion, surgical revascularization, intra-arterial thrombolytic infusion or vasodilators, or systemic anticoagulation may be considered.
- SMA thrombosis: emergent surgical revascularization
- Mesenteric venous thrombosis: if peritoneal sx (laparotomy + infarcted bowel resection), if no peritoneal sx (anticoagulate-heparin)

b. Mesenteric Thrombosis
- Thrombotic occlusion of the mesenteric venous system involving major trunks or smaller branches and leading to intestinal infarction in its acute form

Etiology
- Hypercoagulable states
- Portal HTN
- Inflammation (pancreatitis, peritonitis [appendicitis, diverticulitis, perforated viscus], IBD, pelvic/intra-abd abscess)
- Intra-abd cancer
- Postop state or trauma
- Thrombosis may begin in small mesenteric branches (e.g., in hypercoagulable states) and propagate to the major venous mesenteric trunks or begin in large veins (e.g., in cirrhosis, intra-abd cancer, surgery) and extend distally. If collateral drainage is inadequate, the intestine becomes congested, edematous, cyanotic, and hemorrhagic and eventually may infarct.

Diagnosis
H&P
- Sx: abd pain (90%), typically out of proportion to the physical findings; N/V (50%), GI bleeding (50% occult, 15% gross)
- Early: abd tenderness/distention, ↓ bowel sounds
- Later: guarding and rebound tenderness, fever, and septic shock
Labs
- CBC (leukocytosis), electrolytes (metabolic acidosis [lactic] indicates bowel infarction), amylase
- Hypercoagulable state evaluation: PT, PTT, protein C/S, factor V Leiden, antithrombin III
Imaging
- Abd CT (diagnostic in 90%): bowel wall thickening, venous dilation, venous thrombus

Treatment
- Anticoagulation or thrombolytic Rx
- Laparotomy if intestinal infarction is suspected
  - Short ischemic segment: resection
  - Long ischemic segment:
    - Nonviable: resection or close
    - Viable: intra-arterial papaverine or thrombectomy followed by "second-look" intervention

13 COLORECTAL NEOPLASIA

a. Colorectal Carcinoma
- Descending colon (40%-42%), rectosigmoid and rectum (30%-33%), cecum and ascending colon (25%-30%), transverse colon [10%-13%]

Etiology
- CRC arises via mutations in microsatellite/chromosomal instability, in germline mutations (basis of inherited syndromes), and in accumulation of somatic mutations in cells (basis of sporadic colon cancer).
- Classification and staging
- Dukes' and UICC classification for CRC:
  - A: Confined to the mucosa-submucosa (I)
  - B: Invasion of muscularis propria (II)

- C: Local node involvement (III)
- D: Distant mets (IV)

Diagnosis

H&P

- Presentation initially nonspecific (weight loss, anorexia, malaise)
- Right-sided sx:
  - Anemia (iron deficiency secondary to chronic blood loss)
  - Dull, vague, uncharacteristic abd pain or pt asx
  - Rectal bleeding often missed as blood mixed w/feces (occult blood)
  - Obstruction/constipation unusual (large lumen)
- Left-sided sx:
  - Change in bowel habits (constipation, diarrhea, tenesmus, pencil-thin stools)
  - Rectal bleeding (bright red blood coating the surface of the stool)
  - Intestinal obstruction is frequent because of small lumen.

Labs

- + Fecal occult blood test
- Microcytic anemia
- ↑ Plasma CEA (poor screening test for CRC as may be ↑ in pts w/ [smoking, IBD, alcoholic liver disease]); normal CEA level does not r/o CRC; main use is to monitor CRC recurrence.
- LFTs

Imaging

- Colonoscopy w/bx (primary assessment tool)
- Virtual colonoscopy (sens/spec detection of polyps >10 mm = 70%-96%, 72%-96%, respectively)
- CT of abd, pelvis, chest (preoperative staging)
- PET scan: accurate in detection of CRC + distant mets; combined PET/CT optimal (colonography) can provide whole-body tumor staging in a single session.

Treatment

- Surgical resection: 70% resectable for cure at presentation; 45% of pts are cured by primary resection.
- Rx mainstay = fluorouracil; addition of leucovorin (folinic acid) enhances fluorouracil effect
- Radiation Rx = useful adjunct to fluorouracil + leucovorin (stage II or III rectal cancers)
- For pts w/standard-risk stage III tumors (e.g., involvement of 1-3 regional lymph nodes), both fluorouracil alone and fluorouracil w/oxaliplatin are reasonable choices. Capecitabine is an alternative to IV fluorouracil as adjuvant Rx for stage III CRC.
- Irinotecan can be used to treat metastatic CRC refractory to other drugs.
- Oxaliplatin, a third-generation platinum derivative, can be used in combination w/ fluorouracil and leucovorin for pts w/metastatic CRC whose disease has recurred or progressed despite Rx w/fluorouracil and leucovorin + irinotecan. Fluorouracil + oxaliplatin should be considered for high-risk pts w/stage III cancers (e.g., >3 involved regional nodes [N2] or tumor invasion beyond the serosa [T4 lesion]).
- The monoclonal Abs cetuximab, panitumumab, and bevacizumab can be used for advanced CRC.
- The liver is generally the initial and most common site of CRC mets. Resection of mets limited to the liver is curative in more than 30% of selected pts. In pts who undergo resection of liver mets, postoperative Rx w/a combination of hepatic arterial infusion of floxuridine and IV fluorouracil improves the outcome at 2 yr.

CRC Screening

- Table 6-5 describes CRC screening and surveillance recommendations.
- Table 6-6 shows hereditary colorectal cancer syndromes.

F. DISORDERS OF THE LIVER

1 APPROACH TO THE PT WITH ABNORMAL LIVER ENZYMES

- Table 6-7 describes typical liver test patterns in hepatocellular necrosis and biliary obstruction.

2 VIRAL HEPATITIS

a. Hepatitis A

- Infection by HAV (27-nm, nonenveloped, icosahedral, [+]-stranded RNA virus) transmitted interpersonally via fecal-oral route (contact w/poorly purified food/ water); IV transmission rare; vertical transmission also reported.

TABLE 6-5 ■ Colorectal Cancer (CRC) Screening and Surveillance Recommendations*

Indication	Recommendations
Average risk	Beginning at age 50 yr: colonoscopy every 10 yr, CT colonography every 5 yr Flexible sigmoidoscopy every 5 yr Double-contrast barium enema every 5 yr (stool blood testing annually or stool DNA testing acceptable but not preferred)
One or two first-degree relatives with CRC at any age or adenoma at age <60 yr	Colonoscopy every 5 yr beginning at age 40 yr, or 10 yr younger than earliest diagnosis, whichever comes first
Hereditary nonpolyposis colorectal cancer	Genetic counseling and screening[†] Colonoscopy every 1 to 2 years beginning at age 25 yr and then yearly after age 40 yr[‡]
Familial adenomatous polyposis and variants	Genetic counseling and testing[†] Flexible sigmoidoscopy yearly beginning at puberty[‡]
Personal history of CRC	Colonoscopy within 1 yr of curative resection; repeat at 3 yr and then every 5 yr if normal
Personal history of colorectal adenoma	Colonoscopy every 3 to 5 yr after removal of all index polyps
Inflammatory bowel disease	Colonoscopy every 1 to 2 yr beginning after 8 yr of pancolitis or after 15 yr if only left-sided disease

*Recommendations proposed by the American Cancer Society and U.S. Multi-Society Task Force on Colorectal Cancer; recommendations for average-risk patients also endorsed by the American College of Radiology.
[†]Whenever possible, affected relatives should be tested first because of potential false-negative results.
[‡]Screening recommendation for individuals with positive or indeterminate tests, as well as for those who refuse genetic testing.
From Andreoli, T E, Benjamin IJ, Griggs RC, Wing EJ: Andreoli and Carpenter's Cecil Essentials of Medicine, 8th ed. Philadelphia, Saunders, 2010.

TABLE 6-6 ■ Hereditary Colorectal Cancer Syndromes

Type	Trait	Gastric	Small Bowel	Colon	Histology	GI Malignancy	Extraintestinal
Familial polyposis	AD	<5%	<5%	100%	Adenoma	100%	—
Gardner	AD	5%	5%	100%	Adenoma	100%	Osteoma, others*
Peutz-Jeghers	AD	25%	95%	30%	Hamartoma	Rare	Perioral pigmentation
Juvenile polyposis	AD	—	—	100%	Inflammatory	?	—
Turcot	AR	—	—	100%	Adenoma	100%	Glioma
Cronkhite-Canada	Nonhereditary	100%	50%	100%	Inflammatory	None	Ectodermal changes
Cowden[†]	AD	—	—	—	Hamartoma	None	Oral papilloma[‡]
Ruvalcaba-Myhre[†]	AD	Yes	Yes	Yes	Hamartoma	None	Macrocephaly, penile macules, mental retardation, SC lipomas

*Soft tissue tumors, sarcomas, ampullary carcinoma, ovarian carcinoma.
[†]Extremely rare.
[‡]Gingival hyperplasia, breast cancer, thyroid cancer.
From Weissleder R, Wittenberg J, Harisinghani M, Chen JW: Primer of Diagnostic Imaging, 5th ed. St. Louis, Mosby, 2011.

Diagnosis

H&P

- Infection w/HAV may have acute or subacute presentation, icteric or anicteric. Severity of illness ↑ w/age (90% infections in children <5 yr may be subclinical).
- A preicteric, prodromal phase (1-14 days); 15% no prodrome. Sx onset usually abrupt and may include anorexia, malaise, N/V, fever, headache, abd pain, chills, myalgias, arthralgias, URI sx, constipation, diarrhea, pruritus, urticaria (less common).
- Jaundice (>70%); icteric phase is preceded by dark urine.
- Bilirubinuria is followed a few days later by clay-colored stools and icterus.

TABLE 6-7 ■ Typical Liver Test Patterns

Test	Hepatocellular Necrosis			Biliary Obstruction			
	Toxic or Ischemic	Viral	Alcohol	Chronic Complete	Chronic Partial	Acute Complete (first 24 hr)	Infiltration (Chronic)
Aminotrans-ferases	50-100x	5-50x	2-5x	1-5x	1-5x	1-50x	1-3x
Alkaline phospha-tase	1-3x	1-3x	1-10x	2-20x	2-10x	May be nl	1-20x
Bilirubin	1-5x	1-30x	1-30x	1-30x	1-5x	Usually nl	1-5x
PT	Prolonged in severe cases, unresponsive to vitamin K			May be prolonged, responsive to vitamin K	Usually nl	Usually nl	Usually nl
Albumin	Nl in acute illness, may be ↓ in chronic illness			Usually nl, but may be ↓ in biliary cirrhosis	Usually nl	Usually nl	Usually nl
Typical disorders	Acetamin-ophen toxicity, shock liver	Acute hepatitis A or B	Alcoholic hepatitis	Pancreatic carcinoma	Sclerosing cholan-gitis	Choledo-cholithiasis	Primary or metastatic carcinoma, *Mycobacte-rium avium-intracellulare* infection

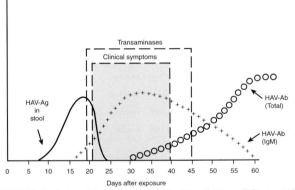

FIGURE 6-2. Serologic test in hepatitis A virus infection. *(From Goldberger E: Treatment of Cardiac Emergencies, 5th ed. St. Louis, Mosby, 1990.)*

Labs (Fig. 6-2)
- Dx confirmed by IgM anti-HAV; detectable in almost all infected pts at presentation and remains (+) for 3 to 6 mo.
- 4x ↑ titer of total Ab (IgM + IgG) to HAV confirms acute infection.
- HAV detection in stool and body fluids by EM
- HAV RNA detection in stool, body fluids, serum, and liver tissue
- ↑ ALT AST (usually >8x nl in acute infection)
- ↑ Bili (usually 5-15x nl)
- Alk phos minimally ↑ but higher level in cholestasis
- Alb and PT generally nl; if ↑ may herald hepatic necrosis

Imaging
- U/S (r/o obstructive jaundice)

Treatment

- Self-limited (supportive care; activity as tolerated)
- Advise to avoid alcohol and hepatotoxic drugs
- Pts w/fulminant hepatitis may require hospitalization/assessment for liver transplantation.

Clinical Pearls

- Reported to public health authorities
- Common illness in internationally traveled/developing countries; preexposure prophylaxis if travel to endemic area (IG 0.02-0.06 mL/kg IM); Lower dose = effective up to 3 mo; higher dose = effective up to 5 mo.
- Postexposure prophylaxis (IG 0.02 mL/kg given IM) if exposure within 2 wk + no previous vaccination; high-risk pts, may vaccinate with immunoglobulin
- Inactivated vaccines HAVRIX or VAQTA safe/immunogenic in adults/children >12 mo w/protective Ab levels reached 94% to 100% 1 mo combined HepA/HepB vaccine TWINRIX also available

b. Hepatitis B

- Infection by HBV (42-nm hepadnavirus w/an outer surface coat [HBsAg], inner nucleocapsid core [HBcAg; HBeAg], DNA polymerase, and partially double-stranded DNA genome) with transmission via parenteral (needle use, tattooing, piercing, acupuncture, blood transfusion, hemodialysis, sexual contact) and perinatal routes

Diagnosis

H&P

- Often nonspecific sx, malaise
- Prodrome:
  - 15% to 20% serum sickness (urticaria, rash, arthralgia) during early HBsAg
  - HBsAg-Ab complex disease (polyarteritis nocosa–arthritis, arteritis, GN)
    - Hepatomegaly (87%) w/RUQ tenderness
    - Hepatic punch tenderness
    - Splenomegaly (10%-15%)
    - Jaundice, dark urine, w/occasional pruritus; fever (when present, precedes jaundice and rapidly declines after icteric phase onset)
    - Spider angiomas: rare; resolve during recovery
    - Rare polyarteritis nodosa, cryoglobulinemia

Labs (Fig. 6-3)

- Acute HBV infection is best confirmed by IgM HBcAb in acute or early convalescent serum or by HB DNA.
  - Generally, IgM present during onset of jaundice
  - Coexisting HBsAg
- HBsAg and IgG-HBcAb during acute jaundice are strongly suggestive of remote HBV infection and another etiology for current illness.
- HBsAb alone is suggestive of immunization response.
- W/recovery, HBeAg is rapidly replaced by HBeAb in 2 to 3 mo, and HBsAg is replaced by HBsAb in 5 to 6 mo.
- In chronic HBV, HBsAg and HBeAg are persistent w/o corresponding Ab.
- In chronic carrier state, HBsAg is persistent, but HBeAg is replaced by HBeAb.
- HBcAb develops in all outcomes.
- HBeAg correlation w/highest infectivity; appearance of HBeAb heralds recovery.
- LFTs:
  - ALT and AST: usually >8x nl at onset of jaundice (low acute ALT/AST ↑ often followed by chronic hepatitis or HCC)
  - ↑ Bili: variably ↑ in icteric viral hepatitis
  - Alk phos: minimally ↑ (1-3× nl) acutely
- Alb and PT: generally nl; if abnl, possible harbinger of impending hepatic necrosis (fulminant hepatitis)
- WBC and ESR: generally nl or mildly ↑

Imaging

- U/S to r/o obstructive jaundice

Treatment

Acute Hepatitis B

- 90% of adults spontaneously clear infection; avoid hepatic metabolized drugs; IV hydration if severe vomiting
- Hospitalization if pt risk dehydration via poor PO intake, PT ↑, bili level >15 to 20 μg/dL, or if hepatic failure

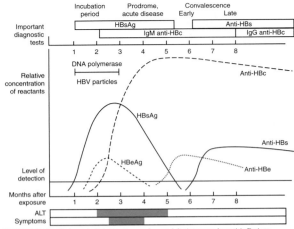

FIGURE 6-3. Serologic and clinical patterns observed during acute hepatitis B virus infection. Patients in whom the hepatitis B infection does not resolve (chronic carrier state) will demonstrate persistence of HBsAg and will not have an elevation of anti-HBs. *(From Ravel R: Clinical Laboratory Medicine, 6th ed. St. Louis, Mosby, 1995.)*

Chronic Hepatitis B
- Rx: determined by e antigen status and viral qualification
  - HbeAg (+): HBV DNA ≥20,000: Rx if ALT ↑ or if biopsy abnl
  - HbeAg (–) : HBV DNA ≥2000: Rx if ALT ↑ or if biopsy abnl
- Documented cirrhosis [(+) or (–) HBeAg] with
  - HBV DNA ≥2000: adefovir 10 mg PO daily or entecavir 0.5 mg PO daily
  - HBV DNA <2000: observe
  - Decompensated cirrhosis (regardless of HBV DNA level): (lamivudine 100 mg PO daily or entecavir 0.5 mg daily) + tenofovir 300 mg PO daily (*dosages for non–HIV-infected pt)

Clinical Pearls
- Virus and HBsAg are present in high titers in blood for 1 to 7 wk before jaundice and for a variable time thereafter.
- Transmission is possible during entire period of HBsAg (and especially during HBeAg) in serum.
- Prevention after exposure:
  - HBV hyperimmune globulin (HBIG) is given immediately after needle stick, within 14 days of sexual exposure, or at birth, followed by HBV vaccination.
  - Standard immune globulin is nearly as effective as HBIG.
- Preventive Rx w/lamivudine for pts who test (+) for HBsAg and are undergoing chemoRx may ↑ the risk for HBV reactivation and HBV-associated morbidity and mortality.

c. Hepatitis C
- Infection via HCV (single-stranded RNA flavivirus) is mostly via the parenteral route (IV drug use 60% new cases, 20%-50% chronic cases). Occupational needle stick exposure from an HCV(+) source has a seroconversion rate of 1.8% (range, 0%-7%).

Diagnosis
H&P
- Sx usually develop 7 to 8 wk after infection (2-26 wk), but 70% to 80% of cases are subclinical.
- 10% to 20% report acute illness w/jaundice and nonspecific sx (abd pain, anorexia, malaise).
- Fulminant hepatitis may rarely occur during this period.

- After acute infection, 15% to 25% have complete resolution (absence of HCV RNA in serum, nl ALT).
- Progression to chronic infection is common (50%-84%); 74% to 86% have persistent viremia; spontaneous clearance of viremia in chronic infection is rare. 60% to 70% of pts will have persistent or fluctuating ALT levels; 30% to 40% w/chronic infection have nl ALT levels.
- 15% to 20% of those w/chronic HCV will develop cirrhosis during a period of 20 to 30 yr; in most others, chronic infection leads to hepatitis and varying degrees of fibrosis.
- 0.4% to 2.5% of pts w/chronic infection develop HCC.
- 25% of pts w/chronic infection continue to have an asymptomatic course w/nl LFTs and benign histology.
- In chronic HCV infection, extrahepatic sequelae include a variety of immunologic and lymphoproliferative disorders (e.g., cryoglobulinemia, membranoproliferative GN, and possibly Sjögren's syndrome, autoimmune thyroiditis, polyarteritis nodosa, aplastic anemia, lichen planus, porphyria cutanea tarda, B-cell lymphoma, others).

Labs (Fig. 6-4)
- Dx is often by exclusion because it takes 6 wk to 12 mo to develop anti-HCV Ab (70% + by 6 wk, 90% + by 6 mo).
- Diagnostic tests include serologic assays for Abs and molecular tests for viral particles.
- Enzyme immunoassay is the test for anti-HCV Ab:
  • The current version can detect Ab within 4 to 10 wk after infection.
  • False (−) rate in low-risk populations is 0.5% to 1%.
  • False (−) also in immune-compromised persons, HIV-1, renal failure, HCV-associated essential mixed cryoglobulinemia.
  • False (+) in autoimmune hepatitis, paraproteinemia, and persons w/no risk factors.
- Recombinant immunoblot is used to confirm + enzyme immunoassays: recommended only in low-risk settings
- Qualitative and quantitative HCV RNA tests using PCR:
  • Lower limit of detection is <100 copies HCV RNA/mL.
  • It is used to confirm viremia and to assess response to Rx.
  • Qualitative PCR is useful in pts w/(−) enzyme immunoassay in whom infection is suspected.
  • Quantitative tests use either branched-chain DNA or reverse transcription PCR; the latter is more sensitive.
- Viral genotyping can distinguish among genotypes 1, 2, 3, and 4, which is helpful in choosing Rx; most of these tests use PCR. (Genotypes 1, 2, 3, and 4 predominate in the United States and Europe [1 is especially common in North America].)

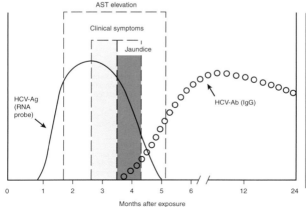

FIGURE 6-4. Hepatitis C virus antigen and antibody. *(From Hollinger FB, Dienstag JL. In Murray PR, et al [eds]: Manual of Clinical Microbiology, 6th ed. Washington, DC, American Society for Microbiology, 1995.)*

- LFTs:
  - ALT and AST may be ↑ > 8× nl in acute infection; in chronic infection, ALT may be nl or fluctuate.
  - Bili may be ↑ 5 to 10× nl.
  - Alb and PT are generally nl; if abnl, may be harbinger of impending hepatic necrosis.
  - WBC and ESR are generally nl.

Imaging
- U/S is useful to r/o obstructive jaundice and to evaluate rapid liver size ↓ during fulminant hepatitis or mass in HCC.

Treatment
Acute Hepatitis C
- HCV PCR detected within 13 days (antibody in >36 days)
- If clear HCV viral load via PCR within 3 to 4 mo (no Rx-supportive care)
Chronic Hepatitis C (persistent HCV viral load)
- Rx duration depends on HCV RNA level:
- Null: no ↓ of 2log10 by wk 12
- Partial: 2log10 ↓ by wk12 but detectable by wk 24
- Nonresponsive: HCV RNA not cleared by wk 24
- Early Virologic Response (EVR): >2log10 ↓ by wk 12, undetectable by wk 24
- Complete EVR: undetectable by wk 12 and 24, but not at wk 4
- Rapid Virologic Response (RVR): undetectable by wk 4, no change during Rx
- Extended Virologic Response (eRVR): undetectable by wk 4 (telaprevir) or wk 8 (boceprevir) and wks 12 and 24
- Relapse: undetectable at Rx end, but detectable within 24 wk s/p Rx
- Sustained Virologic Response (SVR): cure; undetectable s/p 24 wk Rx
- Rx options depend on **Genotype:**
  - **FOR ALL** genotypes, primary Rx: (PEG-IFN Alfa 2a 180 μg SC/wk or PEG-IFN Alfa 2b 1.5 μg/kg SC/wk) + (ribavirin 400 mg qAM + [if < 75 kg: 600 mg qPM; if >75 kg: 600 mg bid])
  - **Genotype 1**
    - Add: telaprevir 750 mg (2 tab) PO tid w/food first 12 wk, then continue without telaprevir for duration of Rx or boceprevir 800 mg (4 cap) PO tid w/food 4 wk after starting primary Rx continued for duration of Rx
    - **Never combine telaprevir/boceprevir or use either as monoRx**
    - If eRVR: Continue Rx 24 wk (telaprevir) or 28 wk (boceprevir); check SVR 48 wk (telaprevir), 52 wk (boceprevir).
    - If not eRVR: Continue Rx 48 wk (telaprevir 12 wk + PEG-IFN/RBV 48 wk) (boceprevir 44 wk + PEG-IFN/RBV 48 wk); check SVR 72 wk.
    - If partial/null response, d/c Rx (failure)
  - Genotypes 2/3
    - If RVR: May shorten Rx 16 to 24 wk; check SVR wk 40 to 48.
    - If EVR: Rx 24 wk; check SVR wk 48.
    - If partial/null response: d/c Rx wk 12 (failure).
  - Genotype 4
    - Rx 48 wk; check SVR at wk 72.
    - If null or partial response, d/c Rx wk 12 or 24, respectively.
- When pt HIV-HCV dually infected pt, monitor interactions between direct-acting antivirals (DAAs) and antiretroviral drugs. Rx duration will likely be the full 48 wk.
- Liver transplantation: May be only option if HCV-related deteriorating cirrhosis exists.

d. Hepatitis D
- Incomplete virus requiring presence of HBV for replication; thus, resolution of HBV infection will result in resolution of HDV infection.

e. Hepatitis E
- Similar to HAV (enteric transmission, acute infection only)
- Despite low overall mortality, infection during third trimester mortality rate ≥25%
- Prevention via good hygiene; avoid dirty water/poorly cooked food.

3 AUTOIMMUNE HEPATITIS

Diagnosis
H&P
- Can manifest asymptomatically → fulminant hepatic failure; most commonly fatigue, pruritus, jaundice, hepatomegaly/splenomegaly

TABLE 6-8 ■ Simplified Diagnostic Criteria for Autoimmune Hepatitis				
Variable	Cutoff	Points	Cutoff	Points
ANA or SMA	≥1:40	1	≥1:80	2
LKM			≥1:40	2
SLA			Positive	2
IgG	≥ULN	1	≥1.1 × ULN	2
Histology	Compatible with AIH	1	Typical of AIH	2
Absence of viral hepatitis			Yes	2
Maximum number of points for all antibodies = 2, total = 8.				
Probable AIH ≥6 points, definite AIH ≥7 points.				

AIH, Autoimmune hepatitis; *LKM,* liver/kidney microsomes; *SLA,* soluble liver antigen; *SMA,* smooth muscle antibody; *ULN,* upper limit of normal.

From Ferri F: Ferri's Clinical Advisor: 5 Books in 1. 2013 edition. Philadelphia, Mosby, 2012.

- Autoimmune findings: arthritis, xerostomia, keratoconjunctivitis, cutaneous vasculitis, and erythema nodosum

Labs
- ↑ ALT and AST (both 2-10× nl)
- Women 4× > risk than men
- Bili and alk phos moderately ↑/nl
- ↑ γ-Globulin (>2.0 g/dL)
- Serum ANA + anti–smooth muscle Ab (64% cases); if (–), p-ANCA helpful
- Liver bx = interface hepatitis (lymphoplasmacytic inflammatory infiltrate extending from portal tract → lobule)
- Table 6-8 describes simplified diagnostic criteria for autoimmune hepatitis.

Imaging
- U/S of liver and biliary tree: r/o obstruction or hepatic mass

Indications for Treatment
- AST >10× nl
- AST >5× nl, w/↑ γ-globulin 2× nl
- Fever, N/V, jaundice
- Histologic features of bridging necrosis or multiacinar necrosis

Treatment
- Prednisone 60 mg PO/day or (prednisone 30 mg + azathioprine 50 mg PO/day); both achieve remission in 80% pts w/combo Rx = less steroid SE
- Taper based on lab response striving for minimum dose needed for maintenance Rx (same regimen 12-18 mo) to ↑ remission rate.
- If liver transplant necessary, 10-yr survival rate 75%

4 CHOLESTATIC LIVER DISEASE

a. Primary Biliary Cirrhosis (PBC)

Diagnosis

H&P
- Typical pt middle-aged female (50 yr); most asx but develop fatigue, pruritus, dry eyes/mouth over 10-yr period

Labs
- (+) Antimitochondrial Ab titer >1:40 (if undetectable, need biopsy)
- ↑ alk phos >1.5× nl (with nl total bili); ↑ AST/ALT <5× nl possible
- **Histology:** *florid duct lesion* (duct obliteration w/granuloma formation = pathognomonic)

Treatment
- Pruritus: cholestyramine (8-24 g qd), sertraline, rifampin
- Hyperlipidemia/malabsorption of fat-soluble vitamins via cholestasis: statin Rx + wt loss and vitamin (especially vitamin D) replacement
- Asymptomatic stage: Follow LFTs q3-4 mo; if alk phos and/or AST >1.5× nl start ursodeoxycholic acid 12 to 15 mg/kg/day (UDCA).
- Liver transplant is only definitive Rx.

b. Primary Sclerosing Cholangitis (PSC)

Diagnosis

H&P
- Mean age 40 yr; 60% men (most asymptomatic, but may have pruritus, abd pain, jaundice)
- ↑ risk cholangiocarcinoma; 2% to 4% pts with IBD develop PSC.

- ↑ Alk phos (3-10× nl); ↑ ALT/AST (2-3× nl); (+) ANA, smooth muscle abs (20%-50%)
- "*Beads on a string*" (segmental bile duct fibrosis w/saccular dilatation of nl areas)
- Cholangiography: MRCP (gold standard); if obstruction, ERCP
- Liver bx: periductal fibrosis, fibro-obliterative cholangiopathy

Staging
- See Table 6-9.

TABLE 6-9 ■ Staging of Primary Sclerosing Cholangitis	
Stage	**Description**
I: Portal	Portal edema, inflammation, ductal proliferation; abnormalities do not extend beyond the limiting plate
II: Periportal	Periportal fibrosis with or without inflammation extending beyond the limiting plate
III: Septal	Septal fibrosis, bridging necrosis, or both
IV: Cirrhotic	Biliary cirrhosis

From: Cameron AM: Current Surgical Therapy, 10th ed. Philadelphia, Saunders, 2011.

Treatment
- Sx relief; liver transplantation

5 COMPLICATIONS OF LIVER DISEASE

a. Cirrhosis
- Defined histologically as the presence of fibrosis/regenerative nodules in the liver

Etiology
- EtOH abuse, secondary to biliary cirrhosis/obstruction of the CBD (stone, stricture, pancreatitis, neoplasm, sclerosing cholangitis), drugs (acetaminophen, INH, MTX, methyldopa), hepatic congestion (CHF, constrictive pericarditis, tricuspid insufficiency, hepatic vein thrombosis, vena cava obstruction), PBC, PSC, chronic hepB/C, Wilson's disease, α_1-antitrypsin deficiency, infiltrative diseases (amyloidosis, glycogen storage diseases, hemochromatosis), jejunoileal bypass, parasitic infections (schistosomiasis), idiopathic portal HTN, congenital hepatic fibrosis, systemic mastocytosis, autoimmune hepatitis, hepatic steatosis, IBD

Diagnosis
H&P
- Jaundice; spider angiomas; ecchymosis; gynecomastia in men; small, nodular liver; ascites; hemorrhoids; testicular atrophy

Labs
- Alcoholic hepatitis and cirrhosis: mild ↑ ALT, AST, usually <500 IU; AST > ALT (ratio >2:3)
- Extrahepatic obstruction: moderate ↑ ALT/AST to levels <500 IU
- Viral, toxic, or ischemic hepatitis: ↑↑ (>500 IU) ALT, AST
- ↑ Alk phos: extrahepatic obstruction, PBC, and PSC
- ↑ Serum LDH: liver mets, hepatitis, cirrhosis, extrahepatic obstruction, congestive hepatomegaly
- ↑ Serum GGTP: alcoholic liver disease, PBC, PSC
- ↑ Serum bili + urinary bili: hepatitis, hepatocellular jaundice, biliary obstruction
- ↓ Serum alb: significant liver disease
- ↑ PT: severe liver damage and poor prognosis
- (+) HBsAg: acute or chronic hepatitis B
- (+) Antimitochondrial Abs: PBC, chronic hepatitis
- ↑ Serum copper, ↓ ceruloplasmin: Wilson's disease
- ↓ α_1-Globulins (α_1-antitrypsin deficiency), ↑ IgA (alcoholic cirrhosis), ↑ IgM (PBC), ↑ IgG (chronic hepatitis, cryptogenic cirrhosis)
- ↑ Serum ferritin, ↑ transferrin saturation: hemochromatosis
- ↑ Blood ammonia: hepatocellular dysfunction
- (+) ANA: autoimmune hepatitis

Imaging
- U/S: detection of gallstones and dilation of CBDs
- CT abd: detection of mass lesions in liver/pancreas; hepatic fat content; identification of idiopathic hemochromatosis; early dx of Budd-Chiari syndrome, dilation of intrahepatic bile ducts; and detection of varices and splenomegaly

- Percutaneous liver bx: evaluation of hepatic filling defects; dx of hepatocellular disease or hepatomegaly; evaluation of persistently abnl LFTs; and dx of hemochromatosis, PBC, Wilson's disease, glycogen storage diseases, chronic hepatitis, autoimmune hepatitis, infiltrative diseases, alcoholic liver disease, drug-induced liver disease, and primary or secondary carcinoma
- Scoring system: Table 6-10

Treatment

- Variable w/etiology. Figure 6-5 summarizes the management of compensated and decompensated cirrhosis.
- Liver transplantation: indicated in otherwise healthy pts (age <65 yr) w/sclerosing cholangitis, chronic hepatitis, cirrhosis, or PBC, w/prognostic information suggesting <20% chance of survival w/o transplantation. Contraindications to liver transplantation are AIDS, most metastatic malignant neoplasms, active substance abuse, uncontrolled sepsis, and uncontrolled cardiac or pulmonary disease.

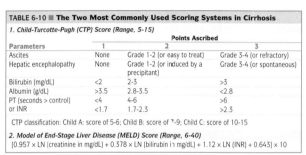

TABLE 6-10 ■ The Two Most Commonly Used Scoring Systems in Cirrhosis

1. Child-Turcotte-Pugh (CTP) Score (Range, 5-15)

		Points Ascribed	
Parameters	1	2	3
Ascites	None	Grade 1-2 (or easy to treat)	Grade 3-4 (or refractory)
Hepatic encephalopathy	None	Grade 1-2 (or induced by a precipitant)	Grade 3-4 (or spontaneous)
Bilirubin (mg/dL)	<2	2-3	>3
Albumin (g/dL)	>3.5	2.8-3.5	<2.8
PT (seconds > control)	<4	4-6	>6
or INR	<1.7	1.7-2.3	>2.3

CTP classification: Child A: score of 5-6; Child B: score of 7-9; Child C: score of 10-15

2. Model of End-Stage Liver Disease (MELD) Score (Range, 6-40)

$$[0.957 \times LN \text{ (creatinine in mg/dL)} + 0.378 \times LN \text{ (bilirubin in mg/dL)} + 1.12 \times LN \text{ (INR)} + 0.643] \times 10$$

From Goldman L, Schafer AI (eds): Goldman's Cecil Medicine, 24th ed. Philadelphia, Saunders, 2012.

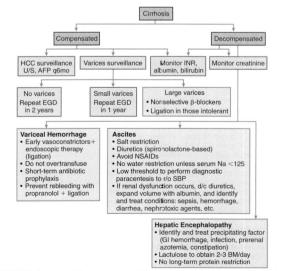

FIGURE 6-5. Summary of the management of compensated and decompensated cirrhosis. *(From Goldman L, Schafer AI [eds]: Goldman's Cecil Medicine, 24th ed. Philadelphia, Saunders, 2012.)*

- Rx of complications of portal HTN (ascites, esophagogastric varices, hepatic encephalopathy, and HRS)

b. Ascites/Paracentesis

Paracentesis

Indications
- Ascites of undetermined etiology
- Evaluation for possible peritonitis
- Relief of abd pain and discomfort caused by tense ascites
- Relief of dyspnea caused by ↑ diaphragm (from ascites)
- Evaluation of possible intra-abd hemorrhage in a pt w/blunt abd trauma
- Institution of peritoneal dialysis

Contraindications
- Bleeding disorders, thrombocytopenia (relative contraindication)
- Bowel distention
- Infection or surgical scars at the site of needle entry
- Acute abdomen
- Distended bladder that cannot be emptied w/Foley catheter

Procedure
1. Have the pt empty the bladder (insertion of a Foley catheter is not recommended but may be necessary in certain pts).
2. To identify the site of paracentesis, first locate the rectus muscle; a good site is approximately 2 to 3 cm lateral to the rectus muscle border in the lower abd quadrants. Avoid the following:
   a. Rectus muscles (↑ risk of hemorrhage from epigastric vessels)
   b. Surgical scars (↑ risk of perforation caused by adhesion of bowel to the wall of the peritoneum)
   c. Areas of skin infection (↑ risk of intraperitoneal infection)
   d. Note: An alternative site is on the linea alba 3 to 4 cm below the umbilicus.
3. Cleanse the area w/povidone-iodine and drape the abd.
4. Anesthetize the puncture site w/1% to 2% lidocaine.
5. Cautiously insert the needle (attached to a syringe) perpendicular to the skin; a small "pop" is felt as the needle advances through the anterior and posterior muscular fascia, and entrance into the peritoneal cavity is evidenced as a sudden "give" (use caution to avoid the sudden thrust forward of the needle). Some physicians use the Z technique to minimize leaks—the needle is inserted through the skin, then moved laterally before entering the peritoneal cavity to avoid a straight shot from skin to peritoneal cavity that is better for leaking fluid.
6. Remove the necessary amount of fluid (generally not more than 1 L, particularly in cirrhotic pts). If it is a therapeutic paracentesis w/plans to remove a significant amount of fluid, one can use an angiocatheter (basically just an IV) to cover the sharp needle during the procedure and to allow the operator to move the catheter around at will (in small increments) to try to restart flow when it stops. Transfusion of alb may be necessary with >4 to 5 L of paracentesis to avoid hemodynamic deterioration.
7. If it is a diagnostic paracentesis, process the fluid as follows:
   a. Tube 1: LDH, glucose, alb levels
   b. Tube 2: protein level, specific gravity
   c. Tube 3: complete blood cell count and diff
   d. Tube 4: save until further notice
8. Draw serum samples for measurement of LDH, protein, and alb.
9. Gram stain, AFB stain, bacterial and fungal cultures, amylase, and TGs should be ordered only when clearly indicated; bedside inoculation of blood culture bottles w/10 to 20 mL of ascitic fluid improves sensitivity in detecting bacterial growth in suspected cases of bacterial peritonitis.
10. If malignant ascites is suspected, consider ascertaining a CEA level on the paracentesis fluid and a cytologic evaluation.

Interpretation of Results
- Peritoneal effusion, like pleural effusion, can be subdivided into exudative or transudative on the basis of its characteristics (Fig. 6-6).
- The *serum-ascites alb gradient (SAAG)* (serum alb level–ascitic fluid alb level) correlates directly w/portal pressure and can also be used to classify ascites (Table 6-11). Pts w/gradients of ≥1.1 g/dL or higher have ascites secondary to portal HTN, and those w/gradients <1.1 g/dL do not; the accuracy of this method is >95%.

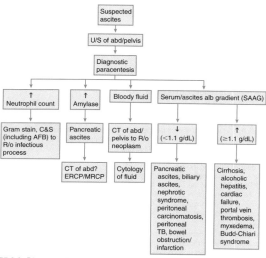

FIGURE 6-6. Diagnostic algorithm for ascites. *(From Ferri FF: Ferri's Best Test: A Practical Guide to Clinical Laboratory Medicine and Diagnostic Imaging, 2nd ed. Philadelphia, Mosby, 2010.)*

TABLE 6-11 ■ Causes of Ascites Based on Normal or Diseased Peritoneum and Serum-to-Ascites Albumin Gradient (SAAG)	
Normal Peritoneum	
Portal Hypertension (SAAG >1.1 g/dL)	Hypoalbuminemia (SAAG <1.1 g/dL)
Hepatic congestion	Nephrotic syndrome
Congestive heart failure	Protein-losing enteropathy
Constrictive pericarditis	Severe malnutrition with anasarca
Tricuspid insufficiency	
Budd-Chiari syndrome	
Liver disease	Miscellaneous Conditions (SAAG <1.1 g/dL)
Cirrhosis	Chylous ascites
Alcoholic hepatitis	Pancreatic ascites
Fulminant hepatic failure	Bile ascites
Massive hepatic metastases	Nephrogenic ascites
	Urine ascites
	Ovarian disease
Diseased Peritoneum (SAAG <1.1 g/dL)	
Infections	Other Rare Conditions
Bacterial peritonitis	Familial Mediterranean fever
Tuberculous peritonitis	Vasculitis
Fungal peritonitis	Granulomatous peritonitis
HIV-associated peritonitis	Eosinophilic peritonitis
Malignant Conditions	
Peritoneal carcinomatosis	
Primary mesothelioma	
Pseudomyxoma peritonei	
Hepatocellular carcinoma	

From Vincent JL, Abraham E, Moore FA, et al (eds): Textbook of Critical Care, 6th ed. Philadelphia, Saunders, 2011.

III

DISEASES AND DISORDERS
6. Gastroenterology

Complications
- Persistent leakage of ascitic fluid
- Hypotension and shock
- Bleeding
- Perforated bowel
- Abscess formation in area of puncture site

c. Varices
- Dilated submucosal veins via portal vein HTN (>10-12 mm Hg), functioning as a shunt between portal and systemic venous circulation; result in severe upper GI hemorrhage (25%-40% cirrhotic pts)

Diagnosis
- EGD (Esophagography with barium noninvasive option)

Labs and W/up
- Anemia (blood loss, nutritional deficiencies, alcohol myelosuppression)
- Thrombocytopenia (hypersplenism, alcohol myelosuppression)
- BUN: often ↑ in setting of upper GI bleeding
- Cr: often ↑ by hypovolemia, monitor for hepatorenal syndrome
- Na⁺: dilutional hyponatremia
- Heme (+) stools (type/crossmatch: in preparation for blood transfusion)
- INR/PT and PTT: may be ↑ in liver disease or impairment
- LFTs: ALT/AST may be nl in cirrhotic pts because of fibrosis, ↑ alk phos, direct hyperbilirubinemia possible if cholestatic liver disease
- Serum alb: Severe liver disease results in hypoalbuminemia.

Treatment
- Hemorrhage: acute hemodynamic resuscitation (pRBC transfusion, correct coagulopathy/thrombocytopenia), SBP prophylaxis (ceftriaxone or norfloxacin), octreotide 2 to 5 days in conjunction with endoscopic Rx
- Ligation (if ↑ risk hemorrhage: Child Pugh B/C or red wale markings on EGD)
- Follow-up surveillance EGD 1 to 3 mo s/p obliteration, then q6-12mo indefinitely
- Primary prophylaxis: nonselective β-blockers (propranolol 20 mg bid or nadolol 40 mg daily)

d. Portal Hypertension
- Portal vein pressure >10 mm Hg

Etiology
- ↑ Resistance to flow (portal/splenic/hepatic vein thrombosis, cirrhosis, schistosomiasis)
- ↑ Portal blood flow (splanchnic arterial vasodilation, arterial-portal venous fistulae)

Imaging
- Duplex-Doppler U/S (CT/MRI/MRA scanning if results unclear)

Treatment
- ↓ HTN directly, minimize volume overload, correct underlying disorders, and prevent complications (most notably SBP and variceal bleeding).

e. Hepatic Encephalopathy (HE)
- Cognitive disturbance via hepatic insufficiency and portosystemic shunting

Etiology
- Precipitating factors in pts w/underlying cirrhosis (UGI bleeding, hypokalemia, hypomagnesemia, analgesic and sedative drugs, sepsis, alkalosis, dietary protein), acute fulminant viral hepatitis, drugs and toxins (INH, acetaminophen-Reye's syndrome, diclofenac, statins, methyldopa, loratadine, propylthiouracil, lisinopril, labetalol, halothane, carbon tetrachloride, erythromycin, nitrofurantoin, troglitazone), shock or sepsis, fatty liver of pregnancy, metastatic carcinoma, HCC, other (autoimmune hepatitis, ischemic veno-occlusive disease, sclerosing cholangitis, heat stroke, amebic abscesses)

Diagnosis
- Requires r/o other causes (medications, metabolic disorders, infectious diseases, intracranial lesions/events). Clinical stages of hepatic encephalopathy are described in Table 6-12. The West Haven criteria is noted here.

West Haven Criteria for Classification of Hepatic Encephalopathy
- Stage 0: nl cognitive function/no abnl detected
- Stage 1: lack of awareness, euphoria/anxiety, ↓ attention/concentration
- Stage 2: lethargy/apathy, altered personality, inappropriate behavior, time disorientation
- Stage 3: somnolence to semistupor, confusion, gross disorientation, bizarre behavior

Stage	Asterixis E	EEG Changes	Clinical Manifestations
I (prodrome)	Slight	Minimal	Mild intellectual impairment, disturbed sleep-wake cycle
II (impending)	Easily elicited	Usually generalized	Drowsiness, confusion, coma/inappropriate behavior, disorientation, mood swings
III (stupor)	Present if patient cooperative	Grossly abnormal slowing of rhythm	Drowsy, unresponsive to verbal commands, markedly confused, delirious, hyperreflexia, positive Babinski's sign
IV (coma)	Usually absent	Appearance of delta waves, decreased amplitudes	Unconscious, decerebrate or decorticate response to pain present (stage IVA) or absent (stage IVB)

TABLE 6-12 ■ Clinical Stages of Hepatic Encephalopathy

From Fuhrman BP, Zimmerman JJ, Carcillo JA, Clark RS, et al (eds): Pediatric Critical Care, 4th ed. Philadelphia, Saunders, 2011.

- Stage 4: Coma, unable to test mental state

PE
- Variable w/the stage and may reveal the following abnormalities:
  - Skin: jaundice, palmar erythema, spider angiomas, ecchymosis, dilated superficial periumbilical veins (*caput medusae*) in pts w/cirrhosis
  - Eyes: scleral icterus, *Kayser-Fleischer rings* (Wilson's disease)
  - Breath: *fetor hepaticus*
  - Chest: gynecomastia in men w/chronic liver disease
  - Abd: ascites, small nodular liver (cirrhosis), tender hepatomegaly (congestive hepatomegaly)
  - Rectal exam: hemorrhoids (portal HTN), guaiac + stool (alcoholic gastritis, bleeding esophageal varices, PUD, bleeding hemorrhoids)
  - Genitalia: testicular atrophy in men w/chronic liver disease
  - Extremities: pedal edema from hypoalbuminemia
  - Neurologic: flapping tremor (*asterixis*), obtundation, coma w/ or w/o decerebrate posturing

Labs
- ALT, AST, bili, alk phos, glucose, Ca, electrolytes, BUN, Cr, alb
- CBC, Plt count, PT, PTT
- Serum/urine toxicology screen (suspected medication/illegal drug use)
- Blood/urine cultures, U/A
- Venous ammonia level (no correlation w/stage HE but helpful in initial evaluation)
- ABGs

Treatment
- Identification and Rx of precipitating factors
- Restriction of protein intake (30-40 g/day) to ↓ toxic protein metabolites
- ↓ Colonic ammonia production:
  - Lactulose 30 mL of 50% solution qid (dose adjusted via clinical response). Ornithine aspartate 9 g tid is also effective.
  - Neomycin 1 g PO q4-6h or given as a 1% retention enema solution (1 g in 100 mL of isotonic saline solution); neomycin should be used w/caution in pts w/renal insufficiency. Metronidazole 250 mg qid may be as effective as neomycin and is not nephrotoxic; however, long-term use can be associated w/ neurotoxicity. Rifaximin 1200 mg/day is a viable alternative to metronidazole.
  - Lactulose + neomycin are used when either agent is ineffective alone.
- Rx of cerebral edema: Cerebral edema is often present in pts w/acute liver failure, and it accounts for nearly 50% of deaths. Monitoring of ICP by epidural, intraparenchymal, or subdural transducers and Rx of cerebral edema w/mannitol (100-200 mL of 20% solution [0.3-0.4 g/kg of BW]) given by rapid IV infusion is helpful in selected pts (e.g., potential transplantation pts). Dexamethasone and hyperventilation (useful in head injury) are of little value in treating cerebral edema from liver failure.

f. Hepatorenal Syndrome (HRS)
Intense renal vasoconstriction resulting from loss of renal autoregulation occurring as a complication of severe liver disease. HRS has 2 types:
- Type 1: progressive renal function impairment (doubling of initial serum Cr >2.5 mg/dL or 50% reduction initial 24-hr CrCl to <20 mL/min in <2 wk)

187

- Type 2: stable/slowly progressive renal function impairment (assoc w/refractory ascites)

Etiology
- HRS may occur after significant ↓ effective blood volume (paracentesis, GI bleeding, diuretics) or in absence of any precipitating factors.

Diagnosis
- Serum Cr >1.5 mg/dL; with no improvement (↓ ≤1.5 mg/dL) after 2 days diuretic withdrawal + albumin volume expansion
- Absence of shock, infection, fluid loss, or current Rx w/nephrotoxic drugs
- Absence of proteinuria (<500 mg/day) or hematuria (<50 RBC/hpf)
- Absence of U/S evidence of obstructive uropathy/parenchymal renal disease
- Urinary Na <10 mmol/L

Treatment
- Volume challenge (↑ MAP) then large-volume paracentesis (↑ CO, ↓ renal venous pressure) recommended to distinguish HRS from prerenal azotemia in pts w/Fe$_{Na}$ <1% [if prerenal azotemia the ↑ renal perfusion pressure/renal blood flow results in prompt diuresis]; volume challenge can be accomplished by 100 g albumin in 500 mL isotonic saline.
- Vasopressin analogues may ↑ renal perfusion by reversing splanchnic vasodilation (hallmark HRS); IV NE + albumin and furosemide may also be effective.
- Rx w/vasoconstrictors 5 to 15 days in attempt to ↓ serum Cr to <1.5 mg/dL:
  - Norepinephrine (0.5-3.0 mg/hr IV)
  - Midodrine (7.5-12.5 mg tid) + octreotide (100 µg SC tid)
  - Terlipressin (0.2-2.0 mg IV q4-12h)
  - Add albumin (1 g/kg IV on day 1, then 20-40 g qd)
- Liver transplantation (most effective Rx) may be indicated pts (<65 yr) w/sclerosing cholangitis, chronic hepatitis w/cirrhosis, or PBC. Contraindications include AIDS, metastatic disease, substance abuse, uncontrolled sepsis, and uncontrolled cardiac/pulmonary disease.

g. Spontaneous Bacterial Peritonitis
Ascitic fluid bacterial culture (+) with absolute polymorphonuclear count ≥250 cells/µL

Management and Treatment
- Third-generation cephalosporin given until culture report finalized
- If SBP + hepatorenal syndrome, concomitant IV alb ↑ survival rate
- Repeat paracentesis (48 hr) should reveal ↓ PMN count, will be ↑ if secondary peritonitis
- Rx secondary peritonitis with norfloxacin (TMP-SMX if fluoroquinolone allergy)
- Prophylaxis with norfloxacin warranted if low-protein ascitic fluid <1 g/dL (10 g/L)

h. Hepatocellular Carcinoma (HCC)
Malignant tumor of the hepatocytes; third leading cause of cancer-related death worldwide (80% HCCs occur in cirrhotic pts; other risk factors = male sex, chronic HepB/C, hemochromatosis, α_1-antitrypsin deficiency)

Diagnosis
H&P
- 33% asx at dx; Abd pain may be initial presentation.
- Sx underlying cirrhosis often present; new ascites, encephalopathy, jaundice/bleeding, paraneoplastic syndromes (hypoglycemia, erythrocytosis, hypercalcemia, severe diarrhea) may be present.

Labs
- ↑ LFTs
- ↑ AFP 70% pts (sens 40%-65%; spec 80%-94%)
- Paraneoplastic syndromes associated w/HCC may cause hypercalcemia, hypoglycemia, and polycythemia.
- HBV DNA level (>10,000 copies/mL) is a strong risk predictor of HCC independent of HBeAg, serum aminotransferase level, and liver cirrhosis.

Imaging
- U/S (optimal for screening q6mo if ↑ risk), CT scan, or MRI
- Percutaneous bx under U/S or CT scan usually is diagnostic. Tissue dx (gold standard); However, HCC reliably diagnosed if
  - Mass >2 cm that shows characteristic arterial vascularization is seen on 2 imaging modalities *or*
  - Single (+) imaging method w/AFP >400 µg/mL

Staging and Treatment
- According to the Barcelona Clinic Liver Cancer staging classification, Rx is determined according to stage.
- Early stage: Liver transplantation is the most effective Rx.
- Ablation (via radiofrequency, transarterial hepatic artery chemoembolization, percutaneous ethanol injection) can be used as bridge to transplantation.
- Nonresectable HCC: sorafenib

i. Fulminant Hepatic Failure (FHF)
Hepatic encephalopathy + jaundice without preexisting liver disease
- Classification:
  - Hyperacute = failure within 1 wk
  - Acute = failure 1 to 4 wk
  - Subacute = failure 4 to 12 wk
- Etiologies: **a**cetaminophen overdose (most common cause), infectious (HepA-E, HSV, CMV, EBV, PB19, varicella), drugs (INH, sulfa, NSAIDs, MDMA, cocaine), autoimmune hepatitis
- Rx: Recognition should prompt immediate referral to liver transplantation center (1-yr survival 73%). Table 6-13 summarizes the management of fulminant hepatic failure.

j. Liver Abscess
Necrotic infection of the liver, usually classified as pyogenic or amebic.

Etiology
- Pyogenic abscess: polymicrobial (streptococcal species [37%], *E. coli* [33%], *Klebsiella pneumoniae* [18%], *Pseudomonas, Proteus, Bacteroides*)
- Sources of pyogenic abscess: biliary disease w/cholangitis, gallbladder disease, diverticulitis, appendicitis, penetrating wounds, hematogenous
- Amebic abscess: *E. histolytica*. Transmission is through fecal-oral contamination w/ invasion of intestinal mucosa and portal system.

TABLE 6-13 ■ Management of Fulminant Hepatic Failure
No Sedation Except for Procedures
Minimal Handling
Enteric Precautions Until Infection Ruled Out
Monitor
Heart and respiratory rate
Arterial BP, CVP
Core/toe temperature
Neurologic observations
Gastric pH (>5.0)
Blood glucose (>4 mmol/L)
Acid-base
Electrolytes
PT, PTT
Fluid Balance
75% maintenance
Dextrose 10%-50% (provide 6-10 mg/kg/min)
Sodium (0.5-1 mmol/L)
Potassium (2-4 mmol/L)
Maintain Circulating Volume with Colloid/FFP Coagulation Support Only If Required
Drugs
Vitamin K
H_2 antagonist
Antacids
Lactulose
N-acetylcysteine for acetaminophen toxicity
Broad-spectrum antibiotics
Antifungals
Nutrition
Enteral feeding (1-2 g protein/kg/day)
PN if ventilated

From Fuhrman BP, Zimmerman JJ, Carcillo JA, Clark RS, et al (eds): Pediatric Critical Care, 4th ed. Philadelphia, Saunders, 2011.

Diagnosis

H&P

- RUQ abd pain, fever, nausea, cough w/pleuritic chest pain, anorexia, jaundice

Labs

- Leukocytosis, + blood cultures (50%), ↑ INR (70%), ↑ alk phos (>90%), ↑ ALT/AST (50%), + stool samples for *E. histolytica* (10%-15%). Serologic testing for *E. histolytica* does not differentiate acute from prior infection.

Imaging

- Abdominal CT (imaging study of choice)
- CXR is abnl in 50% of cases: ↑ right hemidiaphragm, pleural effusion, subdiaphragmatic air fluid levels.
- U/S (80%-95% sensitivity)
- CT or U/S-guided aspiration (50% sterile) in suspected pyogenic abscess.

Treatment

- Medical management (amebic liver abscess) versus percutaneous drainage under CT or U/S guidance + IV abx (pyogenic liver abscess)
- Empiric broad spectrum abx recommended until culture results available:
  - Piperacillin-tazobactam (4.5 g q6h), ticarcillin-clavulanate (3.1 g q4h), or ampicillin-sulbactam (3 g q6h)
  - Imipenem (500 mg IV q6h), meropenem (1 g q8h), or ertapenem (1 g qd)
  - If PCN allergy: clindamycin 600 to 900 mg IV q8h w/an AG
  - Duration of abx Rx: 4 to 6 wk
  - **Pyogenic** abscess: metronidazole (500 mg IV q8h) + quinolone (Cipro 400 mg IV q12h or levofloxacin 500 mg IV qd)
  - **Amebic** abscess: metronidazole 750 mg PO tid × 10 days followed by paromomycin 500 mg tid × 7 days
  - Dehydroemetine 1 mg/kg/day IM × 5 days then chloroquine 1 g/day × 2 days; then 500 mg/day for 2 to 3 wk (alternative to metronidazole)

6 VASCULAR DISORDERS OF THE LIVER

a. Budd-Chiari Syndrome

Hepatic venous outflow obstruction anywhere from small hepatic veins to suprahepatic IVC in the absence of right-sided heart failure or constrictive pericarditis

- Primary BCS = endoluminal obstruction (thromboses/webs)
- Secondary BCS = obstruction from nonvascular invasion (malignant/parasitic masses) or extrinsic compression (tumor, abscess, cysts)

Etiology

- Hypercoagulable state and/or underlying risk factor for thromboses (80%), myeloproliferative disease (50%), Behçet's disease, infection, malignancy (<5%), PNH, abd trauma, UC, celiac disease, dacarbazine

Diagnosis

H&P

- Fulminant/acute (uncommon): severe RUQ abd pain, fever, N/V, jaundice, hepatomegaly, ascites, ↑ serum aminotransferases, ↓ coagulation factors, and encephalopathy. Early recognition and Rx are essential to survival.
- Subacute/chronic (more common): vague abd discomfort, gradual progression to hepatomegaly, portal HTN w/ or w/o cirrhosis; late-onset ascites, LE edema, esophageal varices, splenomegaly, coagulopathy, HRS; asx (15% cases)
- Ascites protein content > 2.5 g/dL and SAAG ≥ 1.1 g/dL = BCS + cardiac disease

Imaging

- Color and pulsed Doppler U/S: (sens >85%) first-line test
- MRI w/gadolinium contrast (second-line test)
- Venography (gold standard); useful if difficult case or precise delineation of venous stenoses required

Treatment

- Lifelong anticoagulation INR 2 to 3 (LMWH → warfarin [Coumadin]) recommended for all
- OCPs contraindicated
- Hepatic vein/IVC angioplasty w/ or w/o stenting if refractory to anticoagulation
- If unresponsive to medical Rx, TIPS insertion recommended
- If unresponsive to TIPS, liver transplant indicated (5-yr survival 70%)
- Rx underlying myeloproliferative or other liver dysfunction

b. Portal Vein Thrombosis

Etiology
- In adults: cirrhosis (common cause), hypercoagulable states, inflammatory diseases, complications of medical intervention: ambulatory dialysis, chemoembolization, liver transplantation, partial hepatectomy, scleroRx, splenectomy, TIPS, infections (appendicitis, diverticulitis, cholecystitis)
- In children: umbilical sepsis

Diagnosis

H&P
- May result in portal HTN → esophageal/GI varices; upper GI hemorrhage (hematemesis or melena) can result from esophageal varices.
- If abd pain is present, mesenteric venous thrombosis should be suspected.

Imaging
- Abd U/S or MRI may show the portal vein thrombosis.
- Esophagogastroscopy (esophageal varices)

Treatment
- Anticoagulation
- Variceal scleroRx or banding
- Surgical mesocaval or splenorenal shunt

7 HEPATIC CYSTS
- Simple cysts (uniform thin wall, no echoic structures) asx, usually occur more in women
- Cysts <4 cm rarely of clinical significance
- If sx (nausea/abd discomfort), r/o cystadenoma (irregularity/internal echoes) via U/S
- **Rx:** Laparoscopic fenestration (simple needle aspiration assoc ↑ recurrence) if cystadenoma as malignant transformation to cystadenocarcinoma possible

8 HEPATIC ADENOMA (HA)
- Sheets of benign hepatocytes without biliary structures/nonparenchymal liver cells
- Assoc use of OCPs
- **Rx:** Resection of HA >5 cm or if pregnancy considered, discontinuation OCP with follow-up imaging if <5 cm

G. METABOLIC LIVER DISEASE

1 ALCOHOLIC HEPATITIS
- Alcohol-induced liver disease: ranges from steatosis (fatty liver) → cirrhosis
  - Steatosis: asx, resolves in 4 to 6 wk with abstinence; continued use (>40 g/day) ↑ risk cirrhosis by 30%

Labs
- ↑ AST (2-6× nl); [AST/ALT ratio 2:3 typical, AST >500/ALT >200 rare]
- Alk phos nl to ↑, bili nl to ↑↑↑, ↑ PT, ↓ GGT
- ↑ CRP, hypophosphatemia, hypomagnesia, CBC (possible leukocytosis w/bandemia or anemia)
- Carbohydrate-deficient transferring (CDT) = reliable marker chronic alcoholism
- Screen to r/o: HbsAg, anti-Hep C, ferritin/transferrin sat, AFP, liver biopsy if necessary

Imaging
- U/S (macrovascular steatosis, hepatocyte ballooning/necrosis, *Mallory's bodies*, perivenular fibrosis, portal/lobular inflammation)

Prognosis
- Maddrey discriminant function (MDF) score: 4.6× (prothrombin time [s] – control prothrombin time [s]) + total bili (mg/dL)
- MDF ≥32 (severe alcoholic hepatitis): short-term mortality risk 50%
- Model for End-Stage Liver Disease (MELD) score (prognostic index based on serum total bili, Cr, and INR): similar implications as MDF score

Treatment
- Lifestyle change, d/c EtOH abuse, vitamin supplementation, caloric monitoring, protein 1.2 to 1.5 g/kg of ideal BW/day (except in encephalopathic pt)
- Indications for initiating Rx (prednisolone 40 mg/day 28 days, 2-wk taper) include: **MDF >30, MELD >20**

2 NONALCOHOLIC FATTY LIVER DISEASE (NAFLD)

Dx of exclusion resulting from insulin resistance/metabolic syndrome with presentation ranging from axs hepatic steatosis → cirrhosis. Pending inflammation and fibrosis is referred to as nonalcoholic steatohepatitis (NASH).

Diagnosis
- Abdominal imaging via U/S, CT, MRI (reveal steatosis but not fibrosis)
- Liver biopsy (confirms NASH)

Treatment
- Lifestyle change, wt loss; monitor LFTs q3-6mo; metformin currently investigational Rx

3 HEREDITARY HEMOCHROMATOSIS

Autosomal recessive disorder (chromosome 6, *HFE* gene missense mutations C282Y/H63D) characterized by ↑ iron accumulation in various organs (adrenals, liver, pancreas, heart, testes, kidneys, pituitary) with hepatic iron overload → organ dysfunction, cirrhosis, and hepatocellular cancer

Diagnosis
H&P
- ↑ Skin pigmentation, hepatomegaly, splenomegaly, hepatic tenderness, testicular atrophy (↓ libido 50% men), amenorrhea (25% women), alopecia, gynecomastia/ascites, fatigue, joint pain, new-onset diabetes, cardiomyopathy, arthropathy
Labs
- Transferrin saturation (iron/TIBC) = best screening test; values >45% indicate need for further testing; values >52% in men and >50% in women suggest hemochromatosis. Serum ferritin is helpful but may be ↑ in inflammatory conditions or malignancy.
- ↑ AST, ALT, alk phos
- Hyperglycemia
- ↓ testosterone, LH, FSH
- Measurement of hepatic iron index (hepatic iron concentration divided by age) in liver bx specimen can confirm dx.
- Genetic testing (HFE genotyping for C282Y/H63D mutations) useful in pts w/liver disease + suspected iron overload (transferrin saturation >40%). Genetic testing should not be performed as part of initial routine evaluation for hereditary hemochromatosis. Once pt confirmed, first-degree relatives should also be screened. Figure 6-7 describes an algorithm for evaluation of possible hereditary hemochromatosis in a person with a (–) family hx.

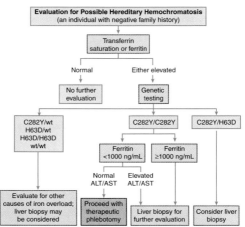

FIGURE 6-7. Algorithm for elevation of possible hereditary hemochromatosis in a person with a negative family history. *(From Goldman L, Schafer AI [eds]: Goldman's Cecil Medicine, 24th ed. Philadelphia, Saunders, 2012.)*

- Pts >40 yr old or serum ferritin level >1000 µg/L ↑ risk cirrhosis

Imaging
- CT or MRI of the liver: useful to r/o other causes + may show iron overload in the liver

Treatment
- Weekly phlebotomies of 1 to 2 U of blood (each w/ ≈250 mg iron) should be continued until ferritin level <50 ng/mL and transferrin saturation <30%. Subsequent phlebotomies PRN to maintain a transferrin saturation <50% and a ferritin level <100 ng/mL.
- Deferoxamine 0.5 to 1 g IM qd or 20 mg SC constant infusion (iron chelating agent) is generally reserved for pts w/severe hemochromatosis w/diffuse organ involvement (liver disease, heart disease) and when phlebotomy is not possible.

4 α₁-ANTITRYPSIN DEFICIENCY
Autosomal codominant deficiency of protease inhibitor α₁-antitrypsin predisposing to early-onset emphysema + hepatic cirrhosis

Diagnosis
- Serum α₁-antitrypsin level, genetic analysis for mutation/allele involvement PFTs (obstructive pattern)
- CXR (emphysematous change at lung bases)
- Chest CT (panacinar emphysema)

H&P
- Early-onset, severe, lower-lobe predominant panacinar emphysema (± bronchiectasis)
- Sx similar to "typical" COPD presentation (dyspnea, cough, sputum production)
- Liver involvement (neonatal cholestasis, cirrhosis, primary hepatocarcinoma)
- Dermatologic manifestation (panniculitis) to 85% deficit in plasma α₁-antitrypsin

Treatment
- Manage acute exacerbations similar to "typical" COPD
- Avoid smoking/factors that would worsen COPD

5 WILSON'S DISEASE
- Rare (1/30,000 newborns) autosomal recessive ↑ hepatic uptake and ↓ biliary excretion of copper

Diagnosis
- Usually pts < 45 yr old; ↓ ceruloplasmin, ↑ urinary copper excretion
- ↑ LFTs
- Liver biopsy (excessive intrahepatic copper)
- Kayser-Fleischer rings
- Neuropsychiatric abnormalities (copper deposition in brain)

Treatment
- Chelating agents (trientine, penicillamine) and low-copper diet

H. DISORDERS OF GALLBLADDER

1 CHOLELITHIASIS
Epidemiology and Demographics
- Incidence ↑ with age (highest in 40s-50s)
- Female sex, pregnancy, FHx, obesity, ileal disease, OCPs, DM
- 90% gallstones = cholesterol/mixed type, black-pigmented stones assoc with chronic hemolytic disease/cirrhosis, brown-pigmented stones assoc with biliary tract infection

Physical Exam and Clinical Findings
- (60%-80%) asx
- If biliary colic: episodic, cramping RUQ pain, may radiate to back/right shoulder

Diagnosis
- Labs nl (unless obstruction: ↑ alk phos, ↑ bili)
- U/S; if unclear HIDA scan (90% accuracy)

Treatment
- Observation recommended for asx gallstones
- If calcified *"porcelain"* gallbladder/stones >3 cm, consider cholecystectomy.

2 ACUTE CHOLECYSTITIS

- Inflammation of the gallbladder

Etiology

- Gallstones (>95% of cases), ischemic damage to the gallbladder, critically ill pt (acalculous cholecystitis), infectious agents (especially in AIDS pts [CMV, Cryptosporidium]), bile duct stricture, neoplasia

Diagnosis

H&P

- Pain/tenderness of right hypochondrium/epigastrium; possibly radiating to infrascapular region. RUQ palpation elicits marked tenderness + stoppage of inspired breath (Murphy's sign). Guarding, fever (33%), jaundice (25%-50%), palpable gallbladder (20%)
- N/V (>70%), fever and chills (>25%), and ingestion of large, fatty meals before onset of pain in the epigastrium and RUQ

Labs

- Leukocytosis (12,000-20,000) >70% of pts, alk phos, ALT, AST, bili; bili elevation >4 mg/dL is unusual and suggests presence of choledocholithiasis.

Imaging

- U/S of gallbladder: presence of stones, dilated gallbladder w/thickened wall and surrounding edema, fluid stranding
- HIDA scan: sensitivity and specificity >90% for acute cholecystitis. Test is reliable only when bili is <5 mg/dL. (+) Test = absence of gallbladder filling within 60 min after the administration of tracer.
- CT of abd: in cases of suspected abscess, neoplasm, or pancreatitis

Treatment

- Cholecystectomy
- Conservative management w/IV fluids and abx (ampicillin-sulbactam 3 g IV q6h *or* piperacillin-tazobactam 4.5 g IV q8h) may be justified in some high-risk pts to convert an emergency procedure into an elective one w/lower mortality.
- ERCP w/sphincterectomy and stone extraction can be performed in conjunction w/laparoscopic cholecystectomy for pts w/choledocholithiasis; 7% to 15% of pts w/cholelithiasis also have stones in the CBD.

Hematology/Oncology 7

A. APPROACH TO THE PATIENT WITH ANEMIA

- Look at reticulocyte count and MCV.
- The reticulocyte count can help distinguish excess RBC destruction or blood loss (↑ reticulocyte count) from ↓ production (↓ reticulocyte count).
- The mean MCV classifies anemia as normocytic, microcytic, or macrocytic.
- A diagnostic algorithm for anemia based on MCV and reticulocyte count is described in Figure 7-1.

1 ANEMIA SECONDARY TO MATURATION DEFECTS OR UNDERPRODUCTION

a. Iron Deficiency Anemia

Etiology

- Blood loss from GI or menstrual bleeding (GU blood loss less often the cause)
- Dietary iron deficiency (rare in adults)
- Poor iron absorption in pts w/gastric or small bowel surgery
- Repeated phlebotomy
- ↑ Requirements (e.g., pregnancy)
- Other: traumatic hemolysis (abnlly functioning cardiac valves), idiopathic pulmonary hemosiderosis (iron sequestration in pulmonary macrophages), PNH (intravascular hemolysis)

Diagnosis

H&P

- Fatigue, dizziness, exertional dyspnea, pagophagia (ice eating), pica. Pt's hx may also suggest GI blood loss (melena, hematochezia, hemoptysis).

Labs

- Vary w/the stage of deficiency: absent iron marrow stores and ↓ serum ferritin → ↓ serum iron, ↑ TIBC → ↓ MCV
- Peripheral smear: microcytic hypochromic RBCs w/a wide area of central pallor, anisocytosis, poikilocytosis
- ↑ RDW (usually <15), ↓ MCV, ↓ serum ferritin level, ↑ TIBC, ↓ serum iron

Treatment

- Ferrous sulfate 325 mg PO qd, parenteral iron, transfusion of PRBCs depending on severity

b. Cobalamin (Vitamin B_{12}) Deficiency

Etiology

- Pernicious anemia (PA): gastric anti–parietal cell Abs in 90% of pts, anti–intrinsic factor Abs in >70% of pts
- Malabsorption, atrophic gastric mucosa, bacterial overgrowth, IBD, meds (PPIs, metformin)

Diagnosis

H&P

- Impaired memory, gait disturbances, paresthesias, and complaints of generalized weakness in advanced stages

Labs

- CBC: macrocytic anemia and leukopenia w/hypersegmented neutrophils
- ↑ MCV, ↓/nl reticulocyte count
- Plasma MMA (P-MMA) (↑) and urinary MMA (↑), total homocysteine level (↑): used for detecting cobalamin deficiency in pts w/nl vitamin B_{12} levels

Treatment

- Traditional Rx of severe cobalamin deficiency consists of IM injections of vitamin B_{12} 1000 μg/wk for 4 wk followed by 1000 μg/mo IM indefinitely.
- PO cobalamin (1000-2000 μg/day) is effective for dietary deficiency and in mild cases of PA because about 1% of PO dose is absorbed by passive diffusion, a pathway that does not require intrinsic factor.

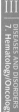

III

DISEASES AND DISORDERS
7. Hematology/Oncology

195

■ Anemia is absent in 20% of pts w/cobalamin deficiency, and macrocytosis is absent in >30% of pts at the time of dx.

c. Folate Deficiency

Etiology

■ Malnutrition (alcoholism), ↑ needs (pregnancy), ↑ cell turnover (sickle cell, psoriasis)

Diagnosis

■ RBC folate *more accurate* (serum folate may be nl after just 1 folate-containing meal)
■ ↑ Homocysteine (>90% sensitivity/specificity) in dx despite nl folate level

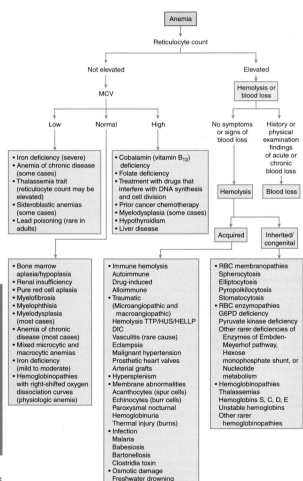

FIGURE 7-1. Algorithm for diagnosis of anemia. *(From Goldman L, Schafer AI [eds]: Goldman's Cecil Medicine, 24th ed. Philadelphia, Saunders, 2012.)*

Treatment

- Folate 1 to 5 mg/day PO
- R/o vitamin B_{12} deficiency before Rx as folate Rx can improve anemia but not B_{12} neuro sx
- If folate deficiency or pregnancy

d. Inflammatory Anemia (Anemia of Chronic Disease [ACD])

Etiology

- Chronic infections (TB, SBE)
- Chronic inflammation (connective tissue disorders, burns)
- Malignant disease (carcinomas, lymphomas)
- Endocrine (hypothyroidism, hypogonadism, hypopituitarism)
- CKD, Chronic liver disease, IBD
- Mechanism: ↓ erythrocyte survival, ↑ uptake and retention of iron within cells of the RES, limited availability of iron for erythroid progenitor cells, iron-restricted erythropoiesis

Diagnosis

Labs

- Normochromic, normocytic, or microcytic anemia
- ↓ Iron and transferrin saturation, ↓ TIBC, and N/↑ ferritin level
- Table 7-1 compares various causes of microcytic anemia.

TABLE 7-1 ■ Lab Differentiation of Microcytic Anemias				
Abnormality	Ferritin	Serum iron	TIBC	RDW
Iron deficiency	↓	↓	↑	↑
Inflammatory anemia	N/↑	↓	↓	N
Sideroblastic anemia	N/↑	↑	N	N
Thalassemia	N/↑	N/↑	N/↓	N/↑

Treatment

- Rx is aimed at identification and Rx of underlying disease.
- Erythropoiesis-stimulating agents (ESAs) (epoetin alfa, epoetin β, and darbepoetin) can be used in pts w/CKD (to ↑ Hgb to max of 11-12 g/dL), in HIV pts undergoing myelosuppressive Rx, and in pts w/cancer who are undergoing chemoRx.

e. Sideroblastic Anemia

Iron-loading anemia secondary to defective heme synthesis

Etiology

- Primary hereditary sideroblastic anemia: inherited as a sex-linked recessive disease
- Secondary acquired sideroblastic anemia: caused by alcohol, isoniazid, pyrazinamide, cycloserine, chloramphenicol, copper deficiency, lead poisoning

Diagnosis

Labs

- Hypochromic anemia (↓ MCV, ↑ RDW)
- Peripheral smear: dimorphic large and small cells revealing "*Pappenheimer bodies*" or siderocytes when stained for iron
- Bone marrow: *ringed sideroblasts*, which represent iron storage in the mitochondria of normoblasts

Treatment

- ESAs
- Avoid alcohol
- Sideroblastic anemia secondary to isoniazid, pyrazinamide, and cycloserine: vitamin B_6 (50-200 mg/day)

2 ACQUIRED HEMOLYTIC ANEMIA

a. Autoimmune Hemolytic Anemia (AIHA)

Premature destruction of RBCs caused by the binding of auto-Abs (IgG [80%], IgM [20%]) or complement to RBCs. AIHA may be idiopathic or associated with other disorders.

Etiology

- Warm AIHA (WAIHA): IgG (often idiopathic or associated w/leukemia, lymphoma, thymoma, myeloma, viral infections, and collagen-vascular disease)
- Cold agglutinin disease (CAD): IgM and complement in majority of cases (often idiopathic, at times associated w/infections [EBV], lymphoma)

- Drug-induced: three major mechanisms:
  - Ab directed against Rh complex (e.g., methyldopa)
  - Ab directed against RBC drug complex (hapten-induced, e.g., PCN)
  - Ab directed against complex formed by drug and plasma proteins; the drug–plasma protein–Ab complex causes destruction of RBCs (innocent bystander, e.g., quinidine)

Diagnosis
H&P
- Pallor, jaundice
- Tachycardia w/flow murmur if anemia is pronounced
- Dyspnea and fatigue: most common presentation
- Pts w/intravascular hemolysis may present w/dark urine and back pain.
- Presence of hepatomegaly or lymphadenopathy suggests an underlying lymphoproliferative disorder or malignant neoplasm.
- Splenomegaly may indicate hypersplenism as a cause of hemolysis.

Labs
- Initial labs: ↑ reticulocyte count, ↑ LFTs (indirect bili, LDH), Coombs' test (+ direct Coombs' = Abs or complement on the surface of RBC; + indirect Coombs' = anti-RBC Abs freely circulating in the pt's serum), ↓ haptoglobin level
- RBC clumping in CAD, falsely ↑ MCV

Imaging
- CXR
- CT of chest and abd: r/o lymphoma

Treatment
- WAIHA: Prednisone 1 mg/kg/day. Consider rituximab, splenectomy, danazol, cyclophosphamide in resistant cases.
- CAD: Avoid cold exposure in pts w/cold Ab.
- Drug-induced AHA: Remove drug, and consider fludarabine.

b. Microangiopathic Hemolytic Anemia
Erythrocyte lysis during travel through the vascular system results in schistocytes or helmet cells on peripheral blood smear.

Differential Diagnosis
- TTP
- HUS
- DIC
- Intravascular foreign devices

Labs
- ↓ Haptoglobin, ↑ LDH
- Hemoglobinuria

Treatment
- Rx varies depending on etiology.
- Plasma exchange may be lifesaving in pts with TTP or HUS.

c. Paroxysmal Nocturnal Hemoglobinuria (PNH)
Acquired clonal stem cell disorder (mutation in PIG-A gene) → episodes of intravascular hemolysis and hemoglobinuria, usually occurring at night

Diagnosis
- CBC (anemia, leukopenia, thrombocytopenia, reticulocytosis)
- ↓ Serum iron saturation, ↓ ferritin
- RBC smear: spherocytes
- (–) Coombs test, (+) Ham test
- ↓ LAP, ↓ haptoglobin, ↑ LDH
- ↑ Urine hemoglobin, urobilinogen, hemosiderin
- Flow cytometry for detection of CD55 and CD59 deficiency on surface of peripheral erythrocytes/leukocytes
- Normoblastic hyperplasia on marrow aspirate or bx

H&P
- First morning urinary void reveals hemoglobinuria with progressive clearing throughout day (25%), bleeding/anemia (30%), and thrombosis (40%).

Treatment
- Anticoagulation in acute thrombotic event: Consider prophylaxis if >50% CD55– or CD59–deficient.
- Eculizumab has shown ↓ transfusion requirements, ↑ quality of life.
- Consider corticosteroids.

III

d. Hemolytic Transfusion Reaction

Acute Hemolytic Transfusion Reaction (AHTR)

Almost always caused by ABO incompatibility between donor and recipient (clerical error)

Physical Exam and Clinical Findings

- Hypotension, fever, kidney failure, pain at transfusion site, DIC

Treatment

- Stop transfusion immediately, recheck specimen for incompatibility, and provide supportive care (fluid resuscitation, vasopressor support, mannitol).

Delayed Hemolytic Transfusion Reaction (DHTR)

Via amnestic response of preformed erythrocyte alloantibody after repeat exposure to erythrocyte antigen outside the ABO system

Physical Exam and Clinical Findings

- 5-10 days s/p transfusion: anemia, jaundice, fever

Treatment

- Supportive care

3 CONGENITAL HEMOLYTIC ANEMIAS

a. Sickle Cell Syndrome

Substitution of the amino acid valine for glutamic acid in the sixth position of the γ-globin chain = Hgb S $\rightarrow$ exposed to low Po_2 $\rightarrow$ RBC sickling $\rightarrow$ stasis of RBCs in capillaries $\rightarrow$ obstruction of blood flow

Diagnosis

H&P

- PE is variable, depending on the degree of anemia and presence of acute vaso-occlusive syndromes or neurologic, CV, GU, and musculoskeletal complications.
- Bones are the most common site of pain. *Dactylitis,* or *hand-foot syndrome* (acute, painful swelling of the hands and feet), is the first manifestation of sickle cell disease in many infants.
- Pneumonia develops during the course of 20% of painful events and can manifest as chest and abd pain. In adults, chest pain may be a result of vaso-occlusion in the ribs and often precedes a pulmonary event. The lower back is also a frequent site of painful crisis in adults.
- The *acute chest syndrome* manifests w/chest pain, fever, wheezing, tachypnea, and cough. CXR reveals pulmonary infiltrates. Common causes include infection (mycoplasma, chlamydia, viruses), infarction, and fat embolism.
- Musculoskeletal and skin abnlities: leg ulcers (particularly on the malleoli) and limb-girdle deformities caused by avascular necrosis of the femoral and humeral heads
- Endocrine abnlities: delayed sexual maturation and late physical maturation, especially evident in boys
- Neurologic abnlities: seizures and MS changes
- Infections: *Salmonella, Mycoplasma,* and *Streptococcus* are common.
- Severe splenomegaly secondary to sequestration often occurs in children before splenic atrophy.

Labs

- Hgb electrophoresis confirms the dx and can identify Hgb variants, such as fetal Hgb and Hgb A_2.
- ↑ Bili and LDH ↓ haptoglobin
- Peripheral blood smear: sickle cells, target cells, poikilocytosis, hypochromia
- ↑ BUN and Cr: in pts w/progressive renal insufficiency
- U/A: hematuria, proteinuria

Imaging

- CXR
- Bone scan or MRI scan in suspected osteomyelitis
- CT or MRI of brain: in pts w/TIA, CVA, seizures, or MS changes
- Transcranial Doppler study: in pts at risk for stroke
- Doppler echocardiography: r/o pulmonary HTN

Treatment

- Avoidance of conditions that may precipitate sickling crisis, such as hypoxia, infections, acidosis, and dehydration
- Maintain adequate hydration (PO or IV).
- Correct hypoxia.
- Ceph and azithromycin + incentive spirometry and bronchodilators in pts w/acute chest syndrome

- Pain relief during the vaso-occlusive crisis
  - Narcotics (e.g., morphine 0.1 mg/kg IV q3-4h or 0.3 mg/kg PO q4h) should be given on a fixed schedule (not PRN for pain), w/rescue dosing for breakthrough pain as needed.
  - Except when contraindications exist, concomitant use of NSAIDs should be standard Rx.
- Indications for transfusion include aplastic crises, severe hemolytic crises (particularly during third trimester of pregnancy), acute chest syndrome, and high risk of stroke.
- Hydroxyurea is indicated for severe disease, typically in pts w/> 3 acute painful crises or episodes of the acute chest syndrome in the previous year.
- Replace folic acid (1 mg PO qd).
- Exchange transfusions: Consider for pts w/acute neurologic signs, in aplastic crisis, or undergoing surgery.
- Allogeneic SCT can be curative in young pts w/symptomatic sickle cell disease; however, the death rate from the procedure is nearly 10%.
- PCN V 125 mg PO bid should be administered by age 2 mo and to 250 mg bid by age 3 yr. PCN prophylaxis can be discontinued after age 5 yr except in children who have had splenectomy.

b. Thalassemia

β-Thalassemia
- β (+)-Thalassemia (suboptimal β-globin synthesis)
- β (0)-Thalassemia (total absence of β-globin synthesis)
- δ-β-Thalassemia (total absence of both δ-globin and β-globin synthesis)
- Lepore hemoglobin (synthesis of small amounts of fused δ-β-globin and total absence of δ- and β-globin)
- Hereditary persistence of fetal hemoglobin (HPHF) (increased hemoglobin F synthesis and reduced or absence of δ- and β-globin)

α-Thalassemia
- Silent carrier (three α-globin genes present)
- α-Thalassemia trait (two α-globin genes present)
- Hemoglobin H disease (one α-globin gene present)
- Hydrops fetalis (no α-globin gene)
- Hemoglobin constant sprint (elongated α-globin chain)

H&P

β-Thalassemia
- Heterozygous β-thalassemia (thalassemia minor): no or mild anemia, microcytosis and hypochromia, mild hemolysis manifested by slight reticulocytosis and splenomegaly
- Homozygous β-thalassemia (thalassemia major): intense hemolytic anemia; transfusion dependency; bone deformities (skull and long bones); hepatomegaly; splenomegaly; iron overload leading to cardiomyopathy, diabetes mellitus, and hypogonadism; growth retardation; pigment gallstones; susceptibility to infection
- Thalassemia intermedia caused by combination of β- and α-thalassemia or β-thalassemia and Hgb Lepore: resembles thalassemia major but is milder

α-Thalassemia
- Silent carrier: no symptoms
- α-Thalassemia trait: microcytosis only
- Hemoglobin H disease: moderately severe hemolysis with microcytosis and splenomegaly
- The loss of all four α-globin genes is incompatible with life (stillbirth of hydropic fetus).

Diagnosis

Labs: β-Thalassemia
- Microcytosis (MCV: 55 to 80 fL)
- Smear: nucleated RBCs, anisocytosis, poikilocytosis, polychromatophilia, Pappenheimer and Howell-Jolly bodies
- Hemoglobin electrophoresis: ↓ hemoglobin A, increased fetal hemoglobin, variable increase in the amount of hemoglobin A_2
- Markers of hemolysis: elevated indirect bilirubin and lactate dehydrogenase, decreased haptoglobin

Labs: α-Thalassemia
- Microcytosis
- Hemoglobin electrophoresis: normal except for the presence of hemoglobin H in hemoglobin H disease

Treatment
- Thalassemia minor: No treatment is indicated, but avoid iron administration for incorrect diagnosis of iron deficiency.
- β-Thalassemia major (and hemoglobin H disease)
  - Transfusion as required together with chelation of iron with desferrioxamine. Deferiprone, an oral chelating agent, can be used as a second-line treatment.
  - Splenectomy for hypersplenism if present
  - Bone marrow transplantation
  - Hydroxyurea may increase the level of hemoglobin F.

c. Glucose-6 Phosphate Dehydrogenase (G6PD) Deficiency
Etiology
- Mutation on X chromosome
- Most common RBC enzyme defect → inability to generate NADPH = hemolysis when exposed to oxidant stress

Diagnosis
H&P
- Episodic hemolysis following exposure to fava beans (Mediterranean G6PD variant) or drugs (nitrofurantoin, dapsone, trimethoprim-sulfamethoxazole) in African variant form
Labs
- Peripheral smear: "*bite*" cells, denatured oxidized hemoglobin (*Heinz bodies*)
- G6PD levels not helpful during acute hemolysis (may be falsely normal because of ↑ G6PD in young reticulocytes)

Treatment
- Removal of offending agent, supportive care

d. Hereditary Spherocytosis
Etiology
- Autosomal dominant
- Most common RBC membrane disorder → spectrin deficiency = loss of erythrocyte surface area → spherocytic shape → trapping and destruction in spleen

Diagnosis
H&P
- Neonatal jaundice, hx anemia, gallstones, splenomegaly
Labs
- Osmotic fragility test with 24-hr incubation = ↑ fragility
- Direct Coombs (–)
- Peripheral smear: spherocytes

Treatment
- Vaccination against meningococcus, pneumococcus, Hib followed by splenectomy in symptomatic pts

B. BONE MARROW FAILURE SYNDROMES

1 APLASTIC ANEMIA
Bone marrow failure is characterized by stem cell destruction or suppression leading to pancytopenia.

Diagnosis
Labs
- CBC: pancytopenia. Macrocytosis and toxic granulation of neutrophils may also be present. Isolated cytopenias may occur in the early stages, ↓ reticulocyte count.
- Additional initial labs: vitamin B_{12} level, RBC folate, HIV, Ham test (r/o PNH) hepatitis serology
- Bone marrow examination: paucity or absence of erythropoietic and myelopoietic precursor cells. Pts w/pure red cell aplasia demonstrate only absence of RBC precursors in the marrow.
- Chromosomal breakpoint analysis to r/o Fanconi anemia in pts <50 yr old

Treatment
- Transplantation of allogeneic marrow (HSCT) or peripheral blood SCT from a histocompatible sibling is preferred initial Rx (cure rate >80%) in pts <40 yr old.
- Immunosuppressive Rx with ATG and cyclophosphamide is indicated in pts who are not candidates for allogeneic bone marrow (long-term survival >60%).

2 PURE RED CELL APLASIA (PRCA)
Bone marrow failure affects erythroblasts (leukocyte and Plt production is normal).

Etiology
- Idiopathic or secondary (thymoma, parvovirus B19, meds [chloramphenicol, phenytoin, INH]), collagen vascular and lymphoproliferative disorders, pregnancy)
- PE: splenomegaly, signs of RA (33% of pts)

Diagnosis
- Flow cytometry: CD57+ T-cells, clonality T-cell receptor gene rearrangement
- Normocytic anemia
- Presence of large granular lymphocytes when PRCA results from large granular lymphocytosis

Treatment
- Removal of offending drugs/Rx secondary condition (IV Ig if parvovirus B19 infection)
- Refractory cases: prednisone, ATG, cyclosporine, cyclophosphamide (first-line agents with response 3-12 wk)
- If sx anemia: erythrocyte transfusion

3 THROMBOCYTOPENIA

Etiology
- ↑ Destruction
  - Immunologic
    - Drugs: quinine, quinidine, digitalis, procainamide, thiazide diuretics, sulfonamides, phenytoin, ASA, PCN, heparin, gold, meprobamate, sulfa drugs, phenylbutazone, NSAIDs, methyldopa, cimetidine, furosemide, INH, cephs, chlorpropamide, organic arsenicals, chloroquine, Plt glycoprotein IIb/IIIa receptor inhibitors, ranitidine, indomethacin, carboplatin, ticlopidine, clopidogrel
    - ITP
    - Transfusion reaction: transfusion of Plts w/plasminogen activator (PLA) in recipients w/o PLA-1
    - Fetal/maternal incompatibility
    - Collagen-vascular diseases (e.g., SLE)
    - AIHA
    - Lymphoreticular disorders (e.g., CLL)
  - Nonimmunologic
    - Prosthetic heart valves
    - TTP
    - Sepsis
    - DIC
    - HUS
    - Giant cavernous hemangioma
- ↓ Production
  - Abnl marrow
  - Marrow infiltration (e.g., leukemia, lymphoma, fibrosis)
  - Marrow suppression (e.g., chemoRx, alcohol, irradiation)
  - Vitamin deficiencies (B_{12}, folate)
  - Hereditary disorders
    - Wiskott-Aldrich syndrome: X-linked disorder characterized by thrombocytopenia, eczema, and repeated infections
    - May-Hegglin anomaly: megakaryocytes but ineffective thrombopoiesis
- Splenic sequestration
- Hypersplenism
- Dilutional (massive transfusion)

Diagnosis
Diagnostic Approach (Fig. 7-2)
- Thorough hx (particularly drug hx)
- PE: Evaluate for presence of splenomegaly (hypersplenism, leukemia, lymphoma).

Labs
- CBC, Coombs, LDH, INR, PTT, Plt Ab, D-dimer, fibrinogen level
- Peripheral blood smear; note Plt size and other abnlities (e.g., fragmented RBCs may indicate TTP or DIC; ↑ Plt size suggests accelerated destruction and release of large young Plt into the circulation, normal smear and ↑ platelet size = ITP).
- Bone marrow: ↑ megakaryocytes suggest accelerated Plt destruction.

4 NEUTROPENIA

Etiology
- Congenital: mild forms not associated with ↑ infection risk; Rx not necessary

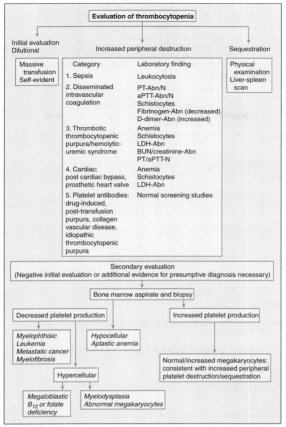

FIGURE 7-2. Evaluation of thrombocytopenia. *(From Goldman L, Schafer AI [eds]: Goldman's Cecil Medicine, 24th ed. Philadelphia, Saunders, 2012.)*

- Acquired: drugs (chemotherapeutic agents, antibiotics [trimethoprim/sulfamethoxazole, cephs, chloramphenicol], anticonvulsants [phenytoin, carbamazepine], NSAIDs, antiarrhythmics [procainamide, amiodarone]), SLE, RA (*Felty syndrome* if splenomegaly present), viral infections (CMV, EBV, HIV), bacterial infections (*S. pneumoniae, N. meningitidis*), rickettsia, vitamin B_{12} and folate deficiencies, myelodysplasia, large granular lymphocytosis, and other malignant disorders
- PE: splenomegaly, signs of RA (*Felty syndrome*)

Diagnosis
- Antineutrophil Ab (if test available)
- Bone marrow exam if suspecting stem cell disorder

Treatment
- Removal of offending drugs/Rx of secondary condition
- Consider G-CSF Rx in severe neutropenia.

C. MYELODYSPLASTIC SYNDROMES

This group of acquired clonal disorders affecting the hematopoietic stem cells is characterized by cytopenias w/hypercellular bone marrow and various morphologic abnlities in the hematopoietic cell lines. Myelodysplastic syndrome cells show abnl (dysplastic) hematopoietic maturation. Marrow cellularity is ↑, reflecting an effective hematopoiesis, but inadequate maturation results in peripheral cytopenias.

CLASSIFICATION

- The French-American-British (FAB) classification is described in Table 7-2.
- The WHO classification includes the following disease subtypes: refractory anemia, refractory anemia w/ringed sideroblasts, refractory cytopenia w/multilineage dysplasia, refractory cytopenia w/multilineage dysplasia and ringed sideroblasts, refractory anemia w/excessive blasts (1, 2), unclassified myelodysplastic syndrome, and myelodysplastic syndrome associated w/isolated deletion (5q).

TABLE 7-2 ■ French-American-British Classification Chart

Subtype	Abbreviation	Peripheral Blood	Bone Marrow
Refractory anemia	RA	Blasts <1%	Blasts <5%
Refractory anemia with ringed sideroblasts	RARS	Blasts <1%	Blasts <5%, and >15% ringed sideroblasts
Refractory anemia with excess blasts	RAEB	Blasts <5%	Blasts 5%-20%
Refractory anemia with excess blasts in transformation	RAEB-T	Blasts >5%	Blasts 20%-30% or Auer rods
Chronic myelomonocytic leukemia	CMML	Monocytes >1 × 10⁹/L	Any of the above
Acute myelogenous leukemia	AML	Blasts >30%	

From Hoffman R et al: Hematology, basic principles and practice, ed 5, Philadelphia 2009, Churchill Livingston.

Diagnosis

H&P
- Splenomegaly, skin pallor, mucosal bleeding, and ecchymosis may be present.
- Fatigue, fever, dyspnea

Labs
- CBC w/diff, HIV, RBC folate, vitamin B_{12} level, bone marrow exam, cytogenetic analysis

Treatment

- ESAs in sx anemia
- Lenalidomide
- Azacitidine
- Decitabine
- Allogeneic stem cell transplantation should be considered in pts <60 yr old.

PROGNOSIS

- Risk of transformation to AML varies w/% of blasts in bone marrow.
- Advanced age, male sex, and deletion of chromosomes 5 and 7 are associated w/ poor prognosis.
- The most important variables in disease outcome are the specific cytogenetic abnlities, the % of blasts in bone marrow, and the number of hematopoietic lineages involved in the cytopenias.

D. MYELOPROLIFERATIVE DISORDERS

1 POLYCYTHEMIA VERA

This myeloproliferative disorder is characterized mainly by erythrocytosis.

Diagnosis (Fig. 7-3)

Clinical Presentation
- Sx associated w/ ↑ blood volume and viscosity or impaired Plt function
  - Impaired cerebral circulation: headache, vertigo, blurred vision, dizziness, TIA, CVA
  - Fatigue, poor exercise tolerance

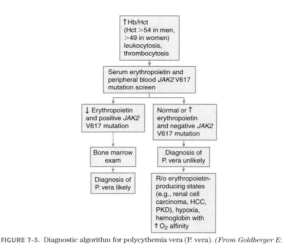

FIGURE 7-3. Diagnostic algorithm for polycythemia vera (P. vera). *(From Goldberger E: Treatment of Cardiac Emergencies, 5th ed. St. Louis, Mosby, 1990.)*

- Pruritus, particularly after bathing (caused by overproduction of histamine)
- Bleeding: epistaxis, UGI bleeding (incidence of PUD)
■ Abd discomfort secondary to splenomegaly, hepatomegaly
■ Nephrolithiasis and gouty arthritis from hyperuricemia
PE
■ Facial plethora, congestion of oral mucosa, ruddy complexion
■ Enlargement and tortuosity of retinal vein
■ Splenomegaly (>75% of pts)
Labs
■ ↑ RBC count, ↑ Hgb/Hct
■ ↑ WBC (often w/basophilia), ↑ Plts (majority of pts)
■ ↑ LAP, serum vitamin B_{12}, and uric acid levels
■ ↓ Serum erythropoietin level
■ + *JAK2* V617F mutation (>95% of pts)
■ N$_l$ O$_2$ sat
■ Bone marrow exam: RBC hyperplasia and absent iron stores

Treatment
■ ASA 81 mg/day
■ Phlebotomy to keep Hct <45%
■ Additional options: hydroxyurea, interferon alfa-2b

Prognosis
■ The median survival time w/o Rx is 6 to 18 mo after dx; phlebotomy extends the average survival time to 12 yr.
■ Prognosis worse in pts >60 yr of age and those who have h/o thrombosis.

2 ESSENTIAL THROMBOCYTHEMIA
↑ Plt count w/o conditions causing secondary thrombocytosis

Epidemiology and Presentation
■ <1% of pts progress to AML.
■ 20%-30% arterial/venous thrombosis. Leukocytosis predicts severity.
■ If + JAK2 V617F mutation (50% pts) is present, then the course is more aggressive.
■ Hemorrhagic sx (40%)

Diagnosis
■ Plt count >600,000/μL on 2 separate occasions 1 mo apart
■ R/o secondary causes (iron deficiency, cancer, infection) in the absence of Philadelphia chromosome (t9:22).

Treatment

- Plt-lowering agents in pt >65 yr old w/hx/↑ risk thrombosis
- Hydroxyurea + low-dose ASA = ↓ risk thrombosis
- Interferon alfa (pregnant pt) or ^{32}P in refractory cases

3 CHRONIC MYELOID LEUKEMIA

This malignant clonal disorder of hematopoietic stem cells is characterized by abnl proliferation and accumulation of immature granulocytes. Philadelphia chromosome, which is chromosome translocation t(9;22)(q34;q11.2), is present in >95% of pts.

Three Major Phases

Chronic Phase (Months to Years)
- Asymptomatic after Rx
- No features of accelerated phase or blast crisis

Accelerated Phase
- Leukocyte count increasingly difficult to control w/standard Rx
- ↑ Blast %
  - >10% in blood or bone marrow
  - >20% blasts plus promyelocytes in blood or bone marrow
  - >20% basophils plus eosinophils in blood
- Progressive anemia or thrombocytopenia
- New cytogenetic abnlities, especially a second Ph chromosome or trisomy 8
- Worsening constitutional sx
- Progressive splenomegaly
- Development of myeloblastomas or myelofibrosis

Blast Crisis
- >30% blasts plus promyelocytes in blood or bone marrow

Diagnosis

H&P
- 40% of pts are asymptomatic, and dx is based solely on an abnl blood count. Common complaints at the time of dx are weakness and discomfort secondary to an enlarged spleen (abd discomfort or pain). Splenomegaly is present in up to 40% of pts at time of dx.

Labs
- WBC count (generally >100,000/mm^3) w/broad spectrum of granulocytic forms, ↓ Hgb/Hct, ↑ Plt
- Bone marrow: hypercellularity w/granulocytic hyperplasia, ratio of myeloid cells to erythroid cells, and number of megakaryocytes. Blasts and promyelocytes constitute <10% of all cells.
- ↑↑ LAP (can distinguish CML from other myeloproliferative disorders)

Treatment
- BCR-ABL inhibitors: imatinib. Nilotinib or dasatinib can be used in pts resistant to or intolerant of imatinib.
- Allogeneic HSCT in pts resistant to BCR-ABL inhibitors

4 PRIMARY MYELOFIBROSIS

This clonal hematopoietic stem cell disorder is characterized by abnl myeloid and megakaryocyte production.

Epidemiology and Presentation
- Fatigue, night sweats, wt loss, abd pain, early satiety, gout, bone pain, pulmonary HTN
- Hepatomegaly
- Extramedullary hematopoiesis (vertebrae, lymph nodes)

Diagnosis
- +*JAK2* mutation (50% pts)
- ↑ LDH, uric acid, alk phos
- Peripheral smear: leukoerythroblastic (L-shifted granulopoiesis, nucleated teardrop RBCs)

Treatment
- If sx anemia: Transfuse.
- Ruxolitinib (JAK inhibitor) Rx in high-risk pts
- Androgen Rx (danazol) for anemia (30% response)
- Hydroxyurea may help constitutional sx (hepatosplenomegaly, thrombocytosis).
- Splenectomy in refractory cases

5 ACUTE MYELOID LEUKEMIA (AML)

This malignant disease is characterized by uncontrolled proliferation of primitive myeloid cells (blasts).

Diagnosis

H&P

- Pts come to medical attention because of the effects of the cytopenias:
  - Anemia: weakness, fatigue
  - Thrombocytopenia: bleeding, petechiae, ecchymosis
  - Neutropenia: infections, fever
  - Hyperleukocytosis: leukostasis with ocular and cerebrovascular dysfunction or bleeding
- PE: skin pallor, bruises, petechiae, hepatosplenomegaly, peripheral lymphadenopathy

Labs

- CBC: anemia, thrombocytopenia. Peripheral WBC count varies from <5000 to >100,000/mm^3.
- Dx requires >20% blast cells in blood or bone marrow.
- Flow cytometry and (+) myeloperoxidase stains distinguish AML from ALL.

Treatment

- Induction chemo: cytarabine + daunorubicin
- Consolidation Rx: high-dose cytarabine in younger pts with favorable risk, intermediate-dose cytarabine in older pts; allogeneic HSCT in pts with high-risk disease
- Sx hyperleukocytosis: leukapheresis, hydroxyurea

Clinical Pearl

- **Acute promyelocytic leukemia (APL)** is a variant of AML (+ 15;17 gene translocation). APL is associated with DIC. Rx by adding all *trans*-retinoic acid (ATRA) to standard chemo = >75% cure. ATRA Rx may result in differentiation syndrome (fever, +/- pulmonary infiltrate, dyspnea hypotension, edema) which is treated with dexamethasone

6 ACUTE LYMPHOBLASTIC LEUKEMIA (ALL)

- Malignancy of B or T lymphoblasts

Diagnosis

H&P

- Skin pallor, purpura, or easy bruising
- Lymphadenopathy or hepatosplenomegaly
- Fever, bone pain, oliguria, weakness, weight loss, change in MS, headaches, cranial nerve palsy

Labs

- CBC: normochromic, normocytic anemia; thrombocytopenia
- Peripheral smear: lymphoblasts
- Dx requires >25% blast cells in bone marrow.
- Flow cytometry and (–) myeloperoxidase stains distinguish ALL from AML.

Treatment

- Intrathecal chemoprophylaxis w/w/o cranial irradiation (because of ↑ risk CNS involvement)
- Prevention of urate nephropathy by vigorous hydration, rasburicase
- Induction Rx: anthracycline, vincristine, L-asparaginase + corticosteroid
- Maintenance chemoRx with multiple agents for 2 to 3 yr to maintain a state of remission
- Allogeneic HSCT in first remission in pts with high-risk disease
- Prognosis is generally poorer in adult disease compared w/childhood disease (30%-40% adult cure rate vs. 80% cure rate in children).

E. MULTIPLE MYELOMA AND RELATED DISORDERS

1 MULTIPLE MYELOMA (MM)

This malignant neoplasm of plasma cells is characterized by overproduction of intact monoclonal immunoglobulin or free monoclonal κ or λ chains.

Diagnosis

- Diagnostic criteria:
  - Presence of >10% plasma cells in bone marrow (or bx of a tissue w/monoclonal plasma cells)

- Monoclonal protein in serum or urine
- Evidence of end-organ damage (**C**a elevation, **R**enal insufficiency, **A**nemia, or **B**one lesions [CRAB])
  - "***Asymptomatic myeloma***": M protein ≥3 g/dL or ≥10% plasma cells on bone marrow but absence of myeloma-related end-organ damage
  - "***Nonsecretory myeloma***": MM w/o detectable monoclonal protein
  - Staging (International Staging System)
    - Stage I: serum β$_2$-microglobulin <3.5 mg/L, serum albumin ≥3.5 g/dL
    - II: not stage I or III
    - III: serum β$_2$-microglobulin >5.5 mg/L

H&P
- Bone pain (58%) (back, thorax) or pathologic Fxs (30%) resulting from osteolytic lesions
- Fatigue (32%) or weakness from anemia secondary to bone marrow infiltration w/ plasma cells
- Recurrent infections from impaired neutrophil function and deficiency of nl immunoglobulins
- N/V related to constipation and uremia
- Delirium resulting from hypercalcemia
- Neurologic complications: spinal cord or nerve root compression, blurred vision from hyperviscosity
- Purpura, epistaxis: from thrombocytopenia
- Peripheral neuropathy: uncommon, seen with coexisting AL amyloidosis (***POEMS syndrome*** [Polyneuropathy, organomegaly, Endocrinopathy, Monoclonal protein, Skin changes])

Labs
- Normochromic, normocytic anemia; ***rouleaux formation*** on peripheral smear
- Hypercalcemia (15% of pts at dx)
- ↑ BUN, Cr, uric acid, and total protein
- Proteinuria secondary to overproduction and secretion of free monoclonal κ or λ chains (***Bence Jones protein***).
- Tall homogeneous monoclonal spike (M spike) on protein IEP (75% of pts). ↑ immunoglobulins are generally IgG (75%) or IgA (15%).
- <20% of pts have flat level of immunoglobulins but light chains in the urine by electrophoresis.
- <3% of pts have nonsecreting myeloma (no ↑ in immunoglobulins and no light chains in the urine) but have other evidence of the disease (e.g., bone marrow exam).
- ↓ AG from the + charge of the M proteins and the frequent presence of hyponatremia in pts w/myeloma
- Hyponatremia, serum hyperviscosity

Imaging
- X-ray films of painful areas: punched-out lytic lesions
- MRI: for suspected spinal compression or soft tissue plasmacytomas
- Bone scans not useful because lesions are not blastic

Treatment
- Treatment strategy is mainly related to age and comorbidities.
- Initiation of induction Rx with thalidomide, lenalidomide, or bortezomib plus HSCT is indicated for pts <65 yr old who do not have substantial heart, lung, renal, or liver dysfunction.
- Autologous stem-cell transplantation with a reduced-intensity conditioning regimen should be considered in older pts or those with coexisting conditions.
- Rx of pts who are not candidates for HSCT (because of age or comorbidities) is with melphalan + prednisone + thalidomide or bortezomib.
- Prompt dx and Rx of infections. Common bacterial agents are *Streptococcus pneumoniae* and *Haemophilus influenzae*. Prophylaxis against *Pneumocystis* w/ TMP-SMZ is indicated in pts receiving chemoRx and high-dose corticosteroid regimens.
- Vaccinate against *S. pneumoniae*, influenza, and *H. influenzae*.
- Rx hypercalcemia w/IV fluids, corticosteroids, bisphosphonates (pamidronate, zoledronate).
- Pain management w/analgesics. RT for painful bone lesions or spinal cord compression. Surgical stabilization of pathologic Fx. Consider vertebroplasty or kyphoplasty for selected vertebral lesions.
- ESAs are given for severe anemia.

Diagnostic Criteria
- Serum M protein concentration <3 g/dL
- <10% plasma cells in the bone marrow
- Absence of anemia/renal insufficiency/hypercalcemia/bone lesions

Treatment
- Rx not indicated. Risk of progression of MGUS to MM is 1%/yr and is related to the level of M protein values and to the type of protein (↑ risk w/higher M protein values and in pts w/IgM and IgA M proteins).
- Monitor serum M protein. If serum M protein is >2 g/dL, repeat electrophoresis every 6 mo.

3 WALDENSTROM'S MACROGLOBULINEMIA

This plasma cell dyscrasia is characterized by production of monoclonal IgM Ab.

Diagnosis

H&P
- Weakness, fatigue, weight loss, fever, night sweats
- Mucosal bleeding, bruising
- Headache, dizziness, vertigo, deafness, and seizures (***hyperviscosity syndrome***)
- Fever, night sweats
- Exam: ecchymoses, purpura, hepatomegaly, splenomegaly, lymphadenopathy, symmetric peripheral neuropathy

Diagnostic Criteria
- Presence of lymphoplasmacytic lymphoma ≥10% of bone marrow cellularity + presence of an IgM M protein

Labs
- CBC w/diff: anemia; WBC count usually nl. Thrombocytopenia may occur.
- Peripheral smear may reveal "stacked coin" rouleaux formations.
- SPEP: homogeneous M spike (monoclonal gammopathy). IEP confirms IgM responsible for the M spike.
- Urine IEP: Monoclonal light chains are usually κ chains.
- Serum viscosity: Sx usually occur when the serum viscosity is 4× nl; this is a classic feature, although present in only 15% of cases.

Treatment
- Plasmapheresis if sx of hyperviscosity
- Rx rituximab ± nucleoside analogues (fludarabine, cladribine) or alkylating agent (chlorambucil, cyclophosphamide)

4 AL AMYLOIDOSIS

Primary amyloidosis (AL) is associated with an underlying clonal plasma cell disorder making an abnormal light chain protein with deposition in multiple organ systems.

Diagnosis
- Histologic confirmation is necessary with a fat pad and bone marrow bx with Congo red staining to establish a diagnosis.
- If a noninvasive fat pad bx does not establish a diagnosis, then bx of the affected organ may be needed.

H&P
- Findings depend on organ system involvement: edema, fatigue, dyspnea, abd pain, dizziness, bleeding.
- Macroglossia, periorbital ecchymoses (raccoon eyes), peripheral neuropathy, tendinopathy

Treatment
- Melphalan and prednisone

F. LYMPHOID MALIGNANCIES

1 NON-HODGKIN'S LYMPHOMA

This comprises a heterogeneous group of malignant neoplasms of the lymphoreticular system.

Diagnosis

H&P
- Asymptomatic lymphadenopathy
- Pruritus, fever, night sweats, wt loss less common than in Hodgkin's disease

- Hepatomegaly and splenomegaly
- One third of NHL originates extranodally. Involvement of extranodal sites can result in unusual presentations (e.g., GI tract involvement can simulate PUD).
- NHL cases associated w/HIV infection occur predominantly in the brain.

Labs
- Labs: CBC, ESR, U/A, LDH, BUN, Cr, serum Ca, uric acid, LFTs, SPEP, HIV, Hep C and Hep B screen. β_2-microglobulin levels should be obtained initially (prognostic value) and serially in pts w/low-grade lymphomas (useful to monitor therapeutic response of the tumor).
- Bone marrow (aspirate and full bone core bx)

Imaging
- CXR (PA and lateral)
- CT scan of abd and pelvis; CT scan of chest if CXR abnl
- PET scan
- Bone scan (particularly in pts w/histiocytic lymphoma)
- Classification and staging
- The WHO classification is described in Table 7-3. NHLs are also subdivided in 3 major groups: low grade (indolent), intermediate (aggressive), and high grade (highly aggressive).
- Staging: The Ann Arbor classification is used to stage NHLs (Table 7-4). Histopathology has greater therapeutic implications in NHL than in Hodgkin's disease.

TABLE 7-3 ■ WHO Classification of Non-Hodgkin's Lymphoma

B-Cell Lymphomas	
Precursor B-cell lymphoma	Precursor B lymphoblastic lymphoma/leukemia
Mature B-cell lymphoma	Chronic lymphocytic leukemia/small lymphocytic lymphoma
	Lymphoplasmacytic lymphoma
	Splenic marginal zone lymphoma
	Extranodal marginal zone B-cell lymphoma of mucosa-associated lymphoid tissue (MALT lymphoma)
	Nodal marginal zone B-cell lymphoma
	Follicular lymphoma
	Mantle cell lymphoma
	Diffuse large B-cell lymphoma
	Mediastinal (thymic) large B-cell lymphoma
	Intravascular large B-cell lymphoma
	Primary effusion lymphoma
	Burkitt's lymphoma/leukemia
T/NK-Cell Lymphomas	
Precursor T-cell lymphoma	Precursor T-cell lymphoblastic leukemia/lymphoma
	Blastic NK-cell lymphoma
Mature T/NK-cell lymphoma	Adult T-cell leukemia/lymphoma
	Extranodal NK/T-cell lymphoma, nasal type
	Enteropathy-type T-cell lymphoma
	Hepatosplenic T-cell lymphoma
	Subcutaneous panniculitis-like T-cell lymphoma
	Mycosis fungoides
	Sézary's syndrome
	Primary cutaneous anaplastic large-cell lymphoma
	Peripheral T-cell lymphoma, unspecified
	Angioimmunoblastic T-cell lymphoma
	Anaplastic large-cell lymphoma

Adapted from Jaffe ES, Harris NL, Stein H, Vardiman JW (eds): World Health Organization Classification of Tumors: Pathology and Genetics. Tumors of Hematopoietic and Lymphoid Tissues. Lyons, France, IARC Press, 2001.

Treatment and Prognosis
- Table 7-5 describes combination chemoRx regimens for NHL. Prognostic indicators are described in Table 7-6.

2 CHRONIC LYMPHOCYTIC LEUKEMIA (CLL)

Definition
- Lymphoproliferative disorder characterized by proliferation and accumulation of mature-appearing neoplastic lymphocytes

TABLE 7-4 ■ Ann Arbor Staging System for Lymphomas

Stage*	Cotswold Modification of Ann Arbor Classification
I	Involvement of a single lymph node region or lymphoid structure
II	Involvement of two or more lymph node regions on the same side of the diaphragm (the mediastinum is considered a single site, whereas the hilar lymph nodes are considered bilaterally); the number of anatomic sites should be indicated by a subscript (e.g., II_3)
III	Involvement of lymph node regions on both sides of the diaphragm: III_1 (with or without involvement of splenic hilar, celiac, or portal nodes) and III_2 (with involvement of para-aortic, iliac, and mesenteric nodes)
IV	Involvement of one or more extranodal sites in addition to a site for which the designation E has been used

*All cases are subclassified to indicate the absence (A) or presence (B) of the systemic symptoms of significant fever (>38.0° C [100.4° F]), night sweats, and unexplained weight loss exceeding 10% of normal body weight within the previous 6 mo. The clinical stage (CS) denotes the stage as determined by all diagnostic examinations and a single diagnostic bx only. In the Ann Arbor classification, the term pathologic stage (PS) is used if a second bx of any kind has been obtained, whether negative or positive. In the Cotswold modification, the PS is determined by laparotomy; X designates bulky disease (widening of the mediastinum by more than one third or the presence of a nodal mass >10 cm), and E designates involvement of a single extranodal site that is contiguous or proximal to the known nodal site.
From Hoffman R, Benz EJ, Shattil SJ, et al (eds): Hematology: Basic Principles and Practice, 5th ed. New York, Churchill Livingstone, 2009.

TABLE 7-5 ■ Combination Chemotherapy Regimens for Non-Hodgkin's Lymphoma

Regimen	Dose	Days of Administration	Frequency
CHOP-R			Every 21 days
Cyclophosphamide	750 mg/m² IV	1	
Doxorubicin	50 mg/m² IV	1	
Vincristine	1.4 mg/m² IV*	1	
Prednisone, fixed dose	100 mg PO	1-5	
Rituximab	375 mg/m² IV	1	
CVP-R			Every 21 days
Cyclophosphamide	1,000 mg/m² IV	1	
Vincristine	1.4 mg/m² IV*	1	
Prednisone, fixed dose	100 mg PO	1-5	
Rituximab	375 mg/m² IV	1	
FCR			Every 28 days
Fludarabine	25 mg/m² IV	1-3	
Cyclophosphamide	250 mg/m² IV	1-3	
Rituximab	375 mg/m²	1	

*Vincristine dose often capped at 2 mg total.
From Goldman L, Schafer AI (eds): Goldman's Cecil Medicine, 24th ed. Philadelphia, Saunders, 2012.

TABLE 7-6 ■ International Prognostic Index for Aggressive Lymphomas*

Risk Group	IPI Score	CR Rate (%)	5-Yr Overall Survival (%)
Low	0, 1	87	73
Low intermediate	2	67	51
High intermediate	3	55	43
High	4, 5	44	26

*One point is given for the presence of each of the following characteristics: age >60 yr, elevated serum LDH level, ECOG performance status ≥2, Ann Arbor stage III or IV, and >2 extranodal sites.
CR, Complete response; ECOG, Eastern Cooperative Oncology Group; IPI, International Prognostic Index.
From Hoffman R, Benz EJ, Shattil SJ, et al (eds): Hematology: Basic Principles and Practice, 5th ed. New York, Churchill Livingstone, 2009.

Diagnosis

H&P
- Clinical presentation varies according to stage of the disease. Some pts come to medical attention because of weakness and fatigue (secondary to anemia) or lymphadenopathy. Many cases are diagnosed on the basis of lab results obtained after routine PE.

Labs
- Proliferative lymphocytosis (>15,000/dL) of well-differentiated lymphocytes is the hallmark of CLL.
- There is monotonous replacement of the bone marrow by small lymphocytes (marrow contains >30% of well-differentiated lymphocytes).

Staging (Table 7-7)

- The pt's prognosis is related to the clinical stage (e.g., the average survival in pts in Rai stage 0 is >120 mo; whereas for Rai stage 4 it is approx 30 mo) and several other adverse factors such as high serum β_2-microglobulin levels (>3.5 mg/L),+ ZAP 70, cytogenetic studies unmutated heavy gene), lymphocyte doubling time (<12 mo), and mutational gene assessment (presence del [17p13][p53]). Overall 5-yr survival is 60%.

TABLE 7-7 ■ Rai Staging Systems in Chronic Lymphocytic Leukemia				
Lymphocytosis	Lymphadenopathy	Hepatomegaly or Splenomegaly	Hemoglobin (g/dL)	Platelets × $10^3/\mu L$
Rai Stage				
0	+	–	–	≥11	≥100
I	+	+	–	≥11	≥100
II	+	±	+	≥11	≥100
III	+	±	±	<11	≥100
IV	+	±	±	Any	<100

From Goldman L, Bennett JC (eds): Cecil Textbook of Medicine, 21st ed. Philadelphia, Saunders, 2000.

Treatment

- Rai stage 0: observation
- Symptomatic pts in Rai stages I and II: fludarabine; local irradiation for isolated symptomatic lymphadenopathy and lymph nodes that interfere w/vital organs
- Rai stages III and IV: rituximab + combination chemo

3 HAIRY CELL LEUKEMIA

Definition

- Lymphoid neoplasm characterized by the proliferation of mature B cells w/ prominent cytoplasmic projections (hairs)

Diagnosis

H&P

- PE: splenomegaly (>90% of cases) secondary to tumor cell infiltration

Labs

- CBC: pancytopenia involving erythrocytes, neutrophils, and Plts
- Peripheral smear: hairy cells (5%-80% of cells in the peripheral blood). The cytoplasmic projections on the cells are redundant plasma membranes.
- Leukemic cells stain + for tartrate-resistant acid phosphatase (TRAP)
- Bone marrow may result in a "dry tap" (because of marrow reticulin).

Treatment

- Cladribine

4 HODGKIN'S LYMPHOMA

This malignant disorder of lymphoreticular origin is characterized histologically by the presence of multinucleated giant cells (**Reed-Sternberg cells**) usually originating from B lymphocytes in germinal centers of lymphoid tissue.

Diagnosis

H&P

- Palpable lymphadenopathy, generally painless, is the most common presenting sx.
- The most common site of involvement is the neck region.
- Fever and night sweats: Fever in a cyclical pattern (days or weeks of fever alternating w/afebrile periods) is known as **Pel-Epstein fever.**
- Wt loss, generalized malaise
- Persistent, nonproductive cough
- Pruritus

Labs

- Dx is confirmed w/lymph node bx.

Staging and Prognostic Risk Factors

- Detailed H&P (w/documentation of "B sx")
- Surgical bx
- Labs (CBC, ESR, BUN, Cr, alk phos, LFTs, alb, LDH, uric acid)
- CT scan of chest, abd, pelvis, neck
- 18-FDG PET scan
- Staging for Hodgkin's disease follows the Ann Arbor staging classification (see Table 7-4).

- Prognostic risk factors are male sex, age >45 yr, leukocyte count >15,000/μL, serum albumin <4 g/dL, Hgb <10.5 g/dL.

Treatment
- Rx is determined by disease stage and not histology (same Rx for all cell types).
- Stage I and II: radiation Rx alone unless a large mediastinal mass is present (mediastinal-to-thoracic ratio ≥1.3); in the latter case, a combination of chemoRx (doxorubicin + bleomycin + vincristine + dacarbazine [ABVD]) and RT may be used.
- Stage IB or IIB: RT is often used, although ABVD chemo is performed in many centers.
- Stage IIIA: Rx is controversial. It varies w/the anatomic substage after splenectomy.
- III₁A and minimum splenic involvement: RT alone may be adequate.
- III₂ or III₁A w/extensive splenic involvement: There is disagreement whether ABVD chemo alone or a combination of chemo and RT is the preferred Rx modality.
- IIIB and IVB: chemoRx w/ or w/o adjuvant RT
- BEACOPP, an intensified regimen consisting of bleomycin, etoposide, doxorubicin, cyclophosphamide, vincristine, procarbazine, and prednisone, has been advocated by some as the new standard for treatment of advanced Hodgkin's lymphoma in place of ABVD, but the long-term clinical outcome did not differ significantly between the two regimens. In addition, with the use of the escalated BEACOPP regimen, the rate of complications is higher (3% treatment-related death, 20% rate of hospitalization, and 3% rate of secondary leukemia). Thus, if the goal is cure with the least overall toxic effects, it is best to favor ABVD Rx, reserving rescue Rx with high-dose chemoRx and autologous HSCT for pts in whom the primary treatment fails.
- Monoclonal Ab Rx: SGN-30 and MDX-060 and rituximab have shown promising results.

G. BLEEDING DISORDERS

1 EVALUATION OF SUSPECTED BLEEDING DISORDER
See Figure 7-4.

2 HEMOPHILIA
This hereditary bleeding disorder is caused by low factor VIII coagulant activity (hemophilia A) or low levels of factor IX coagulant activity (hemophilia B). Spontaneous acquisition of factor VIII inhibitors (acquired hemophilia) is rare.

Diagnosis
- ↑ PTT
- ↓ Factor VIII: C level distinguishes hemophilia A from other causes of ↑ PTT.
- Nl factor VIII antigen, PT, fibrinogen level, and bleeding time
- ↓ Factor IX coagulant activity levels in pts w/hemophilia B
- Coagulation factor activity measurement is useful to correlate w/disease severity: The nl range is 50 to 150 U/dL; 5 to 20 U/dL indicates mild disease, 2 to 5 U/dL indicates moderate disease, and <2 U/dL indicates severe disease w/spontaneous bleeding episodes.

Treatment
Hemophilia A
- Plasma derived and recombinant factor VIII concentrates are effective in controlling spontaneous and traumatic hemorrhage in severe hemophilia. Recombinant factor VIII is w/o added human serum alb (↑ risk of transmission of infectious agents).
- Desmopressin (causes release of factor VIII:C) may be used in preparation for minor surgical procedures in pts w/mild hemophilia.
- Aminocaproic acid is used for persistent bleeding that is unresponsive to factor VIII concentrate or desmopressin.
Hemophilia B
- Factor IX concentrates

3 VON WILLEBRAND'S DISEASE (vWD)
This most common autosomal bleeding disorder (mild form: codominant, severe form: recessive) results from deficiency of vWF (type I, 85% of cases) or qualitative protein abnormality (type II, 15% cases). Type III is a rare autosomal recessive (severe deficiency of vWF) disorder.

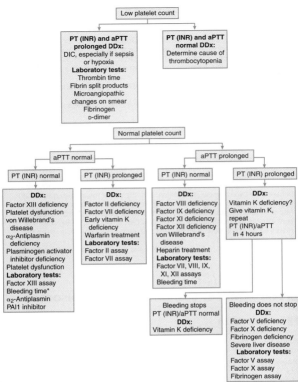

FIGURE 7-4. Differential diagnosis of bleeding disorders. *In many labs, "bleeding time" is no longer available and has been replaced with PFA-100. *(From Cluster JW, Rau, RE: The Harriet Lane Handbook, 18th ed. St. Louis, Mosby, 2009.)*

Diagnosis

H&P

- Hx mucocutaneous bleeding
- Women (menorrhagia, postpartum hemorrhage)

Labs

- ↑ Bleeding time, PFA-100 assay
- ↓ **vWF Ag <30 IU/dL** ("low" vWF 30-50 IU/dL), ↓ vWF activity (measured by ristocetin cofactor assay)
- ↓ Factor VIII:C
- vWF Type II A (absent ristocetin cofactor)
- vWF Type II B (↑ ristocetin agglutination)

Treatment

- Type 1 (mild) vWD: DDAVP
- Types 2, 3 vWD: infusion vWF-containing factor VIII concentrate

4 COAGULOPATHY OF LIVER DISEASE

- Liver disease = ↑ PT, APTT (TCT may also ↑) → coagulopathy, hypofibrinogenemia, dysfibrinogenemia, thrombocytopenia
- Splenomegaly → thrombocytopenia (may be refractory to transfusion)

214

- D-dimer clearance impaired, ↑ Plt consumption (analogous to DIC)
- ↑ INR but pt not autocoagulated and has ↑ risk of DVT
- **Rx:** FFP + vitamin K (correct coagulopathy)

5 DISSEMINATED INTRAVASCULAR COAGULATION (DIC)

This acquired thromboembolic disorder is characterized by generalized activation of the clotting mechanism → microangiopathic hemolysis and intravascular formation of fibrin → thrombotic occlusion of small and midsize vessels.

Etiology
- Infections (e.g., gram(−) sepsis, RMSF, malaria, viral or fungal infection)
- Obstetric complications (e.g., dead fetus, amniotic fluid embolism, toxemia, abruptio placentae, septic abortion, eclampsia)
- Tissue trauma (e.g., burns, hypothermia-rewarming)
- Neoplasms (e.g., adenocarcinomas [GI, prostate, lung, breast], acute promyelocytic leukemia)
- Quinine, cocaine-induced rhabdo
- Liver failure
- Acute pancreatitis
- Transfusion reactions
- Respiratory distress syndrome
- Other: SLE, vasculitis, aneurysms, polyarteritis, cavernous hemangiomas

Diagnosis
- Peripheral blood smear generally shows RBC fragments (schistocytes) and ↓ Plt count.
- Coagulation factors are consumed at a rate in excess of the capacity of the liver to synthesize them, and Plts are consumed in excess of the capacity of the bone marrow megakaryocytes to release them.
- Diagnostic characteristics of DIC are ↑ PT, PTT, TT, fibrin split products, D-dimer; ↓ fibrinogen level, thrombocytopenia.
- Coagulopathy secondary to DIC must be differentiated from that secondary to liver disease or vitamin K deficiency.
- Vitamin K deficiency: ↑ PT and nl PTT, TT, Plt count, and fibrinogen level; PTT may be ↑ in severe cases.
- Liver disease: ↑ PT and PTT; TT and fibrinogen are usually nl unless severe disease is present; Plts are usually nl unless splenomegaly is present.
- Factors V and VIII are ↓ in DIC, but they are nl in liver disease w/coagulopathy.

Treatment
- Correct and eliminate underlying cause (e.g., antimicrobial Rx for infection).
- Replacement Rx w/FFP and Plt in pts w/significant hemorrhage:
  - FFP 10 to 15 mL/kg can be given w/goal of normalizing INR.
  - Plt transfusions are given when Plt count is <10,000 (or higher if major bleeding is present).
- Cryoprecipitate 1 U/5 kg is reserved for hypofibrinogen states.
- Antithrombin III Rx may be considered as a supportive therapeutic option in pts w/ severe DIC. Its modest results and substantial cost are limiting factors.
- Heparin Rx at a dose lower than that used in venous thrombosis (300-500 U/hr) may be useful in selected cases to neutralize thrombin (e.g., DIC associated w/acute promyelocytic leukemia, purpura fulminans, acral ischemia).

6 VITAMIN K DEFICIENCY

Vitamin K is required for generation of active factors II, VII, IX, and X.

Etiology
- Malabsorption syndromes, liver disease, poor dietary intake, and hereditary combined deficiencies of the vitamin K–dependent proteins, including prothrombin, factor VII, factor IX, and factor X

Lab
- ↑ PT (INR) that corrects after a 1:1 mix w/nl pooled plasma

Treatment
- Mild deficiency: PO vitamin K_1 100 to 150 mg qd. INR begins to normalize after 12 hr and should normalize completely in 48 hr. Vitamin K can also be given SC (poorly absorbed in edematous pts) and IV (risk of anaphylaxis).
- Severe deficiency and active bleeding or requiring invasive procedures: The administration of vitamin K should be preceded by the infusion of FFP.

H. PLATELET DISORDERS

1 IMMUNE (IDIOPATHIC) THROMBOCYTOPENIC PURPURA (ITP)

In this autoimmune disorder, Ab-coated or immune complex–coated Plts are destroyed prematurely by the reticuloendothelial system, resulting in peripheral thrombocytopenia.

Etiology
- Drugs commonly implicated: quinidine, heparin, abx (linezolid, vancomycin, sulfonamides, rifampin), Plt inhibitors (tirofiban, abciximab, eptifibatide), cimetidine, NSAIDs, thiazide diuretics, antirheumatic agents (gold salts, penicillamine), acetaminophen, and chemotherapeutic agents (cyclosporine, fludarabine, oxaliplatin)

Diagnosis
H&P
- Children: generally present w/sudden onset of bruising and petechiae from severe thrombocytopenia
- Adults: insidious presentation; dx often made on incidental routine labs
- Petechiae, purpura, epistaxis, or heme(+) stool from GI bleeding in pts w/severe thrombocytopenia

Labs
- CBC, Plt count, and peripheral smear: Plts are ↓ but nl or larger in size.
- Direct assay for Plt-bound Ab (+ predictive value 80%-83%)
- Additional labs: HIV, ANA, TSH, LFTs, bone marrow exam

Imaging
- CT of abd in pts w/splenomegaly (r/o lymphoma)

Treatment
- Asymptomatic pts w/Plts >30,000/mm³: observation
- Pts w/neurologic sx, internal bleeding, or those undergoing emergency surgery: methylprednisolone 30 mg/kg/day IV plus IVIG (1 g/kg/day for 2-3 days) and infusion of Plts
- Adults w/Plts <20,000/mm³ and those who have counts <50,000/mm³ and significant mucous membrane bleeding: prednisone 1 to 2 mg/kg qd, continued until the Plt count is normalized, then slowly tapered off
- Adults w/severe thrombocytopenia or bleeding: high-dose Ig (IgG 0.4 g/kg/day IV, infused on 3-5 consecutive days) or high-dose parenteral glucocorticoids (methylprednisolone 30 mg/kg/day)
- Rituximab: useful in ITP resistant to conventional Rx
- Splenectomy: Consider in adults w/Plts <30,000/mm³ after 6 wk of medical Rx or after 6 mo if >20 mg of prednisone/day is required to maintain Plts >30,000/mm³.
- Plt transfusion: only in case of life-threatening hemorrhage
- Eltrombopag and romiplostim: Rx of chronic ITP refractory to corticosteroids, immunoglobulins, or splenectomy

2 HEPARIN-INDUCED THROMBOCYTOPENIA (HIT)

Immunologic drug reaction caused by Plt-activating IgG Abs that recognize complexes of Plt factor 4 (PF4) and heparin. It is associated w/venous or arterial thrombosis.

Diagnosis and Treatment
- HIT usually develops within 5 to 10 days after heparin exposure. It may develop earlier (within 2 days) in pts w/previous exposure. It may also occur up to 3 wk after exposure to heparin secondary to high titers of Plt-activating IgG induced by heparin (delayed-onset HIT). Risk of HIT > with UFH than LMWH.
- This dx should be differentiated from early, benign, transient thrombocytopenia that can occur w/heparin Rx. Factors favoring immune thrombocytopenia are as follows:
  - ↓ in Plt count to <100,000/mm³ or >50% of baseline value
  - The falling Plt count generally occurs after 5 days of heparin Rx or earlier if the pt had recent exposure to heparin.
  - Screening can be performed w/ELISA HIT test, which detects the presence of all Ig classes (IgA, IgG, IgM) w/specificity for antigens present on a complex of PF4/heparin. The dx can be confirmed w/ELISA IgG-HIT test, which is more specific for type II HIT. The "4T score" in Table 7-8 can be used to determine probability of HIT and the treatment approach.

TABLE 7-8 ■ A Diagnostic and Treatment Approach to Heparin-Induced Thrombocytopenia

Suspicion of HIT Based upon the "4 Ts"	Score	Pretest Probability Score Criteria		
		2	1	0
Thrombocytopenia	☐	Nadir 20-100, or >50% platelet fall	Nadir 10-19, or 30%-50% platelet fall	Nadir <10, or <30% platelet fall
Timing of onset of platelet fall	☐	Day 5-10, or ≤ day 1 with recent heparin*	> Day 10 or timing unclear (but fits with HIT)	≤ Day 1 (no recent heparin)
Thrombosis or other sequelae	☐	Proven thrombosis, skin necrosis, or ASR†	Progressive, recurrent, or silent thrombosis; erythematous skin lesions	None
O**T**her cause of platelet fall	☐	None evident	Possible	Definite
Total Pretest Probability Score	☐	Periodic reassessment as new information can change pretest probability (e.g., positive blood cultures)		

Total Pretest Probability Score		
High	Moderate	Low
8 | 7 | 6	5 |4	3 | 2 | 1 | 0
Stop heparin‡, give alternative non-heparin anticoagulant argatroban¶ or lepirudin# or danaparoid** (or bivalirudin†† or fondaparinux‡‡)	Physician judgment	Continue (LMW) heparin

Positive test for HIT antibodies: continue nonheparin anticoagulant until platelet count recovery	← HIT test →	Negative test for HIT antibodies: consider continuing or switching back to (LMW) heparin##
Thrombosis*** If HIT, continue nonheparin anticoagulant until platelet count recovery, then **cautious coumarin overlap**¶¶	← Imaging studies for lower limb DVT††† →	No thrombosis If HIT, consider anticoagulating until platelet count recovery, even if no thrombosis apparent (± coumarin¶¶)

*Recent heparin indicates exposure within the past 30 days (2 points) or past 30-100 days (1 point).

†ASR, acute systemic reaction following IV heparin bolus (see Table 7-4).

‡Stop all heparin, including catheter "flushes" and possibly heparin-coated catheters.

¶Argatroban: approved (U.S., Canada) for isolated HIT and HIT complicated by thrombosis (2 µg/kg/min IV, adjusted to 1.5-3.0x patient's baseline APTT or the mean of the laboratory normal range); reduce dose for hepatobiliary compromise: may increase INR more than the other direct thrombin inhibitors, thus requiring care in managing coumarin overlap (see footnote ¶¶).

#Lepirudin: approved (United States, Canada, European Union, elsewhere) for treatment of thrombosis complicating HIT (±0.4 mg/kg IV bolus, then 0.15 mg/kg/hr adjusted to 1.5-2.5x patient's baseline APTT or mean of the laboratory normal range); used (off-label) also to treat isolated HIT (0.1 mg/kg/hr, adjusted by APTT); to avoid overdosing and anaphylaxis, it may be preferable to omit the bolus, and begin as IV infusion except when facing life- or limb-threatening thrombosis); reduce dose for renal insufficiency.

**Danaparoid: usual IV bolus, 2250 U (body weight 60-75 kg) followed by infusion (400 U/hr for 4 hr, then 300 U/hr for 4 hr, then 200 U/hr, adjusted by anti-factor Xa levels); this therapeutic-dose regimen is appropriate both for isolated HIT and for HIT complicated by thrombosis (although the dose is higher than approved in some jurisdictions); withdrawn from U.S. market (2002).

††Bivalirudin: no HIT dosing, IV infusion 0.15 mg/kg/hr adjusted by APTT; limited experience (off-label).

‡‡Fondaparinux: dosing for HIT not established; limited experience (off-label).

¶¶Delay coumarin pending substantial platelet count recovery (at least >100, preferably >150); begin coumarin in low doses, with at least 4-5 day overlap, stopping alternative anticoagulant when INR therapeutic for 2 days and platelets recovered.

##Depending on physician confidence in the laboratory's ability to rule out HIT antibodies (usually, negative PF4-dependent enzyme immunoassay and/or washed platelet activation assay performed by an experienced laboratory).

***Some thrombi may require special treatment (e.g., thrombectomy for large limb artery thrombosis).

†††Routine ultrasound of lower limb veins recommended because many pts w/HIT have subclinical DVT.

Adapted from Warkentin TE, Aird WC, Rand JH: Platelet-endothelial interactions: sepsis, HIT, and antiphospholipid syndrome. Hematology Am Soc Hematol Educ Program 497-519, 2003.

3 THROMBOTIC THROMBOCYTOPENIC PURPURA (TTP)

Rare disorder characterized by thrombocytopenia (often accompanied by purpura) and microangiopathic hemolytic anemia; neurologic impairment, renal dysfunction, and fever may also be present.

Etiology
- It is caused in some pts by an acquired deficiency of a circulating metalloproteinase and can also be caused in very rare cases by a hereditary deficiency of ADAMTS13.
- Many drugs, including clopidogrel, PCN, antineoplastic agents, OCPs, quinine, and ticlopidine, have been associated w/TTP.
- Other precipitating causes include infectious agents, pregnancy, malignant neoplasms, allogeneic bone marrow transplantation, and neurologic disorders.

Diagnosis
H&P
- Most pts present w/nonspecific constitutional sx (weakness, nausea, abd pain, vomiting).
- Purpura (secondary to thrombocytopenia), jaundice, pallor (secondary to hemolysis), mucosal bleeding, fever
- Fluctuating levels of consciousness (secondary to thrombotic occlusion of the cerebral vessels)
- Renal failure and neurologic events are usually end-stage features.

Labs
- Severe anemia and thrombocytopenia (Plt count <50,000 or >50% ↓ from previous count)
- ↑ BUN and Cr, ↑ reticulocyte count, indirect bili, LDH, ↓ haptoglobin
- U/A: hematuria (red cells and red cell casts in urine sediment), proteinuria
- Peripheral smear: severely fragmented RBCs (schistocytes); >4% RBC fragments in the peripheral blood
- No laboratory evidence of DIC (nl FDP, fibrinogen)
- The ADAMTS13 level is not necessary, and metalloproteinase deficiency need not be proved for dx of TTP.

Treatment
- Discontinue potential offending agents.
- Daily plasma exchange w/replacement of 1.0 to 1.5× the predicted plasma volume of the pt continued for ≥2 days after the Plt count returns to >150,000/cm^3.

4 HEMOLYTIC-UREMIC SYNDROME (HUS)

Definition
Syndrome characterized by nonimmune hemolytic anemia, thrombocytopenia, and severe renal failure secondary to endothelial damage by Shiga toxin–producing *Escherichia coli* serotype O157:H7 or *Shigella* species.

Diagnosis
H&P
- Usually preceded by bloody diarrhea (90% of cases)

Labs
- Anemia, thrombocytopenia, ↑ BUN, and creat
- Peripheral smear: schistocytes, burr cells, and helmet cells
- Stool cultures for *E. coli* O157:H7 + in >90% of cases

Treatment
- Plasma exchange or infusion started within 24 hr after dx
- Abx should be avoided

5 HELLP SYNDROME

This variant of preeclampsia is the most frequently encountered microangiopathy of pregnancy. HELLP is an acronym for **H**emolysis, **E**levated **L**iver enzymes, and **L**ow **P**latelet count. There are 3 classes:
- Class 1: Plt 50,000/mm^3
- Class 2: Plt >50,000 to 100,000/mm^3
- Class 3: Plt >100,000/mm^3

Diagnosis
H&P
- RUQ pain, edema

Labs
- Abnl peripheral smear w/schistocytes
- ↑ LFTs (ALT, AST), nl PT, PTT, low Plts

- Mg sulfate, BP control (hydralazine, labetalol)
- Pregnancies 34 wk or class 1 HELLP → delivery, either vaginal or abd, within 24 hr is the goal.
- Preterm fetus → corticosteroid Rx to enhance fetal lung maturation

I. THROMBOTIC DISORDERS

1 HYPERCOAGULABLE STATE

This inherited or acquired condition is associated w/risk of thrombosis.

Etiology (Table 7-9)

Inherited

- **Factor V Leiden (FVL) mutation**
  - Autosomal dominant mutation w/low penetrance
  - Causes activated protein C resistance (APCR); 90% of APCR is caused by FVL mutation
  - Most common genetic risk factor for venous thrombosis; accounts for thrombosis in 40%-50% of inherited cases
  - OCP use in heterozygous carriers is associated w/an 8-fold ↑ risk of thrombosis compared w/noncarriers and a 35-fold ↑ risk of thrombosis compared w/ noncarriers not using OCP.
  - Probably low risk of recurrent thrombotic events
  - May be associated w/CVD in select high-risk subgroups
- **Prothrombin G20210A mutation (PGM)**
  - Autosomal dominant mutation w/↓ penetrance
  - OCP use in heterozygous carriers is associated w/a 1 × 6↑ risk of thrombosis compared w/noncarriers not using OCP.
  - Probably low risk of recurrent thrombotic events
  - May be associated w/CVD in select high-risk subgroups and young pts w/ischemic strokes
- **Protein C, protein S, antithrombin deficiency**
  - Autosomal dominant inheritance; many mutations identified for each of these conditions
  - ↓ Level or abnl function
  - First episode of thrombosis usually in young adults
  - ↑ Risk of recurrent thrombosis
- **Protein C and protein S**
  - Lifetime risk of thromboembolic event up to 50%
  - Homozygous condition very rare, usually associated w/lethal thrombosis in infancy
  - Associated w/warfarin-induced skin necrosis, which occurs secondary to depletion of vitamin K–dependent anticoagulant factors sooner than procoagulant factors in the first few days of Rx
- **Antithrombin deficiency (ATD)**
  - Most thrombogenic of the identified inherited factors; lifetime risk of thromboembolic event up to 70%
  - Homozygous condition very rare, probably not compatible w/nl fetal development

TABLE 7-9 ■ Hypercoagulable Conditions				
	Prevalence in General Population (%)	Prevalence in Population with Thrombosis (%)	A/V Events	Relative Risk of Thrombosis
FVL mutation	5% of whites; rare in nonwhites	12%-40%	√	Heterozygous: 3-7 Homozygous: 80
Prothrombin G20210A mutation	3% of whites; rare in nonwhites	6%-18%	√	3
AT deficiency	0.02%	1%-3%	√	20-50
PC deficiency	0.2%-0.4%	3%-5%	√	7-15
PS deficiency	0.03%-0.1%	1%-5%	√	5-11
Antiphospholipid antibody syndrome	1%-2%	5%-21%	√ + A	2-11
Hyperhomocysteinemia	5%-7%	10%	√ + A	3
Elevated factor VIII level	11%	25%		5

A, Arterial; AT, antithrombin; FVL, factor V Leiden; PC, protein C; PS, protein; V, venous.
From Ferri F: Ferri's Clinical Advisor 2010. Philadelphia, Mosby, 2010.

- Rarely, arterial thrombosis can occur.
- Recurrent thrombotic events reported in up to 60% of pts
- Can cause heparin resistance

■ **↑ Factor VIII level**
- May be an important risk factor for thrombosis in African American populations
- Risk of recurrent thrombosis
- Genetic etiology suspected but not yet identified

■ **Other possible causes:** dysfibrinogenemias, thrombin activatable fibrinolysis inhibitor, plasminogen deficiency, factor IX and factor XI levels

Acquired

■ **APS**
- Most common cause of acquired thrombophilia
- Can manifest as arterial or venous thrombosis, recurrent pregnancy loss, and adverse pregnancy outcomes
- Thromboembolic events in up to 30% of pts; high risk of recurrent thrombosis (up to 70% reported)
- See the next section, "Antiphospholipid Syndrome," for more information.

■ **Hyperhomocysteinemia**
- Can be inherited (most commonly an autosomal recessive mutation in methylene tetrahydrofolate reductase gene) but more often secondary to poor dietary intake. Deficiency of folate, vitamin B_6, or vitamin B_{12} accounts for two thirds of cases.
- May be associated w/VTE, atherosclerotic disease (CV, cerebrovascular, and peripheral vascular), and possibly adverse pregnancy outcomes

■ **Conditions associated w/ risk of thrombosis**
- Prior thrombosis
- Trauma
- Chronic medical illness: CHF, DM, obesity, nephrotic syndrome, IBD, PNH, HUS/TTP, DIC, sickle cell anemia
- Pregnancy (6× risk of thrombosis compared w/nonpregnant women), post partum, OCP (3-5× risk of thrombosis w/use, risk w/third-generation OCP), HRT (2× risk of thrombosis w/use), tamoxifen, raloxifene
- Immobilization, travel
- Surgery (especially orthopedic), central venous catheters
- Hyperviscosity syndromes
- Myeloproliferative disorders
- Malignancy: disease or Rx related
- HIT and thrombosis
- Cigarette smoking
- IV drug use

■ *Thrombophilia testing*
- AT, protein C, protein S, and fibrinogen levels are not accurate during acute thrombotic event and should be obtained later than 4 wk post anticoagulation Rx discontinuation.
- Screening for FVL and PGM can be performed anytime.
- Testing criteria should target the following higher risk groups: age ≤40 yr, idiopathic thromboembolism, + family hx (first-degree relative), thromboembolism of unusual sites, pts with warfarin skin necrosis (↑ risk protein C deficiency), pts planning future pregnancies, very young pts with purpura fulminans.

2 ANTIPHOSPHOLIPID SYNDROME

This syndrome is characterized by arterial or venous thrombosis or pregnancy loss and the presence of antiphospholipid Abs (APL).

The syndrome is referred to as *"primary APS"* when it occurs alone and as *"secondary APS"* in association w/SLE, other rheumatic disorders, or certain infections or medications. *"Catastrophic APS"* is APS + disseminated microvascular thrombosis + multiorgan failure.

Diagnosis
■ APS Abs can be detected transiently in up to 5% of asymptomatic adults.
Diagnostic criteria of APS include at least one clinical criteria and at least one of the following lab criteria:

Clinical Features
■ Venous, arterial, or small-vessel thrombosis *or*
■ Morbidity w/pregnancy (fetal death at >10 wk gestation; *or* premature births before 34 wk gestation secondary to eclampsia, preeclampsia, or severe placental

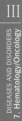

insufficiency; *or* three or more unexplained consecutive spontaneous abortions <10 wk gestation)

Labs

- Anticardiolipin Ab (IgG or IgM ACL in medium or high titers) *or*
- β2-glycoprotein I Ab (IgG or IgM ACL in high titers) *or* lupus anticoagulant found on >2 occasions, at least 12 wk apart

Treatment

- **+ APL w/ venous thrombosis:** initial anticoagulation w/heparin, then lifelong warfarin Rx, INR 2.0 to 3.0. Consider higher target INR (3-4) in pts with recurrent thromboembolism on warfarin.
- **+ APL w/arterial thrombosis**
  - Cerebral arterial thrombosis: ASA 325 mg qd or warfarin
  - Noncerebral arterial thrombosis: warfarin
- **Catastrophic APS:** Combination of anticoagulation, corticosteroids, and IVIG or plasma exchange
- Prophylaxis for asymptomatic pts w/+ APL w/o previous thrombosis:
  - No routine prophylaxis is recommended.
  - Questionable whether ASA 81 mg qd is effective
  - Antithrombotic prophylaxis for major surgery, prolonged immobilization, and pregnancy
- Note on warfarin or UFH monitoring:
  - In pts with APS Ab that artificially ↑ PT/INR, when using warfarin, monitor INR by measuring chromogenic factor X levels.
  - In pts with APS ab that ↑ APTT, when using UFH, use anti-Xa assay to monitor UFH or change over to LMWH.

3 VENOUS THROMBOEMBOLISM (DVT)

Presence of thrombi in the deep veins of the extremities or pelvis

Diagnosis

H&P

- Pain and swelling of the affected extremity
- In LE DVT: leg pain on dorsiflexion of the foot (**Homans' sign**)
- Exam may be unremarkable in early DVT.
- Clinical prediction rules can be used to establish pretest probability of DVT. The **Wells' prediction rules** for DVT are described in Table 7-10. These rules perform better in younger pts w/o h/o DVT and in those w/o comorbidities. In younger pts w/o associated comorbidities and a low pretest probability by Wells' criteria and a (−) high-sensitivity D-dimer test result, the dx of DVT can be reasonably excluded.

Labs

- Baseline PT (INR), APTT, and Plt count should be obtained on all pts before anticoagulation is started.
- D-dimer assay by ELISA: DVT can be ruled out in pts who are clinically unlikely to have DVT and have a (−) D-dimer test result. D-dimer can also be combined w/U/S. The combination of a nl D-dimer w/a nl compression venous U/S is useful to exclude DVT and to eliminate the need for repeated U/S at 5 to 7 days. Figure 7-5 describes an algorithm for the Dx of DVT.

TABLE 7-10 ■ Wells' Clinical Assessment Model for the Pretest Probability of Lower Extremity DVT	
	Score
Active cancer (treatment ongoing or within previous 6 mo or palliative)	1
Paralysis, paresis, or recent plaster immobilization of the lower extremities	1
Recently bedridden >3 days or major surgery within 4 wk	1
Localized tenderness along the distribution of the deep venous system	1
Entire leg swollen	1
Calf swelling >3 cm asymptomatic side (measured 10 cm below tibial tuberosity)	1
Pitting edema confined to the symptomatic leg	1
Collateral superficial veins (nonvaricose)	1
Alternative diagnosis as likely as or greater than that of DVT	−2

In patients with symptoms in both legs, the more symptomatic leg is used. Pretest probability is calculated as the total score: high, >3; moderate, 1-2; low, <0.
From Crawford MH, DiMarco JP, Paulus WJ (eds): Cardiology, 2nd ed. St. Louis, Mosby, 2004.

Imaging
- Compression U/S (see Figure 7-5)

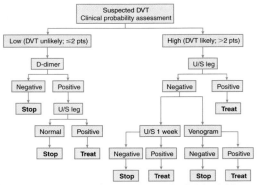

SUSPECTED DVT

FIGURE 7-5. Integrated strategy for diagnosis of DVT by using clinical probability assessment, measurement of D-dimer, and ultrasonography of legs as primary diagnostic tests. If clinical probability is low (i.e., DVT unlikely and D-dimer negative), no further investigations are required. If D-dimer is positive, proceed to ultrasonography of legs; then either treat or stop investigations. If clinical probability is high (i.e., DVT likely), D-dimer measurement need not be carried out; proceed directly to ultrasonography of legs. If negative, options are to repeat ultrasound in 1 week or in some cased to perform an ascending venogram. *(From Vincent JL, Abraham E, Moore FA, et al [eds]: Textbook of Critical Care, 6th ed. Philadelphia, Saunders, 2011.)*

Treatment
- Rapidly acting anticoagulants (LMWH, fondaparinux, or UFH) followed by warfarin Rx ≥5 days and until therapeutic INR (2-3) has been achieved with warfarin. Discontinue parenteral Rx after INR ≥2 has been achieved for at least 24 hr. Alternatives to warfarin may include dabigatran (direct oral thrombin inhibitor) and rivaroxaban (oral factor Xa inhibitor).
- Outpt treatment of DVT is appropriate for pts without prior DVT, thrombophilic conditions, or substantial comorbidity, but not for those who are pregnant or are likely to not to adhere to Rx.
- Exclusions from outpt treatment of DVT include pts with potential high complication risk (e.g., hemoglobin <7, Plt count <75,000, guaiac(+) stool, recent CVA or noncutaneous surgery, noncompliance).
- Insertion of an IVC filter to prevent PE is recommended in pts with contraindications to anticoagulation (e.g., hemorrhagic stroke, active internal bleeding, pregnancy), HIT in a pt with an active VTT/PE, recurrent PE despite adequate anticoagulant Rx, emergency surgery in a pt with DVT, presence of free-floating ileofemoral, lower IVC thrombosis (incipient embolization), and chronic pulmonary (thromboembolic) HTN with limited pulmonary reserve.
- Thrombolytic Rx (streptokinase) can be used in rare cases in pts with extensive iliofemoral venous thrombosis and a low risk of bleeding. There are concerns about hemorrhagic complications related to the large doses of thrombolytics required in systemic thrombolysis for DVT (2%-10% risk of major hemorrhagic complications).
- Other treatment modalities for DVT include surgical thrombectomy and catheter-directed thrombolysis (CDT). Thromboreduction by surgical thrombectomy is effective but invasive and expensive. CDT is also invasive, carries a bleeding risk, and requires ICU admission.

Duration of Anticoagulant Rx
  Rx duration varies w/the cause of DVT and risk factors.
- Rx for 3 mo: pts w/reversible risk factors (low-risk group). ↑ D-dimer level measured after 3 mo of anticoagulation in pts w/unprovoked DVT or persistent thrombosis on duplex imaging should favor a longer duration of Rx.

- Anticoagulation for 3 to 6 mo: pts w/idiopathic venous thrombosis or medical risk factors for DVT (intermediate-risk group)
- Indefinite anticoagulation: pts w/DVT associated w/active cancer; pts w/inherited thrombophilia (e.g., deficiency of protein C or S Ab), APS, and recurrent episodes of idiopathic DVT (high-risk group)

Anticoagulation Monitoring

- Warfarin: INR should be obtained daily when warfarin is initially administered concomitantly with rapidly acting anticoagulants. ts mean half-life is 32 to 40 hr; therefore, full impact of a dose change will take several days. Metabolism is also influenced by meds that affect cytochrome P-450 and dietary vitamin K content.
- UFH: A heparin dosage regimen is described in Box 7-1.

Box 7-1 • Heparin Dosage Regimens

1. Weight-Based Nomogram

The initial dose is a bolus of 80 U/kg body weight, followed by an infusion starting at a rate of 18 U/kg/hr. The APTT is measured every 6 hr, and the heparin dose is adjusted as follows.

Measured Value	Adjustment
PTT <35 sec (<1.2 × control value)	80 U/kg as bolus, then infusion rate by 4 U/kg/hr
APTT 35-45 sec (1.2-1.5 × control value)	40 U/kg as bolus, then infusion rate by 2 U/kg/hr
APTT 46-70 sec (>1.5-2.3 × control value)	No change
APTT 71-90 sec (>2.3-3 × control value)	↓ Infusion rate by 2 U/kg/hr
APTT >90 sec (>3 × control value)	Stop infusion for 1 hr, then ↓ infusion rate by 3 U/kg/hr

2. 5,000-U Bolus Dose, Followed by 1,280 U/hr

APTT (sec)	Bolus (U)	Stop Infusion (min)	Rate of Change (mL/hr)	Repeat APTT
<50*	5,000	0	+3	In 6 hr
50-59	0	0	+3	In 6 hr
60-85	0	0	0	Next morning
85-95	0	0	−2	Next morning
96-120	0	30	−2	In 6 hr
>120	0	60	−4	In 6 hr

3. Intravenous Dose-Titration Nomogram for APTT

The starting dose is a 5,000-U bolus, followed by 40,000 U/24 hr (if the patient has a low risk of bleeding) or 30,000 U/24 hr (if there is a high risk of bleeding).

| | Intravenous Infusion† | | |
APTT (sec)	Rate of Change (mL/hr)	Change in Dose (U/24 hr)	Additional Action
≤45	+6	+5,760	Repeat APTT in 4-6 hr
46-54	+3	+2,880	Repeat APTT in 4-6 hr
55-85	0	0	None‡
86-110	−3	−2,880	Stop heparin for 1 hr; repeat APTT 4-6 hr after restarting heparin Rx
>110	−6	−5,760	Stop heparin for 1 hr; repeat APTT 4-6 hr after restarting heparin Rx

*If the APTT is subtherapeutic despite a heparin dose of at least 1,440 U/hr (36 mL/hr) at any time during the first 48 hours of therapy, the response to an APTT of <50 sec is a bolus of 5,000 U and a rate increase of 5 mL/hr.

†A heparin sodium concentration of 20,000 U in 500 mL is equal to 40 U/mL.

‡During the first 24 hours, repeat the APTT in 4 to 6 hr. Thereafter, the APTT is determined once daily, unless the value is in the therapeutic range.

Note: 1 mL/hr = 40 U/hr.

Reprinted with permission from Ginsberg JS: Management of venous thromboembolism. N Engl J Med 335:1821, 1996.

- LMWH/fondaparinux: No monitoring is needed but it is renally excreted; therefore, ↓ dose in renal insufficiency.
- Dabigatran, rivaroxaban: No monitoring is necessary.

Anticoagulation Reversal
- Warfarin: vitamin K, 10 mg IV over 1 hour
  - Prothrombin complex concentrate 25 to 50 units/kg IV
  - Recombinant human factor VIIa, 25 to 90 µg/kg IV
- UFH: protamine 1 mg/100 U UFH, infused slowly (<5 mg/min)
- LMWH: protamine 0.5 to 1 mg/1 mg enoxaparin or 100 IU dalteparin

Direct Thrombin Inhibitors
- Activated prothrombin complex concentrates, 50 to 100 U/kg IV
- Oral activated charcoal or hemodialysis for dabigatran

J. ONCOLOGIC URGENCIES AND EMERGENCIES

1 TUMOR LYSIS SYNDROME

Syndrome characterized by rapid development of ↑ uric acid, ↑ K^+, ↑ PO_4^-, and ↓ Ca^{2+} due to leukemic cell death secondary to chemoRx (often seen w/high-grade lymphoma, ALL, AML chemoRx)

Treatment

IV hydration with normal saline and administration of allopurinol to lower uric acid level

Pts w/ ↑↑ serum uric acid level may be treated w/recombinant urate oxidase (rasburicase) which converts uric acid to soluble allantoin with faster onset than allopurinol.

2 SUPERIOR VENA CAVA SYNDROME

Definition

This set of sx results when a mediastinal mass (lung cancer [80% of all cases] lymphoma [15%]) compresses the SVC or the veins that drain into it.

The pathophysiologic mechanism of the syndrome involves the pressure in the venous system draining into the SVC, thus producing edema of the head, neck, and UEs. Sx develop during a period of 2 wk in 30% of pts.

Diagnosis

H&P
- Clinical presentation: dyspnea, chest pain, cough, dysphagia, syncope
- PE: chest wall vein distention, neck vein distention, facial edema, UE swelling, cyanosis

Imaging
- CXR
- Chest CT scan or MRI
- Venography: warranted only when an intervention (e.g., stent or surgery) is planned

Treatment
- Management is guided by severity of sx and the underlying etiology.
- Emergency RT is indicated in critical situations, such as respiratory failure or CNS signs associated w/ICP.
- Rx of the underlying malignant disease: RadioRx, systemic/chemoRx
- Percutaneous self-expandable stents can be placed under local anesthesia w/ radiologic manipulation in selected pts to bypass the obstruction.

3 BRAIN METASTASES

Epidemiology and Physical Findings
- >50% of adult intracranial tumors
- Headache 40%-50% (if posterior fossa mets, may result in obstructive hydrocephalus)
  - Cognitive dysfunction (30%-45%)
  - Seizures/hemiparesis (30%-40%)
  - Acute CVA (5%-10%)
- 20% brain mets dx synchronously or before primary tumor found

Imaging and Labs
- LP contraindicated because of ↑ ICP
- Brain bx necessary if unknown primary tumor

- MRI with/without contrast = imaging study of choice
- MRI spectroscopy and PET used to delineate tumor, nontumor, radiation necrosis

Treatment
- Steroids used to $\downarrow$ peritumoral edema and $\uparrow$ ICP
- Pts with no hx seizure, prophylaxis not necessary
- Anticoagulants to prevent venous thromboembolic disease
- Whole brain radiation and stereotactic radiosurgery (SRS) for chronic cases

A. HIV/AIDS

Powel H. Kazanjian

THE ASYMPTOMATIC HIV-INFECTED PATIENT

Natural Hx, Testing, and Case Definition

- Acute infection occurs 2 to 6 wk from the time of viral transmission.
  - It most often is a self-limited mononucleosis-like illness: pharyngitis, rash, splenomegaly, and lymphadenopathy, occasionally w/hepatitis and aseptic meningitis.
  - The p24 antigen and the HIV PCR are detected; HIV serology first becomes (+) 1 mo later.
- HIV viral Ab screening tests include:
  - Enzyme immuno assay (EIA): A (-) EIA excludes infection except during the acute phase following primary infection (window period) before seroconversion occurs. A (+) EIA is confirmed by western blot. Combination of (+) EIA and (+) western blot has 99.5% sensitivity and 99.9% specificity.
  - Rapid serologic screening HIV antigen–coated gelatin or latex particle agglutination assays: They are less sensitive and specific than standard ELISA tests.
  - Western blot confirmatory test: performed when EIA is (+). It identifies specific viral antigens.
  - Tests are (+) when both core and envelope antigens are present.
  - Indeterminate when either antigen is present: A false(+) result occurs if unchanged during 6 mo.
  - An FDA-approved at-home HIV screening test is also available. It uses swabs of oral fluids from upper and lower gums. A positive test requires confirmatory testing in the office. Negative home tests should be repeated within 3 months.
- Early stage (CD4 cells >400/mm^3): Diffuse lymphadenopathy may be present. Levels of viral replication, 10^9 copies/day, occur at this stage even though the pt remains asymptomatic.
- Middle stage (CD4 cells, 200-400/mm^3)
  - *Mycobacterium tuberculosis* infections, recurrent herpes zoster, persistent mucocutaneous herpes simplex infections, and recurrent bacteremias caused by *Streptococcus pneumoniae* and *Salmonella* spp occur.
  - Kaposi's sarcoma, oral candidiasis, and hairy leukoplakia appear.
- AIDS: advanced HIV infection (CD4 cell count <200/mm^3). The classic opportunistic infections PCP, cerebral toxoplasmosis, cryptococcosis occur when CD4 cell count is <200/mm^3; infections with CMV and MAC occur when CD4 cell count is <50/mm^3.

Management Strategies

- Initial testing: CD4 cell count and HIV viral load (VL) are measured q3-6mo to guide decisions about antiretroviral use and prophylaxis against PCP and MAC infection.
- Other testing: This identifies latent infections that may become reactivated because of loss of T-cell function but can be prevented by the use of specific agents.
  - Serology to *Toxoplasma gondii* (IgG): Clinical infection may be prevented by TMP-SMZ used as prophylaxis for PCP.
  - VDRL test: LP should be performed in pts w/a confirmatory specific test (FTA). Rx w/IM benzathine PCN if the CSF formula is nl, and IV PCN × 10 days if the CSF VDRL test is reactive or CSF pleocytosis, protein, or hypoglycorrhachia is present.
  - PPD skin test showing induration of ≥5 mm, or pts w/exposure to someone w/ active TB: Treat w/INH 300 mg/day for 9 mo or, in case of INH-induced hepatitis, rifampin 600 mg PO qd (only for those not receiving PIs or NRTIs) × 4 mo.
- Immunizations: Pts should receive the annual influenza vaccine each fall. Pneumococcal polysaccharide vaccine is recommended for all pts w/HIV infection and is most effective in those w/CD4 counts >200. Invasive pneumococcal infections occur w/↑ frequency in HIV-infected pts; these pts should be revaccinated every 5 yr. Hepatitis B vaccination is recommended for pts who have no evidence of prior infection. They should also receive hepatitis A vaccine.

Prophylactic Agents

- PJP prophylaxis if CD4 cell level is <200/mm^3
  - TMP-SMZ (1 DS qd): most effective agent. It also provides protection against infections with *T. gondii*, *Nocardia* spp, and enteric pathogens.
  - Adverse reactions to TMP-SMZ (GI distress, fever, rash, and leukopenia): occur in 40%. Discontinuation of drug may be necessary.
  - Dapsone indicated w/TMP-SMZ rash; 30% w/TMP-SMZ toxicity develop reaction to dapsone.
  - Aerosolized pentamidine, 300 mg/mo, and atovaquone, 750 mg bid, are third-line agents.
- Prophylaxis against MAC in pts w/CD4 cell counts <50/µL Azithromycin 1200 mg weekly is the most effective agent.
- Prophylaxis for several opportunistic infections can be discontinued if there has been a sustained CD4 cell count ↑ >200 associated w/ART (PCP, toxoplasmosis, cryptococcosis) and 100 for MAC for more than 3 to 6 mo.
- Prophylaxis against toxoplasmosis if CD4 cell count <100/µL and positive serology: TMP-SMZ (IDS qd).
- Prophylaxis against tuberculosis if TST>5 mm or + GRA: INH, 300 mg/day × 9 months.

Antiretroviral Therapy (ART)

- Rx goals are maximal and durable suppression of VLs (<50 copies/mL), restoration of immunologic function (CD4 cell count), prevention of HIV disease progression, and prevention of transmission to an uninfected partner.
- Agents in six separate drug classes are now available: NRTIs, NNRTIs, PIs, fusion inhibitors, co-receptor inhibitors, and integrase inhibitors.
- The standard regimen is two NRTIs (TNF/3TC) plus an NNRTI (efavirenz [Sustiva] or rilpivirine), ritonavir-boosted PI agent (darunavir, lopinavir, atazanavir, fosamprenavir), or an integrase inhibitor (raltegravir, elvitegravir).
- ART should be offered to all pts with HIV infection regardless of CD4 count and HIV VL. The rationale for early Rx is that the disorders associated with long-term viral replication—coronary artery disease, bone demineralization, renal disease, and possibly neurocognitive changes—may be averted or delayed if HIV VL is reduced with ART. ART at this stage may prevent transmission to an uninfected partner.
- Indications for initiation of ART according to DHHS guidelines are: symptomatic HIV infection, CD4 cell count <500/µL, history of AIDS-defining opportunistic infection or malignancy, presence of HIV-associated nephropathy, active co-infection with hepatitis B or C virus, pregnancy (to prevent perinatal transmission).
- After initiation of ART, measure CD4 counts and V_s at 1 and 4 mo. The criteria used to assess initial ART efficacy are as follows:
  - >1.0 log ↓ in HIV VL within 4 wk and undetectable VL (HIV RNA <50 copies/mL) within 4 mo
- Pts should be evaluated q3mo at first to assess VL responses. In adherent pts with undetectable HIV VL, pts may be evaluated q6mo. A new regimen should be initiated in pts whose initial regimen has failed (rebound viremia).
- CD4 counts on an average boost to 250 cells above baseline value within 1 to 2 yr of Rx; failure to achieve this boost in adherent pts with undetectable VL does not indicate ART failure and does not warrant changing the regimen.
- Drug resistance testing should be performed when there is ART failure; a new regimen should be selected on the basis of antiviral hx and absence of mutations to ART-included agents on resistance testing. Once resistance develops to an agent in one class, cross-resistance to other drugs in the same class frequently occurs.
- An ideal regimen should include preferably three agents from two separate drug classes to which the virus retains susceptibility. Agents frequently included in a new regimen include the following:
  - Raltegravir (400 mg bid) or elvitegravir: integrase inhibitors
  - Maraviroc inhibits viral binding to co-receptor CCR5. A viral tropism assay must be first measured before initiation to ensure that the virus is an R5 strain.
  - Etravirine (200 bid): an NNRTI to which certain NNRTI-resistant strains (K103N mutants) remain susceptible
  - Darunavir/ritonavir (600/100 bid): a PI to which certain PI-resistant strains remain susceptible
- NRTI agents and their toxicities
  - Zidovudine (Retrovir, AZT) 300 mg bid with lamivudine (Epivir, 3TC) 150 mg bid (Combivir). Transient myalgias, headache, and fatigue are common. Hematologic toxicity (leukopenia and anemia) is related to HIV disease status.

- Tenofovir (TNF, Viread) 300 mg/day in combination w/emtricitabine (FTC) 200 mg/day (Truvada). Nephrotoxicity is the major adverse reaction, w/declines in GFR of 8%.
- Abacavir (Ziagen) 300 mg bid; combined w/3TC (Epzicom, 1 tablet qd). Risk of abacavir hypersensitivity ↑ to 8% in pts w/HLA-B5701 genotype. Testing for the haplotype is indicated before starting abacavir.
- Zalcitabine (Hivid, ddC) 0.75 mg tid. It is rarely used because of relative lack of potency and tid schedule.
- Didanosine (Videx, ddI) 200 mg bid, or 400 mg enteric-coated tablet once qd. It is rarely used because of toxicities: pancreatitis (10%); peripheral neuropathy (15%).

■ NNRTI agents and their toxicities
- Efavirenz (Sustiva) 600 mg every night used in combination with Truvada (Atripla, once daily): Transient neurologic or psychiatric sx—insomnia, dizziness, or impaired concentration—occur in 50% of pts. The sx may progress and require discontinuation of the drug. Delusions and acute depression may also occur. Transient rash may also occur but rarely requires discontinuation of the drug.
- Rilpivirine (25 mg once daily) used in combination with Truvada (Complera, once daily). It may cause rash and is particularly effective in people whose baseline VL <100,000 copies.
- Etravirine 200 mg bid. It is used primarily as a second-line drug in pts who have resistance to Sustiva. Rash occurs as with nevirapine.
- Nevirapine (Viramune) 200 mg bid. Rash occurs in 10% of pts. Nevirapine should not be used in women w/CD4 cell counts >250 and men w/CD4 cell counts >400 because of risks of severe hepatotoxicity in this setting.

■ PIs (in combination w/low-dose ritonavir) and their toxicities
- The PIs have multiple drug interactions that result from their elimination by P-450 CYP3A.
- Metabolic complications associated w/all PI agents
  - Older agents in this class (ritonavir in high dose, Kaletra) led to insulin resistance, fat accumulation, lipoatrophy, lipid disturbances; these have a reduced incidence with newer agents (darunavir).
  - Serum cholesterol and lipid abnlties may occur. In addition to dietary changes (↑ fiber content of the diet along w/↓ the amount of saturated and hydrogenated fat), Rx w/statins may be necessary.

■ Ritonavir (Norvir) (100 mg bid), a potent inhibitor of CYP3A4, is used to boost the concentration of a PI agent with which it is used. The particular PI agent would include:
- Darunavir/R (Prezista) 600/100 bid. This agent is effective as a first-line agent or a second-line agent. It has a favorable lipid altering profile.
- Atazanavir (Reyataz)/ritonavir 300 mg PO qd/100 mg qd: A first-line PI agent because it does not lead to significant changes in cholesterol or TGs.
- Fosamprenavir/ritonavir 1400/200 qd. It has efficacy comparable to that of other PIs.
- Lopinavir/ritonavir (Kaletra) 400 mg bid/100 mg bid or 800/200 mg qd. This is now a second-line agent because it causes lipid abnlities.
- Saquinavir/ritonavir (1000 mg bid/100 mg bid) and indinavir/ritonavir 800 mg bid/100 mg bid and nelfinavir (Viracept) 1250 mg bid are no longer used because they are not as potent as the preceding agents.

■ Integrase inhibitors
- Raltegravir (Isentress) 400 bid. This is a potent regimen in combination with Truvada with minimal side effects.
- Elvitegravir used in combination with cobicistat (to boost level) and Truvada (Stribild, once daily). It is a potent once daily regimen with minimal side effects.

Postexposure Prophylaxis (PEP)

■ PEP for occupational exposures: The transmission rate of HIV after an exposure w/o antiviral use is low—0.3%. Truvada/raltegravir is indicated for pts w/ high-risk exposures (visible blood on device causing injury from a known HIV-infected person w/high VL), preferably within 24 hr of exposure for a 1-mo duration.

■ PEP for nonoccupational exposures: The same regimen should be considered in high-risk nonoccupational exposures, including sexual encounters when an uninfected person has a sexual encounter with an HIV-infected person without using proper barrier precautions.

Preexposure Prophylaxis (PrEP)

■ Truvada should be considered in selected situations for uninfected persons who have high-risk encounters with known HIV-infected persons. PrEP is effective only when taken regularly.

HIV in Pregnancy

■ The goals of ART in pregnant women are to provide Rx for the mother and to ↓ vertical transmission (in utero or perinatally). Rx should be initiated during the second trimester.

■ Efavirenz is not recommended for women in their first trimester of pregnancy.

■ Possible strategies to improve adherence
  • Several strategies can be used to improve adherence, which is critical to maintain >95% to prevent resistance and to maintain durability of the regimen.
  • Depression or substance abuse should be treated before Rx is initiated (except when antiretroviral Rx is urgently needed), and tools such as pill boxes, alarms, and charts should be provided.

Treatment of Symptomatic Pts w/AIDS-Defining Illness

■ The use of ART in pts w/active opportunistic infections may be complicated by the immune reconstitution inflammatory syndrome (IRIS). IRIS usually involves constitutional sx along w/local reactions 1 to 2 mo after ART. Nonetheless, when both infections are diagnosed simultaneously, particular antimicrobial Rx for the opportunistic infection diagnosed should be started immediately and HAART should not be delayed, especially in pts w/low CD4 cell counts. IRIS may be managed w/anti-inflammatory agents while maintaining both the particular antimicrobial agent and ART Rx.

Fungal Disorders

■ *Candida* infection (thrush) may involve mucous membranes of the mouth.
  • Dx: by clinical appearance—whitish patches w/erythematous base; KOH preparation may demonstrate budding yeast and pseudohyphae.
  • DDx: herpes simplex and aphthous ulcers (painful), oral hairy leukoplakia (as a result of EBV)
  • Rx: clotrimazole troches 5×/day × 10 days; refractory cases fluconazole 100 mg PO × 10 days

■ Esophagitis/oropharyngeal candidiasis is usually present when there is odynophagia or dysphagia.
  • DDx: EBV, CMV, giant esophageal ulcers, and cancer, which should be considered in those pts not responding to antifungal Rx
  • Rx: fluconazole 100 mg PO bid × 3 wk

■ *Cryptococcus (neoformans)* infection
  • Pts may have headache, fever, ΔMS, meningismus (only 30%) w/cranial nerve palsies; *Cryptococcus* may disseminate to lungs, skin, blood, liver, and prostate. Nuchal rigidity may be absent. Dx is made by spinal fluid analysis; head CT scan should be performed first. Spinal WBC, glucose, and protein levels may all be nl. Cryptococcal antigen is the most sensitive (>1:16 in 95% cases). Serum cryptococcal antigen is reactive in >90% of pts w/CNS involvement.
  • Initial Rx is w/amphotericin B (0.7 mg/kg/day) for 2 wk w/adjunctive flucytosine (100 mg/kg/day), unless preexisting cytopenias prohibit its use. Serum flucytosine levels must be monitored. Maintenance PO fluconazole Rx (200-400 mg/day) prevents relapse and may be withdrawn when ART-restored CD4 is >200.

■ Coccidioidomycosis
  • After initial Rx for coccidioidomycosis, lifelong suppressive Rx is recommended w/fluconazole 400 mg PO qd or itraconazole 200 mg PO bid.
  • Recommendations for discontinuation of secondary prophylaxis (long-term maintenance Rx) in a pt w/a CD4 count >100 receiving ART are not available.
  • Fluconazole and itraconazole have potential teratogenicity in pregnant women. Consider amphotericin B (preferred), especially during the first trimester. All HIV(+) women receiving azole Rx for coccidioidomycosis should maintain birth control precautions.

■ Histoplasmosis
  • Initial Rx for disseminated histoplasmosis is amphotericin B for 1 to 2 wk followed by long-term maintenance Rx w/itraconazole 200 mg PO bid.
  • Discontinuation of long-term maintenance may be considered if the ART-restored CD4 count is >200.
  • Itraconazole has teratogenicity and embryotoxicity and should not be offered during pregnancy. Rx w/amphotericin B is preferred during the first trimester. HIV-infected women receiving azole Rx should maintain effective birth control measures.

- Pneumocystis infection
  - Pts have SOB and nonproductive cough w/few findings on exam; CXR usually has an interstitial infiltrate but may be nl in initial stages.
  - Dx is usually made by sputum induction or by BAL, w/visualization by monoclonal Ab, methenamine silver stain, or PCR.
  - PO regimens: Rx in mild cases (Po₂, >70; A-a gradient, <35 mm Hg) for a 3-wk course.
  - TMP-SMZ (Bactrim DS, Septra DS) 15 mg/kg/day in three divided doses
  - TMP-dapsone: trimethoprim 15 mg/kg/day and dapsone 100 mg/day (need to r/o G6PD deficiency w/dapsone)
  - Primaquine and clindamycin: primaquine (also need to exclude G6PD deficiency) 30 mg/day and clindamycin 450 mg PO qid
  - Atovaquone (may be less effective than TMP-SMZ) 750 mg PO tid
  - IV regimens if moderate to severe (Po₂ <70 mm Hg or A-a gradient >35 mm Hg)
  - TMP-SMZ 15 mg TMP/kg/day in three individual doses
  - Pentamidine 3 mg/kg/day; may need to observe for hypotension, pancreatitis, hypoglycemia, and azotemia
  - Trimetrexate 45 mg/m² once qd for pts intolerant of or refractory to TMP-SMZ or pentamidine; must be given w/leucovorin
  - Adjunctive corticosteroid Rx: indicated when PO₂ is <70 mm Hg or A-a gradient is >35 mm Hg to prevent early deterioration of oxygenation by ↓ inflammation. There is a risk of reactivation of latent infection (CMV, histoplasmosis, TB) w/steroid use.

Mycobacterial Infections

- *M. tuberculosis* may cause pulmonary involvement, extrapulmonary involvement, or both. Extrapulmonary TB may involve meningitis, lymphadenitis, or peritonitis. W/more advanced disease (CD4 <200), there may be atypical CXR findings (e.g., nonapical involvement).
  - Caution is required for the use of TB meds and ART. Rifampin should be substituted w/rifabutin w/the use of PIs and NNRTIs. Saquinavir hard-gel should not be given w/rifabutin; PIs (indinavir, nelfinavir, amprenavir) require dosage modifications.
  - HIV-infected pregnant women w/(+) PPD test reaction or exposure to active TB should be considered for chemoprophylaxis. Isoniazid w/pyridoxine is the recommended Rx.
- *Mycobacterium avium-intracellulare* complex (MAC)
  - Sx are fever, night sweats, and wasting. Dissemination may involve lymph nodes, liver, and bone marrow, causing marrow suppression, diarrhea w/abd pain, gastroenteritis, and, rarely, pulmonary involvement. Dx is made by blood culture (special lysis-centrifugation technique), which takes an average of 3 wk; cultures of tissue or bone marrow are rarely necessary to make the dx.
  - Combination Rx w/at least two agents:
    - Clarithromycin 500 mg PO bid (azithromycin, 500 mg/day PO, is alternative)
    - Ethambutol 15 mg/kg/day PO. Addition of a third agent (rifabutin) may be considered.
    - Medications to be considered in pts who have had relapsing disease are rifabutin, ciprofloxacin, and amikacin. Rifabutin 300 mg/day or ciprofloxacin 500 to 750 mg bid can be used as third agents.
  - **Primary prophylaxis** (CD4 count <50/μL, d/c when CD4 count >100): azithromycin 1200 mg PO weekly or clarithromycin 500 mg PO bid

Bacterial Infections

- Pts w/HIV may develop infections from *S. pneumoniae, Haemophilus influenzae,* or *Pseudomonas aeruginosa.* Fever w/productive cough and lobar infiltrates may occur. Functional humoral response to *S. pneumoniae* may be impaired, leading to recurrent infections caused by these pathogens. Other pathogens include the following:
  - *Salmonella* spp: recurrent bacteremia; treat w/ampicillin, TMP-SMZ, ciprofloxacin, or third-generation cephalosporin, based on sensitivities and clinical presentation; GI sx may not be present. Avoid raw or undercooked eggs, poultry, meat, and seafood.
  - *Listeriosis:* in HIV-infected individuals who are severely immunosuppressed. Soft cheeses and ready-to-eat foods (hot dogs, cold cuts) should be avoided or heated until steaming hot.
  - *Sinusitis:* It may be a routine bacterial infection or involve *P. aeruginosa* or fungi.
  - *Bacillary angiomatosis:* an infection involving skin, w/red lesions that can be mistaken for Kaposi's sarcoma; can involve viscera (liver, spleen, bone); caused by *Rochalimaea henselae* or *Rochalimaea quintana;* treat w/erythromycin or

doxycycline. Other potential bacterial pathogens in HIV are *Rhodococcus equi,* which may cause cavitating pneumonia, and *Nocardia.*

Viral Infections

■ Herpes simplex
  • May involve mucous membranes, cause genital herpes, or cause rectal or perirectal infection, resulting in proctitis.
  • Initial Rx: acyclovir 200 mg PO 5×/day × 10 days; recurrent episodes may need Rx w/400 mg PO 3 to 5×/day × 7 days or until clinically resolved. IV foscarnet or cidofovir can be used for acyclovir-resistant isolates of HSV.

■ Hepatitis C
  • Pts w/HIV infection should be tested for HCV by enzyme immunoassay. If test result is (+), confirm w/RIBA or PCR for HCV RNA.
  • Pts w/HCV and HIV should receive vaccination for hepatitis A if they are (−) for hepatitis A Abs.
  • Pts w/HIV-HCV co-infection are at risk for chronic liver disease and should be evaluated for Rx by providers w/experience in treating both HIV and HCV.

■ CMV: Infection from this virus may cause illness involving the retina, GI tract (including esophagus, colon), and CNS.
  • Chorioretinitis may develop in 25% of AIDS pts and also may be unilateral, w/viremia involving other organs; the pt usually reports ↓ vision or "floaters"; ophthalmologic evaluation may be necessary to confirm dx.
  • Esophagitis: Deep ulcerations are seen, confirmed by the presence of inclusion bodies by bx.
  • Colitis: usually associated w/diarrhea, weight loss, and fever. It occurs in approximately 10% of AIDS pts.
  • CNS encephalitis or polyradiculopathy (areflexic paraplegia)
  • Rx: Three agents are available. Rx may be discontinued if ART-restored CD4 cell counts are >200.
  • Retinitis: Ganciclovir implant is effective in delaying progression of disease; PO valganciclovir is used to prevent systemic manifestations of disease.
  • Ganciclovir: induction dose, 5 mg/kg bid × 14 days, followed by 5 mg/kg/day indefinitely for retinitis. It may cause granulocytopenia or neutropenia related to dose, which is compounded by the use of AZT and possibly by other antiretroviral medications.
  • Foscarnet: induction dose, 60 mg/kg q8h IV for 2 to 3 wk; dosing depends on CrCl and requires adjustment. Maintenance Rx is 90 to 120 mg/kg q24h.
  • Cidofovir: 5 mg/kg weekly for 2 wk, then every other week as maintenance

■ Progressive multifocal leukoencephalopathy: demyelinating disease most often involving posterior cortex of brain, resulting in slowly progressive cognitive impairments. Clinical and radiologic improvement or, in some cases, complete resolution may occur w/ART-associated restoration of CD4 cell counts.

Parasitic Infections

■ Toxoplasmosis
  • Sx of *Toxoplasma* encephalitis: headache, fever, encephalopathy, focal neurologic deficits. Pneumonia, myocarditis, and retinal involvement occur less often.
  • Dx is usually presumptive, based on multifocal ring-enhancing and hypodense mass lesions on CT, (+) toxoplasmic IgG serology, and a clinical and radiologic response to antitoxoplasmic Rx. Other causes of CNS mass lesions in AIDS pts include CNS lymphoma, fungal infection *(Aspergillus, Cryptococcus),* tuberculoma, bacterial abscess.
  • Rx
  • Pyrimethamine + sulfadiazine: pyrimethamine 100 to 200 mg loading dose, followed by 50 mg/day PO; sulfadiazine 1 to 1.5 g PO q6h as initial Rx, followed by a maintenance dose of pyrimethamine 25 mg/day, sulfadiazine 500 mg q6h
    • Clindamycin: 600 to 1200 mg IV or 600 mg PO q6h (2.4 g/day) and pyrimethamine 50 mg/day PO
    • Atovaquone, TMP-SMZ, and macrolides may have anti-*Toxoplasma* properties and can be considered alternative Rxs.

■ Cryptosporidiosis: protozoal infection causing watery diarrhea, abd pain, and dehydration, particularly worse in pts w/CD4 counts <50. Dx is made by a modified AFB stain of stool. There is no effective Rx for HIV-infected pts, although nitazoxanide has been used in immunocompetent pts. Azithromycin, when taken for MAC prophylaxis, may ↓ the risk for cryptosporidiosis.

■ Isosporiasis: another protozoal infection w/a presentation similar to that of

Cryptosporidium infection, w/oocysts found in routine stain of stool. Rx w/Bactrim 1 DS tablet qid × 10 days is followed by maintenance.

■ Microsporidiosis: also similar to *Cryptosporidium* infection, w/oocysts found in special modified trichrome stain of stool. Rx w/albendazole (400 mg bid) is effective only against certain species; atovaquone is effective against others.

Malignant Neoplasms

■ Malignant neoplasms may be occurring more frequently, as prognosis has been improved w/ART and prevention of opportunistic infections w/prophylactic Rx. The following have been listed as AIDS-defining malignant neoplasms:

• Kaposi's sarcoma: found most often in HIV-infected homosexual men and less frequently (<5%) in pts in other HIV risk groups. The lesions from Kaposi's sarcoma may be multifocal, involving skin (79%), lymph nodes (70%), GI tract (45%), and lungs (10%). Rx is based on extent of involvement; Rx w/ intralesional vinblastine and w/radiation Rx is recommended for localized or small numbers of lesions, and chemoRx w/vincristine and vinblastine, etoposide, or bleomycin for aggressive and disseminated disease. Use of many interleukins (e.g., interleukin-4), tumor necrosis factor, and pentoxifylline is investigational.

• Non-Hodgkin's lymphoma: a B-cell tumor associated w/EBV; most often extranodal; 30% may occur in pts w/CD4 cell counts >200; GI tract, CNS, bone marrow, or liver (or other viscera in smaller percentages) is also affected. Combination chemotherapy regimen (CHOP, M-BACOD, MACOP-B, CHOP-R, ACVBP) have approximately 50% response. Dose-limiting multiagent Rx is myelosuppression.

• Primary CNS lymphoma: Most cases occur in pts w/CD4 counts <200, but one third occur w/CD4 counts >200. Most are unifocal ring-enhancing mass lesions that cause focal neurologic deficits or seizures. Brain bx establishes dx.

• AIDS-related cervical cancer: associated w/HPV. It often occurs in pts w/multiple sexual partners and is possibly related to primary association of HIV to cancer development.

■ Other cancers associated w/HIV infection

• Hodgkin's lymphoma: may occur in a pt who is an IV drug user or who has STD. EBV may be linked to both Hodgkin's disease and NHL; pts usually present w/ disseminated stage III or stage IV disease involving bone marrow (50%) or liver and lungs.

• Anal carcinoma: associated w/HPV and impaired immunity. Homosexual men are at risk.

AIDS-Related Cachexia

■ Megestrol acetate can ↑ appetite and food intake in pts w/AIDS-related weight loss. It can result in a statistically significant weight gain and in pt-reported improvement in overall sense of well-being.

B. HOSPITAL-ACQUIRED INFECTIONS

Infections associated with health care that occur >48 hr after admission (≥33% of HAIs are preventable via handwashing/hygiene)

MOST COMMON SOURCES

Urinary tract infections (UTIs) (32%), surgical wound and other soft tissue infections (22%), pneumonia (15%), bloodstream infections (14%)

Methicillin-Resistant *Staphylococcus aureus* (MRSA)
■ Health-care–associated MRSA strains typically multiresistant
■ Community-acquired associated with soft tissue (boils, rash, "spider bite")

Vancomycin-Resistant *Enterococcus faecium* (VREF)
■ 80% of VREF isolated are also ampicillin resistant.

Norovirus
■ Sudden onset of nausea, vomiting, and/or diarrhea
■ Disinfection with bleach

Diagnosis

Labs
■ Cultures (urine, blood, sputum, soft tissue)

Treatment
■ Consider aggressive isolation to restrict spread of MRSA, VREF, multidrug-resistant Gram(–) rods (MDR-GNRs).

C. PNEUMONIA

Infection involving lung parenchyma

Diagnosis
H&P
- Fever, tachypnea, chills, tachycardia, cough
- Streptococcal pneumonia: high fever, shaking chills, pleuritic chest pain, cough, and copious production of purulent sputum
- Elderly or immunocompromised pts may present w/only minimal sx (e.g., low-grade fever, confusion)
- Crackles and ↓ breath sounds
- Percussion dullness: pleural effusion
- **Prognosis prediction: CURB-65** (**C**: confusion, **U**: BUN >19 mg/dL, **R**: RR >30 min, **B**P <90/60 mm Hg, age ≥**65** yr). If score = 1, OK outpt Rx; if score >1, hospitalize (higher score, higher mortality).

Imaging (chest x-ray: PA + lateral)
- Segmental lobe infiltrate: pneumococcal pneumonia
- Diffuse infiltrates: *Legionella pneumophila, Mycoplasma pneumoniae,* viral pneumonias, *Pneumocystis jiroveci,* miliary TB, aspiration, aspergillosis

Treatment
- Macrolides (azithromycin or clarithromycin) or levofloxacin for empiric outpt Rx; cefotaxime or a β-lactam/β-lactamase inhibitor can be added in pts w/more severe presentation who insist on outpt Rx. Duration of Rx: 7 to 14 days.
- In pts admitted to general medical ward: second- or third-generation cephalosporin (ceftriaxone, ceftizoxime, cefotaxime, or cefuroxime) + a macrolide (azithromycin or clarithromycin) or doxycycline. An antipseudomonal quinolone (levofloxacin or moxifloxacin) may be substituted in place of the macrolide or doxycycline.
- Empiric Rx in ICU pts: IV β-lactam (ceftriaxone, cefotaxime, ampicillin-sulbactam) + an IV quinolone (levofloxacin, moxifloxacin) or IV azithromycin
- In hospitalized pts at risk for *P. aeruginosa* infection: antipseudomonal β-lactam (cefepime or piperacillin-tazobactam) + an AG + an antipseudomonal quinolone or macrolide
- In pts w/suspected MRSA: vancomycin or linezolid

Clinical Pearls
- Causes of slowly resolving or nonresolving pneumonia: difficult-to-treat infections: viral pneumonia, *Legionella*, pneumococci, or staphylococci w/impaired host response; TB, fungi, neoplasia (lung, lymphoma, mets), CHF, PE, immunologic/idiopathic: Wegener's granulomatosis, pulmonary eosinophilic syndromes, SLE,
- Drug toxicity (e.g., amiodarone)

ASPIRATION PNEUMONIA ± LUNG ABSCESS
- **Etiology:** 35% anaerobes, 26% Gram(+) cocci, 25% *Klebsiella pneumoniae*
- **Rx:** piperacillin-tazobactam 3.375 g IV q6h or 4-hr infusion of 3.375 g q8h or (ceftriaxone 1 g IV q24h + metronidazole 500 mg IV q6h)

MYCOPLASMA PNEUMONIAE
Diagnosis
H&P
- Nonexudative pharyngitis (common), rhonchi or rales, w/o evidence of consolidation (common) in lower lung zones; associated w/bullous myringitis
Imaging
- CXR: predilection for lower lobe involvement (upper lobes <25%), w/radiographic abnlity frequently out of proportion PE; small pleural effusions (30%)
Treatment
- Azithromycin (500 mg initially, then 250 mg qd × 4) or clarithromycin (500 mg bid). Levofloxacin (Levaquin) (alternative Rx agent) not be used in young children.

CYSTIC FIBROSIS ACUTE EXACERBATION OF PULMONARY SYMPTOMS
- Rx *P. aeruginosa:* tobramycin (3.3 mg/kg q8h or 12 mg/kg IV q24h) + ceftazidime 50 mg/kg IV q8h to max of 6 g/day
- Rx *S. aureus:* methicillin-sensitive *S. aureus* (MSSA) (oxacillin/nafcillin 2 g IV q4h), MRSA (vancomycin 1 g q12h)

D. ABSCESS

1 BREAST ABSCESS/MASTITIS

Diagnosis

H&P

- Painful erythematous induration occasionally w/draining through the overlying skin or nipple opening
- 10% to 30% of breast abscesses are lactational *(S. aureus);* may continue breastfeeding
- Subareolar abscess (anaerobes, staph, strep) notorious for recurrence/fistula formation
- Acute mastitis may → breast abscess if untreated.

Labs

- C&S of abscess aspirate

Imaging

- If mammogram or U/S required but prevented by discomfort, perform after Rx.

Treatment

- I&D with bx of abscess cavity wall to r/o carcinoma

Mastitis with/without Abscess

- No MRSA
  - Outpt: dicloxacillin 500 mg PO qid or cephalexin 500 mg PO qid
  - Inpt: nafcillin/oxacillin 2 g IV q4h
- MRSA possible
  - Out-pt: TMP-SMX-DS tabs 1 to 2 PO bid or if susceptible clindamycin 300 mg PO qid
  - Inpt: vancomycin 1 g IV q12h; if >100 kg, 1.5 g IV q12h

Breast Implant Infection

- Acute: vancomycin 1 g IV q12h; if >100 kg, 1.5 g IV q12h
- Chronic: Await culture results.

2 LUNG ABSCESS

Etiology

- Aspiration is the most common factor.
- 90% of abscesses are caused by anaerobic microorganisms (*Bacteroides fragilis, Fusobacterium, Peptostreptococcus*).
- In most cases, anaerobic infection is mixed w/aerobic or facultative anaerobic organisms (*S. aureus, Escherichia coli, K. pneumoniae, P. aeruginosa*).
- Immunocompromised hosts may become infected w/*Aspergillus, Mycobacteria, Nocardia,* and *Rhodococcus equi.*

Diagnosis

H&P

- Fever, cough, sputum production (purulent w/foul odor), hemoptysis
- Dullness to percussion, whispered pectoriloquy and bronchophony

Labs

- Blood tests nonspecific/rarely helpful: CBC w/leukocytosis, blood cultures, sputum Gram stain and culture
- Fiberoptic bronchoscopy with use of bronchial brushings or BAL fluid helpful to obtain dx bacteriologic cultures

Imaging

- CXR: cavitary lesion w/an air-fluid level
- Chest CT: localize and size lesion, assist in differentiating from other processes

Treatment

- PCN 1 to 2 million U IV q4h until improvement, followed by PCN V K 500 mg qid for at least 3 wk
- Metronidazole given w/PCN at doses of 7.5 mg/kg IV q6h followed by PO 500 mg bid to qid
- Clindamycin (if concerned about PCN resistance) 600 mg IV q8h, then by 300 mg PO q6h

Clinical Pearls

- Risk factors: alcoholism, seizure disorder, CVA w/dysphagia, poor oral hygiene, bronchiectasis, obstructive lung lesions, esophageal disorders, drug abuse
- Cure rate >95% w/appropriate abx
- Necrotizing pneumonia is similar to lung abscess but differs in size (<2 cm in diameter) and number (usually multiple suppurative cavitary lesions).

3 LIVER ABSCESS

Pyogenic (most common in United States) or amebic (most common worldwide via *Entamoeba histolytica*).

Etiology

■ Pyogenic = polymicrobial (*K. pneumoniae* [43%], *E. coli* [33%], *Streptococcus* spp [37%], *P. aeruginosa*, *Proteus* spp, *Bacteroides* spp [24%], *Fusobacterium* spp, *Actinomyces* spp., Gram[+] anaerobes, and *S. aureus*). Arising from cholangitis (40%-60%), gallbladder disease, diverticulitis/appendicitis spread via portal circulation, penetrating wounds, cryptogenic, portal pyemia, incidence ↑ DM/metastatic cancer

Diagnosis

■ W/up should focus on differentiating between amebic and pyogenic causes.
■ Features suggesting an amebic cause include travel to an endemic area, single abscess rather than multiple abscesses, subacute onset of sx, and absence of conditions predisposing to pyogenic liver abscess, as highlighted in "Etiology."
■ Lab studies are not specific but are useful as adjunctive tests.
■ Imaging cannot differentiate between the two, and bacteriologic cultures may be sterile in 50% of the cases.

H&P

■ Fever, RUQ abdominal pain, nausea, jaundice, hepatomegaly

Labs

■ CBC: leukocytosis
■ LFTs: alk phos ↑ (95%-100%); AST/ALT ↑ (50%); ↑ bilirubin (28%-30%); ↓ alb
■ PT (INR): prolonged (70%)
■ Blood cultures: (+) in 50% cases
■ Aspiration (50% sterile)
■ Stool samples for *E. histolytica* trophozoites (+ in 10%-15% of amebic liver abscess cases)
■ Serologic testing for *E. histolytica* does not differentiate acute from old infections.

Imaging

■ U/S (80%-100% sensitivity in detecting abscesses) shows a round or oval hypoechogenic mass.
■ CT scan (imaging study of choice)
■ CXR: abnl (50%). It may reveal ↑ right hemidiaphragm, subdiaphragmatic air-fluid levels, pleural effusions, and consolidating infiltrates.

Treatment

■ Serologic tests for amebiasis should be done on all pts.
  • If sero(−): surgical drainage or percutaneous aspiration warranted
  • If sero(+) amebiasis: Rx tissue agent (metronidazole 750 mg PO tid × 10 days) + luminal agent (paromomycin 10 days or diiodohydroxyquin 20 days) required even if stool (−)
■ Aspiration of hepatic amebic abscesses not required unless poor Rx response/pyogenic cause
■ Empiric broad-spectrum Abxs recommended initially until culture results are available.
  • Metronidazole (500 mg IV q8h) + fluoroquinolone (ciprofloxacin 400 mg IV q12h or levofloxacin 500 mg IV daily)
  • Piperacillin-tazobactam (4.5 g q6h), ticarcillin-clavulanate (3.1 g q4h), or ampicillin-sulbactam (3 g q6h)
  • Imipenem (500 mg IV q6h), meropenem (1 g q8h), or ertapenem (1 g daily)
  • If PCN allergy: clindamycin 600 to 900 mg IV q8h + aminoglycoside
  • Rx duration 4 to 6 wk with IV abxs used for wk 1 to 2 or until favorable clinical response, followed by PO abxs (e.g., metronidazole 500 mg PO q8h plus ciprofloxacin 500 mg PO q12h)
  • Third-generation cephalosporins should not be used for empiric Rx because of risk of the emergence of β-lactamase–producing bacteria.

4 PELVIC ABSCESS

Etiology

■ Mixed flora of anaerobes, aerobes, and facultative anaerobes (*E. coli*, *B. fragilis*, *Prevotella* species, aerobic streptococci, *Peptococcus*, *Peptostreptococcus*)

Diagnosis

H&P

■ Abd or pelvic pain, fever, nausea, abnl bleeding, vaginal d/c

- CBC w/diff; aerobic and anaerobic cultures of blood, cervix, urine, peritoneal cavity (if entered) before starting abx; pregnancy test in all women of childbearing age

Imaging
- CT of pelvis (study of choice)
- U/S also excellent modality (>90% sensitivity)
- Surgical diagnostic options: CT-guided drainage, laparoscopy w/drainage and irrigation, transvaginal colpotomy (midline abscess), laparotomy

Treatment
- Decision on whether pt requires immediate surgery (uncertain dx or suspicion of rupture) or management w/IV abx, w/surgery reserved for pts w/inadequate clinical response
- Clindamycin 900 mg IV q8h + gentamicin 5 to 7 mg/kg q24h or 1.5 mg/kg q8h
- Alternatives: ampicillin-sulbactam 3 g IV q6h, or cefoxitin 2 g IV q6h, + doxycycline 100 mg IV q12h

5 PERIRECTAL ABSCESS

Etiology
- Polymicrobial aerobic (*S. aureus*, *Streptococcus* species, *E. coli*) and anaerobic bacteria (*B. fragilis*, *Peptostreptococcus* species, *Prevotella* species, *Fusobacterium* species)

Diagnosis

H&P
- Localized perirectal or anal pain, often worsened w/movement or straining; perirectal erythema or mass by inspection or palpation
- Many pts have predisposing conditions (DM, malignant neoplasm/leukemia, immune deficiency, steroid Rx, recent surgery).

Labs
- CBC w/diff; local aerobic and anaerobic cultures; blood cultures if toxic, febrile, or immunocompromised

Imaging
- Sigmoidoscopy in selected cases
- Imaging (pelvic CT) usually not indicated unless extensive disease, abscess, or immunocompromised pt

Treatment
- I&D; débridement if necrotic tissue, r/o need for fistulectomy
- Local wound care: packing, Sitz baths
- Outpt abx—PO
  - Amoxicillin/clavulanic acid 875 to 1000 mg bid
  - Ciprofloxacin 750 mg PO q12h + metronidazole 500 to 750 mg PO q8h *or*
  - Clindamycin 150 to 300 mg PO q8h
- Inpt abx—IV
  - Ampicillin-sulbactam (Unasyn) 1.5 to 3 g IV q6h
  - Cefotetan 1 to 2 g IV q8h
  - Piperacillin-tazobactam 3.375 g IV q6-8h
  - Imipenem 500 to 1000 mg IV q8h

6 PERITONSILLAR ABSCESS

Infection located between the capsule of the palatine tonsil and the superior constrictor muscle of the pharynx

Etiology
- Peritonsillar abscess is a complication of tonsillitis.
- Group A β-hemolytic streptococcus is the most common bacterial cause, accounting for 15% to 30% of cases in children and 5% to 10% of cases in adults.
- Less common aerobic causes are *S. aureus*, *H. influenzae*, *Neisseria* species.
- The most common anaerobic organism is *Fusobacterium*.

Diagnosis

H&P
- Sore throat, which may be severe; dysphagia and odynophagia; otalgia; foul-smelling breath
- Facial swelling, drooling, headache, fever, trismus
- Hoarseness, muffled voice (also called "hot potato voice")
- Tender submandibular and anterior cervical lymph nodes, tonsillar hypertrophy, contralateral deflection of the uvula, stridor

- Rapid strep antigen-detecting testing and throat swab C&S
- Aspiration of the abscess for C&S

Imaging
- CT soft tissue of neck

Treatment
- Empiric abx Rx
  - PO: amoxicillin-clavulanic acid 875 mg bid, PCN VK 500 mg qid + metronidazole 500 mg qid, or clindamycin 600 mg bid
  - IV: ampicillin-sulbactam 3 g q6h or clindamycin 900 mg q8h
- Steroids may be helpful in reducing sx and speeding recovery.
- Tonsillectomy: 3 to 6 mo after dx
- Although rare, in adults and children w/peritonsillar abscess and h/o recurrent pharyngitis or peritonsillar abscess, the specialist may proceed w/tonsillectomy (a quinsy or "hot" tonsillectomy) directly after prescribing the pt IV abx.

Clinical Pearl
- Complications: airway obstruction, lung abscess or aspiration pneumonia, GN, rheumatic fever, erosion into carotid sheath, and extension of infection into tissues of the deep neck or posterior mediastinum.

7 RETROPHARYNGEAL ABSCESS

Soft tissue infection of the retropharyngeal space (middle [anteriorly] and deep [posteriorly] layers of the deep cervical fascia)

Etiology
- *Streptococcus pyogenes* (group A streptococcus [GAS]), *S. aureus,* and respiratory anaerobes (*Fusobacterium, Prevotella,* and *Veillonella* species), *Haemophilus* (occasional)
- In young children, infection via lymphatic spread from a pharyngeal/sinus septic focus
- In adults, infection via local penetrating trauma (e.g., chicken bones or after instrumentation) or odontogenic sepsis and peritonsillar abscess (rare)

Diagnosis

H&P
- Insidious onset fever, irritability, drooling, a muffled voice (dysphonia), or possibly nuchal rigidity
- Possible intense dysphagia/drooling/odynophagia, or element of respiratory distress from edema and inflammation of the airway (stridor and/or tachypnea)
- Unwillingness to move the neck because of discomfort (prominent presenting feature; especially if febrile/irritable child) causing pt to present holding neck stiffly or w/torticollis
- Trismus is unusual.
- Possible midline/unilateral swelling of posterior pharyngeal wall; mass may be fluctuant to the examining finger (care must be taken to avoid abscess rupture into airway)

Imaging
- CT of soft tissues of the neck
- MRI of neck w/gadolinium (↑ sensitivity than CT)

Treatment
- PCN (2-4 million U IV q4h) + metronidazole (1-g IV loading dose then 500 mg IV q6h) or ampicillin-sulbactam (50 mg/kg/dose IV q6h) or clindamycin (600-900 mg IV q8h)
- Surgical: drainage indicated if large hypodense area or pt unresponsive to IV Rx alone

Clinical Pearl
- Complications are numerous and could be fatal (airway obstruction, septicemia, internal jugular vein thrombosis-*Lemierre's syndrome*, carotid artery rupture, acute necrotizing mediastinitis). Aspiration w/resultant pneumonia may complicate retropharyngeal abscess if rupture of the abscess occurs and empties into the airway.

E. SKIN/SOFT TISSUE/BONE/JOINT INFECTIONS

1 CELLULITIS

Superficial inflammatory condition of the skin characterized by erythema, warmth, and tenderness of the area involved

Etiology

- Group A β-hemolytic streptococci (may follow streptococcal URI)
- Staphylococcal cellulitis
- *H. influenzae*
- *Vibrio vulnificus:* ↑ incidence pts w/liver disease (75%) and in immunocompromised hosts (corticosteroid use, DM, leukemia, renal failure)
- *Erysipelothrix rhusiopathiae:* handlers of poultry, fish, or meat
- *Aeromonas hydrophila:* contaminated open wound in fresh water
- Fungi *(Cryptococcus neoformans),* Gram(−) rods *(Serratia, Enterobacter, Proteus, Pseudomonas):* immunocompromised granulopenic pts

Diagnosis

H&P

- Erysipelas: superficial spreading, warm, erythematous lesion distinguished by indurated and ↑ margin; lymphatic involvement + vesicle formation common
- Staphylococcal cellulitis: area erythematous, hot/swollen; differentiated from erysipelas by nonelevated poorly demarcated margin; local tenderness/regional adenopathy common (85% cases occur on legs and feet)
- *H. influenzae* cellulitis (children, face; adults, neck/upper chest): area blue red/purple red
- *Vibrio vulnificus* (critically ill pt in septic shock): larger hemorrhagic bullae, cellulitis, lymphadenitis, myositis

Labs

- In severe cases, CBC w/diff, Gram stain/culture (aerobic and anaerobic), blood cultures, ASO titer (in suspected streptococcal disease)

Treatment

Extremities, Nondiabetic (Leg Elevation Helpful)

- Inpt: PCN G 1 to 2 million U IV q6h or cefazolin 1 g IV q8h
- *If PCN allergy: vancomycin 15 mg/kg IV q12h
- If afebrile: PCN V K 500 mg PO qid ac and hs × 10 days
- Outpt: PCN V K 500 mg PO qid ac and hs × 10 days
- *If PCN allergy: azithromycin 500 mg PO × 1, then 250 mg PO daily × 4 days

Facial, Erysipelas

- Primary: vancomycin 1 g IV q12h; if >100 kg, 1.5g IV q12h
- Alternate: daptomycin 4 mg/kg IV q24h or linezolid 600 mg IV q12h

Orbital Cellulitis (S. pneumoniae, H. influenzae, S. aureus, anaerobes, GAS)

- **Dx:** image orbit (CT or MRI); ↑ risk cavernous sinus thrombosis
- **Rx:** nafcillin 2 g IV (or if MRSA → vancomycin 30 to 50 mg/kg/day in two to three divided doses to achieve trough 15 to 20 μg/mL) + ceftriaxone 2 g IV q24h + metronidazole 1 g IV q12h
- *If PCN/cephalosporin allergy:* vancomycin + levofloxacin 750 mg IV once daily + metronidazole IV

Staphylococcus Cellulitis

- PO: dicloxacillin 250 to 500 mg qid
- IV: nafcillin 1 to 2 g q4-6h
- Cephalosporins (cephalothin, cephalexin, cephradine) also provide adequate antistaphylococcal coverage except for MRSA.
- Use vancomycin 1.0 to 2.0 g IV qd or linezolid 0.6 g IV q12h in pts allergic to PCN or cephalosporins and in pts w/MRSA. Daptomycin (Cubicin), 4 mg/kg IV given over 30 min q24h, is also effective. Other agents that may be effective against some strains of MRSA include quinupristin-dalfopristin (Synercid) and TMP-SMZ.

Haemophilus influenzae Cellulitis

- PO: cefixime or cefuroxime
- IV: cefuroxime or ceftriaxone

Vibrio vulnificus

- Doxycycline 100 mg IV bid + ceftazidime 2 g IV q8h or IV ciprofloxacin 400 mg bid. Mild cases can be treated w/PO abx (doxycycline 100 mg bid + ciprofloxacin 750 mg bid).
- IV support and admission into ICU (mortality rate >50% in septic shock)

Erysipelothrix

- PCN

Aeromonas hydrophila

- Aminoglycosides
- Chloramphenicol
- Complicated skin and skin structure infections in hospitalized pts can be treated w/daptomycin (Cubicin) 4 mg/kg IV q24h.

Clinical Pearls
- Cellulitis occurs most frequently in pts with DM, immunocompromised hosts, and pts w/venous and lymphatic compromise.
- Frequently found near skin breaks (trauma, surgical wounds, ulcerations, tinea infections)

2 METHICILLIN-RESISTANT *STAPHYLOCOCCUS AUREUS*

Diagnosis
H&P
- CA-MRSA: can manifest with skin infection; red bump, pustule, or boil; erythema, swelling; edema, often fluctuant and very painful
- HA-MRSA: bacteremia; infection associated with IV device
  - Catheters (pneumonia), skin (cellulitis), bone (osteomyelitis), endocarditis, abscesses, pneumonia (nosocomial)

W/up
- Culture of wound, abscess, blood, sputum; r/o colonization; culture of nares or axillae
- Radiographs or CT scan of suspected organ
- Echocardiogram if endocarditis suspected

Treatment
- CA-MRSA: PO TMP-SMX-DS, doxycycline, minocycline, clindamycin (linezolid expensive)
- HA-MRSA: IV vancomycin (15-20 mg/kg IV q8-12h), linezolid (600 mg), daptomycin, telavancin
- Abscess surgically drained
  - Telavancin 10 mg/kg IV per day is bactericidal against MRSA.
  - Ceftaroline (fifth-generation cephalosporin) is also effective against MRSA.
  - Pts with MRSA colonization may have re-exposure or may be unable to eradicate colonized state. Eradication may be attempted via PO agents (rifampin, tetracycline, and minocycline) or mupirocin ointment to nares/infected skin sites.

3 TOXIC SHOCK SYNDROME (TSS)
Acute febrile illness resulting in multiple organ system dysfunction caused most commonly by a bacterial exotoxin

Etiology
- Menstrually associated TSS: 45% of cases associated w/tampons, diaphragm, or vaginal sponge use
- Non–menstruating-associated TSS: 55% of cases associated w/puerperal sepsis, post–cesarean section endometritis, mastitis, wound or skin infection, insect bite, PID, and postoperative fever
- Causative agent: *S. aureus* infection of a susceptible individual (10% of population lacking sufficient levels of antitoxin Abs) that liberates the disease mediator TSST-1 (exotoxin)
- Other causative agents: coagulase(–) streptococci producing enterotoxins B or C, and exotoxin A producing group A β-hemolytic streptococci

Diagnosis
H&P
- Fever (>38.9° C), myalgia, headache, photophobia, rigors/arthralgia, conjunctivitis
- Diffuse macular erythrodermatous rash that desquamates 1 to 2 wk after disease onset in survivors
- Orthostatic to severe hypotension and ARF
- GI sx: vomiting, diarrhea, abd tenderness
- Respiratory sx: dysphagia, pharyngeal hyperemia, strawberry tongue
- GU sx: vaginal d/c, vaginal hyperemia, adnexal tenderness
- End-organ failure (ARF, hepatic failure)
- CV sx: DIC, pulmonary edema, ARDS, endomyocarditis, heart block

Labs
- Pan culture (cervix/vagina, throat, nasal passages, urine, blood, CSF, wound) for *Staphylococcus, Streptococcus,* or other pathogenic organisms
- Electrolytes to detect hypokalemia, hyponatremia
- CBC w/diff, PT, PTT
- Total Protein, AST, ALT, hypocalcemia, BUN/Cr, hypophosphatemia, LDH, CPK
- U/A: WBC (>5/hpf), proteinemia, microhematuria
- ABGs (assess respiratory function and acid-base status)
- Serology (RMSF, Lyme disease, rubeola, and leptospirosis)

Imaging
- CXR
- U/S, CT scan, MRI: if abd/pelvic abscess suspected

Treatment
- Aggressive fluid resuscitation (maintenance of circulating volume, CO, BP)
- Search for localized infection/nidus: I&D, débridement, removal of tampon or vaginal sponge
- Consider central hemodynamic monitoring: Swan-Ganz catheter and A-line for surveillance of hemodynamic status and response to Rx
- Foley catheter to monitor hourly urine output
- Possible MAST trousers as temporary measure
- Staphylococcal: nafcillin or oxacillin 2 g IV q4h or (if MRSA, vancomycin 1 g IV q12h + clindamycin 600 to 900 mg IV q8h + IVIG 1 g/kg day 1, then 0.5 g/kg days 2 and 3)
- Streptococcal: PCN G 24 million U/day IV in divided doses + clindamycin 900 mg IV q8h or ceftriaxone 2 g IV q24h + clindamycin 900 mg IV q8h
- Doxycycline added if RMSF is being considered
- *IVIG associated with ↓ in sepsis-related organ failure: dose = 1 g/kg day 1, then 0.5 g/kg days 2 and 3
- Acute ventilator management if severe respiratory compromise
- Renal dialysis for severe renal impairment
- Surgical intervention as indicated (i.e., ruptured tubo-ovarian abscess, wound abscess, mastitis)
- Isotonic crystalloid (NS solution) for volume replacement following "7-3" rule
- Electrolyte replacement (K^+, Ca^+)
- PRBC, coagulation factor replacement, or FFP to treat anemia or D&C
- Vasopressor Rx for hypotension refractory to fluid volume replacement (i.e., dopamine 2-5 mg/kg/min)

4 DIABETIC FOOT INFECTIONS

Etiology
- Staphylococci/streptococci
- Most often s/p trauma via neuropathy, vascular insufficiency, and immunodeficiency

Diagnosis
Clinical Findings
- Mild (<2 cm: purulence/inflammation, pain, superficial warmth/erythema/induration)
- Moderate (>2 cm: gangrene, deep tissue abscess, spread to lymph/muscle/joint/tendon)
- Severe (limb-threatening, fever, tachycardia, hypotension, kidney injury, ∆MS, leukocytosis)

W/up
- Assessment for possible arterial insufficiency, bone involvement
- Wound care with cleansing, débridement, and off-loading of pressure

Treatment
- All diabetic pts should have at least annual foot examination assessing ↓ sensation, ulcers, calluses, foot deformities, pain, abnl pain response, and peripheral pulses.
- Ulcers that are clinically uninfected should not be Rx with abx.
- Abx should cover Gram(+) staph/strep.
- Severe infection (limb-threatening) requires surgical evaluation and initial broad-spectrum abx.

5 NECROTIZING FASCIITIS

Deep-seated infection of SC tissue resulting in progressive destruction of fascia and fat

Etiology
- Prior surgery
- Trauma
- Causative organisms: streptococci, clostridia, mixed flora (polymicrobic: aerobic + anaerobic [*Meleney's synergistic gangrene* if *S. aureus* + anaerobic strep]), CA-MRSA

Diagnosis
H&P
- Diffuse swelling of an arm or leg, followed by the appearance of bullae filled w/clear fluid (can appear maroon or violaceous)
- Systemic sx may include shock and organ failure.

- Incision and probing of site, Gram stain, C&S

Imaging
- CT or MRI of affected extremity

Treatment
- Surgical débridement, Gram stain/culture, in addition to abx
- If strep or clostridia: PCN G 24 million U/day div q4-6h IV + clindamycin 900 mg IV q8h
- If polymicrobial: imipenem or meropenem
- Add vancomycin or daptomycin if MRSA suspected

6 MUSCLE ("GAS GANGRENE")
- Primary Rx: clindamycin 900 mg IV q8h + PCN G 24 million U/day divided q4-6h IV
- Alternative Rx: ceftriaxone 2 g IV q12h or erythromycin 1 g q6h IV
- Surgical débridement essential; hyperbaric O_2 possible adjunctive Rx (efficacy variable)

7 BITES
Animal Bites
- Dog bites < likely to become infected than cat bites

Management
- Adequate wound irrigation/débridement + abx if infected wound
- Need for tetanus and rabies prophylaxis determined
- Abx prophylaxis needed: immunocompromised, wound near joint/bone, crush injury, edematous wound
- Rx cat bite *(Pasteurella multocida):* amoxicillin-clavulanate (875/125 mg PO bid or 500/125 mg PO tid) or doxycycline 100 mg PO bid
- Rx dog bite *(Pasteurella canis):* amoxicillin-clavulanate (875/125 mg PO bid or 500/125 mg PO tid) or clindamycin 300 mg PO qid + fluoroquinolone

Human Bites
- Early: amoxicillin-clavulanate 875/125 mg PO bid × 5 days; late: ampicillin-sulbactam 1.5 g IV q6h or cefoxitin 2 g IV q8h
- *If PCN allergy: clindamycin + (ciprofloxacin or TMP-SMX)
- Débridement with wound cleaning/irrigation **essential**
- Prophylactic therapy for persons bitten by others with HIV and/or hepatitis B
- Clenched-fist injuries require radiographic evaluation, possibly hospitalization.

8 OSTEOMYELITIS
Infection of bone and bone marrow

Etiology
- *S. aureus*: most common
- Gram(−) bacilli: *Salmonella, E. coli, Pseudomonas, Klebsiella*
- *Salmonella:* sickle cell disease
- *Pseudomonas:* IV drug addicts; puncture wounds in sneakers
- Coagulase(−) staphylococci or *Propionibacterium:* foreign body
- Anaerobes: infected decubitus ulcers in sacrum
- *Bartonella henselae:* HIV infection
- *P. multocida* or *Eikenella corrodens:* human or animal bites

Diagnosis
- Tenderness over the bone and limitations of movement of the involved extremity
- Definitive dx via isolation of infective organism from bone or joint fluid obtained either by surgery or multiple percutaneous needle bx
- MRI: most accurate imaging study
- Doppler studies: in pts w/PVD to determine vascular adequacy

Treatment
- Hematogenous osteomyelitis empiric Rx
  - MRSA possible: vancomycin 1 g IV q12h; if >100 kg, 1.5 g IV q12h
  - MRSA unlikely: nafcillin or oxacillin 2 g IV q4h
  - Allergy/toxicity: TMP-SMX 8 to 10 mg/kg per day divided IV q8h or linezolid 600 mg IV/PO q12h
- Contiguous osteomyelitis **without** vascular insufficiency empiric Rx
  - Primary: ciprofloxacin 750 mg PO bid or levofloxacin 750 mg PO q24h
  - Alternative: ceftazidime 2 g IV q8h or cefepime 2 g IV q12h

- Contiguous osteomyelitis **with** vascular insufficiency
  - No empiric Rx unless acutely ill; débride ulcer and submit bone for histology and culture, selecting abx based on results. Rx for 6 wk.
- Chronic osteomyelitis
  - Surgical débridement important, immobilization of affected bone (plaster, traction) if bone is unstable.

9 SEPTIC ARTHRITIS

Etiology
- *S. aureus*, β-hemolytic strep, and Gram(–) bacilli
- Gonococcus

Diagnosis
- Acute onset of a swollen painful joint, ↓ range of motion, erythema, ↑ warmth around the joint
- Joint aspiration, Gram stain and C&S of synovial fluid (synovial fluid leukocyte count is usually >50,000 cells/mL^3 w/a diff count of 80% or more PMNs)
- Joint x-ray, CT scan, technetium and gallium scans

Treatment
- At risk for STD, Gram stain(–): ceftriazone 1g IV q24h
- At risk for STD, Gram stain(+): vancomycin 1 g IV q12h; if >100 kg, 1.5 g IV q12h
- No risk for STD: all empiric choices guided by Gram stain
  - Vancomycin + third-generation cephalosporin 10 to 14 days
  - Vancomycin + (ciprofloxacin or levofloxacin) 10 to 14 days
  - Acute, polyarticular: ceftriaxone 1 g IV q24h
  - S/p intra-articular injection: no empiric Rx (arthroscopy for C&S, crystals, washout; Rx based on culture results × 14 days assuming no foreign body present)
- Infected prosthetic joint
  - Cultures pending: no empiric Rx, need C&S results; may ↑ culture yield via sonication
  - *S. pyogenes*/viridans strep: débridement + prosthesis retention; PCN G or ceftriaxone IV × 4 wk
  - Methicillin-sensitive *Staphylococcus epidermidis* (MSSE)/MSSA: (nafcillin/oxacillin 2 g IV q4h + rifampin 300 mg IV/PO bid) or (vancomycin 1 g IV q12h + rifampin 300 mg IV/PO bid) or (daptomycin 6 mg/kg IV q24h + rifampin 300 mg IV/PO bid) × 6 wk
  - Methicillin-resistant *Staphylococcus epidermidis* (MRSE)/MRSA: (vancomycin 1 g IV q12h + rifampin 300 mg IV/PO) × 6 wk
  - *P. aeruginosa*: ceftazidime 2 g IV q8h + (ciprofloxacin 750 mg IV/PO bid or levofloxacin 750 mg IV/PO q24h)

10 SEPTIC BURSITIS

Inflammation with infection of a bursa (thin-walled sac lined with synovial tissue facilitating movement of tendons/muscles over bony prominences)

Etiology
- Acute trauma or repetitive injury
- Infection: from hematogenous seeding or spread from contiguous infection (septic bursitis)
- Crystal diseases (e.g., gout, pseudogout)
- Systemic arthritis (i.e., rheumatoid arthritis)

Diagnosis
H&P
- Swelling, when bursitis is superficial (olecranon, prepatellar)
- Local tenderness at site of bursa; pain with joint movement and rest
- Peribursal erythema and warmth (septic bursitis)
- Referred pain

W/up
- Bursal fluid aspiration: Send for Gram stain and culture and sensitivity (C&S) cell count and diff; and crystal analysis.

Imaging
- Plain radiography: R/o foreign body penetration and other potential/coexisting bone/joint problems.
- MRI (extent of soft tissue involvement)
- Musculoskeletal U/S can aid visualization of bursae and guide aspiration/injection.

Treatment
- Avoidance of direct pressure or irritation (joint protection) with rest, ice, elevation, and physical Rx for acute phase

- Septic
  - If MSSA: nafcillin or oxacillin 2 g IV q4h or dicloxacillin 500 mg PO qid
  - If MRSA: vancomycin 15 to 20 mg/kg IV q8-12h or linezolid 600 mg PO bid
  - 7 days of abx may be sufficient for immunocompetent pt undergoing one-stage bursectomy because immunosuppression (not Rx duration) ↑ recurrence risk.
  - Drainage + aspiration of purulent fluid with a large-bore needle (if there is no rapid clinical response, incision and drainage are indicated)
- Nonseptic: aspiration of bursal fluid or blood from acute trauma
- Chronic pain may warrant steroid injection into bursa (40 mg triamcinolone mixed with 1-3 mL lidocaine, depending on size of bursa).
- NSAIDs PRN

Clinical Pearls
- In pts with RA, acute bursitis should be considered septic bursitis until proven otherwise.
- Scapulothoracic bursitis is underrecognized and undertreated. It results from friction between the superomedial angle of the scapula and adjacent second and third ribs. Crepitus, snapping, and tenderness are suggestive findings; it can also cause chest wall pain.
- Sterile bursae should not undergo I&D because a chronic draining sinus tract may develop.
- Pts with crystal-induced bursitis should be investigated for underlying metabolic/hematologic disease (gout, hemochromatosis, hyperparathyroidism-calcium pyrophosphate deposition disease).

11 SKIN INFESTATIONS

a. Scabies (Sarcoptes scabiei)

Diagnosis
- Via clinical presentation + mites, eggs, or mite feces
- Intense pruritus (especially nocturnal) 1 to 4 wk after the primary infestation (in web spaces of the hands, wrists, buttocks, scrotum, penis, breasts, axillae, and knees) from acquired sensitivity to the mite or fecal pellets
- Skin exam: burrows, tiny vesicles, excoriations, inflammatory papules

Treatment
- Permethrin 5% cream massaged into the skin from head to soles of feet. Remove 8 to 14 hr later by washing.
- PO ivermectin single dose (150-200 mg/kg)
- Topical corticosteroid creams for secondary eczematous dermatitis
- AIDS and HTLV-infected (CD4 <150 per mm^3) pts: permethrin 5% cream daily × 7 days, then 2 × wk until cured

b. Bed bugs

Etiology
- Cimex hemipterus/Cimex lectularius: nocturnal feeding via saliva containing nitrophorin (anticoagulant interfering with factor Xa, inhibiting Plt aggregation)

Diagnosis
- Firm, purpuric/erythematous macules, papules, urticaria, or bullae may be present.
- Bite may have a central hemorrhagic punctum; it is generally on areas of exposed skin.
- Insect has poor attachment mechanism; thus person-person transmission is unlikely.
- Victim may observe a linear series of three bites ("breakfast, lunch, and dinner").
- W/up begins with hx and physical for clinical sx and environmental findings.
- Bites are histologically similar to other insect bites (perivascular infiltrate of lymphocytes, histiocytes, eosinophils, and mast cells within upper dermis).

Treatment
- Topical glucocorticoids/systemic antihistamines if severe pruritus
  - Triamcinolone cream 0.1%. Apply thin film to affected areas bid.
  - Chlorpheniramine 4 mg PO hs (adults), 2 mg PO hs (children)
- Multi-insecticides (because of resistance) may be effective in eradication; consult pest control.
  - Use permethrin spray for clothing and bedsheets or bednets.
  - Deltamethrin and chlorfenapyr are two common insecticides used.

c. Lice (Pediculosis)

- **Head lice Rx:** Permethrin 1% lotion to shampooed/dried hair 10 min. Repeat in 9 days.
- **Pubic lice Rx** ("crabs"): Permethrin 1% lotion to clean/dried hair 10 min. Repeat in 9 days.
- **Body lice Rx:** No abx; lice in clothing, thus discard. If not possible, apply 1% malathion powder to clothing.

F. FEVER OF UNKOWN ORIGIN (FUO)

Table 8-1 describes definitions and major features of the four subtypes of FUO.

G. SEXUALLY TRANSMITTED DISEASES

1 CHLAMYDIA *TRACHOMATIS* INFECTION

- This most common bacterial STI in United States results in urethritis, epididymitis, cervicitis, and acute salpingitis, but often asx in women. In men, sx include urethritis, mucopurulent d/c, dysuria, urethral pruritus.

Diagnosis

H&P

- Clinical manifestations may be similar to those of gonorrhea: mucopurulent endocervical d/c w/edema, erythema, and easily induced endocervical bleeding caused by inflammation of endocervical columnar epithelium. Less frequent manifestations may include bartholinitis, urethral syndrome w/dysuria and pyuria, perihepatitis *(Fitz-Hugh-Curtis syndrome)*.

Labs

- Cell culture (single culture sensitivity 80%-90%), but it is labor intensive/takes 48-96 hr. It is not suited for large screening programs.
- Nonculture methods
  - DFA, EIA, DNA probes, PCR
  - W/the exception of PCR, the other tests are probably less specific than cell culture and may yield false(+) results.
- Because this is an intracellular organism, purulent d/c is not an appropriate specimen. An adequate sample of infected cells must be obtained.

Treatment

- Evaluation and Rx of sex partners
- NGU, urethritis, cervicitis, conjunctivitis (except for LGV)
  - Primary: azithromycin 1g PO × 1 *or* doxycycline 100 mg PO bid × 7 days
  - Alternatives: erythromycin base 500 mg PO qid × 7 days *or* levofloxacin 500 mg q24h × 7 days
- Pregnancy: erythromycin base 500 mg PO qid × 7 days *or* amoxicillin 500 mg PO tid ×7 days
  - Note: Doxycycline and ofloxacin/levofloxacin are contraindicated in pregnancy.
- Recurrent/persistent urethritis: metronidazole 2 g PO × 1

Clinical Pearl

- Assume concomitant gonorrhea co-infection: PO ceftriaxone 125 mg IM single dose + azithromycin 1 g PO single dose will treat both.

2 *NEISSERIA GONORRHOEAE* INFECTION

This second most commonly reported bacterial sexually transmitted infection manifests as urethritis, cervicitis, or salpingitis. Infection may be asx (12%-15% men, 50%-80% women), differing between male and female pts in course/severity.

Diagnosis

- Gram(−) intracellular diplococci diagnostic in male urethral smears, 60% to 70% false(+) in female cervical/urethral smears. Culture, nucleic acid hybridization tests, and nucleic acid amplification tests (NAATs >99% specificity) require endocervical (female)/urethral (male) swab, or urine testing.
- Culture on Thayer-Martin medium (sensitivity ≥95%)
- Concomitant *Chlamydia* as well as serologic testing for syphilis on all pts
- Offer of HIV counseling and testing to all pts

H&P

- Male pts: purulent d/c from anterior urethra with dysuria appearing 2 to 7 days after infecting exposure. Pts may have rectal infection causing pruritus, tenesmus, and d/c or may be asx.

Feature	Classic FUO	Health Care-Associated FUO	Immune-Deficient FUO	HIV-Related FUO
Definition	≥38.0°C, >3 wk, >2 visits or 1 wk in hospital	≥38.0°C, >1 wk, not present or incubating on admission	≥38.0°C, >1 wk, negative cultures after 48 hr	≥38.0°C, >3 wk for outpatients, >1 wk for inpatients, HIV infection confirmed
Patient location	Community, clinic, or hospital	Acute care hospital	Hospital or clinic	Community, clinic, or hospital
Leading causes	Cancer, infections, inflammatory conditions, undiagnosed, habitual hyperthermia	Health care-associated infections, postoperative complications, drug fever	Majority caused by infections, but cause documented in only 40%-60%	HIV (primary infection), typical and atypical mycobacterial infection, CMV infection, lymphomas, toxoplasmosis, cryptococcosis, immune reconstitution inflammatory syndrome (IRIS)
History emphasis	Travel, contacts, animal and insect exposure, medications, immunizations, family history, cardiac valve disorder	Operations and procedures, devices, anatomic considerations, drug treatment	Stage of chemotherapy, drugs administered, underlying immunosuppressive disorder	Drugs, exposures, risk factors, travel, contacts, stage of HIV infection
Examination emphasis	Fundi, oropharynx, temporal artery, abdomen, lymph nodes, spleen, joints, skin, nails, genitalia, rectum or prostate, lower limb deep veins	Wounds, drains, devices, sinuses, urine	Skin folds, IV sites, lungs, perianal area	Mouth, sinuses, skin, lymph nodes, eyes, lungs, perianal area
Investigation emphasis	Imaging, biopsies, sedimentation rate, skin tests	Imaging, bacterial cultures	CXR, bacterial cultures	Blood and lymphocyte count; serologic tests; CXR; stool examination; biopsies of lung, bone marrow, and liver for cultures and cytologic tests; brain imaging
Management	Observation, outpatient temperature chart, investigations, avoidance of empiric drug treatments	Depends on situation	Antimicrobial treatment protocols	Antiviral and antimicrobial protocols, vaccines, revision of treatment regimens, good nutrition
Time course of disease	Months	Weeks	Days	Weeks to months
Tempo of investigation	Weeks	Days	Hours	Days to weeks

TABLE 8-1 ■ Summary of Definitions and Major Features of the Four Subtypes of Fever of Unknown Origin

Adapted from Mandell GL, Bennett, JE, Dolin R (eds): Mandell, Douglas, and Bennett's Principles and Practice of Infectious Diseases, 7th ed. Philadelphia, Churchill Livingstone, 2010, p 780. From Kliegman RM, Stanton B, St. Geme J, et al (eds): Nelson Textbook of Pediatrics, 19th ed. Philadelphia, Saunders, 2011.

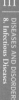

III

DISEASES AND DISORDERS
8. Infectious Diseases

- Female pts: initial urethritis or cervicitis may occur days after exposure, frequently mild; uterine invasion (20%) after menstrual period with sx of endometritis, salpingitis, or pelvic peritonitis. Pts may have purulent d/c or inflamed Skene's or Bartholin's glands.
- Acute gonococcal PID: fever, abd and adnexal tenderness, in absence of purulent d/c. Disseminated gonococcal infection may manifest with various skin lesions.

Treatment
- Uncomplicated infections of the cervix, urethra, and rectum
  - Ceftriaxone 250 mg IM + azithromycin 1 g PO *or* doxycycline 100 mg PO bid for 7 days
- Alternative regimens
  - Cefixime 400 mg PO + azithromycin 1 g PO *or* doxycycline 100 mg PO bid for 7 days + test of cure at 1 wk
  - Cephalosporin allergy: azithromycin 2 g PO + test of cure at 1 wk
- Uncomplicated gonococcal infections of the pharynx
  - Ceftriaxone 250 mg IM + azithromycin 1 g PO *or* doxycycline 100 mg PO bid for 7 days
  - Pregnant pts require test of cure (reculture 4-7 days s/p Rx).
  - All sexual partners should be identified, examined, tested, and receive presumptive Rx.
  - This is a reportable disease.

3 PELVIC INFLAMMATORY DISEASE (PID)
- Spectrum of inflammatory disorders of the upper genital tract
  - Endometritis, salpingitis, tubo-ovarian abscess, or pelvic peritonitis
  - Resulting from an ascending lower genital tract infection
  - Not related to obstetric or surgical intervention
  - Most common cause of female infertility and ectopic pregnancy

Risk Factors
- Adolescent sexually active females <20 yr; multiple sexual partners; hx gonococcal PID

Diagnosis
H&P
- Fever, lower abdominal pain, dysuria, dyspareunia
- Abnl vaginal d/c and/or uterine bleeding
- Nausea and vomiting (suggestive of peritonitis)
- RUQ tenderness (perihepatitis): 5% of cases
- Cervical motion tenderness and adnexal tenderness/mass
- Clinical dx of sx of PID (PPV 65%-90%) compared with laparoscopy: oral temp >38.3°C (101°F), abnl cervical or vaginal d/c, ↑ ESR/CRP, cervical infection *(N. gonorrhoeae/C. trachomatis)*, leukocytosis with ↑ WBC on saline microscopy of vaginal fluid Gram stain endocervical exudate: >30 PMN cells/hpf (chlamydial/gonococcal)
- Endocervical cultures for *N. gonorrhoeae* and *C. trachomatis*
- Fallopian tube aspirate or peritoneal exudate culture if laparoscopy performed
- β-hCG to r/o ectopic pregnancy
- Definitive criteria: laparoscopic abnlities, histopathologic evidence of endometritis on biopsy (warranted in women undergoing laparoscopy without visual evidence of salpingitis), transvaginal U/S (thickened fluid-filled tubes with/without free pelvic fluid/tubo-ovarian complex)

Treatment
- Empiric Rx: sexually active young women experiencing pelvic/lower abd pain without other cause and with ≥1 of the following present on pelvic examination: uterine tenderness, adnexal tenderness, cervical motion tenderness
- Outpt Rx if: temp <38°C, WBC <11,000 per mm³, minimal evidence peritonitis, active bowel sounds and able to tolerate PO intake: ([ceftriaxone 250 mg IM or IV × 1] [±metronidazole 500 mg PO bid × 14 days] + [doxycycline 100 mg PO bid × 14 days] *or* [cefoxitin 2 g IM with probenecid 1 g PO; both as single dose] + [doxycycline 100 mg PO bid with metronidazole 500 mg PO bid; both × 14 days])
- Hospitalize if: tubo-ovarian abscess, pregnant, immunodeficient, unable to tolerate/follow/respond to outpt regimens
- Inpt Rx: ([cefotetan 2 g IV q12h or cefoxitin 2 g IV q6h] + [doxycycline 100 mg IV/PO q12h]) *or* ([clindamycin 900 mg IV q8h] + [gentamicin 2 mg/kg loading dose, then 1.5 mg/kg q8h or 4.5 mg/kg once per day]), then doxycycline 100 mg PO bid × 14 days

- Essential to evaluate and Rx male sex partners. Offer HIV testing.
- Repeat testing of all women dx with chlamydia/gonorrhea is recommended 3 to 6 mo s/p Rx.
- Pts should abstain from sexual intercourse until Rx completed and until partners asx.

4 GENITAL WARTS

Benign epidermal lesions caused by human papillomavirus (HPV); more commonly types 6 or 11 (90%)

Diagnosis
- Based on clinical findings. Suspect lesions should be biopsied.
- Screening for cervical cancer with cytology (Pap smear or liquid-based cytology) at age 21 yr or s/p first sexual encounter with annual cytology recommended until at least three nl results obtained; colposcopy + biopsy if cervical squamous cell change

H&P
- Flesh-colored papule with a rough surface obscuring nl skin lines → hyperkeratotic appearance with black surface dots or cauliflower-like appearance

Treatment
- Imiquimod (5% cream): thin layer at bedtime, washed off after 6 to 10 hr, 3 × wk for max 16 wk
- Podofilox (0.5% gel or solution): bid × 3 days, no Rx 4 days, with use up to four such cycles
- IFN alfa-2b (regimens from drug labels specific for external genital and/or perianal condylomata acuminata): injection 1 million IU intc lesion base, 3 × weekly alternating days up to 3 wk; max five lesions/course
- IFN alfa-N3: injection 0.05 mL into lesion base, up to 0.5 mL per session, 2 × wk up to 8 wk
- Sinecatechins (15% ointment): 0.5 cm strand each wart 3 × days, until healing, up to 16 wk

5 VAGINITIS

- Table 8-2 decribes diagnostic features and management of vaginal infections.
- Candidiasis (pH <4.5, pruritic, thick, cheesy d/c)
  • Rx: fluconazole 150 mg PO × 1 or itraconazole 200 mg PO bid × 1 day
- Trichomoniasis (pH >4.5, copious, foamy d/c)
  • Rx: [metronidazole (2 g PO × 1) or (500 mg PO bid)] or tinidazole 2 g PO × 1
  • *Treat male sexual partners (2 g metronidazole single dose)
- Bacterial vaginosis (pH >4.5, malodorous d/c)
  • Rx: [metronidazole (0.5 g PO bid × 7 days) or (intravaginal gel 1 x/day × 5 days)] or tinidazole 2 g PO once daily × 3 days

6 GENITAL ULCERS

Differential Diagnosis
- Herpes genitalis
- Syphilis
- Condyloma acuminatum
- Chancroid
- LGV
- Granuloma inguinale
- Neoplastic lesion
- Trauma

a. Syphilis
- Systemic infectious disease caused by *Treponema pallidum*
- "Latent syphilis" (seroreactivity w/o other evidence of disease)
- "Tertiary syphilis" (gummatous and CV syphilis)

Diagnosis
H&P
- Primary infection: ulcer or chancre at site of infection
- Secondary infection: rash, mucocutaneous lesions, and adenopathy
- Tertiary infection: cardiac, neurologic, ophthalmic, auditory, or gummatous lesions
Labs
- Darkfield examinations and DFA tests of lesion exudate or tissue
- Presumptive dx is possible w/the use of two types of serologic tests for syphilis: (1) nontreponemal (e.g., VDRL and rapid plasma reagin) and (2) treponemal (e.g., FTA-ABS and microhemagglutination assay for Ab to *T. pallidum*). The use of one type of test alone is not sufficient for dx.

TABLE 8-2 ■ Diagnostic Features and Management of Vaginal Infections

	No Infection	Yeast Vaginitis	Trichomoniasis	Bacterial Vaginosis
Etiology	—	Candida albicans and other yeasts	Trichomonas vaginalis	Gardnerella vaginalis, anaerobic bacteria, mycoplasma
Typical symptoms	None	Vulvar itching, irritation, ↑ discharge	Malodorous frothy discharge, vulvar itching	Malodorous, slightly ↑ discharge
Discharge				
Amount	Variable; usually scant	Scant to moderate	Profuse	Moderate
Color	Clear or white	White	Yellow green	Usually white or gray
Consistency	Nonhomogeneous, floccular	Clumped; adherent plaques	Homogeneous	Homogeneous, low viscosity; smoothly coats vaginal walls
Vulvar/vaginal inflammation	No	Yes	Yes	No
pH of vaginal fluid	Usually <4.5	Usually <4.5	Usually >5.0	Usually >4.5
Amine ("fishy") odor with 10% KOH	None	None	May be present	Present
Microscopy	Normal epithelial cells; Lactobacillus predominates	Leukocytes, epithelial cells, yeast, mycelia, or pseudomycelia in 40%–80% of cases	Leukocytes; motile trichomonads seen in 50%–70% of symptomatic patients, less often if asymptomatic	Clue cells, few leukocytes; Lactobacillus outnumbered by profuse mixed flora (nearly always including G. vaginalis plus anaerobes)
Usual treatment (see Formulary)	None	Oral fluconazole; intravaginal azoles	Metronidazole or tinidazole	Oral/intravaginal metronidazole or clindamycin
Management of sex partners	None	None	Treatment recommended	None

From Tschudy MM, Arcara KM: The Harriet Lane Handbook, 19th ed. Philadelphia, Mosby, 2012.

Treatment

- **Early** (primary, secondary, latent <1 yr): PCN G benzathine 2.4 million U IM × 1 or azithromycin 2 g PO × 1
- **More than 1-yr duration** (latent, CV, gumma): PCN G benzathine 2.4 million U IM q wk × 3 wk or doxycycline 100 mg PO bid × 4 wk
- **Neurosyphilis:** aqueous crystalline PCN G 18 to 24 million U/day, administered as 3 to 4 million U IV q4h × 10 to 14 days, or procaine PCN 2.4 million U IM/day + probenecid 500 mg PO qid both for 10 to 14 days
- **Congenital syphilis:** aqueous crystalline PCN G 50,000 U/kg/dose IV q12h × first 7 days of life then q8h ×10 days, or procaine PCN G 50,000 U/kg/dose IM/day × 10 days
- **PCN-allergic pts w/primary or secondary syphilis:** doxycycline 100 mg PO bid × 14 days, or tetracycline 500 mg PO qid × 14 days, or ceftriaxone 1 g IM or IV × 8 to 10 days
- **Latent syphilis in PCN-allergic pts:** doxycycline 100 mg PO bid or tetracycline 500 mg qid for 28 days
- Tetracyclines are contraindicated in pregnancy. If the pt is pregnant and PCN allergic, she must be desensitized.

b. Herpes Simplex Virus (HSV) Infection

After the primary infection, the virus enters the nerve endings in the skin directly below the lesions and ascends to the dorsal root ganglia, where it remains in a latent stage until it is reactivated.

Diagnosis

H&P

- Primary infection
  - Sx occur 3 to 7 days after contact.
  - Constitutional sx include low-grade fever, headache and myalgias, regional lymphadenopathy, and localized pain.
  - Pain, burning, itching, and tingling last several hours.

- Grouped vesicles usually w/surrounding erythema appear and generally ulcerate or crust within 48 hr.
- The vesicles are uniform in size (differentiating it from herpes zoster vesicles, which vary in size).
- During the acute eruption, the pt is uncomfortable; urinary retention may occur in severe cases.
- Lesions generally last 2 to 6 wk and heal w/o scarring.

■ Recurrent infection
- It is generally caused by alteration in the immune system, fatigue, stress, menses, or local skin trauma.
- The prodromal sx (fatigue, burning and tingling of the affected area) last 12 to 24 hr.
- A cluster of lesions generally evolves within 24 hr from a macule to a papule and then vesicles surrounded by erythema; the vesicles coalesce and subsequently rupture within 4 days, revealing erosions covered by crusts.
- The crusts are generally shed within 7 to 10 days, revealing a pink surface.
- The most frequent location of the lesions is on the penile shaft or glans penis and the labia (HSV-2).

Labs

■ DFA slide tests will provide a rapid dx.
■ Viral culture (definitive dx); results in 1 to 2 days. Lesions/cervical samples should be sampled during the vesicular/early ulcerative stage.
■ Pap smear will detect HSV-infected cells in cervical tissue from women w/o sx.
■ Serologic tests for HSV: IgG and IgM serum Abs. Abs to HSV occur in 50% to 90% of adults.

Treatment

Genital Herpes

■ **Primary episode:** acyclovir 400 mg PO tid × 7 to 10 days or valacyclovir 1000 mg PO bid × 7 to 10 days or famciclovir 250 mg PO tid × 7 to 10 days
■ **Episodic recurrence:** acyclovir 800 mg PO bid × 2 days or famciclovir 1000 mg bid × 1 day or valacyclovir 500 mg PO bid × 3 days; if HIV pt, acyclovir 400 mg PO tid × 5 to 10 days or famciclovir 500 mg PO bid × 5 to 10 days or valacyclovir 1 g PO bid × 5 to 10 days
■ **Chronic daily suppression** (↓ frequent sx outbreak 70%-80% if >6 recurrences/yr): acyclovir 400 mg PO bid or famciclovir 250 mg PO bid or valacyclovir 1 g PO q24h; if HIV pt, acyclovir 400 to 800 mg PO bid or famciclovir 500 mg PO bid or valacyclovir 500 mg PO bid
■ **Oral labial, normal host** (start Rx with prodrome [tingling/burning] before lesion formation): valacyclovir 2 g PO q12h × 1 day or famciclovir 500 mg PO bid × 7 days or acyclovir 400 mg PO q4h × 5 days; Topical (penciclovir 1% cream q2h × 4 days, acyclovir 5% cream q3h × 7 days)
■ **Oral labial, immunocompromised:** acyclovir 5 mg/kg IV q8h × 7 days or famciclovir 500 mg PO bid × 7 days or valacyclovir 500 mg PO bid × 5 to 10 days; acyclovir-resistant HSV, IV foscarnet 90 mg/kg IV q12h × 7 days
■ **Herpes whitlow:** acyclovir 400 mg tid PO × 10 days

Clinical Pearl

■ >85% of adults have serologic evidence of HSV-1 infection. The seroprevalence of adults w/HSV-2 in the United States is 25%; however, only ~20% of these pts recall having sx of HSV infection.

c. Chancroid *(Haemophilus ducreyi)*

Diagnosis

H&P

■ One to three extremely painful ulcers accompanied by tender inguinal lymphadenopathy (especially if fluctuant); chancroid typically soft in comparison with the hard, painless chancre of syphilis.
■ May manifest with inguinal bubo and several ulcers
■ In women: initial lesion in the fourchette, labia minora, urethra, cervix, or anus; inflammatory pustule or papule that ruptures, leaving a shallow, nonindurated ulceration, usually 1- to 2-cm diameter with ragged, undermined edges
■ Unilateral lymphadenopathy (50% pts) developing 1 wk later
■ R/o syphilis (RPR, VDRL) in women because of the consequences of inappropriate Rx if pregnant
■ Darkfield microscopy, HSV cultures, *H. ducreyi* culture

Treatment

■ Primary: ceftriaxone 250-mg IM single dose *or* azithromycin 1-g PO single dose

- Alternative: ciprofloxacin 600 mg bid PO × 3 days *or* erythromycin base 500 mg qid PO × 7 days
- As HIV(+) pts have Rx failure with single dose azithromycin, evaluate s/p 7 days Rx.
- Test all pts for HIV and syphilis.
- Rx of sex partners if evidence of disease or have had sex with pt within 10 days of presentation

d. Lymphogranuloma venereum (LGV)
STD caused by *C. trachomatis*, serovars L₁, L₂, or L₃.

Diagnosis
- Serology; biopsy contraindicated because of the risk of sinus tract development
- *C. trachomatis* culture, direct immunofluorescence, or nucleic acid detection
- Mild leukocytosis with lymphocytosis or monocytosis, ↑ ESR
- VDRL and HIV screening to r/o other STDs
- CT scan (suspected retroperitoneal adenitis)

H&P
- First stage (incubation period 3-21 days)
  - Primary lesion: papule, shallow ulcer
  - Herpetiform lesion at site of inoculation (most common)
  - Women: posterior wall, fourchette, or vulva (most common)
  - **Spontaneous healing without scarring**
- Second stage (1-4 wk after primary lesion)
  - Inguinal syndrome: inguinal adenopathy (unilateral 70% cases)
  - Sx: painful, extensive adenitis (bubo) and suppuration with numerous sinus tracts
  - "*Groove sign*" (femoral/inguinal node involvement ~20%, men)
  - Female involvement deep iliac/retroperitoneal lymph nodes possible pelvic mass
- Third stage (anogenital syndrome)
  - Subacute: proctocolitis
  - Late: tissue destruction/scarring, sinuses, abscesses, fistulas, strictures, elephantiasis

Treatment
- Primary: doxycycline 100 mg PO bid ×21d
- Alternative: erythromycin 500 mg PO qid × 21 days *or* azithromycin 1 g PO q wk × 3 wk

7 MALE GENITAL TRACT INFECTIONS

a. Balanitis
- **Rx:** metronidazole 2 g PO × 1 or fluconazole 150 mg PO × 1

b. Epididymo-orchitis
- **Rx age <35 yr:** ceftriaxone 250 mg IM × 1 + doxycycline 100 mg PO bid × 10 days
- **Rx age >35 yr/homosexual men** (insertive partners in anal intercourse)
  - Primary: levofloxacin 500 to 750 mg IV/PO once daily or ciprofloxacin 500 mg PO bid 10 to 14 days
  - Alternative: ampicillin-sulbactam 3 g IV q6h or piperacillin-tazobactam 3.375 g q6h

H. INFECTIOUS GI SYNDROMES

1 *CLOSTRIDIUM DIFFICILE* INFECTION (CDI)
Diarrhea and bowel inflammation associated with abx use. Sx range from fulminant diarrhea to leukocytosis associated with pseudomembranous colitis, mild to severe acute diarrhea, short-term colonization seen typically in health care facilities, and recurrent CDI with 60 days occurring in 20% to 30% of cases.
- Highest-incidence pseudomembranous colitis: cephalosporins
- Highest-incidence CDI: clindamycin (10% pseudomembranous colitis)
- ↑ Emergence of an epidemic virulent strain (NAP1/BI/027)

Risk Factors
- Administration of abxs: can occur with any abx
- Prolonged hospitalization
- Advanced age
- Abd surgery
- Underlying disease (malignancy, renal failure, debilitated status)
- Hospitalized, tube-fed pts
- PPI and H₂ blocker Rx

Diagnosis

- Sx: diarrhea, fever, and abdominal cramps after abx use

Labs

- Stool assay for *C. difficile* toxins A and B (sensitivity of 85%, specificity of 100%).
- Fecal leukocytes: generally present in stool samples
- CBC (leukocytosis). Sudden ↑ in WBC to >30,000/mm³ may be indicative of fulminant colitis.

Treatment

- WBC <15,000; no ΔCr
  - Primary: metronidazole 500 mg PO tid or 250 mg qid × 10 to 14 days
  - Alternative: vancomycin 125 mg PO qid × 10 to 14 days; teicoplanin 400 mg PO bid × 10 days
- Sicker: WBC >15,000, ≥50% ↑ Cr
  - Primary: vancomycin 125 mg PO qid × 10 to 14 days
- Alternative: fidaxomicin 200 mg PO bid × 10 days
- Post-Rx relapse:
  - First relapse: metronidazole 500 mg PO tid × 10 days
  - Second relapse: vancomycin 125 mg PO qid × 10 to 14 days, then taper (wk 1, bid; wk 2, q24h; wk 3, qod; then q third day for five doses)
- Postop ileus (toxic megacolon)
  - Primary: metronidazole 500 mg IV q6h + vancomycin 500 mg q6h via NG tube
- Fecal transplantation (intestinal microbiota transplantation [IMT]): eradication rate = 94%. Infusing intestinal microorganisms (in a suspension of healthy donor stool) into the intestine of a sick pt via enema, gastroscope/colonoscope, or nasojejunal tube restores the microbiota.
- Recurrence after initial episode is 20% to 25% regardless of initial abx; each recurrence ↑ risk of repeat episodes (65% chance of recurrence after three CDI episodes). Recurrent CDI is usually a relapse rather than re-infection, regardless of the time between episodes.

2 *SALMONELLA* INFECTION

- An estimated 1 million cases/yr of nontyphoidal salmonellosis occur in the United States.
- Approximately 500 cases of *Salmonella typhi* infection are reported each yr.
- Raw produce and contact with live poultry are central vehicles for salmonellosis.

Infections

- Localized to GI tract (gastroenteritis)
- Systemic (typhoid fever)
- Localized outside of GI tract

Diagnosis

- Gastroenteritis
  - Incubation period: 12 to 48 hr
  - Nausea, vomiting
  - Diarrhea, abdominal cramps
  - Fever
  - Bacteremia: occurs mostly in the immunocompromised host or those with underlying conditions, including HIV infection
  - Self-limited illness lasting 3 or 4 days
  - Colonization of GI tract persistent for months, especially in those treated with abxs

Typhoid Fever

- Incubation period of few days to several wk
- Prolonged fever, often with a stepwise-increasing temperature pattern
- Myalgias
- Headache, cough, sore throat
- Malaise, anorexia
- Abdominal pain
- Hepatosplenomegaly
- Diarrhea or constipation early in the course of illness
- ***Rose spots*** (faint, maculopapular, blanching lesions) sometimes seen on chest or abd

Infections Outside GI Tract

- Can occur in virtually any location
- Usually occur in pts with underlying diseases
- Endocarditis, endovascular infections are caused by seeding of atherosclerotic plaques or aneurysms

- Hepatic or splenic abscesses in pts with underlying disease in these organs
- Urinary tract infections in pts with renal TB or schistosomiasis
- Salmonellae a frequent cause of Gram(–) meningitis in neonates
- Osteomyelitis in children with hemoglobinopathies (particularly sickle cell disease)

Diagnosis
- Typhoid fever
  - Cultures of blood, stool, urine. Repeat if initially (–).
  - Blood cultures are more likely to be (+) early in the course of illness.
  - Stool and urine cultures are more commonly (+) in the second and third wk of illness.
  - Highest yield is with bone marrow biopsy cultures: 90% (+).
  - Serology using Widal's test is helpful in retrospect, showing a fourfold ↑ in convalescent titers.
- Gastroenteritis: stool cultures
- Extraintestinal localized infection
  - Blood cultures
  - Cultures from the site of infection

Labs
- Neutropenia is common.
- Transaminitis is possible.
- Culture to grow organism from blood, body fluids, biopsy specimens.

Treatment
- Adequate hydration and electrolyte replacement in people with diarrhea
- *Typhoid fever*
  - Ciprofloxacin 500 mg PO bid or 400 mg IV bid for 14 days
  - Ceftriaxone 2 g IV qd for 14 days
  - If sensitive, may switch Rx to TMP/SMX 1 to 2 DS tabs PO bid or amoxicillin 2 g PO q8h to complete 14 days
  - Dexamethasone 3 mg IV initially, followed by 1 mg IV q6h for eight doses for pts with shock or ΔMS
- *Gastroenteritis*
  - Usually not indicated for gastroenteritis alone because this illness generally self-limited
  - May prolong the carrier state
  - Prophylactic Rx for pts who are at high risk of developing complications from bacteremia (neonates, pts w/hemoglobinopathies, atherosclerosis, aneurysms, prosthetic devices, immunocompromised)
- Rx should be considered for those with persistently (+) stool cultures and for food handlers.
- Suggested regimens for eradication of carrier state
  - Ciprofloxacin 500 mg PO bid for 4 wk
  - TMP-SMX-DS 1 to 2 tab PO bid for 6 wk (if susceptible)
  - Amoxicillin 2 g PO q8h for 6 wk (if susceptible)

3 *CAMPYLOBACTER* INFECTION

Etiology
- *Campylobacter jejuni* (most commonly assoc. with gastroenteritis)

Clinical Findings
- Diarrhea, fever, abd pain onset several days after bacterial ingestion
- Grossly bloody stools (<10%), occult blood (35%)
- Late complications: reactive arthritis, GBS

Diagnosis
- Stool culture

Treatment
- Typically self-limiting
- Macrolide indicated (high fever, frequent or bloody stools, pts at extremes of age/with comorbid conditions/immunocompromised or sx >7 days)
- Table 8-3 compares major food-borne pathogens.

4 *SHIGELLA* INFECTION
Caused by one of several species of *Shigella* (most common cause of bacillary dysentery in the United States). *Shigella sonnei* is the most commonly isolated species in the United States, and it usually causes mild watery diarrhea. Direct person-to-person

TABLE 8-3 ■ Major Food-Borne Microbes by the Principal Presenting Gastrointestinal Symptom in Immunocompetent Adults

	Organism	Source/Vehicles	Incubation Period	Diagnosis	Recovery
Vomiting	Staphylococcus aureus	Prepared food (e.g., sandwiches)	2-4 hr	Diagnosis usually clinical for all organisms	<24 hr
	Bacillus cereus	Rice, meat	1-6 hr		2-3 days
	Norovirus	Shellfish, prepared food	24-48 hr		2-3 days
Watery diarrhea	Clostridium perfringens	All by contaminated food and water	8-22 hr	Stool culture	2-3 days
	Enterotoxigenic Escherichia coli (ETEC)		24 hr		1-4 days
	Enteric viruses		Variable		Variable
	Cryptosporidium parvum and Cryptosporidium hominis		5-28 days		7-14 days
	Cyclospora cayetanensis		7 days		Weeks to months
	Yersinia enterocolitica		2-14 hr		1-22 days
	Vibrio cholerae		Hours-6 days		2-3 days
Diarrhea with blood (dysentery)	Campylobacter jejuni	Cattle and poultry: meat and milk	48-96 hr	Stool culture	3-5 days
	Nontyphoidal Salmonella	Cattle and poultry: eggs, meat	12-48 hr		3-6 days, may be up to 2 wk
	Enterohemorrhagic E. coli (usually serotype O157:H7)*	Cattle: meat, milk	12-48 hr		10-12 days
	Shigella spp.	Contaminated food and water	24-48 hr		7-10 days
	Vibrio parahaemolyticus	Contaminated seafood	2-48 hr		1-12 days
Nongastrointestinal manifestations	Clostridium botulinum Paralysis from neuromuscular blockade	Environment: bottled or canned food	18-24 hr	Toxin in food or feces	10-14 days
	Listeria monocytogenes Meningitis	Contaminated packaged chilled foods	Up to 6 wk	CSF culture	Variable

*A low threshold for suspecting E. coli O157 infection in gastroenteritis is vital because this infection can have serious complications; 1%-15% of infections progress to hemolytic uremic syndrome (acute kidney injury, hemolytic anemia, thrombocytopenia). Antibiotics are contraindicated in E. coli O157 infection.

Adapted from Ballinger A: Kumar & Clark's Essentials of Clinical Medicine, 6th ed. Edinburgh, Saunders, 2012.

transmission is thought to be the most common route. Outbreaks occur among men who have sex with men (direct or indirect oral-anal contact).

Diagnosis

H&P

- Incubation period ranging from 1 to 7 days (average = 3 days)
- Mild illness that is usually self-limited, resolving in a few days
- Fever, watery, or bloody diarrhea
- Dysentery (abdominal cramps, tenesmus, and numerous, small-volume stools with blood, mucus, and pus)
- Descending intestinal tract illness, reflecting infection of small bowel first and then the colon
- Extraintestinal manifestations rare
- Bacteremia more common in children; in adults, has been described in pts with AIDS, the elderly, and pts with DM
- Hemolytic-uremic syndrome (HUS), usually as the initial illness seems to be resolving
- Reactive arthritis, sometimes as part of Reiter's syndrome

Labs

- Total WBCs may be ↓, nl, or ↑. Leukemoid reactions can occur in children.
- Stool should be cultured from fresh samples, because the yield is ↑ by processing the specimen soon after passage. The best yield is from the mucoid part of the stool.
- Serology is available but rarely useful.
- PCR may be diagnostic.
- Fecal leukocyte preparation may show WBCs.

Imaging

- Abdominal films may suggest megacolon or perforation in rare, severe cases.

Treatment

- Adequate hydration/electrolyte replacement
- Abxs
  - For children: IV ceftriaxone (50 mg/kg/day) for severe disease. For PO Rx, one can use SMX/TMP or ampicillin for 5 days for susceptible strains. Azithromycin can be used for 5 days when susceptibilities are still not known or in areas of high resistance (12 mg/kg for the first day, then 6 mg/kg/day for 4 days).
  - For adults: Pending susceptibilities, ciprofloxacin 500 mg PO bid for 5 days should be used. If susceptible, can also use SMX/TMP one DS PO bid for 5 days. Azithromycin is a second alternative.

Clinical Pearls

- *Shigella* is one cause of "gay bowel syndrome."
- Illness is worsened by agents that ↓ intestinal motility.
- Food handlers, child care providers, and health care workers should have a (–) stool culture documented following Rx.

5 VANCOMYCIN-RESISTANT ENTEROCOCCI (VRE)

80% of *Enterococcus faecium* organisms are VRE; 69% of *Enterococcus faecalis* organisms are VRE. They are most commonly transmitted from one pt to another by health care workers whose hands have become contaminated inadvertently with feces or fluids of a person carrying the organism. VRE are not airborne but can survive on surfaces for several weeks.

Risk Factors

- Prior antimicrobial Rx, especially vancomycin
- Prolonged hospitalization
- Chronic medical conditions, renal failure
- Invasive devices
- ICU stay
- Colonization: VRE colonize the GI tract and can be found on skin, perirectal swab culture, or stool culture.

Diagnosis

H&P

- Pts may be asx and have GI colonization associated with diarrhea. In hospitalized pts, infection is associated with colonization and can cause wound infections, bacteremia, abscesses (intra-abd), and, rarely, pneumonia and UTIs.

Labs

- VRE rectal culture

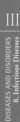

- VRE stool culture
- Blood, urine, and wound cultures

Treatment
- If colonization: Rx not recommended
- In pts w/sx: linezolid, quinupristindalfopristin, and daptomycin

Clinical Pearl
- Association between VRE colonization and CDI is reported in pts with hematologic malignancies.

6 PARASITIC INFECTIONS

a. Amebiasis
Caused by the protozoal parasite *E. histolytica*. Transmission is by the fecal-oral route. Infection is usually localized to the large bowel, particularly the cecum, where a localized mass lesion (ameboma) may form. In extraintestinal infection, the organism invades the bowel mucosa and gains access to the portal circulation. Incidence is highest in institutionalized pts and sexually active homosexual men. Although primarily an infection of the colon, amebiasis may cause extraintestinal disease (liver abscess).

Diagnosis
- Three stool specimens over 7 to 10 days to exclude the dx (sensitivity 50%-80%)
- Concentration/staining specimen (Lugol's iodine or methylene blue) ↑ dx yield
- Available culture (rarely necessary in routine cases)

H&P
- Approximately 20% of cases sx (diarrhea [may be bloody], abd/back pain)
- Abdominal tenderness in 83% of severe cases
- Fever in 38% of severe cases
- Hepatomegaly, RUQ tenderness, and fever in almost all pts with liver abscess (may be absent in fulminant cases)

Labs
- Stool examination is generally reliable.
- Mucosal biopsy is occasionally necessary.
- Serum Ab may be detected and is particularly sensitive and specific for extraintestinal infection or severe intestinal disease.

Imaging
- Abdominal sonography or CT scan to diagnose liver abscessTreatment
- Metronidazole (750 mg PO tid × 10 days) in mild to severe intestinal infection and amebic liver abscess. It may be administered IV when necessary.
- Follow with iodoquinol (650 mg PO tid × 20 days) to eradicate persistent cysts.
- For asymptomatic pts with amebic cysts on stool examination, use iodoquinol or paromomycin (500 mg PO tid × 7 days).
- Avoid antiperistaltic agents in severe intestinal infections to avoid risk of toxic megacolon.
- Liver abscess is generally responsive to medical management, but surgical intervention is indicated for extension of liver abscess into pericardium or for toxic megacolon.

b. *Giardia* Infection
Intestinal and/or biliary tract infection caused by the protozoal parasite *Giardia lamblia*, which frequently contaminates fresh water sources worldwide

Diagnosis
- Stool specimen (three specimens yield 90% sensitivity) or duodenal aspirate for microscopic examination to establish dx and exclude other pathogens
- Immunoassays for *Giardia* sp antigens in stool samples (85% to 98% sensitive and 90% to 100% specific)

H&P
- Diarrhea, flatulence, cramps, bloating, nausea.
- Fever in <30%
- Chronic diarrhea, malabsorption, and weight loss

Treatment
Adult and Pediatric
- Metronidazole 250 mg PO tid × 5 to 7 days (in children: 5 mg/kg tid × 7 days). Avoid in pregnancy.
- Tinidazole (a congener of metronidazole): 2-g single dose (50 mg/kg in children)
- Nitazoxanide: aged 12 to 47 mo: 100 mg bid × 3 days; aged 4 to 11 yr: 200 mg bid × 3 days

- Paromomycin 25 to 30 mg/kg/day in three doses for 5 to 10 days
- Other alternatives: furazolidone: 100 mg qid × 7 to 10 days in adults, 2 mg/kg qid × 10 days in children; and albendazole: 400 mg qid × 5 days in adults, 15 mg/kg/day × 5 to 7 days (max: 400 mg) in children

c. *Cryptosporidium* Infection
Infection w/the intracellular protozoan parasite *Cryptosporidium parvum*
Diagnosis
H&P
- Acute GI illness, especially associated w/HIV infection or w/travel and water-borne outbreaks. Sx are usually limited to GI (diarrhea, severe abd pain, impaired digestion, dehydration, N/V).

Labs
- Stool evaluation: characteristic oocyst by modified AFB stain
- May be seen in mucosal surfaces of GI lumen by bx

Treatment
- May be self-limited in nl host, often requiring hydration. Antidiarrheal agents Pepto-Bismol, Kaopectate, and loperamide may give symptomatic relief.
- Nitazoxanide 500 mg PO bid × 3 days. Nitazoxanide elixir is approved in children 1 to 11 yr old.
- Biliary cryptosporidiosis can be treated w/antiretroviral Rx in the setting of HIV infection.

7 PERITONITIS

a. Primary (SBP)
- 1-yr risk SBP in pt with ascites/cirrhosis ~30%
- Prevention via TMP-SMX-DS 1 tab PO 5 days/wk or ciprofloxacin 750 mg PO q wk
- Dx: (+) culture ≥250 neutrophils/μL ascitic fluid

Treatment
- At least for 5 days (duration unclear; longer if pt bacteremic)
- Albumin 1.5 g/kg IV at dx + 1 g/kg day 3 may ↓ renal impairment
- Cefotaxime 2 g IV q8h (q24h if life-threatening) or piperacillin-tazobactam 3.375 g q6h or 4.5 g q8h or 4-hr infusion of 3.375 g q8h or ceftriaxone 2 g IV q24h
- If resistant *Klebsiella/E. coli* species (ESBL[+]), then: ciprofloxacin 400 mg q12h + levofloxacin 750 mg q24h + moxifloxacin 400 mg q24h

b. Secondary (Bowel Perforation, Ruptured Appendix/Diverticula)
- Mild to moderate disease
  - Surgery to control source
  - Rx: piperacillin-tazobactam 3.375 g IV q6h *or* ticarcillin-clavulanate 3.1 g q6h *or* ciprofloxacin 400 mg IV q12h or (levofloxacin 750 mg IV q24h + metronidazole 1 g IV q12h)
- Severe life-threatening disease
- Surgical source control and management imperative
- Rx: Imipenem-cilastatin 500 mg IV q6h or meropenem 1g IV q8h or doripenem 500 mg IV q8h (1-hr infusion) or ([ampicillin + metronidazole] + [ciprofloxacin 400 mg IV q8h or levofloxacin 750 mg IV q24h])

I. CENTRAL NERVOUS SYSTEM INFECTIONS

1 LUMBAR PUNCTURE (LP)
Procedure
1. Perform a careful ophthalmoscopic examination; if ICP or a CNS space-occupying lesion is suspected, CT scan of the head should be done before LP.
2. Place the pt in a lateral decubitus position w/spine flexed (draw shoulders forward and bring thighs toward the abd; maximal flexion of the spine helps open up the interspace and improves chances of a successful procedure). If the pt is able to, LP can also be performed w/the pt sitting upright, ideally leaning over a tray table.
3. Identify the L4-5 interspace (imaginary line connecting the iliac crests).
4. Clean the area w/povidone-iodine solution.
5. Anesthetize the skin and SC tissues w/1% to 2% lidocaine.

6. Gently introduce the spinal needle (w/bevel turned upward) in the L4-5 interspace in a horizontal direction and w/slight cephalad inclination. Point toward the umbilicus. A drop in resistance may be felt as the needle penetrates the dura.
7. Measure opening pressure (nl is 100-200 mm Hg [10-20 cm Hg]).
   a. If the pressure is ↑, instruct the pt to relax and ensure that there is no abd compression or breath holding (straining and pressure on the abd wall will ↑ CSF pressure).
   b. If the pressure is markedly ↑, remove only 5 mL of spinal fluid and remove the spinal needle immediately.
8. Collect 5 to 10 mL of spinal fluid in four collection tubes (2 mL/tube).
9. Measure closing pressure, then remove the manometer and stopcock, and then replace stylet before removing the spinal needle; apply pressure to the puncture site w/sterile gauze for a few minutes.
10. Instruct the pt to remain in a horizontal position for approximately 4 hr to minimize post-LP headache (caused by CSF fluid leakage through the puncture site).
11. Process the CSF fluid.
    a. Tube 1: protein, glucose
    b. Tube 2: Gram stain of the centrifuged specimen
    c. Tube 3: Save the fluid until further notice.
    d. Tube 4: cell count (total and diff)
12. Consider additional tests (if indicated).
    a. Bacterial cultures are performed in suspected bacterial meningitis.
    b. Assay for cryptococcal antigen is used in immunocompromised pts.
    c. Countercurrent immunoelectrophoresis or latex agglutination is used to detect specific polysaccharide bacterial antigens *(Neisseria meningitidis, H. influenzae, S. pneumoniae)* in the CSF of pts w/inconclusive Gram stain findings (e.g., pts w/partially treated meningitis).
    d. Oligoclonal banding and assay for myelin basic protein are useful to diagnose MS.
    e. VDRL, AFB stain, Wright stain of sediment, India ink preparation, Lyme titer Ab, fungal or viral cultures, and cytologic examination should be ordered only when specifically indicated.
    f. The most sensitive technique for rapid dx of tuberculous meningitis is PCR assay. Bacteriologic methods are inadequate for early dx because there are generally too few organisms in the CSF for identification by direct smear, and identification w/cultures takes 6 to 8 wk.
    g. Rapid dx of herpes simplex encephalitis (when suspected) can be accomplished by nested PCR assay of CSF.
    h. Enterovirus-specific reverse transcriptase PCR assay of CSF fluid is useful for rapid dx of enteroviral meningitis.

Interpretation of Results
1. Appearance of the fluid:
   a. Clear is nl.
   b. Yellow color (xanthochromia) in the supernatant of centrifuged CSF within 1 hour or less after collection is usually the result of previous bleeding (subarachnoid hemorrhage); it may also be caused by ↑ CSF protein, melanin from meningeal melanosarcomas, or carotenoids.
   c. Pinkish color is usually the result of a bloody tap; the color generally clears progressively from tubes 1 to 4 (the supernatant is usually crystal clear in traumatic taps).
   d. Turbidity usually indicates the presence of leukocytes (bleeding introduces approximately 1 WBC to 500 RBCs into the CSF).
2. CSF pressure: ↑ Pressure can be seen in pts w/meningitis, meningoencephalitis, pseudotumor cerebri, mass lesions, and intracerebral bleeding.
3. Cell count: In the adult, the CSF is nlly free of cells (although up to 5 mononuclear cells/mm^3 is considered nl); the presence of granulocytes is never nl.
   a. Neutrophils are seen in cases of bacterial meningitis, early viral meningoencephalitis, and early tuberculous meningitis.
   b. ↑ Lymphocytes are seen in tuberculous meningitis, viral meningoencephalitis, syphilitic meningoencephalitis, fungal meningitis, Lyme disease, SLE, listeriosis.

4. Protein: Serum proteins are generally too large to cross the nl blood-CSF barrier; however, CSF protein is seen w/meningeal inflammation, traumatic tap, CNS synthesis, tissue degeneration, obstruction to CSF circulation, and GBS.
5. Glucose
   a. ↓ Glucose is seen w/bacterial meningitis, tuberculous meningitis, fungal meningitis, subarachnoid hemorrhage, and some cases of viral meningitis.
   b. A mild ↑ in CSF glucose level can be seen in pts w/very ↑ serum glucose levels.
Note: Table 8-4 describes CSF abnlities found in various CNS conditions.

TABLE 8-4 ■ **Cerebrospinal Fluid Abnormalities in Various CNS Conditions**

	Appearance	Glucose (mg/dL)	Protein (mg/dL)	Cell Count (cells/mm³) and Cell Type	Pressure (mm Hg)
Normal	Clear	50-80	20-45	<6 lymphocytes	100-200
Acute bacterial meningitis	Cloudy	↓↓	↑↑	↑↑ PMNs	↑↑
Aseptic (viral) meningitis	Clear/cloudy	nl	↑	↑, usually mononuclear cells; may be PMNs in early stages	nl/↑
Hemorrhage	Bloody/xanthochromic	nl/↓	↑	↑↑ RBCs	↑
Neoplasm	Clear/xanthochromic	nl/↓	nl/↑	nl/↑ lymphocytes	↑↑
Tuberculous meningitis	Cloudy	↓	↑	PMNs (early) lymphocytes (later)	↑
Fungal meningitis	Clear/cloudy	↓	↑	↑ monocytes	↑
Neurosyphilis	Clear/cloudy	nl	↑	↑ monocytes	nl/↑
Guillain-Barré syndrome	Clear/cloudy	nl	↑↑	nl/↑ lymphocytes	nl

2 BACTERIAL MENINGITIS

Etiology

- **S. pneumoniae:** adults and elderly pts. Predisposing factors include blunt head trauma, otitis media, pneumonia, sickle cell disease, and CSF leaks; mortality rate is 30%; permanent neurologic sequelae occur in 50% of survivors.
- **N. meningitidis:** young adults and children, especially those w/complement deficiencies
- **H. influenzae:** preschool-age children. Predisposing factors in adults include head trauma, otitis media, and sinusitis.
- **Listeria monocytogenes:** elderly and immunosuppressed pts (lymphoma, corticosteroids, dialysis pts, organ transplant recipients)
- **Gram(−) bacilli:** neonates (acquired in passage through birth canal), elderly debilitated pts, neutropenic pts, and in postcranial surgery
- **S. aureus:** diabetic pts and pts w/S. aureus pneumonia or cancer

Diagnosis

H&P

- Classic presentation consists of fever, headache, lethargy, confusion, and nuchal rigidity; these manifestations are not always present, particularly in infants, elderly, and immunocompromised pts.
- **Kernig's sign:** pain in the lower back or posterior thigh when the knee is extended while the pt is lying in the supine position and the hip is flexed at a right angle
- **Brudzinski's sign:** rapid flexion of the neck elicits involuntary flexing of the knees in a supine position
- ΔMS (confusion, lethargy)
- Bulging fontanelle, poor feeding, vomiting, and respiratory distress in infants
- Petechial-purpuric rash that develops on the trunk, LEs, mucous membranes, conjunctiva, and occasionally the palms and soles is suggestive of meningococcal meningitis but can also be present in viral meningitis and other types of bacterial meningitis.
- Papilledema is unusual and should raise the suspicion of brain abscess or mass lesion.
- Seizures (up to 40% of pts in the first wk of illness). Cranial nerve palsies (most notably sensorineural hearing loss) may also be present early in the course of illness.

Labs
- WBC usually reveals leukocytosis w/left shift; however, leukopenia can also be present; peripheral lymphocytosis is usually suggestive of a viral cause (aseptic meningitis).
- Blood cultures (abx Rx should not be delayed until all cultures are obtained if pt is very ill)
- LP: CSF exam
  - Opening pressure >100 to 200 mm Hg
  - WBC <5 to >100 mm^3
  - Neutrophilic predominance: >80%
  - Gram stain of CSF: + in 60% to 90%
  - CSF protein: >50 mg/dL
  - CSF glucose: <40 mg/dL
  - Culture: (+) in 65% to 90% cases
  - CSF bacterial antigen: 50% to 100% sensitivity
  - E-test for susceptibility of pneumococcal isolates

Treatment
- The goal is empiric Rx, then CSF exam within 30 min. I the pt has a focal neurologic deficit, give empiric Rx, then head CT, then LP.

Empiric Rx: CSF Gram Stain (−) Immunocompetent
- *1 mo to 50 yr (S. pneumoniae, meningococci, H. influenzae now uncommon)*
  - (Cefotaxime 2 g IV q4-6h or ceftriaxone 2 g IV q12h) + (dexamethasone 0.15 mg/kg IV q6h × 2-4 days; first dose before or with first dose abx to block TNF production) + vancomycin 15 mg/kg IV q8h (trough level 15-20 μg/mL)
  - *If severe β-lactam allergy: See the next subsection, on empiric Rx for (+) Gram stain, for alternative agents to cover suspected pathogens.
- *>50 yr or alcoholism/chronic disease (S. pneumoniae, Listeria, Gram[−] bacilli)*
  - Ampicillin 2 g IV q4-6h + (ceftriaxone 2 g IV q12h or cefotaxime 2 g IV q4-6h) + vancomycin 15 mg/kg IV q8h (trough level 15-20 μg/mL) + (dexamethasone 0.15 mg/kg IV q6h × 2-4 days; first dose before or with first dose abx)
  - *If severe β-lactam allergy: See the next subsection, on empiric Rx for (+) Gram stain, for alternative agents to cover suspected pathogens.
- Post-neurosurgery/ventriculostomy/lumbar catheter; penetrating trauma w/o basilar skull fracture (S. epidermidis, S. aureus, facultative aerobic Gram[−] bacilli; P. aeruginosa and Acinetobacter baumannii)
  - Vancomycin 15 mg/kg IV q8h (trough level 15-20 μg/mL) + (cefepime or ceftazidime 2 g IV q8h)
  - *If severe PCN/cephalosporin allergy, substitute either aztreonam 2 g IV q6-8h or ciprofloxacin 400 mg IV q8-12h
  - *If IV Rx inadequate: intraventricular daily doses vancomycin 10 to 20 mg; amikacin 30 mg; tobramycin 5 to 20 mg; gentamicin 4 to 8 mg; colistin 10 mg; polymyxin B 5 mg
  - *Trauma w/basilar skull fracture (S. epidermidis, H. influenzae, S. pyogenes)*
    - Vancomycin 15 mg/kg IV q8h (trough level 15-20 μg/mL) + (ceftriaxone 2 g IV q12h or cefotaxime [Cefotax] 2 g IV q6h) + (dexamethasone 0.15 mg/kg IV q6h × 2-4 days; first dose with or before first abx dose)

Empiric Rx: CSF Gram Stain (+)
- Gram(+) diplococci *(S. pneumoniae)*
  - Primary: (cefotaxime 2 g IV q4-6h OR ceftriaxone 2 g IV q12h) + vancomycin 15 mg/kg IV q8h (trough level 15-20 μg/mL) + (timed dexamethasone 0.15 mg/kg IV q6h × 2-4 days)
  - Alternatives: meropenem 2 g IV q8h or moxifloxacin 400 mg IV q24h
- Gram(−) diplococci *(N. meningitidis)*
  - Primary: (cefotaxime 2 g IV q4-6h or ceftriaxone 2 g IV q12h)
  - Alternatives: PCN G 4 million U IV q4h or ampicillin 2 g IV q4h or moxifloxacin 400 mg IV q24h or chloramphenicol 1 g IV q6h
- Gram(+) bacilli or coccobacilli *(L. monocytogenes)*
  - Primary: ampicillin 2 g IV q4h ± gentamicin 2 mg/kg loading dose then 1.7 mg/kg IV q8h
  - *If PCN allergic: TMP-SMX 5 mg/kg (TMP comp) q6-8h or meropenem 2 g IV q8h
- Gram(−) bacilli *(H. influenzae, P. aeruginosa)*
  - Primary: (ceftazidime or cefepime 2 g IV q8h) ± gentamicin 2 mg/kg IV first dose then 1.7 mg/kg IV q8h
  - Alternatives: ciprofloxacin 400 mg IV q8-12h; meropenem 2 g IV q8h; aztreonam 2 g IV q6-8h. Consider adding IV gentamicin to β-lactam or ciprofloxacin if resistance.

Prophylaxis for _H. influenzae_
- Nonpregnant adults: rifampin 600 mg q24h × 4 days
- Household: If one unvaccinated contact is ≤4 yr old, give rifampin to all contacts except pregnant women.
- Child care facilities: If one case occurs and unvaccinated children who attend are ≤2 yr old, consider prophylaxis + vaccinate; if ≥2 cases occur in 60 days and unvaccinated children attend, provide prophylaxis for all children and personnel.

Prophylaxis for _N. meningitidis_
- Close contact: ceftriaxone 250 mg IM × 1 dose or rifampin 600 mg PO q12h × four doses

3 VIRAL MENINGITIS

Acute febrile illness with signs and sx of meningeal irritation, usually with a lymphocytic pleocytosis of the CSF and (–) CSF bacterial stains and cultures

Etiology
- Enterovirus: 85% to 95% of all cases

Diagnosis
- CSF examination
  - Usually shows pleocytosis
  - Lymphocytic predominance (neutrophils in early stages)
  - Opening pressure: 200 to 250 mm Hg
  - WBC: 100 to 1000 mm³
  - ↑ CSF protein
  - ↓ or nl CSF glucose
  - (–) Gram stain, cultures, CIE, latex agglutination
  - Viral cultures or serologic testing may be diagnostic.
  - PCR for HSV, West Nile, or enterovirus (which could shorten duration of abx Rx and hospitalization if bacterial meningitis was suspected)

_H&P_
- Fever, headache, nuchal rigidity, photophobia, myalgias

Imaging
- CT scan or MRI: If cerebral edema, focal neurologic findings develop.

Treatment
- No specific antiviral Rx for most viruses. Rx is supportive unless HSV is detected, which would be treated with IV acyclovir: 10 mg/kg q8hr in adults; up to 20 mg/kg q8hr in children <12 yr old.

4 ENCEPHALITIS

a. Herpes simplex encephalitis

Acute febrile syndrome with evidence of meningeal involvement and cerebellar, cerebral, or brainstem function derangement

Diagnosis
- LP: pleocytosis, usually lymphocytic (although neutrophils may be seen early on), ↑ CSF protein, nl or ↓ CSF glucose, RBCs, and xanthochromia
- Selected tests on CSF fluid in viral encephalitis are described in Table 8-5.
- EEG changes showing periodic high-voltage sharp waves in the temporal regions and slow wave complexes
- Temporal lobe involvement
- PMR that amplifies DNA from the CSF
- Classic herpetic skin lesions may be present.

_H&P_
- Initially, fever and evidence of meningeal irritation
- Headache and stiff neck
- Later, development of signs of cortical dysfunction: lethargy, coma, stupor, weakness, seizures, facial weakness, as well as brainstem findings
- Cerebellar findings: ataxia, nystagmus, hypotonia, myoclonus, cranial nerve palsies, and abnl tendon reflexes

Treatment
- Supportive care
- Avoidance of infusion of hypotonic fluids to minimize the risk of hyponatremia
- For pts who develop seizures: anticonvulsant Rx
- Acyclovir 30 mg/kg/day IV total dose divided in q8h intervals 14 days
- Short courses of corticosteroids to control brain edema and prevent herniation

TABLE 8-5 ■ Selected Tests for Viral Encephalitis

Organism/Syndrome	Test	Comment
West Nile Virus		
West Nile encephalitis	IgM in CSF	Diagnostic of CNS invasive disease or acute flaccid paralysis
Herpes Simplex Virus Type 1		
Herpes simplex encephalitis	PCR in CSF CSF-serum antibody ratio	Sensitive and specific in the acute phase Useful 2 wk-3 mo after onset
Herpes Simplex Virus Type 2		
Neonatal encephalitis	PCR in CSF	Confirmatory, high sensitivity
Relapsing meningitis	PCR in CSF	Sensitive and specific in first 3 days of illness
Varicella-Zoster Virus		
Meningoencephalitis	PCR in CSF	Confirmatory when used with clinical and spinal fluid findings; sensitivity unclear
Epstein-Barr Virus		
EBV encephalitis	PCR in CSF	Suggests CNS invasion by virus
JC Virus		
Progressive multifocal leukoen-cephalopathy	PCR in CSF	Diagnostic but incompletely (70%) sensitive
Cytomegalovirus		
CMV ventriculitis	PCR in CSF	Sensitive and specific

From Goldman L, Schafer AI: Goldman's Cecil Medicine, ed 24, Philadelphia, 2011 Saunders.

b. West Nile Virus (WNV) Encephalitis
Infected mosquito vector in midsummer to midautumn (maximum mosquito intensity)

Diagnosis

H&P
- Initial phase of illness is nonspecific, with abrupt onset of fever accompanied by malaise, eye pain, anorexia, headache, and, occasionally, rash and lymphadenopathy. Less commonly, myocarditis, hepatitis, or pancreatitis may occur.
- In approximately 1 in 150 cases, especially among elderly pts, severe neurologic sequelae (ataxia, CN palsies, optic neutitis, seizures, myelitis, polyradiculitis) occur.

Labs
- CBC, electrolytes (hyponatremia common)
- LP: lymphocytic pleocytosis with nl level of glucose and ↑ level of protein
- CSF WNV IgM Ab level: rare false(+) results in people recently vaccinated against Japanese encephalitis or yellow fever viruses

Imaging
- CT or MRI studies of the brain to r/o mass lesions and cerebral edema

Treatment
- IV hydration, ventilator support may be necessary.
- No specific Rx is established (ribavirin and INF alfa-2b have in vitro activity; IVIG under study).

5 BRAIN ABSCESS

Etiology
- Contiguous focus of infection (55% of cases): paranasal sinus infection (streptococci, *Bacteroides, Haemophilus, Fusobacterium*); otitis media/mastoiditis (streptococci, Enterobacteriaceae, *Bacteroides, Pseudomonas*); dental sepsis (*Fusobacterium, Bacteroides, Streptococcus*); penetrating head injury (*S. aureus, Clostridium*); postoperative (*S. epidermidis, S. aureus*)
- Hematogenous spread (25% of cases): endocarditis (*S. aureus,* viridans strep); CHD (streptococci, *Haemophilus* species); UTI (Enterobacteriaceae, Pseudomonadaceae); lung (strep, *Actinomyces, Fusobacterium*); intra-abd (strep, Enterobacteriaceae, anaerobes)
- Immunocompromised host: *Toxoplasma,* fungi, *Nocardia, Listeria,* Enterobacteriaceae
- Cryptogenic (unknown source): 20%

Diagnosis

H&P

- Classic triad: fever, headache, and focal neurologic deficits depending on location (50% of cases)
- Papilledema (25%)

Labs

- ↑ WBC (60% of pts), ↑ ESR
- Blood cultures most often (–) (90%)
- LP contraindicated in pts w/suspected abscess because of ↑ ICP (20% die or suffer neurologic decline)
- Gram stain/culture of material aspirated at surgical drainage approaching 100%

Imaging

- MRI of brain with and without gadolinium
- CT w/IV contrast if MRI contraindicated

Treatment

- If abscess <2.5 cm and pt is neurologically stable and conscious, start abx and observe.
- Empiric abx Rx: varies w/abscess, location, suspicion of primary source, presence of single or multiple abscesses, pt's underlying medical condition (e.g., HIV, immunocompromised status)
- Otitis media/mastoiditis: cefotaxime 2 g q4h IV or ceftriaxone 2 g q12h IV plus metronidazole 7.5 mg/kg q6h IV or 15 mg/kg q12h IV
- Dental infection: PCN G 6 million U q6h plus metronidazole 7.5 mg/kg q6h IV
- Head trauma or after cranial surgery: third-generation cephalosporin (cefotaxime 2 g IV q6h or ceftriaxone 2 g IV q12h) + metronidazole 7.5 mg/kg q6h or 15 mg/kg IV q12h and nafcillin 2 g IV q4h or vancomycin (30 mg/kg IV in two divided doses adjusted for renal function)
- Hematogenous spread (CHD, endocarditis, urinary tract, lung, intra-abd): nafcillin or vancomycin plus metronidazole plus third-generation cephalosporin (cefotaxime 2 g IV q6h or ceftriaxone 2 g IV q12h)
- Duration of abx Rx: 4 to 8 wk, w/repeated neuroimaging to ensure adequate Rx (imaging suggested every wk for first 2 wk of Rx, then every 2 wk until abx finished, and then every 2 to 4 mo for 1 yr to monitor for disease recurrence)
- Indications for surgical intervention
  - Collect specimens for C&S.
  - Reduce mass effect.
- Stereotactic bx or aspirate of abscess if surgically feasible
- Timing and choice of surgery depend on
  - Primary infection source
  - Number and location of the abscesses
  - Whether the procedure is diagnostic or therapeutic
  - Neurologic status of the pt
- Hyperosmolar agents such as mannitol may be indicated if pt is still suffering from sx of ICP after abx and other Rx.

6 SPINAL EPIDURAL ABSCESS (SEA)

Etiology

- Pyogenic bacteria account for the majority of cases in the United States. The most common causative organism is *S. aureus*. Immigrants from TB-endemic areas may present w/TB SEAs. Fungi and parasites can also cause this condition. Most posterior EAs are thought to originate from distant focus (e.g., skin and soft tissue infections); anterior EAs are commonly associated w/diskitis or vertebral osteomyelitis. No source found in approximately one third of cases.
- Associated predisposing conditions include DM, alcoholism, cancer, AIDS, and chronic renal failure, or after epidural anesthesia, spinal surgery or trauma, or IV drug use. No predisposing condition is noted in 20% of pts.

Diagnosis

H&P

- Fever, malaise, and back pain are the most consistent early sx; pain is often focal.
- As the disease progresses, root pain can occur, followed by motor weakness, sensory changes, bladder and bowel dysfunction, and paralysis.
- Damage to the spinal cord can be caused by direct compression of the spinal cord, vascular compromise, bacterial toxins, and inflammation.

Labs
- WBC ↑ or nl, ↑ ESR, blood cultures ([+] in 60% of pts)
- CSF cultures ([+] in 19%), but LP unnecessary and may be contraindicated
- CT-guided aspiration or open bx recommended to determine causative organism; abscess content culture (+) in 90%

Imaging
- MRI w/gadolinium; CT scan w/contrast may show the abscess but is less sensitive than MRI.
- CT myelogram for suspected cord compression

Treatment
- Surgical decompression
- Abx directed at the most likely organism. If MRSA is possible: vancomycin 1 g IV q12h. If MRSA is unlikely: nafcillin or oxacillin 2 g IV q4h.
- If the organism is unknown, broad coverage against staphylococci, streptococci, and Gram(–) bacilli should be initiated. The regimen can be adjusted according to culture results. Rx should continue for at least 4 to 6 wk.

7 SUBDURAL EMPYEMA

Etiology
- Usually from paranasal sinusitis (40%-50% cases)
- Polymicrobial (aerobic strep, staph, Gram[–] bacilli, anaerobic strep)

Diagnosis
- MRI (may detect empyemas at base of brain, along falx cerebri, or in posterior fossa, all of which are difficult to see on CT)

H&P
- May be rapidly progressive with sx (headache) via ↑ ICP, meningeal irritation/cortical inflammation

Treatment
- Medical and surgical emergency
  - Medical Rx: **Empiric abx** ([cefotaxime 2 g IV q4h or ceftriaxone 2 g IV q12h] + metronidazole 7.5 mg/kg q6h or 15 mg/kg IV q12h])
  - Surgical Rx: **Craniotomy** (lower mortality rate than limited drainage procedure [burr holes], which is otherwise preferable in septic shock/parafalcine collections or children with subdural empyema secondary meningitis)

J. URINARY TRACT INFECTIONS

1 CYSTITIS

Diagnosis
- **Dysuria**, urgency, frequency, suprapubic pain, or hematuria

Treatment
- Acute uncomplicated UTI (cystitis-urethritis) in female pts
  - **Primary:** TMP-SMX-DS bid × 3 days (sulfa allergy: nitrofurantoin 100 mg PO bid × 5 days or fosfomycin 3 g PO once) + phenazopyridine (Pyridium)
  - **Alternative:** ciprofloxacin 250 mg bid × 3 days or levofloxacin 250 mg q24h × 3 days
- ***7-day Rx recommended in pregnancy**
- ↑ **Risk for STD:** azithromycin 1 g PO once or doxycycline 100 mg bid × 7 days (pelvic exam for vaginitis/HSV, urine ligase chain reaction (LCR)/PCR for gonococcus and *C. trachomatis*)
- **Recurrent** (≥3 infections/yr): Eradicate infection, then take TMP-SMX 1 single-strength tab PO q24h long term.

2 PYELONEPHRITIS

- Infection of the upper urinary tract

Etiology
- Gram(–) bacilli: *E. coli* and *Klebsiella* spp in >95% of cases
- Resistant Gram(–) organisms or fungi: hospitalized pts w/indwelling catheters
- Gram(+) organisms: enterococci
- *S. aureus:* hematogenous spread

Diagnosis

H&P
- Fever, flank pain, dysuria, hematuria

■ CBC w/diff, blood cultures, U/A, urine C&S, BUN, Cr, Gram stain of urine

Imaging
■ Renal U/S: if obstruction or closed space infection suspected
■ CT scan: suspected abscess, calculi

Treatment
■ Stable pt w/sensitive pathogens: ciprofloxacin (500 mg bid × 7 days); clinical success higher for 7 days of ciprofloxacin than for 14 days of TMP-SMX
■ Severe/complicated infection: ampicillin 1 to 2 g IV q4-6h + AGs; alternative regimen: ceftazidime 2 g IV q8h or piperacillin 3 g IV q6h
■ Prompt drainage w/nephrostomy tube placement for obstruction
■ If male pt, look for obstructive uropathy or other complicating pathology.

3 PERINEPHRIC ABSCESS
■ Usual etiology: *S. aureus* bacteremia

Treatment
■ Drainage, surgical, or image-guided aspiration
■ If MSSA: nafcillin/oxacillin 2 g IV q24h or cefazolin 1 g IV q8h
■ If MRSA: vancomycin 1 g IV q12h or daptomycin 6 mg/kg IV q24h

4 PROSTATITIS
■ Inflammation of the prostate gland. There are four major categories:
• Acute bacterial prostatitis (type I)
• Chronic bacterial prostatitis (type II)
• Chronic prostatitis/pelvic pain syndrome (type III): subdivided into type IIIA (inflammatory) and type IIIB (noninflammatory)
• Asymptomatic inflammatory prostatitis (type IV)

Etiology
■ Acute bacterial prostatitis: usually Gram(−) infection of the prostate gland from the ascent of bacteria in the urethra
■ Chronic bacterial prostatitis: exacerbation of sx of BPH caused by the same mechanism as in acute bacterial prostatitis
■ Chronic prostatitis/chronic pain syndrome
• Type IIIA: sx of prostatic inflammation associated w/the presence of WBCs in prostatic secretions w/no identifiable bacterial organism. *Chlamydia* infection may be etiologically implicated in some cases.
• Type IIIB: refers to sx of prostatic inflammation w/no or few WBCs in the prostatic secretion. The cause is unknown. Spasm in the bladder neck or urethra may be responsible for the sx.

Diagnosis
H&P
■ Acute bacterial prostatitis: sudden or rapidly progressive onset of
• Dysuria, frequency, urgency
• Perineal pain that may radiate to the back, the rectum, or the penis
■ Hematuria or a purulent urethral d/c, urinary retention, fever, chills, and signs of sepsis can also be part of the clinical picture.
■ Chronic bacterial prostatitis: characterized by (+) culture of expressed prostatic secretions. It may cause sx such as suprapubic, low back, or perineal pain and mild urgency, frequency, and dysuria w/urination; it may be associated w/recurrent UTIs.
■ Chronic prostatitis/chronic pain syndrome: manifested w/pain in the pelvic region >3 mo. Sx also can include pain in the suprapubic region, low back, penis, testes, or scrotum.

Labs
■ U/A, urine C&S
■ Cell count and culture of expressed prostatic secretions
■ CBC and blood cultures if fever, chills, or signs of sepsis exist

Treatment
■ **Acute uncomplicated <35 yr:** ceftriaxone 250 mg IM × 1 or cefixime 400 mg PO × 1 then doxycycline 100 mg bid × 10 days
■ **Chronic bacterial:** TMP-SMX-DS 1 tab PO bid × 1 to 3 mo
■ **Chronic prostatitis/chronic pain syndrome:** α-blocking agents controversial
■ A brief course of NSAIDs may be tried until urine localization cultures are completed.

K. TICK-BORNE DISEASES

1 LYME DISEASE

Multisystem disease caused by a spirochete (*Borrelia burgdorferi*) transmitted by the bite of an *Ixodes* tick (most commonly belonging to the species *scapularis*)

Diagnosis

H&P

- The clinical manifestations vary w/stage of disease
- **Early localized stage:** usually manifested by a characteristic expanding annular skin lesion (**erythema chronicum migrans [ECM]**). It typically occurs 3 to 30 days after the tick bite as a centrifugally expanding, erythematous annular patch giving a bull's-eye appearance.
- **Early disseminated stage:** follows stage I by days or wk (incubation period 3-6 wk). Pts may experience attacks of joint swelling and pain in large joints, neurologic complications (aseptic meningitis, encephalitis, cranial neuritis), cardiac abnlities (AV block, myocarditis), and various other multisystem manifestations.
- **Late stage:** incubation period of months to years. It is manifested by inflammatory arthritis affecting large joints (particularly the knee) and chronic cutaneous and neurologic sequelae (encephalopathy, encephalomyelitis); chronic Lyme arthritis is associated w/HLA-DR4 and HLA-DR2 alleles.
- **Post-Lyme syndrome:** nonspecific headaches, fatigue, arthralgias

Labs

- Western blot dx criteria: IgM (2/3 [+] kilodaltons: 23, 39, 41) IgG (5/10 [+] kilodaltons: 18, 21, 28, 30, 39, 41, 45, 58, 66, 93)

Treatment

- Postexposure prophylaxis (*Ixodes*-infected tick bite in endemic area): doxycycline 200 mg PO once with food within 72 hr of bite
- Erythema migrans (early): doxycycline 100 mg PO bid or amoxicillin 500 mg PO tid or cefuroxime axetil 500 mg PO bid or erythromycin 250 mg PO qid all for 14 to 21 days
- Carditis: ceftriaxone 2 g IV q24h or cefotaxime 2 g IV q4h or PCN G 3 million U IV q4h or doxycycline 100 mg PO bid or amoxicillin 500 mg PO tid all for 14 to 21 days
- Facial nerve paralysis: doxycycline 100 mg PO bid or amoxicillin 500 mg PO tid × 14 to 21 days
- Meningitis, encephalitis: ceftriaxone 2 g IV q24h × 14 to 28 days or PCN G 20 million U IV q24h in divided doses or cefotaxime 2 g IV q8h × 14 to 28 days
- Arthritis: doxycycline 100 mg PO bid or amoxicillin 500 mg PO tid × 30 to 60 days or PCN G 20 to 24 million U/day IV × 14 to 28 days
- Pregnant women: avoid doxycycline; amoxicillin 500 mg PO tid × 21 days
- *If PCN allergic + pregnant: azithromycin 500 mg PO q24h × 7 to 10 days
- Post-Lyme syndrome: supportive care, no abx

2 EHRLICHIOSIS AND ANAPLASMOSIS

Zoonotic infection of granulocytes that is caused by an *Ehrlichia* species (*Ehrlichia chaffeensis* and *Anaplasma phagocytophilum*)

Diagnosis

H&P

- Both human monocytic ehrlichiosis (HME) and human granulocytic anaplasmosis (HGA) manifest with headaches, myalgias, and fatigue following 1- to 2-wk incubation.
- Skin lesions (maculopapular rash) are more common in HME (30%).
- Complications include hepatitis, interstitial pneumonitis, renal and respiratory failure, meningoencephalitis (more common with HME [20%]).

Labs

- Giemsa-stained smear demonstrating morulae of the organism within granulocytes (seen in 20% of pts)
- CBC: progressive leukopenia and thrombocytopenia w/nadir near day 7
- LFTs: ALT, AST, LDH, alk phos
- Serologic testing may not be (+) for 2 to 4 wk after onset of symptoms

Treatment

- Doxycycline: 100 mg bid 10 to 14 days for adults. Rifampin: 300 mg bid 7 to 10 days can be used in pregnancy.

3 BABESIOSIS

A tick-transmitted protozoan disease caused by intraerythrocytic parasites of the genus *Babesia*

Diagnosis

H&P

- Clinical presentation: incubation period 1 to 4 wk, or 6 to 9 wk in transfusion-associated disease. Pts have gradual onset of fever, chills, diaphoresis, headache, myalgia, arthralgia, fatigue, and dark urine.
- PE: petechiae, frank or mild hepatosplenomegaly, and jaundice. Infection w/*Babesia divergens* produces a more severe illness w/a rapid onset of sx and parasitemia progressing to massive intravascular hemolysis and AKI.

Labs

- Babesial DNA by PCR on whole blood specimen is the preferred diagnostic method.
- Examination of Giemsa- or Wright-stained thick and thin blood films may reveal intraerythrocytic parasites (*tetrad* or *Maltese cross* composed of four daughter cells attached by cytoplasmic strand) but needs to be differentiated from falciparum malaria.

Treatment

- Combination of atovaquone 750 mg q12h and azithromycin 500 mg on day 1 and 250 mg/day thereafter for 7 days is preferred Rx.
- Combination of quinine sulfate 650 mg PO tid + clindamycin 600 mg PO tid (1.2 g parenterally) is taken for 7 to 10 days for severe disease.
- Exchange transfusions in addition to antimicrobial Rx are successful Rx of severe infections in asplenic pts associated w/high levels of *Babesia microti* or *B. divergens* parasitemia.

4 ROCKY MOUNTAIN SPOTTED FEVER (RMSF)

Tick-borne febrile illness caused by infection with *Rickettsia rickettsii*. In the United States *R. rickettsii* is transmitted mainly by the American dog tick *(Dermacentor variabilis)* and the Rocky Mountain wood tick *(Dermacentor andersoni)*.

Diagnosis

H&P

- Incubation (3-12 days) with initial sx: fever, headache, malaise, myalgias
- **Rash** (88%; but <50% in first 72 hr): blanching erythematous macules **spreading from distal extremities** (wrists/ankles) **to trunk.** Lesions may evolve into papules → nonblanching (petechiae/palpable purpura).
- GI sx: nausea, vomiting, abdominal pain, may mimic "acute abd" (e.g., appendicitis, cholecystitis), mild hepatitis
- Cardiopulmonary: interstitial pneumonitis, myocarditis
- Renal: prerenal azotemia, interstitial nephritis, GN
- Neurologic involvement: encephalitis (confusion, lethargy, delirium), ataxia, convulsion, CN palsy, speech impediment, hemi/paraparesis, spasticity

W/up

- CBC w/diff, LFTs
- Ab titers for *R. rickettsii* (indirect fluorescent Ab test): dx requiring fourfold ↑ 2 wk apart thus not helpful in care of pt despite sensitivity/specificity ~100%
- Timely dx via immunohistologic demonstration of *R. rickettsii* in skin biopsy specimens

Treatment

- Doxycycline 100 mg PO/IV bid × 7 days or 2 days after temp nl. Avoid in pregnancy. May use a 200-mg loading dose.
- Chloramphenicol 50-75 mg/kg/day in four divided doses. This is preferred in pregnancy.
- 3% to 18% of pts present with fever, rash, hx tick bite. Because of the ↑ risk of mortality, empiric doxycycline is recommended.

L. FUNGAL INFECTIONS

1 SYSTEMIC CANDIDIASIS

Etiology

- *Candida albicans:* Together with *Candida glabrata,* they account for 70% to 80% of *Candida* organisms in invasive candidiasis.

- *Candida parapsilosis:* This is associated with indwelling vascular catheters and prosthetic devices.
- *Candida tropicalis:* This occurs especially in leukemic pts.

Risk Factors
- Prolonged hospitalization and ICU stay
- Use of broad-spectrum abxs
- Prolonged indwelling of catheters, especially central venous catheters
- Acute and chronic renal failure
- Surgery requiring general anesthesia
- Cancer (e.g., solid neoplasms)
- Transplantation (bone marrow or solid organ)
- Recent chemoRx/radiation Rx
- Use of immunosuppressive drugs
- Parenteral alimentation
- Use of internal prosthetic devices

Diagnosis

H&P
- Fever unresponsive to broad-spectrum abxs
- Hx of prolonged indwelling IV catheter
- A personal hx of any of the foregoing risk factors
- Physical findings: fever, hypotension, malaise, tachycardia, ΔMS

Specific Diseases
- Candidemia
  - *Candida spp* isolated from at least one blood culture
  - Most common form of invasive candidiasis
  - PE: fever, macronodular skin lesions, septic shock, candida endophthalmitis
- Disseminated candidiasis
  - Seen in pts with neutropenia
  - Associated with multiple deep organ infections or organ failure
  - Blood culture (−)
  - Fever not responding to broad-spectrum abxs
  - PE: discrete erythematous or palpable rash, sepsis/septic shock
- Endophthalmitis
  - Iatrogenic/accidental fungal infection of the eye (exogenous) or hematogenous seeding of the eye (endogenous)
  - Starting as choroidal lesion, progressing to vitreitis and endophthalmitis and eventually blindness
  - PE: fever. Funduscopic exam shows large and off-white "cottonball-like" lesions with indistinct borders.
- *Candida* infection of the CNS
  - Exogenous and endogenous forms
  - Commonly found in long-term ICU pts
  - May manifest as meningitis, mycotic aneurysms, ΔMS
  - PE: fever, neck rigidity, confusion, and coma
- Candidal musculoskeletal infections
  - Previously uncommon; now relatively common probably because of the ↑ frequency of candidemia and disseminated candidiasis
  - Knee and vertebral column involvement (especially lumbosacral vertebral disks and vertebral bodies)
  - PE: tenderness over involved area, fever, erythema, bone deformity, weight loss, and sometimes a draining fistulous tract
- Candidal infections of the heart
  - May manifest as infective endocarditis, myocarditis, or pericarditis
  - PE: fever, hypotension, tachycardia, new or changing murmur
- Hepatosplenic candidiasis (chronic systemic candidiasis)
- Seen in pts with hematologic malignancy and neutropenia; usually develops during recovery from a neutropenic state (normally after undergoing myeloablative chemoRx)
- PE: low-grade fever, right upper quadrant pain, palpable/tender liver, splenomegaly, and rarely jaundice
- *Candida* peritonitis
  - Associated with GI surgery, peritoneal dialysis
  - Clinical manifestations including fever, chills, abdominal pain; nausea vomiting, constipation
  - PE: abdominal distention, abdominal pain, absent bowel sounds

III

DISEASES AND DISORDERS
8. Infectious Diseases

- Other forms of invasive candidiasis
  - *Candida* splenic abscess
  - *Candida* cholecystitis
  - Renal candidiasis

Labs
- Candidemia/disseminated candidiasis
  - Blood cultures helpful but low (+) yield
  - Serum (1,3) β-D-glucan detection assay; high specificity and high (+) predictive value
- Hepatosplenic candidiasis (focal)
  - ↑ Serum alk phos

Imaging
- U/S is useful for diagnosing hepatosplenic abscess. "Bull's-eye or target lesions" are observed in the liver and spleen.
- CT scanning may be used to diagnose hepatosplenic candidiasis as well as intra-abc or renal abscesses.
- Echo is useful to rule in or out *Candida* endocarditis.

Treatment
- Rx depends on whether the patent is neutropenic or not.
  - **Neutropenic adult pts:** fluconazole 800 mg as loading dose then 400 mg/day for at least 2 wk after clinical improvement or (–) blood culture. Amphotericin B is equally efficacious.
  - **Non-neutropenic adult pts:** An echinocandin is the drug of choice (e.g., caspofungin 70 mg IV loading dose then 50 mg/day IV or micafungin 100 mg/day IV or anidulafungin 200 mg IV loading dose then 100 mg IV all for at least 2 wk after clear blood culture and after clinical improvement).
- **Oropharyngeal candidiasis (non-AIDS pts):** fluconazole 100 to 200 mg day or nystatin suspension qid or clotrimazole troches 10 mg 5 × daily all for 7 to 14 days
- **Oropharyngeal candidiasis (AIDS pts):** fluconazole 100 to 200 mg/day × 7 to 14 days
- **Vulvovaginitis:** topical azole Rx: butoconazole 2% cream (5 g) q24h hs × 3 days or clotrimazole 100-mg vaginal tabs (2 hs × 3 days)
- Fluconazole 150 mg PO × 1 day or itraconazole 200 mg PO bid × 1 day

Rx of Disseminated Candidiasis
- Fluconazole 400 mg (6 mg/kg daily IV or PO) or if unstable pt: amphotericin B 0.5 to 0.7 mg/kg/day

Rx of Disseminated Candidiasis with End-Organ Infection
- Rx is the same as for candidemia in non-neutropenic pts. In most cases, Rx is prolonged for at least 4 to 6 wk.
- The echinocandins comprise the first-line Rx.

Surgical Care
- Drainage
- Removal of any foreign bodies
- Surgical débridement
- Organ-specific care (e.g., valve replacement for endocarditis, splenectomy for splenic abscess, or vitrectomy for fungal endophthalmitis)

2 HISTOPLASMOSIS

Definition

Infection caused by the fungus *Histoplasma capsulatum*. It is characterized by a primary pulmonary focus w/occasional progression to *chronic pulmonary histoplasmosis (CPH)* or various forms of dissemination. *Progressive disseminated histoplasmosis (PDH)* may manifest w/a diverse clinical spectrum, including adrenal necrosis, pulmonary and mediastinal fibrosis, and ulcerations of the oropharynx and GI tract. In those pts co-infected w/HIV, it is a defining disease for AIDS.

Diagnosis

Labs
- Demonstration of the organism *(H. capsulatum)* on culture from body fluid or tissues to make definitive dx
- Especially high yield in pts w/AIDS
- Characteristic oval yeast cells in neutrophils w/Giemsa stain from peripheral smear
- Preparations of infected tissue w/Gomori's silver methenamine for revealing yeast forms, especially in areas of caseation necrosis

- Serologic tests, including complement-fixing (CF) Abs and immunodiffusion assays
- Detection of *Histoplasma* antigen in urine: may be influenced by infections w/*Blastomyces* and *Coccidioides*

Treatment
- No drug Rx is required for asymptomatic pulmonary disease.
- Itraconazole is used for mild infection.
- Amphotericin B is used for moderately severe to life-threatening disease or continued illness as a result of primary failure or relapse with itraconazole Rx.
- In pts w/AIDS: lifelong suppressive Rx w/either itraconazole, given 200 mg PO qd, or IV amphotericin B at a dose of 50 mg once weekly. A triazole compound, posaconazole (400 mg PO bid), may be useful in refractory cases, but clinical experience is limited.

3 ASPERGILLOSIS

Illness caused by an infection w/the *Aspergillus* species. *Aspergillus fumigatus* is the usual cause, *Aspergillus flavus* is the second most important species, particularly in invasive disease of immunosuppressed pts and in lesions beginning in the nose and paranasal sinuses.

Diagnosis
H&P
- Clinical presentation is variable, but most pts present w/cough, fever, dyspnea, hemoptysis.

Invasive Aspergillosis
- Definitive dx requires demonstration of tissue invasion as seen on a bx specimen or a (+) culture from the tissue obtained by an invasive procedure such as transbronchial bx.
- CXR and CT scan may reveal cavity formation.

Allergic Bronchopulmonary Aspergillosis
- Lab: peripheral eosinophilia. Galactomannan antigen immunoassay is useful for dx of aspergillus in serum, CSF, BAL. PCR and β-D-glucan assay can also be used.
- CXR: variable from small patchy, fleeting infiltrates (commonly in upper lobes) to lobar consolidation or cavitation. Most pts eventually develop central bronchiectasis.

Treatment
- Invasive aspergillosis
  - Voriconazole 6 mg/kg IV q12h for two doses, then 4 mg/kg q12h PO. Rx for adults is 200 mg bid or 4 mg/kg bid.
  - Caspofungin in pts who fail to respond to or are unable to tolerate other antifungal drugs. The recommended dosage is 70 mg on the first day and 50 mg qd thereafter given as a single dose IV over 1 hr.
  - Allergic bronchopulmonary aspergillosis: prednisone (0.5-1 mg/kg PO) until the CXR has cleared, followed by alternate-day Rx at 0.5 mg/kg PO for 3 to 6 mo, then gradually tapered. Itraconazole is added to corticosteroids (corticosteroid-sparing effect).
  - Aspergillomas: surgical resection/arterial embolization for those pts w/severe hemoptysis or life-threatening hemorrhage. For those pts at risk for marked hemoptysis w/inadequate pulmonary reserve, consider itraconazole 200 to 400 mg/day PO.

4 BLASTOMYCOSIS

Systemic pyogranulomatous disease caused by a dimorphic fungus, *Blastomyces dermatitidis*. It exists in warm, moist soil that is rich in organic material. Widely disseminated disease is most common in immunocompromised hosts, especially those with AIDS. Initial infections result from inhalation of conidia into the lungs, although primary cutaneous blastomycosis has been reported after dog bites.

Diagnosis
H&P
- Acute infection: <50% symptomatic, median incubation 30 to 45 days. Sx are nonspecific and mimic influenza or bacterial infection with abrupt onset of myalgias, arthralgias, chills and fever; transient pleuritic pain, cough that is initially nonproductive. Resolution within 4 wk is usual.
- Sx and signs of chronic pneumonia include productive cough, hemoptysis, pleuritic chest pain, weight loss, low-grade pyrexia.

- Cutaneous infection is most common. It may occur with or without pulmonary disease. Two different lesions are seen:
  - *Verrucous:* Beginning as a small, papulopustular lesion on exposed body areas, it may develop into an eschar with peripheral microabscesses.
  - *Ulcerative:* SC nodules (cold abscesses) and rarely cutaneous inoculation blastomycosis may occur.

Labs
- Dx established by isolation of *B. dermatitidis* on culture

Treatment
- Oral itraconazole for 6 to 12 mo for mild to moderate disease
- Amphotericin B × 2 wk followed by oral itraconazole for 6 to 12 mo for moderately severe to severe disease

5 MUCORMYCOSIS

Definition

Mucormycosis is a fungal infection by *Zygomycetes fungi.* Infection is seen in association with underlying conditions, including DM especially with ketoacidosis, hematologic malignancies, stem cell or solid organ transplants, severe burns or trauma, Rx with deferoxamine or iron overload states, steroid Rx, immunodeficiency states (e.g., AIDS), injection drug use, and malnutrition. Immunocompetent hosts may become infected in tropical climates.

Diagnosis
- Established by tissue biopsy and culture

H&P
- Rhinocerebral–rhino-orbital–paranasal syndrome may manifest with fever, facial and orbital pain, headache, diplopia, loss of vision, facial or orbital cellulitis, facial anesthesia, cranial nerve dysfunction, black nasal d/c, epistaxis, and seizure. Physical findings in this situation include proptosis; chemosis; nasal, palatal, or pharyngeal necrotic ulcerations; and retinal infarction. Thrombosis of the cavernous sinus or internal carotid artery may occur. This form of mucormycosis is found most commonly in pts with DM, primarily in the presence of acidosis, and in pts with leukemia and neutropenia.
- Pulmonary mucormycosis can manifest with pneumonia, lung abscess, pulmonary infarction, pleurisy, pleural effusion, hemoptysis, chills, and fever. This form of mucormycosis is found most commonly in immunocompromised neutropenic hosts after chemoRx for hematologic malignancies.

Treatment
- Aggressive surgical débridement of involved tissues and antifungal Rx with liposomal amphotericin B 5 to 10 mg/kg/day

6 CRYPTOCOCCOSIS
- Infection caused by the fungal organism *C. neoformans*

Diagnosis

H&P
- >90% of pts present w/meningitis; almost all have fever and headache. Meningismus, photophobia, and ∆MS are seen in approximately 25%.
- Most common infections outside the CNS:
  - Lungs (fever, cough, dyspnea)
  - Skin (cellulitis, papular eruption)
  - Lymph nodes (lymphadenitis)

Labs
- Culture and India ink stain (60%-80% sensitive in culture-proven cases), examination of the CSF in all cases when CNS involvement is suspected
- Blood and serum cryptococcal antigen assay (>90% sensitivity and specificity)
- Culture and histologic examination of bx material
- HIV

Imaging
- CT scan or MRI of the head: if focal neurologic involvement is suspected
- CXR: to exclude pulmonary involvement

Treatment
- Primary cutaneous infection: fluconazole
- Disseminated infection or immunocompromised host: Rx w/IV amphotericin B (0.8 mg/kg/day) w/flucytosine 37.5 mg/kg

- After stabilization (usually several weeks), consider fluconazole (200-400 mg qd PO) for additional 6 to 8 wk. Voriconazole, a newer imidazole, also has activity against most isolates.
- Alternative: IV fluconazole for initial Rx in pts unable to tolerate amphotericin B
- If symptomatic ICP: therapeutic LP or intraventricular shunt

7 COCCIDIODOMYCOSIS

Infectious disease caused by the fungus *Coccidioides immitis*. It is usually asymptomatic and characterized by a primary pulmonary focus with infrequent progression to chronic pulmonary disease and dissemination to other organs.

Diagnosis

H&P

- The clinical manifestations vary widely according to the host, the severity of the illness, and location of dissemination.
- Asx infection or illness is consistent with a nonspecific URI in at least 60%.
- Sx of primary infection—cough, malaise, fever, chills, night sweats, anorexia, weakness, and arthralgias (desert rheumatism)—occur in the remaining 40% within 3 wk of exposure.
- Erythema nodosum and erythema multiforme are more common in women.
- Disseminated or extrapulmonary disease occurs in approximately 0.5% of acutely infected pts.
- Early signs of probable dissemination are fever, malaise, hilar adenopathy, and ↑ ESR persisting in the setting of primary infection.
- Musculoskeletal involvement includes bone lesions, often unifocal; rib, long bone, and vertebral lesions are common.
- Meningeal involvement includes headache, fever, weakness, confusion, lethargy, cranial nerve defects, seizures; meningeal signs often minimal or absent.
- Cutaneous involvement consists of variable lesions—pustules, papules, plaques, nodules, ulcers, abscesses, or verrucous proliferative lesions.

Labs

- CBC to reveal eosinophilia, especially with erythema nodosum
- Definitive dx based on demonstration of the organism by culture from body fluids or tissues
  - Greatest yield with pus, sputum, synovial fluid, and soft tissue aspirations, varying with the degree of dissemination
  - Possible (+) cultures of blood, gastric aspirate, pleural effusion, peritoneal fluid, and CSF, but less frequently obtained
- Serologic evaluations
  - Latex agglutination and complement fixation
  - ↑ Serum complement-fixing Ab (CFA) titers ≥1:32 strongly correlated with disseminated disease, except in meningitis, which has lower titers
  - Meningeal disease: CFA detected in CSF, except with high serum CFA titers secondary to concurrent extraneural disease
  - ELISA against a 33-kDa spherule antigen to detect and monitor CNS disease

Treatment

- Severe disease: Fluconazole, ketoconazole, or itraconazole is given for 3 to 6 mo.
- For pulmonary infections, Rx with either fluconazole or itraconazole, given for 6 to 12 wk, appears to be = in efficacy.
- Amphotericin B is the classic Rx for disseminated extraneural disease; the dose is 0.6 to 1 mg/kg/day, qd for the first wk then 0.8 mg/kg every other day, for a total dose of 1 to 2.5 g or until clinical and serologic remission is accomplished.
  - Local instillation into body cavities such as sinuses, fistulas, and abscesses has been adjunct to Rx.
  - Duration of Rx for extraneural disease is undefined but probably ~1 yr.
- With meningeal disease, fluconazole 400 to 1000 mg PO q24h is given indefinitely.

8 SPOROTRICHOSIS

Granulomatous disease caused by skin inoculation with the dimorphic fungus *Sporothrix schenckii*

Diagnosis

- The Dx should be considered in individuals who are occupationally exposed to soil, decaying plant matter, and thorny plants (gardeners, horticulturists, farmers) who present with chronic nonhealing ulcers or lesions with or without associated arthritis or pulmonary sx.
- Isolation of the fungus from any site is considered diagnostic of infection.

Treatment

- **Cutaneous:** itraconazole 200 mg/day × 2 to 4 wk after all lesions resolved (usually 3-6 mo)
- **Osteoarticular:** itraconazole 200 mg PO bid × 12 mo
- **Pulmonary:** lipid amphotericin B 3 to 5 mg/kg IV
- **Meningeal or disseminated:** lipid amphotericin B 5 mg/kg IV once daily × 4 to 6 wk, then (if improved) itraconazole 200 mg PO bid for 12 mo

9 TINEA

Tinea Corporis

Caused by the genera *Trichophyton* and *Microsporum*

Diagnosis

H&P

- Erythematous plaques have a half-moon shape and a scaling border.
- The acute inflammation tends to move down the inner thigh and usually spares the scrotum; in severe cases the fungus may spread onto the buttocks.
- Itching may be severe.
- An important diagnostic sign is the **advancing well-defined border with a tendency toward central clearing.**
- Single or multiple annular lesions have an advancing scaly border; the margin is slightly raised, reddened, and may be pustular.
- The central area becomes hypopigmented and less scaly as the active border progresses outward.
- The trunk and legs are primarily involved.

Labs

- Microscopic examination of hyphae (wet mount preparation and KOH solution): Dermatophytes appear as translucent branching filaments (hyphae) with lines of separation appearing at irregular intervals.

Treatment

- Butenafine or terbinafine cream qd for 14 days
- Systemic Rx (PO fluconazole, PO terbinafine × 4 wk) reserved for severe cases

Tinea Cruris

- Caused by the genera *Trichophyton, Epidermophyton,* and *Microsporum. Trichophyton rubrum* and *Epidermophyton floccosum* are the most common infecting agents.

Labs

- Microscopic examination

Treatment

- Butenafine or terbinafine cream qd for 14 days
- Systemic Rx (PO fluconazole, PO terbinafine × 4 wk) reserved for severe cases

Onychomycosis

Treatment

- Terbinafine 250 mg PO q24h × 6 wk for fingernails, 12 wk Rx for toenails

M. VIRAL INFECTIONS

1 INFLUENZA

Infection with influenza type A or B virus. Seasonal influenza can include the H1N1 virus. Severe acute respiratory syndrome (SARS) is a similar respiratory illness caused by a coronavirus called SARS-associated coronavirus (SARSCoV).

H&P

- "Classic flu" is characterized by abrupt onset of fever, headache, myalgias, anorexia, and malaise after a 1- to 2-day incubation period.
- Clinical syndromes are similar to those produced by other respiratory viruses, including pharyngitis, common colds, tracheobronchitis, bronchiolitis, and croup.
- Respiratory sx such as cough, sore throat, and nasal d/c are usually present at the onset of illness, but systemic sx predominate.
- Elderly pts may experience fever, weakness, and confusion without any respiratory complaints.
- Acute deterioration to status asthmaticus may occur in pts with asthma.
- Influenza pneumonia: Rapidly progressive cough, dyspnea, and cyanosis may occur after typical flu onset. This may be caused by primary influenza pneumonia or secondary bacterial pneumonia (often pneumococcal or staphylococcal infection).

Diagnosis

- Diagnostic tests available for influenza include viral cultures, serology, rapid diagnostic (antigen) testing, RT-PCR, and IFA.
- Virus isolation from nasal or throat swab or sputum specimens is the most rapid diagnostic method in the setting of acute illness.
- Commercial rapid influenza diagnostic tests (RIDTs) are available. They can detect influenza virus antigens within 15 min of testing. Rapid flu test should be collected as early as possible, ideally within 4 days of onset. False(−) results are common during the flu season. A (−) test result does *not* exclude dx of influenza.

Treatment

- Supportive care: antipyretics. Avoid use of aspirin in children because of the association with Reye's syndrome.
- Abxs are indicated if bacterial pneumonia is proven or suspected.
- Amantadine is *not* recommended because of resistant isolates.
- Neuraminidase inhibitors block release of virions from infected cells, resulting in shortened duration of sx and ↓ in complications; they are effective against both influenza A and B.
- Zanamivir, administered via inhaler
  - For Rx, 10 mg (2 inhalations of 5 mg each) twice daily for 5 days
  - For prevention in households, 10 mg (2 inhalations of 5 mg each) once daily for 17 days
- Oseltamivir: 75 mg PO bid × 5 days
- For prevention, 75 mg PO once daily for a minimum of 2 wk in an outbreak setting or 7 days after exposure for an adult

2 HERPES SIMPLEX (HSV)

HSV-1 is associated primarily with oral infections, and HSV-2 causes mainly genital infections. However, either type can infect any site. After the primary infection, the virus enters the nerve endings in the skin directly below the lesions and ascends to the dorsal root ganglia, where it remains in a latent stage until it is reactivated.

H&P

Primary Infection

- Sx occur from 3 to 7 days after contact (respiratory droplets, direct contact).
- Constitutional sx include low-grade fever, headache and myalgias, regional lymphadenopathy, and localized pain.
- Pain, burning, itching, and tingling last several hr.
- Grouped vesicles, usually with surrounding erythema, appear and generally ulcerate or crust within 48 hr.
- The vesicles are uniform in size (differentiating it from herpes zoster vesicles, which vary in size).
- During the acute eruption the pt is uncomfortable; involvement of lips and inside of mouth may make it unpleasant for the pt to eat; urinary retention may complicate involvement of the genital area.
- Lesions generally last from 2 to 6 wk and heal without scarring.

Recurrent Infection

- This is generally caused by alteration in the immune system; fatigue, stress, menses, local skin trauma, and exposure to sunlight are contributing factors.
- The prodromal sx (fatigue, burning and tingling of the affected area) last 12 to 24 hr.
- A cluster of lesions generally evolves within 24 hr from a macule to a papule, and then vesicles surrounded by erythema; the vesicles coalesce and subsequently rupture within 4 days, revealing erosions covered by crusts.
- The crusts are generally shed within 7 to 10 days, revealing a pink surface.
- The most frequent location of the lesions is on the vermilion border of the lips (HSV-1), the penile shaft or glans penis and the labia (HSV-2), buttocks (seen more frequently in women), fingertips (herpetic whitlow), and trunk (may be confused with herpes zoster).
- Rapid onset of diffuse cutaneous herpes simplex (eczema herpeticum) may occur in certain atopic infants and adults. It is a medical emergency, especially in young infants, and should be promptly treated with acyclovir.
- Herpes encephalitis, meningitis, and ocular herpes can occur in pts with immunocompromised status and occasionally in nl hosts.

Diagnosis

Labs

- Direct immunofluorescent Ab slide tests provide a rapid dx.

- Viral culture is the most definitive method for dx; results are generally available in 1 or 2 days. The lesions should be sampled during the vesicular or early ulcerative stage; cervical samples should be taken from the endocervix with a swab.
- Pap smear will detect HSV-infected cells in cervical tissue from women without sx.
- Serologic tests for HSV

Treatment
- See the earlier section on genital herpes under "Genital ulcers."

N. TUBERCULOSIS

DEFINITION
Infection of the lung and, occasionally, surrounding structures, caused by the bacterium *M. tuberculosis*

Diagnosis

W/up
- Sputum for AFB stains
- CXR
- PPD
  - Recent conversion from (−) to (+) reaction within 3 mo of exposure is highly suggestive of recent infection.
  - Single (+) PPD reaction is not helpful diagnostically.
  - (−) PPD reaction: Never r/o acute TB.
  - Be certain that (+) PPD reaction does not reflect "booster phenomenon" (prior [+] PPD reaction may become [−] after several years and return to [+] only after second repeated PPD; repeat second PPD within 1 wk), which thus may mimic skin test conversion.
  - (+) PPD reaction is determined as follows:
    - Induration after 72 hr of intradermal injection of 0.1 mL of 5 tuberculin units (TU) PPD
    - 5-mm induration if HIV(+) (or other severe immunosuppressed state affecting cellular immune function), close contact of active TB, fibrotic chest lesions
    - 10-mm induration if in high–medical risk groups (immunosuppressive disease or Rx, renal failure, gastrectomy, silicosis, diabetes), foreign-born high-risk group (Southeast Asia, Latin America, Africa, India), low socioeconomic groups, IV drug addict, prisoner, health care worker
      - 15-mm induration if ↓ risk
- QuantiFERON test (QFT-G) is a blood test that measures interferon response to specific *M. tuberculosis* antigens. It may assist in distinguishing true (+) reactions of individuals w/latent TB from PPD reactions related to nontuberculous mycobacteria, prior bacillus Calmette-Guérin (BCG) vaccination, or difficult-to-interpret skin test results from persons w/dermatologic conditions or immediate allergic reactions to PPD.

Labs
- Sputum for AFB stains and culture. Induce sputum if pt is not coughing productively.
- Sputum from bronchoscopy is used if there is a high suspicion of TB w/(−) expectorated induced sputum for AFB.
- (+) AFB smear is essential before or shortly after Rx to ensure subsequent growth for definitive dx and sensitivity testing.
- Consider lung bx if sputum (−), especially if infiltrates are predominantly interstitial.
- AFB stain(−) sputum may grow *M. tuberculosis* subsequently.

CXR
- Primary infection reflected by a calcified peripheral lung nodule w/a calcified hilar lymph node
- Reactivation pulmonary TB
  - Necrosis
  - Cavitation (especially on apical lordotic views)
  - Fibrosis and hilar retraction
  - Bronchopneumonia
  - Interstitial infiltrates
  - Miliary pattern
- Many of preceding features may also accompany progressive primary TB.

Treatment

- Compliance (rigid adherence to Rx regimen) is the chief determinant of success. Supervised directly observed Rx (DOT) is recommended for all pts and is mandatory for unreliable pts.
- Table 8-6 describes current regimens for Rx of drug-susceptible TB. Dosages and side effects of anti-TB drugs are described in Table 8-7.
- Drug resistance (often multiple drug resistance [MDRTB]) by
  - Prior Rx
  - Acquisition of TB in developing countries
  - Homelessness
  - AIDS
  - Imprisonment
  - IV drug addiction
  - Known contact w/MDRTB
- Preventive Rx for PPD conversion only (infection w/o disease)
  - Must be certain that CXR is nl and pt has no sx of TB
  - INH 300 mg qd for 9 to 12 mo; at least 12 mo if HIV(+)
  - Most important groups
    - HIV(+) and other severely immunocompromised pts
    - Close contacts of active TB pt
    - Recent converters
    - Pts with old TB on CXR
    - IV drug addicts
    - Pts w/a medical risk factor
    - Residents and natives of, or travellers to, a high-risk foreign country
    - Homeless pts
  - Infants are generally given prophylaxis immediately if they have recent contact with an active TB pt (even if the infant's PPD reaction is [−]), then retested w/ PPD in 3 mo (continuing INH if PPD reaction becomes [+] and stopping INH if PPD reaction remains [−]).
  - Pts w/a long-term, stable PPD reaction (several years) are given INH prophylaxis generally only if they are <35 yr old.
    - INH toxicity may outweigh benefit.
    - Individualize decision.
  - Preventive Rx for suspected INH-resistant organisms is unclear.
  - All contacts (especially close household contacts and infants) should be properly tested for PPD conversions during 3 mo after exposure.
  - Those w/(+) PPD reaction should be evaluated for active TB and properly treated or given prophylaxis.

TABLE 8-6 ■ Current Regimens for Treatment of Drug-Susceptible Tuberculosis

Regimen	Initial Phase	Continuation Phase
Daily or 5 days/wk[*]	8 wk of INH, RIF, PZA, ± EMB	18 wk of INH and RIF
Intermittent[†]	(a) 2 wk of daily INH, RIF, PZA, and EMB (or SM); then 6 wk of INH, RIF, PZA, EMB biw or tiw	18 wk of INH and RIF biw
	(b) 8 wk of tiw INH, RIF, PZA, and EMB (or SM)	18 wk of INH and RIF tiw

biw, Twice weekly; EMB, ethambutol; INH, isoniazid; PZA, pyrazinamide; RIF, rifampin; SM, streptomycin; tiw, thrice weekly.

[*]The daily regimen is employed when patients self-administer their drugs. There is enough redundancy that if patients miss some of their doses, the outcome will remain acceptable.

[†]The intermittent regimens are intended for directly observed therapy (DCT). Regimen (a) entails a total of 62 doses and has yielded more than 95% success rates for the past 22 yr in Denver, Colorado. Regimen (b) involves 78 doses and has also resulted in success rates of approximately 95% in Hong Kong, where it is the standard regimen.

Adapted from Vincent JL, Abraham E, Moore FA, et al: Textbook of Critical Care, 6th ed. Philadelphia, Saunders, 2011.

Drug	Daily Dosage	Twice- or Thrice-Weekly Dosage	Adverse Effects
Isoniazid	5 mg/kg oral (max: 300 mg)	900 mg biw 600 mg tiw	Hepatitis, peripheral neuritis, drug-induced lupus, seizures, and hypersensitivity with rash and fever; drug interactions with phenytoin (Dilantin) and disulfiram; pyridoxine can decrease neurotoxicity
Rifampin	10 mg/kg oral (max: 600 mg)	10 mg/kg 600 mg biw 600 mg tiw	Orange body secretions, flulike syndrome, hepatitis, pruritus, thrombocytopenia, nausea, anorexia, diarrhea, renal failure, and multiple drug interactions
Rifabutin*	10 mg/kg oral (max: 300 mg)	5 mg/kg	Neutropenia, uveitis, hepatotoxicity, orange discoloration of body fluids
Rifapentine†	10 mg/kg *once weekly* (max: 600 mg)		Similar to rifampin
Pyrazinamide	15-30 mg/kg oral (max: 2 g)	30-35 mg/kg	Hyperuricemia, hepatitis, rash, nausea, and anorexia
Ethambutol	25 mg/kg initial 2 mo, then 15 mg/kg oral	50 mg/kg biw 30 mg/kg tiw	Optic neuritis and GI discomfort

biw, Twice weekly; tiw, thrice weekly.

*Rifabutin and rifapentine are considered first-line agents when intolerance to rifampin precludes its use or concerning drug interactions exist.

†Rifapentine is only used in once-weekly dose in HIV-negative patients with noncavitary and uncomplicated disease. It is not approved for use in children.

Adapted from Vincent JL, Abraham E, Moore FA, et al: Textbook of Critical Care, 6th ed. Philadelphia, Saunders, 2011.

Nephrology 9

A. RENAL FLUID AND ELECTROLYTE FORMULAS

- See Box 9-1.

B. WATER BALANCE

- See Box 9-2.

C. REPLACEMENT FLUIDS

- See Table 9-1.

D. ACID-BASE DISORDERS

1 APPROACH TO ACID-BASE DISORDERS

- Figure 9-1 illustrates the diagnostic approach to determining acid-base status.
- Table 9-2 describes acid-base abnlities and appropriate compensatory responses for simple disorders.
- Figure 9-2 illustrates the acid-base nomogram.
- Box 9-3 describes causes of mixed disturbances associated with metabolic acidosis.

Box 9-1 • Renal Fluid and Electrolyte Formulas

Calculation of Creatinine Clearance (C_{Cr})

$$C_{Cr} \text{ (male)} = \frac{(140 - age) \times wt \ (in \ Kg)}{Serum \ creatinine \times 72}$$

$$C_{Cr} \text{ (female)} = 0.85 \times C_{Cr} \text{ (male)}$$

Calculation of Fractional Excretion of Sodium (FE_{Na})

$$FE_{Na} \ (\%) = \frac{Quantity \ of \ Na^+ \ excreted}{Quantity \ of \ Na^+ \ filtered} \times 100$$

or

$$FE_{Na} \ (\%) = \frac{U/P_{Na} \times 100}{U/P_{Cr}}$$

or

$$FE_{Na} \ (\%) = \frac{U_{Na} \times V}{P_{Na} \times \left(U_{Cr} \times V/P_{Cr}\right)} \times 100$$

or

$$FE_{Na} \ (\%) = \frac{U_{Na} \times P_{Cr}}{P_{Na} \times U_{Cr}} \times 100$$

where U_{Na} is urine sodium concentration, V is urine flow rate, P_{Na} is plasma sodium concentration, U_{Cr} is urine creatinine concentration, and P_{Cr} is plasma creatinine concentration.

Box 9-1 • Renal Fluid and Electrolyte Formulas—cont'd

Sodium Formulas

Serum sodium correction in hyperglycemia:

$$Na^+_{euglycemic} = Measured\ Na^+ + 0.028\ (glucose - 100)$$

Estimated sodium deficit in hyponatremia:

$$Na^+\ deficit\ (mEq) = 0.6 \times body\ weight \times \left(desired\ plasma\ Na^+ - current\ plasma\ Na^+\right)$$

Estimated sodium excess in hypernatremia:

$$Na^+\ excess\ (mEq) = 0.6\ body\ weight\ (kg) \times \left(current\ plasma\ Na^+ - 140\right)$$

Serum sodium correction in hyperlipidemia and hyperproteinemia:

$$Decrease\ (mEq/L)\ serum\ Na^+\ in\ hyperlipidemia = plasma\ lipids\ (mg/dL) \times 0.002$$

$$Decrease\ (mEq/L)\ serum\ Na^+\ in\ hyperproteinemia = increment\ of\ total\ protein > 8\ g/dL \times 0.25$$

Potassium Formulas

Diagnostic equations for hyperkalemia:

Fractional excretion of potassium (FEK)	$\dfrac{\left(U_K/S_K \times 100\%\right)}{\left(U_{Cr}/S_{Cr}\right)}$	FEK <10% indicates renal cause FEK >10% indicates extrarenal cause Values can be increased in cases of chronic renal failure
Transtubular potassium gradient	$\dfrac{\left[\dfrac{(U_K)}{\left(U_{osm}/S_{osm}\right)}\right]}{S_K}$ *or* $\dfrac{U_K \times S_{osm}}{S_K \times U_{osm}}$	Gradient <6-8 indicates renal cause Gradient >6-8 indicates extrarenal cause Values can be increased in cases of chronic renal failure

Osmolality Formulas

$$Calculated\ osmolality = 2\left(Na^+ + K^+\right) + \frac{Glucose}{18} + \frac{BUN}{2.8}$$

$$Effective\ osmolality = 2\left(Na^+\right) + \frac{Glucose}{18}$$

$$Osmolal\ gap = Measured\ osmolality - calculated\ osmolality$$

U_K, Urine potassium; S_K, serum potassium; U_{Cr}, urine creatinine; S_{Cr}, serum creatinine; U_{osm}, urine osmolality; S_{osm}, serum osmolality.

2 METABOLIC ACIDOSIS

Etiology

- Metabolic acidosis w/AG (AG acidosis). The mnemonic MUDPILES is useful to remember the causes of AG acidosis:
  - Methanol
  - Uremia
  - DKA, alcoholic ketoacidosis (AKA), starvation ketoacidosis (SKA)

To estimate the amount of TBW, the following formula is frequently used:

$$TBW = Body\ weight\ (kg) \times 60\%$$

The water deficit of a pt can be estimated by the following equation:

$$Water\ deficit = 0.6 \times body\ weight\ in\ kg \times ([P_{Na}/140 - 1])$$

where P_{Na} is plasma sodium concentration.
Alternatively, the free water deficit from the osmolality can be calculated as the following:

$$H_2O\ deficit\ (L) = Total\ body\ weight\ (kg) \times 0.6 \left(1 - \frac{nl\ osm}{observed\ osm}\right)$$

To calculate the free water clearance based on the osmolar clearance, the following formula can be used:

$$Free\ water\ clearance = Urine\ volume - osmolar\ clearance$$

where the osmolar clearance is calculated as:

$$Osmolar\ clearance = \frac{Urine\ osmolarity \times urine\ volume}{Plasma\ osmolality}$$

TABLE 9-1 ■ Replacement Fluids

Fluids	Na (mEq/L)	K (mEq/L)	Cl (mEq/L)	HCO₃⁻ (mEq/L)	Ca (mEq/L)	Kcal/L
½ Nl saline	77	—	77	—	—	—
Nl saline	154	—	154	—	—	—
D₅W	—	—	—	—	—	170
D₁₀W	—	—	—	—	—	340
Lactated Ringer's solution	130	4	109	28*	3	9
Extracellular fluid	141	4	—	27	5	—

From Nguyen TC, Abilez OJ (eds): Practical Guide to the Care of the Surgical Patient: The Pocket Scalpel. Philadelphia, Mosby, 2009.

*Lactate converted to HCO₃⁻ in liver.

- Paraldehyde, phenformin (or metformin)
- Iron, isoniazid
- Lactic acidosis (cyanide, H_2S, CO, methemoglobin)
- Ethylene glycol
- Salicylates
- Metabolic acidosis w/nl AG (hyperchloremic acidosis)
  - RTA (including acidosis of aldosterone deficiency)
  - Intestinal loss of HCO_3^- (diarrhea, pancreatic fistula)
  - Carbonic anhydrase inhibitors (e.g., acetazolamide)
  - Dilutional acidosis (as a result of rapid infusion of HCO_3^--free isotonic saline)
  - Ingestion of exogenous acids (ammonium chloride, methionine, cystine, CaCl)
  - Ileostomy
  - Ureterosigmoidostomy
  - Drugs: amiloride, triamterene, spironolactone, β-blockers

Diagnosis (Fig. 9-3)
- Measurement of urinary AG ($U_{Na+} + U_{K+} - U_{Cl-}$) and urinary pH is useful in the ddx of hyperchloremic metabolic acidosis:
  - (−) Urinary AG suggests GI loss of HCO_3^-.
  - (+) Urinary AG suggests altered distal urinary acidification.
  - ↓ Urinary pH and ↑ plasma K^+ in pts w/(+) urinary AG suggest selective aldosterone deficiency.
  - Urinary pH >5.5 and ↑ plasma K^+ suggest hyperkalemic distal RTA.
  - Urinary pH >5.5 and nl/↓ plasma K^+ indicate classic RTA.

Treatment
- Correct the underlying cause (e.g., DKA, diarrhea, uremia).

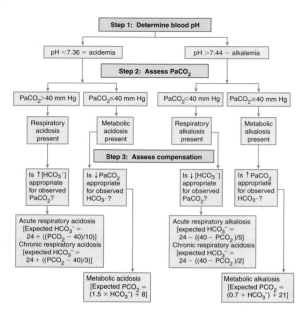

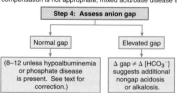

FIGURE 9-1. Determining acid-base status. *(From Cameron AM: Current Surgical Therapy, 10th ed. Philadelphia, Saunders, 2011.)*

3 RENAL TUBULAR ACIDOSIS (RTA)

- Disorder characterized by an inability to excrete H^+ or inadequate generation of new HCO_3^-. Four types:
  - **Type 1 (classic, distal RTA):** abnlity in distal hydrogen secretion resulting in hypokalemic hyperchloremic metabolic acidosis
  - **Type 2 (proximal RTA):** ↓ proximal HCO_3^- reabsorption resulting in hypokalemic hyperchloremic metabolic acidosis
  - **Type 3 (RTA of glomerular insufficiency):** normokalemic hyperchloremic metabolic acidosis as a result of impaired ability to generate sufficient NH_3 in the setting of ↓ GFR (<30 mL/min). This type of RTA is described in older textbooks and is considered by many not to be a distinct entity.
  - **Type 4 (hyporeninemic hypoaldosteronemic RTA):** aldosterone deficiency or antagonism resulting in ↓ distal acidification and ↓ distal Na^+ reabsorption w/subsequent hyperkalemic hyperchloremic acidosis

Etiology

- Type 1 RTA: autoimmune disorders, PBC and other liver diseases, meds (amphotericin, NSAIDs), SLE, SS, genetic disorders (Ehlers-Danlos syndrome,

TABLE 9-2 ■ Acid-Base Abnormalities and Appropriate Compensatory Responses for Simple Disorders

Primary Acid-Base Disorders	Primary Defect	Effect on pH	Compensatory Response	Expected Range of Compensation	Limits of Compensation
Respiratory acidosis	Alveolar hypoventilation ($\uparrow$ P_{CO_2})	$\downarrow$	$\uparrow$ Renal HCO_3^- reabsorption (HCO_3^- $\uparrow$)	Acute: $\Delta[HCO_3^-] = +1$ mEq/L for each $\uparrow$ ΔP_{CO_2} of 10 mm Hg	$[HCO_3^-] = 38$ mEq/L
				Chronic: $\Delta[HCO_3^-] = +4$ mEq/L for each $\uparrow$ ΔP_{CO_2} of 10 mm Hg	$[HCO_3^-] = 45$ mEq/L
Respiratory alkalosis	Alveolar Hyperventilation ($\downarrow$ P_{CO_2})	$\uparrow$	$\downarrow$ Renal HCO_3^- reabsorption (HCO_3^- $\downarrow$)	Acute: $\Delta[HCO_3^-] = -2$ mEq/L for each $\downarrow$ ΔP_{CO_2} of 10 mm Hg	$[HCO_3^-] = 18$ mEq/L
				Chronic: $\Delta[HCO_3^-] = -5$ mEq/L for each $\downarrow$ ΔP_{CO_2} of 10 mm Hg	$[HCO_3^-] = 15$ mEq/L
Metabolic acidosis	Loss of HCO_3^- or gain of $H+$ ($\downarrow$ HCO_3^-)	$\downarrow$	Alveolar hyperventilation to $\uparrow$ pulmonary CO_2 excretion ($\downarrow$ P_{CO_2})	$P_{CO_2} = 1.5[HCO_3^-] + 8 \pm 2$ $P_{CO_2} =$ last 2 digits of pH $\times$ 100 $P_{CO_2} = 15 + [HCO_3^-]$	$P_{CO_2} = 15$ mm Hg
Metabolic alkalosis	Gain of HCO_3^- or loss of $H+$ ($\uparrow$ HCO_3^-)	$\uparrow$	Alveolar hypoventilation to $\downarrow$ pulmonary CO_2 excretion ($\uparrow$ P_{CO_2})	$P_{CO_2} = +0.6$ mm Hg for $\Delta[HCO_3^-]$ of 1 mEq/L. $P_{CO_2} = 15 + [HCO_3^-]$	$P_{CO_2} = 55$ mm Hg

Adapted from Bidani A, Tauzon DM, Heming TA: Regulation of whole body acid-base balance. In: DuBose TD, Hamm LL, editors. Acid-Base and Electrolytes Disorders: A Companion to Brenner and Rector's The Kidney. Philadelphia, Saunders, 2002, pp. 1-21.

From Vincent JL, Abraham E, Moore FA, et al (eds): Textbook of Critical Care, 6th ed. Philadelphia, Saunders, 2011.

Marfan syndrome, hereditary elliptocytosis), toxins (toluene), disorders w/ nephrocalcinosis (hyperparathyroidism, vitamin D intoxication, idiopathic hypercalciuria), tubulointerstitial disease (obstructive uropathy, renal transplantation)
- Type 2 RTA: Fanconi's syndrome, primary hyperparathyroidism, MM, medications (acetazolamide)
- Type 4 RTA: DM, sickle cell disease, Addison's disease, urinary obstruction

Diagnosis

Labs

- ABGs: metabolic acidosis, with nl AG
- Serum K^+ $\downarrow$ in RTA types 1 and 2, nl in type 3, and high in type 4
- Minimum urine pH >5.5 in RTA type 1 and <5.5 in types 2, 3, and 4
- Urinary AG 0 or (+) in all types of RTA

Treatment

- Type 1 and type 2: PO $NaHCO_3$ (1-2 mEq/kg/day in type 1 RTA, 2-4 mEq/kg/day in type 2 RTA) titrated to correct acidosis
- K^+ supplementation in hypokalemic pts
- Type 4 RTA: furosemide to lower $\uparrow$ K^+ levels and $NaHCO_3$ to correct significant acidosis. Fludrocortisone 100 to 300 μg/day can be used to correct mineralocorticoid deficiency.

4 RESPIRATORY ACIDOSIS

Etiology

- Pulmonary disease (COPD, severe pneumonia, pulmonary edema, interstitial fibrosis)

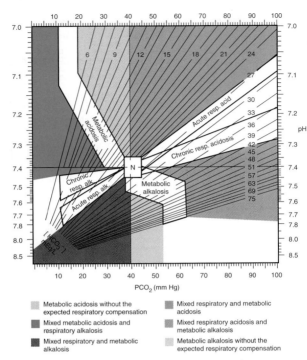

FIGURE 9-2. Map for acid-base disorders. *(From Ferri F: Practical Guide to the Care of the Medical Patient, 8th ed. St. Louis, Mosby, 2011.)*

Legend:
- Metabolic acidosis without the expected respiratory compensation
- Mixed metabolic acidosis and respiratory alkalosis
- Mixed respiratory and metabolic alkalosis
- Mixed respiratory and metabolic acidosis
- Mixed respiratory acidosis and metabolic alkalosis
- Metabolic alkalosis without the expected respiratory compensation

The labeled uncolored areas may represent either a pure primary disturbance or a complex mixed disturbance.

- Airway obstruction (foreign body, severe bronchospasm, laryngospasm)
- Thoracic cage disorders (pneumothorax, flail chest, kyphoscoliosis)
- Defects in muscles of respiration (myasthenia gravis, hypokalemia, muscular dystrophy)
- Defects in PNS (amyotrophic lateral sclerosis, poliomyelitis, GBS, botulism, tetanus, organophosphate poisoning, spinal cord injury)
- Depression of respiratory center (anesthesia, narcotics, sedatives, vertebral artery embolism or thrombosis, ICP)
- Failure of mechanical ventilator

Diagnosis
- Figure 9-4 is a diagnostic algorithm.

Treatment
- Correction of the underlying etiology

5 METABOLIC ALKALOSIS

Etiology
- Divided into chloride-responsive (urinary chloride <20 mEq/L) and chloride-resistant (urinary chloride level >20 mEq/L) forms

Chloride Responsive
- Vomiting
- NG suction

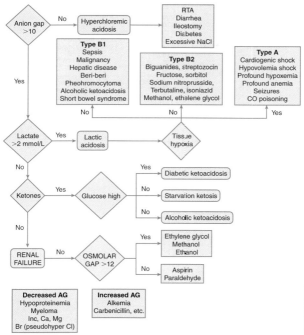

METABOLIC ACIDOSIS

Anion gap >10 → No → Hyperchloremic acidosis → RTA / Diarrhea / Ileostomy / Diabetes / Excessive NaCl

Type B1
Sepsis
Malignancy
Hepatic disease
Beri-beri
Pheochromocytoma
Alcoholic ketoacidosis
Short bowel syndrome

Type B2
Biguanides, streptozocin
Fructose, sorbitol
Sodium nitroprusside
Terbutaline, isoniazid
Methanol, ethylene glycol

Type A
Cardiogenic shock
Hypovolemia shock
Profound hypoxemia
Profound anemia
Seizures
CO poisoning

Anion gap >10 → Yes → Lactate >2 mmol/L → Yes → Lactic acidosis → Tissue hypoxia (No / No / Yes)

Lactate >2 mmol/L → No → Ketones → Yes → Glucose high → Yes → Diabetic ketoacidosis
Glucose high → No → Starvation ketosis
Glucose high → No → Alcoholic ketoacidosis

Ketones → No → RENAL FAILURE → No → OSMOLAR GAP >12 → Yes → Ethylene glycol / Methanol / Ethanol
OSMOLAR GAP >12 → No → Aspirin / Paraldehyde

Decreased AG
Hypoproteinemia
Myeloma
Inc, Ca, Mg
Br (pseudohyper Cl)

Increased AG
Alkemia
Carbenicillin, etc.

FIGURE 9-3. Diagnostic approach to metabolic acidosis. *(From Vincent JL, Abraham E, Moore FA, et al [eds]: Textbook of Critical Care, 6th ed. Philadelphia, Saunders, 2011.)*

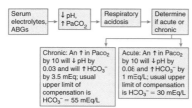

Serum electrolytes, ABGs → ↓ pH, ↑ PaCO₂ → Respiratory acidosis → Determine if acute or chronic

Chronic: An ↑ in PaCO₂ by 10 will ↓ pH by 0.03 and will ↑ HCO₃⁻ by 3.5 mEq; usual upper limit of compensation is HCO₃⁻ = 55 mEq/L

Acute: An ↑ in PaCO₂ by 10 will ↓ pH by 0.08 and ↑ HCO₃⁻ by 1 mEq/L; usual upper limit of compensation is HCO₃⁻ = 30 mEq/L

FIGURE 9-4. Diagnostic algorithm for respiratory acidosis. *(From Ferri FF: Ferri's Best Test: A Practical Guide to Clinical Laboratory Medicine and Diagnostic Imaging, 2nd ed. Philadelphia, Mosby, 2010.)*

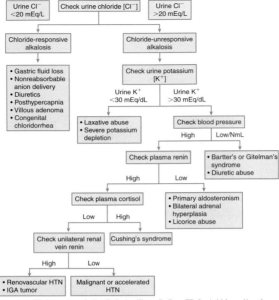

FIGURE 9-5. Workup of metabolic alkalosis. *(From DuBose TD Jr: Acid-base disorders. In: Brenner BM [ed]: Brenner and Rector's The Kidney, 8th ed. Philadelphia: Saunders, 2008, p. 513.)*

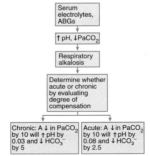

FIGURE 9-6. Diagnostic algorithm for respiratory alkalosis. *(From Ferri FF: Ferri's Best Test: A Practical Guide to Clinical Laboratory Medicine and Diagnostic Imaging, 2nd ed. Philadelphia, Mosby, 2010.)*

- Diuretics
- Posthypercapnic alkalosis
- Stool losses (laxative abuse, cystic fibrosis, villous adenoma)
- Massive blood transfusion
- Exogenous alkali administration

Chloride Resistant
- Hyperadrenocorticoid states (Cushing's syndrome, primary hyperaldosteronism, secondary mineralocorticoidism [licorice, chewing tobacco])
- Hypomagnesemia
- Hypokalemia
- Bartter's syndrome

Diagnosis
- Figure 9-5 describes the w/up of metabolic alkalosis.

Treatment
- Chloride-responsive forms: saline administration and correction of accompanying hypokalemia
- Chloride-resistant forms: correction of underlying cause and associated K^+ depletion

6 RESPIRATORY ALKALOSIS

Etiology
- Hypoxemia (pneumonia, PE, atelectasis, high-altitude living)
- Drugs (salicylates, xanthines, progesterone, epinephrine, thyroxine, nicotine)
- CNS disorders (tumor, CVA, trauma, infections)
- Psychogenic hyperventilation (anxiety, hysteria)
- Hepatic encephalopathy
- Gram(–) sepsis
- Hyponatremia

III

DISEASES AND DISORDERS
9. Nephrology

- Sudden recovery from metabolic acidosis
- Assisted ventilation

Diagnosis
- Figure 9-6 describes a diagnostic algorithm for respiratory alkalosis.

Treatment
- Rx is aimed at its underlying cause; symptomatic pts w/psychogenic hyperventilation often require some form of rebreathing apparatus (e.g., paper bag, breathing 5% CO_2 by mask).

E. DISORDERS OF SODIUM HOMEOSTASIS

1 HYPONATREMIA

Etiology
Isovolemic
- SIADH
- Water intoxication (e.g., schizophrenic pts, primary polydipsia, Na^+-free irrigant solutions, multiple tap-water enemas, dilute infant formulas). These entities are rare and often associated w/a deranged ADH axis.
- Renal failure
- Reset osmostat (e.g., chronic active TB, carcinomatosis)
- Glucocorticoid deficiency (hypopituitarism)
- Hypothyroidism
- Thiazide diuretics, NSAIDs, carbamazepine, amitriptyline, thioridazine, vincristine, cyclophosphamide, colchicine, tolbutamide, chlorpropamide, ACEIs, clofibrate, oxytocin, SSRIs, amiodarone
Hypovolemic
- Renal losses (diuretics, partial urinary tract obstruction, salt-losing renal disease)
- Extrarenal losses: GI (vomiting, diarrhea), extensive burns, third spacing (peritonitis, pancreatitis)
- Adrenal insufficiency
Hypervolemic
- CHF
- Nephrotic syndrome
- Cirrhosis
- Pregnancy
- Isotonic hyponatremia (nl serum osmolality)
- Pseudohyponatremia (↑ serum lipids and serum proteins). Newer Na^+ assays eliminate this problem.
- Isotonic infusion (e.g., glucose, mannitol)
- Hypertonic hyponatremia (serum osmolality)
- Hyperglycemia: each 100 mg/dL ↑ in blood glucose level above nl ↓ plasma Na^+ concentration by 1.6 mEq/L
- Hypertonic infusions (e.g., glucose, mannitol)

Diagnosis
- Figure 9-7 shows a diagnostic algorithm for hyponatremic pts.

Treatment
Isovolemic Hyponatremia
- SIADH: fluid restriction unless acutely symptomatic
- Acute symptomatic pt: hypertonic 3% to 5% saline solution infusion; give 200 to 500 mL slowly, followed by fluid restriction to 750 mL/day for 24 to 48 hr. Hypertonic saline can be combined w/furosemide to limit Rx-induced expansion of the ECF volume.
Hypovolemic Hyponatremia
- 0.9% NS infusion
Hypervolemic Hyponatremia
- Na^+ and water restriction. The combination of captopril and furosemide is effective in pts w/hyponatremia resulting from CHF.
Chronic Hyponatremia
- Correction of chronic hyponatremia should be kept at a rate <10 mEq/L (mmol/L) in any 24-hr period to prevent myelinolysis, a neurologic disorder that can occur after rapid correction of hyponatremia. Initially named **central pontine**

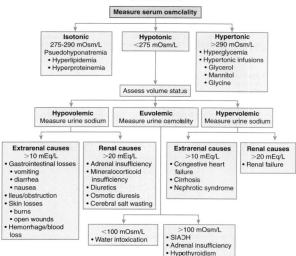

HYPONATREMIA

Measure serum osmolality

Isotonic
275-290 mOsm/L
Pseudohyponatremia
• Hyperlipidemia
• Hyperproteinemia

Hypotonic
<275 mOsm/L

Hypertonic
>290 mOsm/L
• Hyperglycemia
• Hypertonic infusions
  • Glycerol
  • Mannitol
  • Glycine

Assess volume status

Hypovolemic
Measure urine sodium

Euvolemic
Measure urine osmolality

Hypervolemic
Measure urine sodium

Extrarenal causes
>10 mEq/L
• Gastrointestinal losses
  • vomiting
  • diarrhea
  • nausea
• Ileus/obstruction
• Skin losses
  • burns
  • open wounds
• Hemorrhage/blood loss

Renal causes
>20 mEq/L
• Adrenal insufficiency
• Mineralocorticoid insufficiency
• Diuretics
• Osmotic diuresis
• Cerebral salt wasting

Extrarenal causes
>10 mEq/L
• Congestive heart failure
• Cirrhosis
• Nephrotic syndrome

Renal causes
>20 mEq/L
• Renal failure

<100 mOsm/L
• Water intoxication

>100 mOsm/L
• SIADH
• Adrenal insufficiency
• Hypothyroidism

FIGURE 9-7. Algorithm for treatment of hyponatremia. *(From Cameron AM: Current Surgical Therapy, 10th ed. Philadelphia, Saunders, 2011.)*

myelinolysis, this disease is now known also to affect extrapontine brain areas and is known as ***osmotic demyelination syndrome***. Manifestations of myelinolysis usually evolve several days after correction of hyponatremia. Typical features are disorders of UMNs, spastic quadriparesis and pseudobulbar palsy, and mental disorders ranging from mild confusion to coma. Death may occur. The motor and localizing signs of myelinolysis differ from those of the generalized encephalopathy that is caused by untreated hyponatremia.

Clinical Pearls
- In general, the serum Na^+ should be corrected only halfway to nl in the initial 24 hr (but not >1 mEq/L/hr) to prevent complications from rapid correction (cerebral edema, myelinolysis, seizures). A slower correction rate is indicated in pts w/ chronic hyponatremia.
- In symptomatic pts w/hyponatremia, an ↑ in the serum Na^+ concentration of 2 mEq/L/hr to a level of 120 to 130 mEq/L is considered safe by some experts; however, less rapid correction may be indicated in pts w/severe or chronic hyponatremia.

2 HYPERNATREMIA

Etiology
- Isovolemic (↓ TBW, nl TBNa, and ECF)
  • DI (neurogenic and nephrogenic)
  • Skin loss (hyperemia), iatrogenic, reset osmostat
- Hypervolemic (TBW, TBNa, and ECF)
  • Iatrogenic (administration of hypernatremic solutions)
  • Mineralocorticoid excess (Conn's syndrome, Cushing's syndrome)
  • Salt ingestion
- Hypovolemic: loss of H_2O and Na^+ (H_2O loss > Na^-)
  • Renal losses (e.g., diuretics, glycosuria)
  • GI, respiratory, skin losses
  • Adrenal deficiencies

Diagnosis
- Figure 9-8 describes a diagnostic and treatment algorithm for hypernatremia.

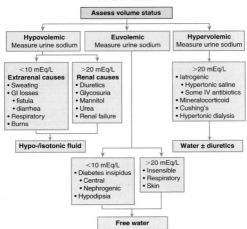

HYPERNATREMIA

FIGURE 9-8. Algorithm for treatment of hypernatremia. *(From Cameron AM: Current Surgical Therapy, 10th ed. Philadelphia, Saunders, 2011.)*

Treatment

Isovolemic Hypernatremia

- Fluid replacement w/D₅W. Correct only half of estimated water deficit in initial 24 hr. The rate of correction of serum Na⁺ should not exceed 1 mEq/L/hr in acute hypernatremia or 0.5 mEq/L/hr in chronic hypernatremia.
- Calculate water deficit in hypernatremic pts.
- H₂O deficit (in liters) = 0.6 × BW (kg) × ([measured Na+/140] − 1)

Hypovolemic Hypernatremia

- Fluid replacement is achieved w/isotonic saline solution.
- The rate of correction of plasma osmolarity should not exceed 2 mOsm/kg/hr.

Hypervolemic Hypernatremia

- Fluid replacement w/D₅W (to correct hypertonicity) is instituted after use of loop diuretics (to ↑ Na⁺ excretion).

F. DISORDERS OF POTASSIUM HOMEOSTASIS

1 HYPOKALEMIA

Etiology

- Cellular shift (redistribution) and undetermined mechanisms
  - Alkalosis (each 0.1 ↑ in pH ↓ serum K⁺ by 0.4-0.6 mEq/L)
  - Insulin administration
  - Vitamin B₁₂ Rx for megaloblastic anemias, acute leukemias
  - **Hypokalemic periodic paralysis:** rare familial disorder manifested by recurrent attacks of flaccid paralysis and hypokalemia
  - Beta adrenergic-Agonists, decongestants, bronchodilators, theophylline, caffeine
  - Barium poisoning, toluene intoxication, verapamil intoxication, chloroquine intoxication
  - Correction of digoxin intoxication w/digoxin Ab fragments (Digibind)
- Renal excretion
  - Drugs: diuretics, including carbonic anhydrase inhibitors (e.g., acetazolamide); amphotericin B; high-dose Na⁺ PCN, nafcillin, ampicillin, or carbenicillin; cisplatin, AGs, corticosteroids, mineralocorticoids, foscarnet Na⁺

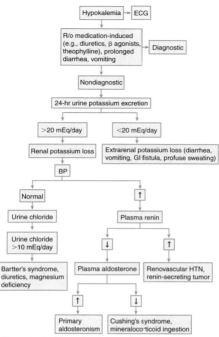

FIGURE 9-9. Diagnostic algorithm for hypokalemia. *(From Ferri FF: Ferri's Best Test: A Practical Guide to Clinical Laboratory Medicine and Diagnostic Imaging, 2nd ed. Philadelphia, Mosby, 2010.)*

- RTA: distal (type 1) or proximal (type 2)
- DKA, ureteroenterostomy
- Mg deficiency
- Postobstruction diuresis, diuretic phase of ATN
- Osmotic diuresis (e.g., mannitol)
- Bartter's syndrome: hyperplasia of juxtaglomerular cells leading to renin and aldosterone, metabolic alkalosis, hypokalemia, muscle weakness, and tetany (seen in young adults)
- Mineralocorticoid activity (primary or secondary aldosteronism), Cushing's syndrome
- Chronic metabolic alkalosis from loss of gastric fluid (renal K^+ secretion)

■ GI loss
- Vomiting, NG suction
- Diarrhea
- Laxative abuse
- Villous adenoma
- Fistulas

■ Inadequate dietary intake (e.g., anorexia nervosa)
■ Cutaneous loss (excessive sweating)
■ High dietary Na^+ intake, excessive use of licorice

Diagnosis
■ Figure 9-9 illustrates a diagnostic algorithm for hypokalemia.
■ Distinguish true K^+ depletion from redistribution (e.g. alkalosis, insulin administration).

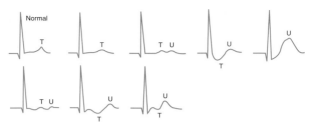

FIGURE 9-10. Variable ECG patterns can be seen with hypokalemia, ranging from slight T wave flattening to the appearance of prominent U waves, sometimes with ST depression or T wave inversion. These patterns are not always directly related to the specific level of serum K^+. *(From Ferri FF: Ferri's Best Test: A Practical Guide to Clinical Laboratory Medicine and Diagnostic Imaging, 2nd ed. Philadelphia, Mosby, 2010.)*

- If the cause of hypokalemia is not apparent (e.g. diuretics, vomiting), measure 24-hr urinary K^+ excretion while pt is receiving regular dietary Na^+ intake.
  - <20 mEq: consider extrarenal K^+ loss
  - >20 mEq: renal K^+ loss
- If renal K^+ wasting is suspected, the following steps are indicated:
  - Measure 24-hr urine chloride.
    - >10 mEq: diuretics, Bartter's syndrome, mineralocorticoid excess (chloride unresponsive)
    - <10 mEq: vomiting, gastric drainage (chloride responsive)
  - Measure BP; if ↑, consider mineralocorticoid excess.
  - Measure serum HCO_3^-: a ↓ level is suggestive of RTA.
- ECG manifestations (Fig. 9-10)
  - Mild hypokalemia: flattening of T waves, ST-segment depression, PVCs, QT interval
  - Severe hypokalemia: prominent U waves, AV conduction disturbances, VT, VF

Treatment
- K^+ replacement
  - PO K^+ replacement is preferred.
  - IV infusion should generally not exceed 20 mEq/hr.
- Monitor ECG and urinary output.
- Identify the underlying cause and treat accordingly.
- IV NS solution is given in chloride-responsive hypokalemia.

2 HYPERKALEMIA

Etiology
- Pseudohyperkalemia
  - Hemolyzed specimen
  - Severe thrombocytosis (Plt count >10^6 mL)
  - Severe leukocytosis (WBC >10^5 mL)
  - Fist clenching during phlebotomy
- ↑ K^+ intake (often in setting of impaired excretion)
  - K^+ replacement Rx
  - ↑ K^+ diet
  - Salt substitutes w/K^+
  - K^+ salts of abx
- ↓ Renal excretion
  - K^+-sparing diuretics (e.g., spironolactone, triamterene, amiloride)
  - Renal insufficiency
  - Mineralocorticoid deficiency
  - Hyporeninemic hypoaldosteronism (DM)
  - Tubular unresponsiveness to aldosterone (e.g., SLE, MM, sickle cell disease)
  - Type 4 RTA
  - ACEIs

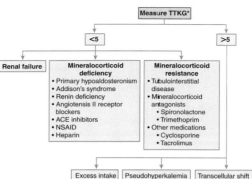

HYPERKALEMIA

Measure TTKG*

< 5 → **Renal failure** | **Mineralocorticoid deficiency**
- Primary hypoaldosteronism
- Addison's syndrome
- Renin deficiency
- Angiotensin II receptor blockers
- ACE inhibitors
- NSAID
- Heparin

| **Mineralocorticoid resistance**
- Tubulointerstitial disease
- Mineralocorticoid antagonists
  - Spironolactone
  - Trimethoprim
- Other medications
  - Cyclosporine
  - Tacrolimus

> 5

Excess intake | **Pseudohyperkalemia** | **Transcellular shift**

*Transtubular gradient = $\dfrac{[K^+]_u \times P_{osm}}{[K^+]_p \times U_{osm}}$

The TTKG is typically <5 when a renal cause of hyperkalemia is present.

FIGURE 9-11. Algorithm for treatment of hyperkalemia. *(From Cameron AM: Current Surgical Therapy, 10th ed. Philadelphia, Saunders, 2011.)*

- Heparin administration
- NSAIDs
- TMP-SMZ
- β-Blockers
- Pentamidine
- Redistribution (excessive cellular release)
  - Acidemia (each 0.1 ↓ in pH ↑ the serum K^+ by 0.4-0.6 mEq/L); lactic acidosis and ketoacidosis cause minimal redistribution.
  - Insulin deficiency
  - Drugs (e.g., succinylcholine, marked digitalis level, arginine, β-adrenergic blockers)
  - Hypertonicity
  - Hemolysis
  - Tissue necrosis, rhabdo, burns
  - Hyperkalemic periodic paralysis

Diagnosis
- R/o pseudohyperkalemia or lab error: Repeat serum K^+ level.
- Obtain ECG; in pts w/suspected pseudohyperkalemia secondary to hemolyzed specimen or thrombocytosis, the ECG will not show any manifestations of hyperkalemia.
- In pts w/thrombocytosis or severe leukocytosis, an accurate serum K^+ level can be determined by drawing a heparinized sample.
- Check pH, correct acidosis (if present).
- Check Ca, Mg, glucose, serum and urine electrolytes, BUN, and Cr levels. Calculate the transtubular K^+ gradient (TTKG). Figure 9-11 provides a diagnostic algorithm for hyperkalemia.
- Monitor ECG: ECG manifestations (Fig. 9-12)
  - Mild hyperkalemia: peaking or tenting of T waves, PVCs
  - Severe hyperkalemia: peaking of T waves, widening of QRS complex, depressed ST segments, prolongation of PR interval, sinus arrest, deep S wave, PVCs, VT, VF, and cardiac arrest

Treatment
- Table 9-3 describes treatment modalities for hyperkalemia.

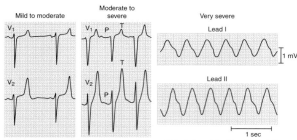

FIGURE 9-12. The earliest ECG change with hyperkalemia is peaking ("tenting") of the T waves. With progressive increases in serum potassium, the QRS complexes widen, the P waves decrease in amplitude and may disappear, and, finally, a sine wave pattern leads to asystole. (*From Ferri FF: Ferri's Best Test: A Practical Guide to Clinical Laboratory Medicine and Diagnostic Imaging, 2nd ed. Philadelphia, Mosby, 2010.*)

TABLE 9-3 ■ Treatment of Hyperkalemia

Treatment	Mechanism	Dosage/Comment	Onset	Duration
Calcium	Stabilizes cardiac cells	10 mL of 10% solution (calcium gluconate or calcium chloride)	Seconds	30-60 min
Insulin (regular)	Shifts K+ into cells	10 U IV + glucose (50 g)	15-30 min	2-4 hr
Albuterol	Shifts K+ into cells	10-20 mg by inhaler over 10 min	20-30 min	2-3 hr
NaHCO₃	Shifts K+ into cells	In cases of acidosis	Delayed	—
Kayexalate with sorbitol	Removes K+ from body	Oral: 15-30 g	4-6 hr	—
		Retention enema: 30-50 g	1 hr	—
Loop diuretics	Removes K+ from body	Intravenous, varies by drug and renal function	1 hr	—
Hemodialysis	Removes K+ from body	Preferred over peritoneal dialysis in acute cases	15-30 min	—

From Vincent JL, Abraham E, Moore FA, et al (eds): Textbook of Critical Care, 6th ed. Philadelphia, Saunders, 2011.

G. DISORDERS OF MAGNESIUM METABOLISM

1 HYPOMAGNESEMIA

Etiology

- GI and nutritional
  - Defective GI absorption (malabsorption)
  - Inadequate dietary intake (e.g., alcoholism)
  - Parenteral Rx w/o Mg
  - Chronic diarrhea, villous adenoma, prolonged NG suction, fistulas (small bowel, biliary)
- Excessive renal losses
  - Diuretics
  - RTA
  - Diuretic phase of ATN
  - Endocrine disturbances (DKA, hyperaldosteronism, hyperthyroidism, hyperparathyroidism), SIADH, Bartter's syndrome, hypercalciuria, hypokalemia
  - Cisplatin, alcohol, cyclosporine, digoxin, pentamidine, mannitol, amphotericin B, foscarnet, MTX
  - Abx (gentamicin, ticarcillin, carbenicillin)
- Redistribution: hypoalbuminemia, cirrhosis, administration of insulin and glucose, theophylline, epinephrine, acute pancreatitis, cardiopulmonary bypass

- Miscellaneous: sweating, burns, prolonged exercise, lactation, "hungry bones" syndrome

Diagnosis

H&P
- Neuromuscular: weakness, hyperreflexia, fasciculations, tremors, convulsions, delirium, coma
- CV: cardiac arrhythmias
- Hypokalemia refractory to K^+ replacement
- Hypocalcemia refractory to Ca replacement

ECG
- Prolonged QT interval, T wave flattening, prolonged PR interval, AF, torsades de pointes

Treatment
- Mild hypomagnesemia: 600 mg oxide PO provides 35 mEq of Mg; dosage is 1 to 2 tablets qd.
- Moderate: 50% solution Mg sulfate (each 2-mL ampule contains 8 mEq or 96 mg of elemental Mg); dosage is one 2-mL ampule of 50% Mg solution q6h PRN.
- Severe (serum Mg level <1 mg/dL) and symptomatic pt (seizures, tetany): 2 g Mg in 20 mL D_5W IV during 60 min; monitor ECG, BP, pulse, respiration, DTRs, and urinary output. An alternative regimen is the administration of 6 g Mg sulfate (49 mEq) in 1000 mL of D_5W during 3 hr, followed by 10 g of Mg sulfate in 2000 mL of 5% dextrose in water during 24 hr.

2 HYPERMAGNESEMIA

Etiology
- Renal failure
- ↓ Renal excretion secondary to salt depletion
- Abuse of antacids and laxatives containing Mg in pts w/renal insufficiency
- Endocrinopathies (deficiency of mineralocorticoid or thyroid hormone)
- ↑ Tissue breakdown (rhabdo)
- Redistribution: DKA, pheochromocytoma
- Other: lithium, volume depletion, familial hypocalciuric hypercalcemia

Diagnosis

H&P
- Clinical manifestations: paresthesias, hypotension, confusion, ↓ DTRs, paralysis, coma, apnea; acute hypermagnesemia suppresses PTH secretion and can produce hypocalcemia.

ECG
- ↓ PR interval, heart block, peaked T waves, QRS duration

Treatment
- Identify and correct the underlying disorder.
- Intracardiac conduction abnlities can be treated w/IV Ca gluconate.
- Prescribe dialysis for severe hypermagnesemia.

H. DISORDERS OF PHOSPHATE METABOLISM

1 HYPOPHOSPHATEMIA

Etiology
- ↓ Intake (prolonged starvation, alcoholism, hyperalimentation, or IV infusion w/o phosphorus)
- Malabsorption
- PO_4^{-3}-binding antacid
- Renal loss
  - RTA
  - Fanconi's syndrome, vitamin D–resistant rickets
  - ATN (diuretic phase)
  - Hyperparathyroidism (primary or secondary)
  - Familial hypophosphatemia
  - Hypokalemia, hypomagnesemia
  - Acute volume expansion
  - Glycosuria, idiopathic hypercalciuria
  - Acetazolamide

- Transcellular shift into cells
  - Alcohol withdrawal
  - DKA (recovery phase)
  - Glucose-insulin or catecholamine infusion
  - Anabolic steroids
  - TPN
  - Theophylline OD
  - Severe hyperthermia; recovery from hypothermia
  - "Hungry bones" syndrome

Treatment
- Mild to moderate hypophosphatemia (>1 mg/dL): Neutra-Phos capsules (250 mg per capsule), 2 capsules tid
- Severe symptomatic hypophosphatemia (<1 mg/dL): IV administration of PO_4^{-3} salts (0.08-0.16 mmol/kg during 6 hr) repeated q6h until serum PO_4^{-3} level is >1.5 mg/dL

2 HYPERPHOSPHATEMIA

Etiology
- Excessive PO_4^{-3} administration
  - PO intake or IV administration
  - Laxatives containing PO_4^{-3} (PO_4^{-3} tablets, PO_4^{-3} enemas)
  - ↓ Renal PO_4^{-3} excretion
  - Acute or chronic renal failure
  - Hypoparathyroidism or pseudohypoparathyroidism
  - Acromegaly, thyrotoxicosis
  - Bisphosphonate Rx
  - Tumor calcinosis
  - Sickle cell anemia
- Transcellular shift out of cells
  - ChemoRx of lymphoma or leukemia, tumor lysis syndrome, hemolysis
  - Acidosis
  - Rhabdo, malignant hyperthermia
- Artifact: in vitro hemolysis
- Pseudohyperphosphatemia: hyperlipidemia, paraproteinemia, hyperbilirubinemia

Treatment
- Administration of Ca^{2+} carbonate (1 g w/each meal, gradually to 8-12 g of Ca carbonate a day) to bind PO_4^{-3} in the gut and to prevent its absorption
- Insulin and glucose infusion (to promote cell phosphate uptake); may be useful when a rapid ↓ in phosphate is needed
- Institution of hemodialysis when renal failure is present

J. ACUTE KIDNEY INJURY (AKI)

DEFINITION
AKI is an increase in serum creatinine or a decline in urine output. The RIFLE and AKIN criteria for AKI are described in Table 9-4.

Etiology
- The causes of AKI can be subdivided into prerenal, intrinsic renal diseases, and postrenal.
- Figure 9-13 describes the causes of each type of AKI and characteristic lab findings.

Labs
- Diagnostic tests to distinguish prerenal and renal AKI are described in Table 9-5.
- Rx: See Rx of CKD.

K. CHRONIC KIDNEY DISEASE (CKD)

Progressive ↓ in renal function (GFR <60 mL/min for >3 mo) with subsequent accumulation of waste products in the blood, electrolyte abnlities, and anemia. The definition criteria for CKD are described in Table 9-6. Table 9-7 gives the classification of CKD based on GFR.

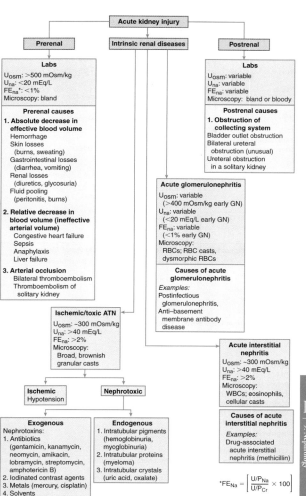

FIGURE 9-13. Acute kidney injury.

TABLE 9-4 ■ RIFLE and AKIN Criteria for Diagnosis of AKI

RIFLE Classification

	GFR Criteria	UO Criteria
Risk	S_{Cr} > 1.5 × baseline or ΔGFR > 25% reduction	UO < 0.5 mL/kg/hr × 6 hr
Injury	S_{Cr} > 2.0 × baseline or ΔGFR > 50% reduction	UO < 0.5 mL/kg/hr × 12 hr
Failure	S_{Cr} > 3.0 × baseline or ΔGFR > 75% reduction or S_{Cr} > 4.0 mg/dL	UO < 0.3 mL/kg/hr × 24 hr or anuria × 12 hr
Loss	Persistent ARF = Complete loss of function for >4 wk	
ESRD	ESRD >3 mo	

AKIN Classification

Stage	S_{Cr} Criteria	UO Criteria
1	ΔS_{Cr} ≥ 0.3 mg/dL (30μmol/L) or S_{Cr} ≥ 1.5, ≤ 2.0 baseline	UO < 0.5 mL/kg/hr × 6 hr
2	S_{Cr} > 2.0, ≤ 3.0 × baseline	UO < 0.5 mL/kg/hr × 12 hr
3	S_{Cr} ≥ 4.0 mg/dL with an acute rise ≥ 0.5mg/dL (50μmol/L) or renal replacement therapy	UO < 0.3 mL/kg/hr × 24 hr or anuria × 12 hr

From Floege J, John RJ, Feehally J (eds): Comprehensive Clinical Nephrology, 4th ed. Philadelphia, Saunders, 2010.
S_{Cr}, Serum creatinine; *UO*, urine output.

TABLE 9-5 ■ Diagnostic Tests to Distinguish Prerenal and Renal AKI

Index	Prerenal Causes	Renal Causes
FE_{Na}*	<1%	>2%
Urine sodium	<10 mmol/L	>40 mmol/L
Urine/plasma osmolality	>1.5	1-1.5
Renal failure index	<1	>2
BUN/creatinine ratio	>20	<10

From Cameron AM: Current Surgical Therapy, 10th ed. Philadelphia, Saunders, 2011.
*Calculation of FE_{Na}: (Urine sodium × Plasma creatinine)/(Plasma sodium × Serum creatinine) × 100
Renal failure index: (Urine sodium × Urine creatinine)/Plasma creatinine

Etiology
- DM (37%), HTN (30%), chronic GN (12%)
- Polycystic kidney disease
- Tubular interstitial nephritis (e.g., drug hypersensitivity, analgesic nephropathy), obstructive nephropathies (e.g., nephrolithiasis, prostatic disease)
- Vascular diseases (renal artery stenosis, hypertensive nephrosclerosis)
- Autoimmune diseases

Diagnosis
H&P
- Skin pallor, ecchymoses
- Edema, leg cramps, restless legs, peripheral neuropathy
- HTN
- Emotional lability and depression, ↓ mental acuity
- The clinical presentation varies with the degree of renal failure and its underlying etiology. Common sx are generalized fatigue, nausea, anorexia, pruritus, sleep disturbances, smell and taste disturbances, hiccups, and seizures.

TABLE 9-6 ■ Criteria for Definition of CKD

Kidney damage for ≥3 mo, as defined by structural or functional abnlities of the kidney, with or without decreased GFR, that can lead to decreased GFR, manifested by any of the following:

    Pathologic abnlities

    Markers of kidney damage, including abnlities in the composition of blood or urine, or abnlities in imaging tests

    GFR <60 mL/min/1.73 m² for ≥3 mo, with or without kidney damage

From Floege J, John RJ, Feehally J (eds): Comprehensive Clinical Nephrology, 4th ed. Philadelphia, Saunders, 2010.

TABLE 9-7 ■ Classification of CKD Based on GFR

CKD Stage*	Definition
1	Nl or increased GFR; some evidence of kidney damage reflected by microalbuminuria, proteinuria, and hematuria as well as radiologic or histologic changes
2	Mild decrease in GFR (89-60 mL/min/1.73 m²) with some evidence of kidney damage reflected by microalbuminuria, proteinuria, and hematuria, as well as radiologic or histologic changes
3	GFR 59-30 mL/min/1.73 m²
3A	GFR 59-45 mL/min/1.73 m²
3B	GFR 44-30 mL/min/1.73 m²
4	GFR 29-15 mL/min/1.73 m²
5	GFR <15 mL/min/1.73 m²; when renal replacement therapy in the form of dialysis or transplantation has to be considered to sustain life

From Floege J, John RJ, Feehally J (eds): Comprehensive Clinical Nephrology, 4th ed. Philadelphia, Saunders, 2010.

Classification of CKD based on GFR was proposed by the Kidney Disease Outcomes Quality Initiative (KDOQI) guidelines and modified by the National Institute for Health and Care Excellence (NICE) in 2008.

*The suffix p is added to the stage in proteinuric pts (proteinuria >0.5 g/24 hr).

Imaging
- Sonographic evaluation of the kidneys reveals smaller kidneys with ↑ echogenicity in CKD.

Treatment
- Table 9-8 describes nutritional recommendations in renal disease.
- Adjust drug doses to correct for prolonged half-lives.
- ACEIs and ARBs are useful in reducing proteinuria and slowing the progression of chronic renal disease, especially in hypertensive diabetic pts. Avoid combinations of ACEIs and ARBs because of the ↑ risk of hyperkalemia, hypotension, and worsening renal failure.
- Initiation of dialysis:
  - Urgent indications: uremic pericarditis, neuropathy, neuromuscular abnlities, CHF, hyperkalemia, seizures
  - Judgment-based indications: CrCl 10 to 15 mL/min; progressive anorexia, weight loss, reversal of sleep pattern, pruritus, uncontrolled fluid gain with HTN, and signs of CHF
  - Initiation of dialysis when the GFR is 10 to 14 mL/min per 1.73 m² does not enhance survival compared with a strategy of symptom-driven initiation or initiation of dialysis at eGFR <7 mL/min per 173 m².
- ESAs to reduce the need for transfusions in pts with anemia. Anemia should not be fully corrected in pts with CKD. Maintaining a target hemoglobin of <10 g/dL or hematocrit 30% to 33% is satisfactory. Targeting higher hemoglobin levels in CKD may ↑ risks for stroke, HTN, and serious cardiovascular events.
- Restrict fluid if significant edema is present. Give diuretics for significant fluid overload (loop diuretics are preferred).
- Correct HTN to at least 130/85 mm Hg with ACEIs (avoid in pts with significant hyperkalemia), ARBs, and/or nondihydropyridine Ca²⁺ channel blockers (verapamil, diltiazem), which can be used in pts intolerant to ACEIs or when other agents are needed to control blood pressure. Systolic BP between 110 and 129 mm Hg may be beneficial in pts with urine protein excretion >1.0 g/day. Systolic BP <110 mm Hg may be associated with a higher risk for kidney disease progression.
- Correct electrolyte abnormalities.
- Lipid-↓ agents are indicated in pts with dyslipidemia; target LDL cholesterol is <100 mg/dL; these agents are shown to ↓ cardiac death and atherosclerosis-mediated cardiovascular events in persons with CKD.
- Control renal osteodystrophy with Ca²⁺ supplementation and vitamin D.
- Dietary PO₄⁻³ restriction effectively reduces serum PO₄⁻³ levels and is recommended in all pts with CKD.
- Kidney transplantation in selected pts improves survival. The 2-yr kidney graft survival rate for living related donor transplantations is >80%, whereas the 2-yr graft survival rate for cadaveric donor transplantation is approximately 70%.

TABLE 9-8 ■ Nutritional Recommendations in Renal Disease

Daily Intake	Predialysis Chronic Renal Failure	Hemodialysis	Peritoneal Dialysis
Protein (g/kg ideal BW) (see KDOQI for estimation of adjusted edema-free BW)	0.6-1.0	1.1-1.2	1.0-1.3
	Level depends on the view of the nephrologist 1.0 for nephrotic syndrome	This is a broad recommendation because protein intake would be individualized for the pt's nutritional status, serum phosphate levels, and dialysis adequacy	
Energy (kcal/kg BW)	35 (<60 yr) 30-35 (>60 yr)	35 (<60 yr) 30-35 (>60 yr)	35 including dialysate calories (<60 yr) 30-35 including dialy-sate calories (>60 yr)
Sodium (mmol) Potassium	<100 (more if salt wasting) Reduce if hyperkalemic	<100 Reduce if hyperkalemic	<100 Reduce if hyperkalemic; potassium restriction is generally not required
	If hyperkalemic, advice will take the form of decreasing certain foods (e.g., some fruits and vegetables) and giving information about cooking methods		
Phosphorus	Reduce; level depends on protein intake Advice will take the form of reducing certain foods (e.g., dairy, offal, some shellfish) and giving information about the timing of binders with high-phosphorus meals and snacks		
Calcium	In CKD stages 3-5, total intake of elemental cal-cium (including dietary calcium) should not exceed 2000 mg/day	Total intake of elemen-tal calcium (including dietary calcium) should not exceed 2000 mg/day	Total intake of elemen-tal calcium (including dietary calcium) should not exceed 2000 mg/day

From Floege J, John RJ, Feehally J (eds): Comprehensive Clinical Nephrology, 4th ed. Philadelphia, Saunders, 2010.
Recommendations are for typical pts but should always be individualized on the basis of clinical, biochemical, and anthropometric indices.

KDOQI, Kidney Disease Outcomes Quality Initiative.

L. GLOMERULAR DISEASE

1 NEPHROTIC SYNDROME

Definition
Table 9-9 describes the definition of nephrotic syndrome. There is primary protein leakage across the glomeruli. The hallmarks of this syndrome are hypoalbuminemia and edema. Common clinical manifestations include hyperlipidemia and coagulation abnlities.

Etiology
- Idiopathic (may be secondary to the following glomerular diseases: minimal-change disease [nil disease, lipoid nephrosis], focal segmental glomerular sclerosis, membranous nephropathy, membranoproliferative glomerular nephropathy)
- Systemic diseases: DM, SLE, amyloidosis, dysproteinemias
- Most children w/nephrotic syndrome have minimal-change disease (this form is also associated w/allergy, NSAIDs, and Hodgkin's disease).
- Focal glomerular disease: associated w/HIV, heroin abuse, obesity. A more severe form of nephrotic syndrome associated w/rapid progression to ESRD within months can also occur in HIV(+) pts and is known as ***collapsing glomerulopathy.***
- Membranous nephropathy can occur w/Hodgkin's lymphoma, carcinomas, SLE, gold Rx.
- Membranoproliferative glomerulonephropathy is often associated w/URIs.
- Table 9-10 summarizes primary renal diseases that manifest as idiopathic nephrotic syndrome.

Diagnosis
H&P
- Typically pts present w/severe peripheral edema, exertional dyspnea, and abd fullness secondary to ascites. Most pts have a significant amount of weight gain.

TABLE 9-9 ■ Nephrotic Syndrome: Definitions

Term	NS Definitions* Adult	Pediatric
Relapse	Proteinuria ≥3.5 g day^{-1} occurring after complete remission has been obtained for >1 mo	Albu-stix 3+ or proteinuria >40 mg m^{-2} h^{-1} occurring on 3 days within 1 wk
Frequently relapsing	2+ relapses within 6 mo	2+ relapses within 6 mo
Complete remission	Reduction of proteinuria to ≤0.20 g day^{-1} and serum albumin >35 gl^{-1}	<4 mg m^{-2} h^{-1} on at least 3 occasions within 7 days serum albumin >35 gl^{-1}
Partial remission	Reduction of proteinuria to between 0.21 g day^{21} and 3.4 g day^{-1} ± decrease in proteinuria of ≥50% from baseline	Disappearance of edema. Increase in serum albumin >35 gl^{-1} and persisting proteinuria >4 mg m^{-2} h^{-1} or >100 m^{-2} day^{-1}
Steroid-resistant	Persistence of proteinuria despite prednisone therapy 1 mg kg^{21} day^{21} × 4 mo	Persistence of proteinuria despite prednisone therapy 60 mg m^{22} × 4 wk†
Steroid-dependent—NS recurs when pts stop or decrease treatment	Two consecutive relapses occurring during therapy or within 14 days of completing steroid therapy	Two relapses of proteinuria within 14 days after stopping or during alternate day steroid therapy

From Floege J, John RJ, Feehally J (eds): Comprehensive Clinical Nephrology, 4th ed. Philadelphia, Saunders, 2010.
NS, Nephrotic syndrome.
*Definition of terms used in idiopathic nephrotic syndrome in adults and children. The definitions were generated by a consensus of the International Society for Kidney Diseases in Children and the German Pediatric Nephrology Society.
†Or persistence of proteinuria despite prednisone therapy 60 mg m^{-2} × 4 wk and three methylprednisolone pulses.

TABLE 9-10 ■ Summary of Primary Renal Diseases That Manifest as Idiopathic Nephrotic Syndrome

	Minimal-Change Nephropathy Syndrome (MCNS)	Focal Segmental Sclerosis	Membranous Nephrotic	Membranoproliferative GN (MPGN)	
				Type I	Type II
Frequency*					
Children	75%	10%	<5%	10%	10%
Adults	15%	15%	50%	10%	10%
Clinical Manifestations					
Age (yr)	2-6	2-10	40-50	5-15	5-15
Sex	2:1 male:female	1.3:1 male:female	2:1 male:female	Male=female	Male=female
Nephrotic syndrome	100%	90%	80%	60%	60%
Asymptomatic proteinuria	0	10%	20%	40%	40%
Hematuria	10%-20%	60%-80%	60%	80%	80%
Hypertension	10%	20% early	Infrequent	35%	35%
Rate of progression to renal failure	Does not progress	10 yr	50% in 10-20 yr	10-20 yr	5-15 yr
Associated conditions	Allergy? Hodgkin's disease, usually none	None			
	Manifestations of nephrotic syndrome	Manifestations of nephrotic syndrome	Renal vein thrombosis, cancer, SLE, hepatitis B virus	None	Partial lipodystrophy
Laboratory Findings	↑ BUN in 15%-30%	↑ BUN in 20%-40%	Manifestations of nephrotic syndrome	Low C1, C4, C3-C9	NI C1, C4, low C3-C9
Immunogenetics	HLA-B8, B12 (3.5)†	Not established	HLA-DRW3 (12-32)†	Not established	C3 nephritic factor
Renal Pathology					Not established

Continued

	Minimal-Change Nephropathy Syndrome (MCNS)	Focal Segmental Sclerosis	Membranous Nephrotic	Membranoproliferative GN (MPGN)	
				Type I	Type II
Light microscopy	Nl	Focal	Thickened	Thickened	Lobulation
Immunofluorescence	Negative	IgM	Fine	Granular	C3 only
Electron microscopy	Foot process fusion	Foot	Subepithelial	Mesangial	Dense deposits
Response of Steroids	90%	15%-20%	May slow progression	Not established	Not established

Modified from Goldman L, Ausiello D (eds): Cecil Textbook of Medicine, 22nd ed. Philadelphia, Saunders, 2004.

C, complement.

*Approximate frequency as a cause of idiopathic nephrotic syndrome. About 10% of cases of adult nephrotic syndrome result from various diseases that usually manifest with AGN.

†Relative risk.

■ HTN
■ Pleural effusion

Labs
■ U/A: proteinuria, oval fat bodies (tubular epithelial cells w/cholesterol esters). The presence of hematuria, cellular casts, and pyuria is suggestive of nephritic syndrome.
■ 24-hr urine protein excretion >3.5 g/1.73 m^3/24 hr
■ Blood chemistries: ↓ alb <3 g/dL, ↓ total protein, ↑ serum cholesterol, ↑ BUN, ↑ Cr

Imaging
■ U/S of kidneys

Treatment
■ ↓-Fat diet, fluid restriction in hyponatremic pts; nl protein intake unless urinary protein loss >10 g/24 hr (some pts may require additional dietary protein to prevent [−] nitrogen balance and significant protein malnutrition). Improved urinary protein excretion and serum lipid changes have been observed w/↓-fat soy protein diet providing 0.7 g of protein/kg/day. However, because of the risk of malnutrition, many nephrologists recommend nl protein intake.
■ Na$^+$ restriction for peripheral edema
■ Monitor for development of peripheral venous thrombosis and renal vein thrombosis (risk related to loss of antithrombin III and other proteins involved in the clotting mechanism).
■ Furosemide for severe edema
■ ACEIs to ↓ proteinuria
■ Anticoagulants as long as nephrotic proteinuria or alb level <20 g/L is present
■ Minimal-change glomerulopathy (MCG): prednisone 1 mg/kg/day; cyclophosphamide or other immunosuppressive agents for relapses
■ Focal segmental glomerulosclerosis (FSGS): corticosteroids or calcineurin inhibitors initially. Many pts eventually require immunosuppressive Rx (cyclophosphamide, mycophenolate mofetil, rituximab).
■ Membranous GN: immunosuppressive Rx (cyclophosphamide/corticosteroids or calcineurin inhibitor) if persistent proteinuria ≥4 g/day; rituximab for Rx failure
■ Membranoproliferative GN (MPGN): corticosteroids with immunosuppressive agents and antiplatelet drugs

2 NEPHRITIC SYNDROME

Definition
Immunologically mediated inflammation involving the glomerulus allows the passage of erythrocytes, leukocytes, and protein into the renal tubule, with resulting hematuria, pyuria, and proteinuria.

Etiology
■ Post–group A β-hemolytic streptococcus infection (other infectious etiologies, including endocarditis and visceral abscess)
■ Collagen-vascular diseases (SLE)

- Vasculitis (granulomatosis with polyangiitis [Wegener's granulomatosis], polyarteritis nodosa). ***Pauci-immune crescenteric GN (PICG)*** is associated with polyangiitis, microscopic polyangiitis, and Churg-Strauss syndrome and manifests with RPGN.
- Idiopathic GN (membranoproliferative, idiopathic, crescentic, IgA nephropathy)
- Goodpasture's syndrome
- Other cryoglobulinemia (Henoch-Schönlein purpura)
- Drug induced (gold, penicillamine)
- Table 9-11 summarizes primary renal diseases that manifest as AGN.

TABLE 9-11 ■ Summary of Primary Renal Diseases That Manifest as AGN				
Diseases	Poststreptococcal GN	IgA Nephropathy	Goodpasture Syndrome	Idiopathic Rapidly Progressive GN
Clinical Manifestations				
Age and sex	All ages, mean 7 yr, 2:1 male	10-35 yr, 2:1 male	15-30 yr, 6:1 male	Adults, 2:1 male
Acute nephritic syndrome	90%	50%	90%	90%
Asymptomatic hematuria	Occasionally	50%	Rare	Rare
Nephrotic syndrome	10%-20%	Rare	Rare	10%-20%
Hypertension	70%	30%-50%	Rare	25%
ARF	50% (transient)	Very rare	50%	60%
Other	Latent period of 1-3 wk	Follows viral syndromes	Pulmonary hemorrhage; iron deficiency anemia	None
Laboratory findings	↑ ASLO titers (70%) Positive streptozyme (95%) ↓ C3-C9; nl C1, C4	↑ Serum IgA (50%) IgA in dermal capillaries	Positive anti-GBM antibody	Positive ANCA in some
Immunogenetics	HLA-B12, D "EN" (9)*	HLA-Bw 35, DR4 (4)*	HLA-DR2 (16)*	None established
Renal Pathology				
Light microscopy	Diffuse proliferation	Focal proliferation	Focal → diffuse proliferation with crescents	Crescentic GN
Immunofluorescence	Granular IgG, C3	Diffuse mesangial IgA	Linear IgG, C3	No immune deposits
Electron microscopy	Subepithelial humps	Mesangial deposits	No deposits	No deposits
Prognosis	95% resolve spontaneously 5% RPGN or slowly progressive	Slow progression in 25%–50%	75% stabilize or improve if treated early	75% stabilize or improve if treated early
Treatment	Supportive	Uncertain (options include steroids, fish oil, and ACEIs)	Plasma exchange, steroids, cyclophosphamide	Steroid pulse therapy

Modified from Kliegman RM, Greenbaum L, Lye P: Practical Strategies in Pediatric Diagnosis and Therapy, 2nd ed. Philadelphia, Saunders, 2004, p. 427.

RPGN, idiopathic rapidly progressive GN.

*Relative risk.

Diagnosis

Labs

- U/A : hematuria (dysmorphic erythrocytes and RBC casts), proteinuria
- Table 9-12 describes various antigens identified in the nephritic syndrome.

Imaging

- CXR: r/o pulmonary congestion, Wegener's granulomatosis, and Goodpasture's syndrome
- Renal U/S: evaluate renal size and determine extent of fibrosis. A kidney size of <9 cm suggests extensive scarring and ↓ likelihood of reversibility.
- Echo: in pts w/new cardiac murmurs or + blood cultures to r/o endocarditis and pericardial effusion
- Angiography or bx of other affected organs if systemic vasculitis is suspected

TABLE 9-12 ■ Antigens Identified in GN

Poststreptococcal GN	Streptococcal pyrogenic exotoxin B (SPEB), plasmin receptor
Anti-GBM disease	α3 type IV collagen (likely induced by molecular mimicry)
IgA nephropathy	Possibly no antigen but rather polymerized polyclonal IgA (? superantigen driven)
Membranous nephropathy	Phospholipase A₂ receptor (idiopathic), neutral endopeptidase (NEP) in podocyte (congenital), HBeAg (hepatitis associated)
Staphylococcus aureus–associated GN	*Staphylococcus* superantigens induce polyclonal response; not necessarily antigen in glomeruli
Membranoproliferative GN	HCV and HBsAg in hepatitis-associated MPGN
ANCA-associated vasculitis	Proteinase 3 (c-ANCA) and myeloperoxidase (p-ANCA) in neutrophils; antibodies to lysosome-associated membrane protein 2 (LAMP-2) on endothelial cells (likely induced by molecular mimicry to fimbriated bacterial antigens)

From Floege J, John RJ, Feehally J (eds): Comprehensive Clinical Nephrology, 4th ed. Philadelphia, Saunders, 2010.

Treatment

- Avoidance of salt if edema or HTN is present
- ↓ Protein intake (≈0.5 g/kg/day) in pts w/renal failure
- Fluid restriction in pts w/significant edema; furosemide PRN
- Avoidance of ↑ K⁺ foods
- Correction of electrolyte abnlities (hypocalcemia, hyperkalemia) and acidosis (if present)
- ACEIs or ARBs for HTN
- Rx of specific cause of nephritic syndrome:
  - **Postinfectious GN (PIGN):** early Rx of bacterial infection may prevent or ↓ severity; supportive care; unproven benefit for use of corticosteroids/immunosuppressants
  - **IgA nephropathy:** ACEIs/ARBs, pulse and oral corticosteroids, alkylating agents (cyclophosphamide, azathioprine) for progressive disease
  - **MPGN:** corticosteroids and immunosuppressive agents; no proven benefit for corticosteroids
  - **Hep C virus–associated GN (HCV-GN):** peginterferon and ribavirin. Add telaprevir or boceprevir for pts with hep C genotype I. Consider rituximab if hep C–related cryoglobulinemia.
  - **Lupus nephritis:** class I, II → ACEIs, ARBs, and corticosteroids; class III, IV, V → immunosuppressive agents
  - **Anti-GBM antibody disease:** plasmapheresis using albumin replacement × 2 wk and cyclophosphamide + corticosteroids × 3 to 6 mo
  - **PICG:** induction with cyclophosphamide and corticosteroids followed by long-term Rx with azathioprine and corticosteroids

M. TUBULOINTERSTITIAL DISORDERS

1 ACUTE TUBULAR NECROSIS

Definition

Acute injury to the tubules of the kidneys. The term *tubulointerstitial nephropathy* refers to damage to the tubules and interstitium. Because these structures are intimately related, initial damage to either one generally progresses to affect the other.

Etiology

- Perfusion deficits (prolonged prerenal failure, shock, hypovolemia, sepsis, pancreatitis, ↓ output states, CABG surgery, aortic aneurysm repair)
- Pigment nephropathy: myoglobinuria (rhabdo), hemoglobinuria
- Contrast agent toxicity
- Drug toxicity: AGs, cisplatinum, pentamidine, lithium, amphotericin
- Crystal-induced ARF: acyclovir, sulfonamides, MTX, oxalate from ethylene glycol ingestion or high doses of vitamin C
- Uric acid deposition in the tumor lysis syndrome
- The acute reductions in GFR lead to an ↑ in Cr (2+ mg/day), a ↓ U/P-to-Cr ratio (<20), oliguric or nonoliguric urinary volumes, threatening hyperkalemia, and pulmonary vascular congestion.

Diagnosis

Labs

- Serial ↑ in Cr and BUN varies w/catabolic rate and protein intake.
- Oliguria or nonoliguria occurs, but at relatively fixed outputs.
- Variable response to high-dose furosemide: may allow diuresis but does not change the underlying lesion.
- Pulmonary vascular congestion and hyperkalemia represent the most important parameters to follow: pulmonary artery catheter may be necessary to monitor fluid status.
- Urinary Na^+ is ↑, generally >30.
- Urinary osmolarity is <350 mOsm/kg.
- Urinary Cr is ↓ in relation to urinary volume, leading to a U/P Cr level <20.
- FE_{Na} >1
- Urinary sediment contains "muddy brown" renal tubular casts.
- Myoglobinuria and serum CPK are ↑ in rhabdo.

Treatment

- Most pts w/ARF recover w/conservative management (fluid monitoring, protein restriction, drug adjustments, and dietary or Kayexalate K^+ control).
- Dialysis, usually temporary, may become necessary.

N. KIDNEY CYSTIC DISORDERS

See Table 9-13.

O. UROLITHIASIS

Presence of calculi within the urinary tract. The five major types of urinary stones are Ca oxalate (>60%), Ca phosphate (10%), uric acid (10%), struvite (< 10%), and cystine (<3%).

Etiology

- Absorption of Ca in the small bowel: type I absorptive hypercalciuria (independent of Ca intake)
- Idiopathic hypercalciuria nephrolithiasis is the most common dx for pts w/Ca stones; the dx is made only if there is no hypercalcemia and no known cause of hypercalciuria.
- ↑ Vitamin D synthesis (e.g., secondary to renal PO_4^{-3} loss: type III absorptive hypercalciuria)
- Renal tubular malfunction w/inadequate reabsorption of Ca and resulting hypercalciuria
- Heterozygous mutations in the *NPT2a* gene resulting in hypophosphatemia and urinary PO_4^{-3} loss
- Hyperparathyroidism w/resulting hypercalcemia
- Uric acid level (metabolic defects, dietary excess)
- Chronic diarrhea (e.g., IBD) w/oxalate absorption
- Type 1 (distal tubule) RTA (<1% of Ca stones)
- Chronic hydrochlorothiazide Rx
- Chronic infections w/urease-producing organisms (e.g., *Proteus, Providencia, Pseudomonas, Klebsiella*). Struvite or Mg ammonium PO_4^{-3} crystals are produced when the urinary tract is colonized by bacteria, thus producing concentrations of ammonia.
- Abnl excretion of cystine
- ChemoRx for malignant neoplasms

Diagnosis

H&P

- Stones may be asymptomatic or may cause sudden onset of flank tenderness.
- Pain may be referred to the testes or labium (progression of stone down the urinary ureter) or may radiate anteriorly over to the abd and result in intestinal ileus.

Labs

- U/A: Hematuria may be present; however, its absence does not exclude urinary stones.

TABLE 9-13 ■ Comparison of Clinical Features of Cystic Kidney Diseases

Disease	Inheritance	Frequency	Gene Product	Age of Onset	Cyst Origin	Renomegaly	Cause of ESRD	Other Manifestations
ADPKD	AD	1:400-1,000	Polycystin-1 Polycystin-2	20s and 30s	Anywhere (including Bowman's capsule)	Yes	Yes	Liver cysts, Cerebral aneurysms, Hypertension, Mitral valve prolapse, Kidney stones, UTIs
ARPKD	AR	1:6,000-10,000	Fibrocystin/poly-ductin	First yr of life	Distal nephron, CD	Yes	Yes	Hepatic fibrosis, Pulmonary hypoplasia, Hypertension
ACKD	No	90% of ESRD pts at 8 yr	None*	Years after onset of ESRD	Proximal and distal tubules	Rarely	No	None
Simple cysts	No	50% in those >40 yr	None*	Adulthood	Anywhere (usually cortical)	No	No	None
Nephronophthisis	AR	1:80,000	Nephrocystins (NPHP1-9)	Childhood or adolescence	Medullary DCT	No	Yes	Retinal degeneration, neurologic, skeletal, hepatic, cardiac malformations
MCKD	AD	Rare	Uromodulin, others	Adulthood	Medullary DCT	No	Yes	Hyperuricemia, gout
MSK	No	1:5,000-20,000	None*	30s	Medullary CD	No	No	Kidney stones, Hypercalciuria
Tuberous sclerosis	AD	1:10,000	Hamartin (TSC1), tuberin (TSC2)	Childhood	Loop of Henle, DCT	Rarely	Rarely	Renal cell carcinoma, Tubers, seizures, Angiomyolipoma, Hypertension
VHL syndrome	AD	1:40,000	VHL protein	20s	Cortical nephrons	Rarely	Rarely	Retinal angioma, CNS hemangioblastoma, renal cell carcinoma, pheochromocytoma
Oral-facial-digital syndrome-1	XD	1:250,000	OFD1 protein	Childhood or adulthood	Renal glomeruli	Rarely	Yes	Malformation of the face, oral cavity, and digits; liver cysts; mental retardation
Bardet-Biedl syndrome	AR	1:65,000-160,000	BBS 1-14	Adulthood	Renal calyces	Rarely	Yes	Syndactyly and polydactyly, obesity, retinal dystrophy, male hypogenitalism, hypertension, mental retardation

From Goldman L, Schafer AI (eds): Goldman's Cecil Medicine, 24th ed. Philadelphia, Saunders, 2012.

ACKD, Acquired cystic kidney disease; CD, collecting duct; DCT, distal convoluted tubule; MCKD, medullary cystic kidney disease; MSK, medullary sponge kidney; TSC, tuberous sclerosis complex; VHL, von Hippel-Lindau.

- Plain films of the abd can identify radiopaque stones (Ca, uric acid stones).
- Unenhanced (non–contrast-enhanced) helical CT scan has a sensitivity of 15% to 100% and a specificity of 94% to 96%.

Treatment
- ↑ Water or other fluid intake (doubling of previous fluid intake unless pt has h/o CHF or fluid overload)
- Specific Rx tailored to the stone type:
  - *Uric acid calculi:* control of hyperuricosuria w/allopurinol 100 to 300 mg/day; urinary pH w/K^+ citrate, 10-mEq tablets tid
  - *Ca stones*
    - Thiazide diuretic in pts w/type I absorptive hypercalciuria
    - ↓ Bowel absorption of Ca w/cellulose PO_4^{-3} 10 g/day in pts w/type I absorptive hypercalciuria
    - Orthophosphates to inhibit vitamin B synthesis in pts w/type III absorptive hypercalciuria
    - K^+ citrate supplementation in pts w/hypocitraturic Ca nephrolithiasis
    - Purine dietary restrictions or allopurinol in pts w/hyperuricosuric Ca nephrolithiasis
  - *Struvite stones*
    - Prolonged use of abx directed against the predominant urinary tract organism may be beneficial to prevent recurrence.
  - *Cystine stones*
    - Hydration and alkalinization of the urine to pH >6.5 with tiopronin or penicillamine
- Surgical Rx in pts w/severe pain unresponsive to medication and pts w/persistent fever or nausea or significant impediment of urine flow:
  - Ureteroscopic stone extraction
  - ESWL for most renal stones
- Rx of ureteral stones:
  - Proximal ureteral stones <1 cm in diameter: ESWL, percutaneous nephro ureterolithotomy, ureteroscopy
  - Proximal ureteral stones >1 cm in diameter: ESWL, percutaneous nephro ureterolithotomy, ureteroscopy
  - Distal ureteral stones <1 cm in diameter (most of these pass spontaneously): ESWL or ureteroscopy
  - Distal ureteral stones >1 cm in diameter: watchful waiting, ESWL, ureteroscopy (after stone fragmentation)

Clinical Pearls
- >50% of pts will pass the stone within 48 hr.
- Stones will recur in 50% of pts within 5 yr if no medical Rx is provided.

III

DISEASES AND DISORDERS
9. Nephrology

10 Neurology

A. DIAGNOSTIC AIDS

1 SPINAL DERMATOMES
- See Figure 10-1.

2 KEY AREAS DETERMINING SENSORY LEVEL
- See Box 10-1.

3 KEY MUSCLES DETERMINING MOTOR LEVEL
- See Box 10-2.

4 GRADING OF MUSCLE STRENGTH
- See Table 10-1.

5 GRADING OF DEEP TENDON REFLEXES
- See Table 10-2.

6 TESTING OF CRANIAL NERVES
- See Table 10-3.

B. EPILEPSY

1 PARTIAL (FOCAL EPILEPSY)
Characterized by focal cortical discharges that provoke seizure sx related to the area of the brain involved. Simple partial seizures do not cause impaired consciousness, whereas complex partial seizures involve an alteration in consciousness.

Etiology
- Temporal lobe epilepsy (most common form epilepsy in adults) manifests as a complex partial seizure.
- Frequent causes of partial seizures are tumor, stroke, CNS infections (cysticercosis, abscesses), AVMs, traumatic brain injury, cortical malformations, and idiopathic/genetic conditions.

Diagnosis
- EEG
- Ambulatory EEG and/or video EEG if diagnostic uncertainty

H&P
- Usually physical/neurologic exam is nl unless the cause is structural abnlity (stroke), wherein neuro exam is consistent with the area of CNS structural damage.
- During partial seizures pts are conscious, unless there is spread of the epileptic focus causing secondary generalization and unresponsiveness. A focal seizure can evolve to a generalized tonic clonic seizure. Table 10-4 describes clinical manifestations of different types of focal seizures and areas of the brain involved.

Imaging
- Head CT to r/o space-occupying lesions. If possible, avoid in children unless an emergency.
- Brain MRI with defined epilepsy protocol should be performed if recurrent seizures.

Treatment
- First unprovoked seizure with nl imaging/EEG/labs generally requires no Rx; recurrent or abnl w/up requires Rx with compliance; avoidance of EtOH and sleep deprivation is essential to prevent recurrence.
- No driving is allowed until seizure freedom in accordance w/local laws/regulations (47% seizure free w/monoRx, 67% w/polyRx).
- Avoid valproic acid (↑ risk teratogenicity) in women of childbearing age and regardless of antiepileptic drug taken; begin folic acid (1-4 mg/day) to prevent neural tube defects.
- Carbamazepine is the traditional initial drug for partial seizures.

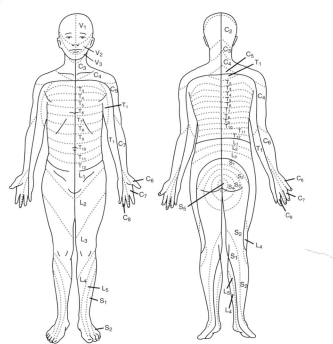

FIGURE 10-1. Spinal dermatomes. *(From Green GM [ed]: The Harriet Lane Handbook: A Manual for Pediatric House Officers, 12th ed. St. Louis, Mosby–Year Book, 1991.)*

Box 10-1 • Key Areas Determining Sensory Level

C2	Occipital protuberance	T6	Sixth intercostal space, xiphisternum
C3	Supraclavicular fossa	T7-9	Intercostal spaces
C4	Top of the acromioclavicular joint	T10	Umbilicus
C5	Lateral side of the antecubital fossa	T11	Intercostal space
C6	Thumb	T12	Inguinal ligament
C7	Middle finger	L1	Upper anterior thigh
C8	Little finger	L2	Midanterior thigh
T1	Medial side of the antecubital fossa	L3	Medial femoral condyle
T2	Apex of the axilla	L4	Medial malleolus
T3	Third intercostal space	L5	Dorsum of the foot at the third metatarsophalangeal joint
T4	Fourth intercostal space, nipple line	S1	Lateral heel
T5	Fifth intercostal space	S2	Popliteal fossa in the midline
		S3	Ischial tuberosity
		S4-5	Perianal area

Box 10-2 • Key Muscles Determining Motor Level

C1-4	Diaphragm
C5	Elbow flexors (biceps)
C6	Wrist extensors
C7	Elbow extensors (triceps)
C8	Finger flexors, distal phalanx
T1	Hand intrinsics (interossei)
T2-L1	Use sensory level and Beevor's sign
L2	Hip flexors (iliopsoas)
L3	Knee extensors (quadriceps)
L4	Ankle dorsiflexors (tibialis anterior)
L5	Long toe extensors (extensor hallucis longus)
S1	Ankle plantar flexors (gastrocnemius)
S2-5	Use sensory level and sphincter ani

TABLE 10-1 ■ Grading of Muscle Strength

Grade	Description
0	Absent muscle contraction
1	Minimal contraction
2	Active movement with gravity eliminated
3	Active movement against gravity only
4	Active movement against gravity and some resistance
5	Normal muscle strength

TABLE 10-2 ■ Grading of Deep Tendon Reflexes

Grade	Description
0	Absent
+	Hypoactive
++	Normal
+++	Brisker than average
++++	Hyperactive, often indicative of disease

TABLE 10-3 ■ Testing of Cranial Nerves

	Cranial Nerves	Action
I	Olfactory	Sense of smell
II	Optic	Vision (visual acuity, visual fields, color)
III	Oculomotor	Extraocular movement, pupillary constriction (oculomotor), elevation of upper lids, abduction of eye
IV	Trochlear	
VI	Abducens	
V	Trigeminal	Mastication; sensory of forehead, face, and jaw
VII	Facial	Facial expression; taste in anterior two thirds of tongue
VIII	Acoustic	Hearing and balance
IX	Glossopharyngeal	Sensory and motor functions of pharynx and larynx
X	Vagus	(gag reflex, position of uvula, swallowing)
XI	Accessory	Shrugging of shoulders, movement of head, motor to trapezius, sternocleidomastoid
XII	Hypoglossal	Motor control of tongue

Seizure Type	Areas of Brain Involved	Clinical Expression
Somatosensory	Postcentral rolandic; parietal	Contralateral intermittent or prolonged tingling, numbness, sense of movement, desire to move, heat, cold, electric shock; sensation may spread to other body segments
	Parietal	Contralateral agnosia of a limb, phantom limb, distortion of size or position of body part
	Second sensory; supplementary sensory-motor	Ipsilateral or bilateral facial, truncal or limb tingling, numbness, or pain; often involving lips, tongue, fingertips, feet
Motor	Precentral rolandic	Contralateral regional clonic jerking, usually rhythmic, may spread to other body segments in jacksonian motor march; often accompanied by sensory symptoms in same area
	Supplementary sensory-motor	Bilateral tonic contraction of limbs causing postural changes; may exhibit classic fencing posture; may have speech arrest or vocalization
	Frontal	Contralateral head and eye version, salivation, speech arrest or vocalization; may be combined with other motor signs (as above) depending on seizure spread
Auditory	Heschl's gyrus—auditory cortex in superior temporal lobe	Bilateral or contralateral buzzing, drumming, single tones, muffled sounds
Olfactory	Orbitofrontal; mesial temporal cortex	Often described as unpleasant odor
Gustatory	Parietal; rolandic operculum; insula; temporal lobe	Often unpleasant taste, acidic, metallic, salty, sweet, smoky
Vertiginous	Occipitotemporal-parietal junction; frontal lobe	Sensation of body displacement in various directions
Visual	Occipital	Contralateral static, moving, or flashing colored or uncolored lights, shapes, or spots; contralateral or bilateral, partial or complete loss of vision
	Temporal; occipitotemporal-parietal junction	Formed visual scenes, faces, people, objects, animals
Limbic	Limbic structures: amygdala, hippocampus, cingulum, olfactory cortex, hypothalamus	Autonomic: abdominal rising sensation, nausea, borborygmi, flushing, pallor, piloerection, perspiration, heart rate changes, chest pain, shortness of breath, cephalic sensation, lightheadedness, genital sensation, orgasm
		Psychic: déjà vu, jamais vu, depersonalization, derealization, dreamlike state, forced memory or forced thinking, fear, elation, sadness, sexual pleasure; hallucinations or illusions of visual, auditory, or olfactory nature
Dyscognitive	Usually bilateral involvement of limbic structures (see above)	Previously known as "complex partial seizures," characterized by a predominant alteration of consciousness or awareness; current definition requires involvement of at least two of five components of cognition: perception, attention, emotion, memory, and executive function

From Goldman L, Schafer AI (eds): Goldman's Cecil Medicine, 24th ed. Philadelphia, Saunders, 2012.

- Lamotrigine and levetiracetam are effective and well tolerated.
- Antiepileptics (lacosamide, oxcarbazepine, ezogabine) may be used by epilepsy specialists.
- Surgery (temporal lobectomy in mesial temporal sclerosis) may be indicated in refractory cases.

2 IDIOPATHIC GENERAL EPILEPSY

Table 10-5 describes a classification and clinical expression of generalized seizures.

Diagnosis
- EEG
- Ambulatory EEG and/or video EEG if diagnostic uncertainty

309

TABLE 10-5 ■ Generalized Seizures: Classification and Clinical Expression		
Seizure Type	Subtype	Clinical Expression
Absence	Typical	Abrupt cessation of activities, with motionless, blank stare and loss of awareness lasting ≈10 sec; the attack ends suddenly, and pt resumes normal activities immediately
	Atypical	Longer duration than typical absence, often accompanied by myoclonic, tonic, atonic, and autonomic features as well as automatisms
	With myoclonias	Absence with myoclonic components of variable intensity
Myoclonic	Myoclonic	Sudden, brief (<100 msec), shocklike, involuntary, single or multiple contractions of muscle groups of various locations
	Myoclonic-atonic	A sequence consisting of a myoclonic followed by an atonic phase
	Myoclonic-tonic	A sequence consisting of a myoclonic followed by a tonic phase
Tonic		Sustained increase in muscle contraction lasting a few seconds to minutes
Clonic		Prolonged, regularly repetitive contractions involving the same muscle groups at a rate of 2-3 cycles/sec
Atonic		Sudden loss or diminution of muscle tone lasting 1-2 sec, involving head, trunk, jaw, or limb musculature
Tonic-clonic		A sequence consisting of a tonic followed by a clonic phase

From Goldman L, Schafer AI (eds): Goldman's Cecil Medicine, 24th ed. Philadelphia, Saunders, 2012.

Labs
- Routine blood w/up (CBC, CMP, glucose, electrolytes), urine tox screen
- LP recommended if suspicion of meningitis

Imaging
- Head CT scan r/o space-occupying lesions; avoid in children unless a neurologic emergency
- MRI of the brain epilepsy protocol performed in all pts with recurrent seizures

Treatment
- First unprovoked seizure with nl imaging/EEG/laboratory w/up requires no Rx; recurrent seizures or pts w/abnl w/up require Rx based on type/etiology.
- Chronic Rx is indicated for more than two unprovoked seizures or in pts with one seizure with abnl w/up.
- Levetiracetam (initial dose 250-500 mg bid, max 1500 mg bid) is an effective and well-tolerated antiepileptic drug for generalized tonic clonic seizures.
- Valproic acid (initial dose 10-15 mg/kg/day div bid, max dose 60 mg/kg/day) is better tolerated than topiramate and more efficacious than lamotrigine in pts w/generalized and unclassified epilepsy types; avoid valproic acid (↑ risk teratogenicity) in women of childbearing age and regardless of antiepileptic drug taken; begin folic acid (1-4 mg/day) to prevent neural tube defects.
- No driving is allowed until seizure freedom in accordance with local laws and regulations.

3 STATUS EPILEPTICUS

Continuous seizure activity lasting ≥5 min or two or more discrete seizures w/incomplete recovery of consciousness between them.

Diagnosis
- *Convulsive* status epilepticus: Pts are unresponsive w/obvious tonic, clonic, or tonic-clonic extremity movements.
- *Nonconvulsive* status epilepticus varies from complete unresponsiveness w/ little or no observable motor activity to confusion and/or repetitive behaviors/ automatisms; confirm dx by video EEG monitoring or paradoxical improvement in ms after low-dose benzodiazepine.

Management
- Figure 10-2 describes a management algorithm for status epilepticus.

C. STROKE

1 TRANSIENT ISCHEMIC ATTACK (TIA)

Transient neurologic deficit resulting from focal brain, spinal cord, or retinal ischemia without acute infarction; sx typically <60 min with full function recovery. TIA is a neurologic emergency because 40% pts w/ischemic stroke experience a prior TIA.

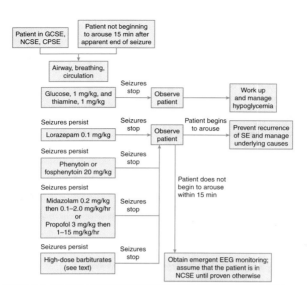

FIGURE 10-2. Management algorithm for status epilepticus. *CPSE,* complex partial status epilepticus; *GSCE,* generalized convulsive status epilepticus; *NCSE,* nonconvulsive status epilepticus; *SE,* status epilepticus. (*From Vincent JL, Abraham E, Moore FA, et al [eds]: Textbook of Critical Care, 6th ed. Philadelphia, Saunders, 2011.*)

Box 10-3 • Characteristics of Carotid Artery Syndrome

Ipsilateral monocular vision loss (amaurosis fugax); the pt often feels as if "a shade" has come down over one eye
Episodic contralateral arm, leg, and face paresis and paresthesias
Slurred speech and transient aphasia
Ipsilateral headache of vascular type
Carotid bruit may be present over the carotid bifurcation
Microemboli, hemorrhages, and exudates may be noted in the ipsilateral retina

---

Box 10-4 • Characteristics of Vertebrobasilar Artery Syndrome

Binocular visual disturbances (blurred vision, diplopia, and total blindness)
Vertigo, N/V, and tinnitus
Sudden loss of postural tone of all four extremities (drop attacks) w/o loss of consciousness
Slurred speech, ataxia, and numbness around lips or face

Etiology
- Cardioembolic
- Large-vessel atherothrombotic disease
- Lacunar disease
- Hypoperfusion w/fixed arterial stenosis
- Hypercoagulable states

Diagnosis
H&P
- Neurologic abnlities are confined to discrete vascular territory (Boxes 10-3 and 10-4).

Imaging
- Head CT, brain MRI, MRA
- Carotid Doppler, echo, ECG
- Telemetry for hospitalized pts

Labs
- CBC w/Plt, PT, PTT
- Glucose, lipid profile, ESR
- CXR; other tests dictated by suspected etiology

Treatment
- Depends on etiology. Table 10-6 describes the characteristics of thrombosis vs embolism. The ABCD2 score can help stratify pts who are at highest risk of subsequent stroke after TIA (Table 10-7). Consider hospital admission for pts with ABCD2 score >3 or those with transient monocular blindness.
- Acute anticoagulation is indicated for new-onset AF and atherothrombotic carotid disease causing recurrent transient neurologic sx, especially before carotid endarterectomy (CEA) or carotid stenting. It is also considered for basilar artery thrombosis, given concern for progression to brainstem stroke w/high morbidity and mortality.
- Antiplatelet therapy should be used to reduce the risk of recurrent TIAs or subsequent stroke. Three antiplatelet agents are commonly used in stroke prevention: aspirin, aspirin/dipyridamole, and clopidogrel. All are reasonable choices, but practitioners should consider their individual pt's comorbidities when selecting an antiplatelet agent.
- Chronic therapy should be aimed at modifying the four major risk factors: BP control, control of dyslipidemia, control of blood sugar, and smoking cessation.

TABLE 10-6 ■ Characteristics of Thrombosis and Embolism

	Thrombosis	Embolism
Onset of sx	Progression of sx during hours to days	Very rapid (seconds)
Hx of previous TIA	Common	Uncommon
Time of presentation	Often during night hours while pt is sleeping. Classically, pt awakens w/a slight neurologic deficit that gradually progresses in a stepwise fashion	Pt is usually awake and involved in some type of activity
Predisposing factors	Atherosclerosis, HTN, diabetes, arteritis, vasculitis, hypotension, trauma to head and neck	AF, mitral stenosis and regurgitation, endocarditis, mitral valve prolapse

TABLE 10-7 ■ ABCD2 Risk of Stroke After a TIA

	Score (points)
Age ≥60 yr	1
BP: ≥140 mm Hg systolic or 90 mm Hg diastolic	1
Clinical features	
Unilateral weakness	2
Speech disturbance without weakness	1
Duration of TIA	
≥60 min	2
10-59 min	1
Presence of diabetes mellitus	1
Two-day risk of stroke is 4.1% with a score 4-5 and 8.1% with a score 6-7.	

Modified from Ballinger A: Kumar & Clark's Essentials of Clinical Medicine, 6th ed. Edinburgh, Saunders, 2012.

2 ISCHEMIC STROKE

Rapid onset of neurologic deficit involving a certain vascular territory secondary to thrombosis or embolism

Diagnosis

H&P
- Clinical presentation varies w/the cerebral vessel involved (Table 10-8).

Imaging
- Immediate CT of the head without contrast or MRI of the brain with stroke protocol to rule out hemorrhage and, if possible, to assess the extent of stroke. CT

TABLE 10-8 ■ Selected Stroke Syndromes

Artery Involved	Neurologic Deficit
Middle cerebral artery	Hemiplegia (UEs and face usually more involved than LEs) Hemianesthesia (hemisensory loss) Hemianopia (homonymous) Aphasia (if dominant hemisphere is involved)
Anterior cerebral artery	Hemiplegia (LEs more involved than UEs and face) Primitive reflexes (e.g., grasp and suck) Urinary incontinence
Vertebral and basilar arteries	Ipsilateral cranial nerve findings, cerebellar findings Contralateral (or bilateral) sensory or motor deficits
Deep penetrating branches of major cerebral arteries (lacunar infarction)	Usually seen in elderly pts with HTN and diabetic pts Four characteristic syndromes are possible: 1. Pure motor hemiplegia (66%) 2. Dysarthria—clumsy hand syndrome (20%) 3. Pure sensory stroke (10%) 4. Ataxic hemiplegia syndrome w/pyramidal tract signs

of brain: area of ↓ density; initial CT scan may be nl because the infarct may not be evident for 2 to 3 days afterward.

Treatment

- IV TPA is the only medical therapy approved by the U.S. FDA for the treatment of acute ischemic stroke.
- The time window for administration is ≤3 hr of symptom onset.
- There are strict criteria for the administration of IV TPA (Box 10-5).
- The protocol is weight based, with 90 mg being the maximum allowable dose.
- The risk of brain hemorrhage with IV TPA is ≈5% in pts w/stroke.
- Multimodal therapy (i.e., thrombectomy and intra-arterial TPA) is sometimes performed.
- Endovascular treatment may be performed for select cases in which IV TPA has failed to recanalize an occluded artery.
- Endovascular intervention may be an option for pts w/systemic contraindications to IV TPA.

Box 10-5 • Inclusion and Exclusion Criteria for IV TPA

Inclusion Criteria
1. Ischemic stroke onset is within 3 hours of drug administration.
2. Measurable deficit is noted on NIH Stroke Scale examination.
3. Pt's CT does not show hemorrhage or nonstroke cause of deficit.
4. Pt's is >18 years old.

Exclusion Criteria (Absolute)
1. Pt's symptoms are minor or rapidly improving.
2. Pt had seizure at onset of stroke.
3. Pt has had another stroke or serious head trauma within the past 3 months.
4. Pt had major surgery within the last 14 days.
5. Pt has known hx of intracranial hemorrhage.
6. Pt has sustained SBP >185 mm Hg.
7. Pt has sustained DBP >110 mm Hg.
8. Aggressive treatment is necessary to lower the pt's BP.
9. Pt has symptoms suggestive of SAH.
10. Pt has had gastrointestinal or urinary tract hemorrhage within the last 21 days.
11. Pt has had arterial puncture at noncompressible site within the last 7 days.
12. Pt has received heparin with the last 48 hours and has elevated PTT.
13. Pt's PT is >15 sec.
14. Pt's Plt count is <100,000 μL.
15. Pt's serum glucose is <50 or >400 mg/dL.

Exclusion Criteria (Relative)
1. Pt has a large stroke with NIH Stroke Scale score >22.
2. Pt's CT shows evidence of large MCA territory infarction (i.e., sulcal effacement or blurring of gray-white junction in greater than one third of MCA territory).

NIH, National Institutes of Health.
Modified from Vincent JL, Abraham E, Moore FA, et al (eds): Textbook of Critical Care, 6th ed. Philadelphia, Saunders, 2011.

- Endovascular intervention is useful only for large, accessible thrombi. Therefore, if a pt w/stroke is a candidate for IV TPA, then he or she should probably receive IV TPA.
- Antiplatelet therapy: Beginning oral or feeding tube administration of aspirin (325 mg/day) ≤48 hours of stroke onset is advised. This will decrease the likelihood of a repeat ischemic stroke. Another oral antiplatelet regimen approved for secondary stroke prophylaxis (e.g., clopidogrel, aspirin plus extended-release dipyridamole) will also suffice and may be superior in the long term.
- ↑ BP is common during acute stroke, and it often subsides without specific Rx. In general, HTN is not treated acutely unless it is extremely high (e.g., >220 mm Hg SBP); unless there is evidence of organ damage caused by the HTN; or unless thrombolysis is being considered, in which case BP needs to ↓ (if it can be safely accomplished) to ~185/110 mm Hg. It is risky to ↓ BP severely the presence of acute ischemic stroke. A 15% to 25% decrease over the first 24 hours is recommended.

3 ACUTE HEMORRHAGIC STROKE

a Intracranial hemorrhage
Neurologic deficit secondary to intracerebral hemorrhage (17% of all strokes)

Etiology
- HTN (50%-60%)
- Cerebral amyloid angiopathy (10%)
- Hemorrhagic infarcts (10%)
- Use of anticoagulants and fibrinolytic agents (10%)
- Brain tumors (5%)
- Vascular malformations (5%)

Diagnosis
H&P
- Neurologic deficits vary w/the area involved (Fig. 10-3 and Table 10-9).
- Signs of ↑ ICP (e.g., bradycardia, ↓ RR, third nerve palsy)

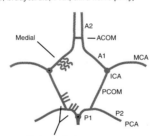

FIGURE 10-3. Circle of Willis. *ACOM,* anterior communicating artery; *MCA,* middle cerebral artery; *PCA,* posterior cerebral artery; *PCOM,* posterior communicating artery. *(From Weissleder R, Wittenberg J, Harisinghani M, Chen JW [eds]: Primer of Diagnostic Imaging, 5th ed. St. Louis, Mosby, 2011.)*

Imaging
- Immediate: CT scanning of the head without contrast is highly sensitive for hemorrhage (area of hemorrhagic infarct appears as a zone of ↑ density).
- MRI of the brain with a gradient echo sequence is also highly sensitive for hemorrhage, including intracerebral microhemorrhages that may not be visible with CT scanning.

Treatment
- Surgery should be performed promptly for cases of cerebellar hemorrhage of >3 cm when the pt is deteriorating clinically or showing brainstem edema or hydrocephalus.
- Surgery for lobar or deep brain clots may be considered for select cases, although the level of evidence for efficacy is not high.
- Pneumatic compression devices should be applied to help prevent DVT.
- Early mobilization for rehabilitation is desirable.

TABLE 10-9 ■ Localizing Signs in Pts w/Intracerebral Hemorrhage

Location of Intracerebral Hemorrhage	Common Neurologic Signs	Examples
Putamen	Both eyes deviating conjugately to the side of the lesion (away from hemiparesis) Pupils normal in size and reacting normally Contralateral hemiplegia present Hemisensory defect noted	Left putaminal hemorrhage
Thalamus	Both eyes deviating downward and looking at the nose Impairment of vertical eye movements present Pupils small (≈2 mm) and nonreactive Contralateral hemisensory loss present	Thalamic hemorrhage
Pons	Both eyes in midposition No doll's-eye movements Pupils pinpoint but reactive (use magnifying glass) Coma common Flaccid quadriplegia noted	Pontine hemorrhage
Cerebellum	Ipsilateral paresis of conjugate gaze (inability to look toward side of lesion) Pupils normal in size and reacting normally Inability to stand or to walk Vertigo and dysarthria present	Cerebellar hemorrhage

Box 10-6 • Suggested Recommended Guidelines for the Treatment of Elevated BP in Pts w/Spontaneous Intracerebral Hemorrhage

1. SBP of >200 mm Hg or MAP of >150 mm Hg: Consider the aggressive reduction of BP with continuous IV infusion, with BP monitoring every 5 min.
2. SBP of >180 mm Hg or MAP of >130 mm Hg with evidence or suspicion of elevated ICP: Consider ICP monitor and reducing BP with intermittent or continuous IV medications to keep cerebral perfusion pressure >60 to 80 mm Hg.
3. SBP of >180 mm Hg or MAP of >130 mm Hg without evidence or suspicion of elevated ICP: Consider a modest reduction of BP (e.g., MAP of 110 mm Hg or target BP of 160/90 mm Hg) with intermittent or continuous IV medications, and clinically reexamine the pt every 15 min.

Modified from Broderick J, Connolly S, Feldmann E, et al: Guidelines for the management of spontaneous intracerebral hemorrhage in adults: 2007 update. Stroke 38:2001-2023, 2007.

- HTN: BP should be quickly lowered by 15% and then gradually and safely brought to the individual pt's target range. In theory, this may diminish expansion of the hematoma. Recommended guidelines for Rx of HTN in pts w/spontaneous hemorrhage are described in Box 10-6.
- Hyperglycemia: A high blood glucose level predicts a worse outcome. Markedly elevated glucose levels should be lowered to <300 mg/dL.
- Seizures: If seizures occur, they should be treated aggressively, including with IV medications, if needed.
- ↑ ICP: This condition should be treated with a graded approach, which may include the elevation of the head of the bed, analgesia/sedation, hyperventilation, and osmotic therapy.
- Antipyretics should be administered for cases that involve fever; in addition, the cause of the fever should be sought.
- Protamine sulfate is used to treat cases of heparin-induced intracerebral hemorrhage.
- Vitamin K is given for warfarin-associated intracerebral hemorrhage. In addition, recombinant factor VIIa and fresh frozen plasma are sometimes used.
- Recommendations for thrombolytic-associated intracerebral hemorrhage treatment include the consideration of the infusion of Plts and cryoprecipitate.

b Subarachnoid Hemorrhage (SAH)

Presence of active bleeding into the subarachnoid space via ruptured congenital aneurysm or AVM

Diagnosis

H&P

- Abrupt onset of severe occipital or generalized headache that radiates into the posterior neck region and is worsened by neck and head movements; often described as "the worst headache" of the pt's life
- Restlessness, vomiting, diminished level of consciousness, syncope
- Focal neurologic signs usually are absent.
- Level of consciousness varies from nl to deeply comatose.
- Fever and nuchal rigidity are present or usually develop within 24 hr.
- Fundi may show papilledema or retinal hemorrhage.
- Cranial nerve abnlities may be noted (e.g., pupillary dilation secondary to oculomotor nerve dysfunction).
- HTN may be present and can lead to an incorrect dx of primary hypertensive emergency.
- Tachycardia and irregular heartbeat may be present (≤91% of pts w/SAH have cardiac arrhythmias).

Imaging and Labs

- CT of brain is (+) in >95% of cases, especially during the acute phase (i.e., 24-48 hr) after the onset of bleeding.
- A CT angiogram or a cerebral angiogram is imperative for determining the origin of the SAH. Angiography may also be extremely useful because it may offer a therapeutic benefit via the coiling of the aneurysm.
- Basic labs should include CBC, chemistry panel, PT, PTT, Plt count, troponin.
- LP is a very important part of the w/up, especially because 3% of pts with normal CT scans show evidence of hemorrhage on LP. An RBC count of >100,000/m^3 strongly suggests SAH. If RBC counts ↓ between the first and fourth tubes, then the tap is most likely traumatic. The presence of xanthochromia or bilirubin in the CSF is a sign of SAH.

Treatment

- Management of SAH varies w/the pt's clinical status (Table 10-10), as well as the location (see Fig. 10-3) and surgical accessibility of the aneurysm.

TABLE 10-10 ■ Glasgow Coma Scale*

Eyes	Motor	Verbal
1. None	1. None	1. None
2. To pain	2. Abnl extension	2. Incomprehensible (groaning)
3. To speech	3. Abnl flexion	3. Inappropriate
4. Spontaneous	4. Flexion (withdrawal)	4. Disoriented, confused
	5. Localizing	5. Oriented
	6. Obeying commands	

*The best score for each response should be documented and communicated in the format described above. Assessment of the best motor score is based on the best response of the arms. For use in individual pts, separate description of the three components of the GCS is strongly recommended. For purposes of classification, the total GCS can be calculated by adding the best score obtained in each category. The GCS should be annotated to indicate confounding factors: *T* signifies an intubated pt; *S*, sedation; *P*, neuromuscular blockade.
From Vincent JL, Abraham E, Moore FA, et al (eds): Textbook of Critical Care, 6th ed. Philadelphia, Saunders, 2011.

- Pts with a depressed level of consciousness may need to be intubated and mechanically ventilated in an ICU setting.
- A lumbar drain or ventriculostomy is required should the pt develop hydrocephalus or ↑ ICP.
- Initial management strategies are geared toward stabilizing the pt and preventing recurrent hemorrhage and hydrocephalus.
- Tight BP control is paramount. This can be done with the use of drips (e.g., nitroprusside) or PRN medications. An SBP 120 to 150 mm Hg is recommended.
- After an aneurysm has been identified, measures to secure it should be undertaken; this can be done by either clipping or coiling the aneurysm. Clipping consists of placing a clip around the neck of the aneurysm and is performed via intra-arterial angiography; it consists of deploying platinum coils inside the aneurysm to cause thrombosis of the aneurysmal sac.
- Pain control is performed with the use of short-acting and less-sedating medications (e.g., codeine, low-dose morphine).
- Seizures occur in ≤3% of pts during the acute phase; however, the use of prophylactic antiepileptics is still controversial.

- Vasospasm, which typically begins around day 3 after the hemorrhage and reaches a peak on day 6 to 8, is the leading cause of death and disability after aneurysm rupture. Nimodipine has been shown to improve outcomes if it is administered between days 4 and 21 after the hemorrhage, even if it does not significantly reduce the amount of vasospasm detected on angiography. After vasospasm develops, "triple H" therapy—to achieve Hypertension, Hypervolemia, and Hemodilution—is used in an attempt to provide adequate cerebral perfusion.

4 SINUS VENOUS THROMBOSIS

Etiology
- *Staphylococcus aureus* (50%-60%), *Streptococcus* (second leading cause), gram(−) rods/anaerobes; sphenoid sinusitis (most common site)

Diagnosis
H&P
- Ptosis, proptosis
- Chemosis
- CN palsies (III, IV, V (VI and VII); VI); VI is most common
- Sensory deficits of the ophthalmic/maxillary branch of the fifth nerve are common.

Labs
- CBC, ESR, blood/sinus cultures (identify infectious primary source)
- LP necessary to r/o meningitis

Imaging
- MRV, MRI w/gadolinium including MR angiography

Treatment
- Rx should take into account the primary source of infection, as well as possible associated complications, such as brain abscess, meningitis, or subdural empyema.
- Broad-spectrum IV abx are used as empiric Rx until a definite pathogen is found. Rx should include a penicillinase-resistant PCN at maximum dose plus a third- or fourth-generation ceph:
  - Nafcillin (or oxacillin) 2 g IV q4h plus either ceftriaxone (2 g q12h) or cefepime (2 g q6h)
  - Metronidazole 500 mg IV q6h should be added if anaerobic bacterial infection is suspected (dental or sinus infection).
  - Vancomycin (1 g q12h w/nl renal function) may be substituted for nafcillin if significant concern exists for infection by MRSA or resistant *Streptococcus pneumoniae*.
- Anticoagulation w/heparin: controversial. Cerebral infarction or ICH should first be ruled out by non–contrast-enhanced CT scan before initiation of heparin Rx. Current recommendation is for early heparinization in pts w/unilateral CST to prevent clot propagation and to ↑ the incidence of septic emboli. Warfarin Rx should be avoided in the acute phase of the illness but should ultimately be instituted to achieve an INR of 2 to 3 and continued until the infection, sx, and signs of CST have resolved or significantly improved.
- Steroid Rx: controversial but may prove helpful in ↓ cranial nerve dysfunction or when progression to pituitary insufficiency occurs. Corticosteroids should be instituted only after appropriate abx coverage. Dexamethasone 10 mg q6h is the Rx of choice.
- Emergency surgical drainage w/sphenoidotomy: indicated if the primary site of infection is thought to be the sphenoid sinus.
- All pts w/CST are usually treated w/prolonged courses (3-4 wk) of IV abx. If there is evidence of complications such as intracranial suppuration, 6 to 8 wk of total Rx may be warranted.
- All pts should be monitored for signs of complicated infection, continued sepsis, or septic emboli while abx Rx is being administered.

5 STROKE PREVENTION: ASYMPTOMATIC CAROTID STENOSIS

Carotid stenosis is narrowing of the arterial lumen within the carotid artery.

Etiology
- Atherosclerosis (most common)
- Aneurysm
- Arteritis
- Carotid dissection
- Fibromuscular displasia

- Postradiation necrosis
- Vasospasm
- Risk factors: HTN, dyslipidemia, DM, and smoking

Diagnosis
- Carotid duplex. If carotid stenosis is suspected on carotid duplex, but results are inconclusive, MRI, CT angiography, or traditional angiography should be obtained to confirm the degree of stenosis.

H&P
- Pts with carotid stenosis are often asymptomatic, but many have presence of a carotid bruit or TIA.

Treatment (Table 10-11)
- CEA and carotid angioplasty and stenting are available.
- **CEA:** The selection of surgical candidates should be guided primarily by the presence or absence of symptoms and the degree of stenosis.

Asymptomatic Pts
- CEA should be considered in asymptomatic pts only if the perioperative risk for stroke and death at the given surgical institution is <3%.
- CEA should be considered in pts between the ages of 40 and 75 yr with an asymptomatic 60% to 99% stenosis if their life expectancy is >5 yr and the perioperative stroke and mortality rates are <3%. However, medical therapy has improved since early trials comparing medical management and revascularization, and many experts are favoring intensified medical management rather than revascularization procedures in pts with ACS.
- All pts undergoing CEA should be started on aspirin (ASA 81 or 325 mg daily) before surgery, and aspirin should be continued indefinitely.

Symptomatic Pts
- CEA is recommended for recently symptomatic pts with 70% to 99% stenosis if their life expectancy is >5 yr and perioperative risk for mortality is <6%.
- CEA is beneficial for recently symptomatic men with 50% to 69% stenosis if their life expectancy is >5 yr and perioperative risk of mortality is <6%. Medical management is recommended for pts with stenosis <50%.
- General medical therapy should be aimed at risk factor reduction. Major risk factors for carotid stenosis are HTN, DM, lipid disorders, and smoking.
- Antiplatelet therapy: Three antiplatelet options are available for pts with carotid stenosis: ASA, ASA plus dipyridamole, and clopidogrel.

TABLE 10-11 ■ Carotid Stenosis Management

Degree of Carotid Stenosis	<50%	50%-69%	70%-99%
Asymptomatic	Medical management	Men: CEA if stenosis >60% and age <75 yr; otherwise, medical management Women: medical management	Men <75 yr: CEA Women: medical management
Symptomatic	Medical management	Men: CEA Women: medical management	Men: CEA Women: CEA

From Ferri F: Ferri's Clinical Advisor: 5 Books in 1. 2013 edition. Philadelphia, Mosby, 2012.

D. HEADACHES

Table 10-12 compares the various types of headache.

1 MIGRAINE (AURA, TRIGGER)

Recurrent headaches are preceded by a focal neurologic sx (migraine w/aura), occur independently (migraine w/o aura), or have atypical presentations (migraine variants). Aura, typically w/visual or sensory sx, develops over 5 to 20 min. In both migraine w/and w/o aura, headache is typically unilateral, pulsatile, and associated with N/V, photophobia, and phonophobia.

Treatment

Acute Abortive Rx
- Triptans (SC, PO, and intranasal) are the drug class of choice for abortive Rx.
- Early administration improves effectiveness.

Prophylactic Rx
- Prophylactic Rx is generally indicated when headaches occur >once/wk or when symptomatic Rxs are contraindicated or not effective. All prophylaxis should be maintained for ≥3 mo before deeming the medication a failure.

TABLE 10-12 ■ Differential Diagnosis of Headache

Headache Type	Genetics	Epidemiology	Characteristic Features	Length	Accompanying Symptoms
Migraine headache	Complex genetics but usually a fhx	More frequent in women	Unilateral, bilateral; throbbing; moderate to severe; worsens with activity	Hours to days	Photophobia, phonophobia, nausea and/or vomiting
Tension-type headache	Usually a fhx	Equally frequent in men and women	Tight bandlike pain; bilateral; pain may be mild to moderate; improves with activity	Hours to days	No nausea or vomiting; small amount of light or sound sensitivity, but not both
Cluster headache	Possibly a fhx	More frequent in men	Unilateral, severe pain in the face	Minutes to hour	Ipsilateral ptosis, miosis, rhinorrhea, eyelid edema, tearing
Paroxysmal hemicrania	Usually no fhx	More frequent in women	Unilateral pain in the face	Minutes	Ipsilateral ptosis, miosis, rhinorrhea, eyelid edema, tearing; responds to indomethacin
Hemicrania continua	No fhx	More frequent in women	Unilateral, continuous headache with episodic stabbing pains	Continuous	Ipsilateral autonomic features: ptosis, miosis, rhinorrhea, eyelid edema, tearing

fhx = family history

From Goldman L, Schafer AI (eds): Goldman's Cecil Medicine, 24th ed. Philadelphia, Saunders, 2012.

- Options include β-blockers (propranolol, timolol, atenolol, metoprolol), tricyclic antidepressants (amitriptyline), and the antiepileptic drug valproic acid.
- Less-established options include Ca^{2+} channel blockers, selective serotonin reuptake inhibitors, and the antiepileptic drugs gabapentin and topiramate. The FDA has approved injection of onabotulinum toxin A (Botox) for prevention of headaches in adult pts with chronic migraines (≥15 headache days/mo for ≥3 mo).

2 TENSION-TYPE HEADACHE (BILATERAL, VICE-LIKE)

Recurrent headaches lasting 30 min to 7 days w/o N/V and w/at least two of the following: pressing or tightening quality (nonthrobbing), mild or moderate intensity, bilateral, and not aggravated by routine physical activity

Treatment
- Relaxation and cognitive-behavioral Rx (especially in adolescents and children), Schultz-type autogenic training (relaxation technique based on passive concentration and body awareness of specific sensations), transcutaneous electrical nerve stimulation, heat

Acute General Treatment
- Nonnarcotic analgesics with limited frequency to prevent drug-induced and/or rebound headache

Chronic Treatment
- Tricyclic antidepressants (amitriptyline 10-150 mg qhs) and SSRIs
- Avoid narcotics, limit NSAIDs, consider indomethacin; if related to cervical muscle spasm, consider a trial of muscle relaxants (e.g., metaxalone [Skelaxin] 400-800 mg tid)

3 CLUSTER HEADACHE (UNILATERAL, LACRIMATION, PERIORBITAL)

Attacks of severe, unilateral orbital, supraorbital, and/or temporal pain lasting 15 to 180 min, occurring from once every other day to eight times/day. Attacks are associated w/one or more of the following, all of which are ipsilateral: conjunctival injection, lacrimation, nasal congestion, rhinorrhea, forehead/facial sweating, miosis, ptosis, and eyelid edema. Most pts are restless or agitated during an attack.

Treatment

Abortive Treatment

- Inhalation of 100% O$_2$ by face mask for 15 min often aborts an attack.
- 75% of users of triptans (sumatriptan, zolmitriptan) are pain free within 20 min.
- Ergotamine (Cafergot), octreotide, intranasal lidocaine, or dihydroergotamine may abort an attack or prevent one if given just before a predictable episode.

Prophylaxis Treatment

- Various medications have been tried without great success, although good responses may be obtained in up to 50% of cases. Examples include:
  - Valproic acid: start at 500 mg/day
  - Topiramate: up to 50 mg bid
  - Verapamil: up to 480 mg/day as tolerated

4 IDIOPATHIC INTRACRANIAL HYPERTENSION (IIH; PSEUDOTUMOR CEREBRI)

Syndrome of ↑ ICP w/o underlying hydrocephalus/mass lesion + nl CSF analysis

Diagnosis

H&P

- Symptoms
  - Headaches: generalized, throbbing, slowly progressive, worse with straining maneuvers, worse in the morning
  - Transient visual obscurations as a brief blurring of vision or scotomata lasting <30 sec; occur frequently with Valsalva maneuver and may be monocular
  - Double vision: most often in the horizontal plane (because of pseudo–sixth nerve palsy)
  - Pulsatile tinnitus: may be initial symptom
  - Photopsia: lights, sparkles in the eyes
  - Pain: mainly retro-orbital; pain may also be located in the shoulders or neck and may be present without a headache; may be associated with Lhermitte's sign.
- Signs
  - Papilledema: in virtually all cases; bilateral but may be asymmetric
  - Sixth nerve palsy: in approximately 10% to 20% of pts
  - Visual field defects: enlarged physiologic blind spot, constricted visual fields
  - Loss of vision: end result of long-standing and untreated IIH

Labs

- CSF analysis: ↑ opening pressure, nl protein, glucose, and cell count
- Hypercoagulability w/up if suspicion of venous sinus thrombosis

Imaging

- Brain MRI r/o underlying structural lesions; empty sella sign often associated w/IIH but not pathognomonic
- Cerebral venography/MRV to evaluate venous flow
- CT (slit-like ventricles)

Treatment

- Weight loss in obese pts
- CPAP if obstructive sleep apnea suspected
- Acetazolamide 250 mg to 4 g/day: ↓ CSF production occurs by inhibition of carbonic anhydrase, occasionally causing anorexia and resultant weight loss.
- Furosemide 40 to 120 mg/day in divided doses: Apparent mechanism of action is by ↓ Na$^+$ transport, leading to ↓ total CSF volume.
- Topiramate 100 to 400 mg/day: This antiepileptic medication, reported to be effective in Rx of IIH, is a weak carbonic anhydrase inhibitor with weight loss as one of its primary side effects.
- Serial LP is attempted in pts with severe headaches resistant to medical Rx. Goal is to ↓ spinal fluid pressure, thus allowing immediate reduction in headache severity. This Rx should be reserved only for the most resistant cases and should be used as a conduit to future surgical intervention.
- Surgical intervention is indicated in cases of Rx failure and progressive visual loss.
- Optic nerve fenestration is preferred for pts with visual loss and easily controlled headaches.
- CSF shunting: This neurosurgical procedure is performed in pts with significant visual deterioration.

DISEASES AND DISORDERS | 10. Neurology

E. MOVEMENT DISORDERS

1 PARKINSON'S DISEASE (PD)

Progressive neurodegenerative disorder characterized clinically by rigidity, tremor, and bradykinesia and pathologically by cytoplasmic eosinophilic inclusions (Lewy bodies) in neurons of the substantia nigra and locus ceruleus and by depigmentation of the brainstem nuclei

Diagnosis
- The four cardinal signs used to diagnose PD are (mnemonic = TRAP):
  - **T**remor (resting, typically 4-6Hz)
  - **R**igidity, of the cogwheel type
  - Bradykinesia/**a**kinesia: slowness of movement
  - **P**ostural instability: failure of postural "righting" reflexes leading to poor balance and falls
- One need not show all four cardinal signs to make a presumptive diagnosis of PD and begin treatment.

Imaging
- MRI of the head may sometimes distinguish between idiopathic PD and other conditions that manifest with signs of parkinsonism.

Treatment
- Physical therapy, pt education and reassurance, treatment of associated conditions (e.g., depression)
- Avoidance of drugs that can induce or worsen parkinsonism: neuroleptics (especially high potency), certain antiemetics (prochlorperazine, trimethobenzamide), metoclopramide, nonselective MAO inhibitors (may induce hypertensive crisis), reserpine, methyldopa

Medical Treatment
- Whether levodopa or dopamine agonists should be the initial treatment remains controversial. In younger pts, agonists are usually the drug of choice; in pts >70 yr, levodopa is typically the drug of choice.
- Levodopa is the cornerstone of symptomatic therapy. It should be used with a peripheral dopa decarboxylase inhibitor (carbidopa) to minimize side effects (nausea, lightheadedness, postural hypotension). The combination of the two drugs is marketed under the trade name Sinemet. Levodopa therapy has been found to reduce morbidity and mortality in pts w/PD.
- Dopamine receptor agonists (Ropinirole and Pramipexole) are not as potent as levodopa, but they are often used as initial treatment in younger pts to attempt to delay the onset of complications (dyskinesias, motor fluctuations) associated with levodopa therapy. In general these drugs cause more side effects than levodopa, including nausea, vomiting, lightheadedness, peripheral edema, confusion, and somnolence. They can also cause impulse control behaviors such as hypersexuality, binge eating, and compulsive shopping and gambling. Presence of these behaviors must be assessed at each visit.
- MAO-B inhibitors (rasagiline, selegiline, amantadine) can be used as monotherapy early in the disease or as adjunctive therapy in later stages. They have milder symptomatic benefit than dopamine agonists or levodopa and are well tolerated and easy to titrate. Concurrent use of stimulants and sympathomimetics should be avoided. Certain food restrictions may apply.
- Anticholinergic agents (trihexyphenidyl, benztropine) are helpful only in treating tremor and drooling in pts w/PD. Potential side effects include constipation, urinary retention, memory impairment, and hallucinations. These drugs should be avoided in elderly pts.

Surgical Options
- Pallidal (globus pallidus interna) and subthalamic deep brain stimulation (DBS; subthalamic nucleus) are currently the surgical options of choice for pts w/ advanced PD; similar improvement in motor function and adverse effects have been reported after either procedure. Compared with ablative procedures, DBS has the advantage of being reversible and adjustable. Thalamic DBS may be useful for refractory tremor. It improves the cardinal motor symptoms, extends medication "on" time, and reduces motor fluctuations during the day. In general pts are likely to benefit from this therapy if they show a clear response to levodopa. Therefore, when considering DBS, pts should be evaluated for motor response to levodopa by stopping levodopa overnight and evaluating motor response before and after a dose of levodopa.

- Surgery is limited to patients with disabling, medically refractory problems, and pts must still have a good response to L-dopa to undergo surgery. DBS results in decreased dyskinesias, fluctuations, rigidity, and tremor.

2 ATAXIA
- Vertebral-basilar artery ischemia
- AIDS
- Diabetic neuropathy
- Vitamin B_{12} deficiency
- MS and other demyelinating diseases
- Meningomyelopathy
- Cerebellar neoplasms, hemorrhage, abscess, infarct
- Nutritional (Wernicke's encephalopathy)
- Paraneoplastic syndromes
- Parainfectious: GBS, acute ataxia of childhood and young adults
- Toxins: phenytoin, alcohol, sedatives, organophosphates
- Wilson's disease (hepatolenticular degeneration)
- Hypothyroidism
- Myopathy
- Cerebellar and spinocerebellar degeneration: ataxia-telangiectasia, Friedreich's ataxia
- Frontal lobe lesions: tumors, thrombosis of anterior cerebral artery, hydrocephalus
- Labyrinthine destruction: neoplasm, injury, inflammation, compression
- Hysteria
- Tabes dorsalis

3 ESSENTIAL TREMOR
Predominantly postural and action tremor that is bilateral and tends to progress slowly during the years in the absence of other neurologic abnlities; most common of all movement disorders

Etiology
- Often inherited (autosomal dominant); sporadic cases w/o an fhx also encountered

Diagnosis
- Pts complain of tremor that is most bothersome when writing or holding something, such as a newspaper, or trying to drink from a cup. It worsens under emotional duress and is made better w/alcohol ingestion.
- Tremor, 4 to 12 Hz, bilateral postural and action tremor of the UEs; may also affect the head, voice, trunk, and legs. Table 10-13 compares essential tremor with cerebellar and parkinsonian tremor.

TABLE 10-13 ■ Distinguishing Features of Parkinsonian, Cerebellar, and Essential Tremor			
Feature	Parkinson's Syndrome	Cerebellar Tremor	Essential Tremor
Present at rest	Yes	No	Yes
Increased tone	Yes	No	No
Decreased tone	No	Yes	No
Postural abnlity	Yes	Yes	No
Head involvement	Yes	Yes	Yes
Intentional component	No	Yes	Yes
Incoordination	No	Yes	No

From Remmel KS, Bunyan R, Brunback R, et al: Handbook of Symptom-Oriented Neurology, 3rd ed. St. Louis, Mosby, 2002.

Treatment
- Propranolol
- Primidone

4 DYSTONIA
A group of disorders characterized by involuntary muscle contractions (sustained or spasmodic) that lead to abnl body movements or postures. It can be generalized or focal, of early (<20 yr) or late onset, and primary or secondary.

Etiology
- Primary dystonia is believed to involve ↓/abnl basal ganglia activity resulting in disinhibition of motor thalamus and cortex, thus producing abnl movement.

- Secondary dystonia results from CNS disease of basal ganglia (stroke, demyelination, hypoxia, trauma, Huntington's disease, Wilson's disease, Parkinson's syndromes, and lysosomal storage diseases).
- Acute dystonia is caused by drugs that block dopamine receptors.
- TD can result from long-term Rx with antiemetics (e.g., phenothiazines), antipsychotics (e.g., haloperidol), levodopa, anticonvulsants, or ergots.

Diagnosis

- Hx (family hx, birth hx, trauma, medication use)
- Physical examination

H&P

- Focal dystonias
  - Neck *(torticollis):* most commonly affected site with a tendency for the head to turn to one side
  - Eyelids *(blepharospasm):* involuntary closure of the eyelids that leads to excessive eye blinking, sometimes with persistent eye closure and functional blindness
  - Mouth *(oromandibular dystonia):* involuntary contraction of muscles of the mouth, tongue, or face
  - Hand *(writer's cramp)*
  - Isolated foot dystonia is very rare and may suggest an underlying parkinsonian disorder or brain structural abnlity.
- Generalized dystonia
  - Affects multiple areas of the body and can lead to marked joint deformities

Labs

- Usually not helpful for dx
- Serum ceruloplasmin if Wilson's disease is suspected

Imaging

- Primary dystonias are generally not associated with structural CNS abnormalities. CT scan or MRI of brain is indicated if a CNS lesion is suspected as a cause of secondary dystonia.
- Electrophysiologic testing can provide support for the dx.

Treatment

Acute Treatment

- For acute dystonic reactions to phenothiazines/butyrophenones, use diphenhydramine 50 mg IV or benztropine 2 mg IV.

Chronic Treatment

- Pharmacologic Rx is often ineffective.
- Slowly withdraw offending agents.
- Diazepam, baclofen, or carbamazepine may be helpful.
- Intrathecal baclofen is most useful for spastic or truncal dystonia.
- Trihexyphenidyl or benztropine may be helpful in up to 50% of tardive dystonias.
- For generalized dystonia, a trial of carbidopa/levodopa may be beneficial and diagnostic of dopa-responsive dystonia (DYT5).
- Injection of botulinum toxin into the affected muscles is the standard Rx.
- Surgical procedures, including denervation, myectomy, rhizotomy, thalamotomy (pallidotomy), or functional stereotactic surgery, may be helpful for severe, refractory cases.
- DBS is becoming more promising, especially for refractory primary generalized dystonias.

5 CHOREA

Etiology

- Pathology to the basal ganglia resulting in a pattern of discrete, randomly occurring jerks or twitches, either generalized or confined to a single body part
- The most common type of chorea is dyskinesia produced by dopamine drugs in pts with PD.
- The most common neurodegenerative choreic disorder is Huntington's disease.

Treatment

- Severity ↓ by dopamine-depleting or D_2 receptor-blocking agents

6 TARDIVE DYSKINESIA (TD)

Syndrome of involuntary movements associated with the long-term use of antipsychotic medication, particularly first-generation antipsychotics. Pts exhibit rapid, repetitive, stereotypic movements that mostly involve the oral, lingual, trunk, and limb areas.

Treatment
- Clozapine has the best evidence for improving the sx of TD, although olanzapine and amisulpride may also be of benefit.

7 MYOCLONUS

Sudden, brief, jerky, "shock-like" involuntary movements that can involve the muscles of the extremities, face, or trunk. (+) Myoclonus is caused by muscle contraction, whereas (–) myoclonus is caused by inhibition of active (such as postural) muscles. Myoclonus is a symptom that can be seen in a number of different neurologic disorders.

Treatment
- Carefully remove or ↓ potentially causative medications.
- For acute Rx of epileptic myoclonus, antiepileptic drugs such as valproic acid, levetiracetam, or clonazepam are helpful.
- Clonazepam, valproic acid, levetiracetam are typically used for all forms of myoclonus, and often combinations of several medications seem to be more effective.

8 TOURETTE'S SYNDROME

Inherited neuropsychiatric disorder characterized by multiple motor and vocal tics that change during the course of the illness. Onset is typically before age 18 yr (new-onset tics can occasionally occur after age 18 yr, but for DSM-IV criteria of TS, they must begin before this age). Tics are sudden, brief, intermittent involuntary or semi-voluntary movements (motor tics) or sounds (phonic or vocal tics) that mimic fragments of nl behavior.

Treatment
- Dopamine-blocking agents may be used to ↓ severity of tics acutely (e.g., haloperidol 0.25 mg PO qhs initially). There are risks of side effects, such as acute dystonic reactions.
- Clonidine: Many choose this as a first-line agent because of fewer long-term side effects. Start at 0.05 mg and slowly titrate to approximately 0.45 mg daily (needs tid/qid dosing). May also help with sx of ADHD.
- Greater improvement in symptom severity among children with Tourette's syndrome and chronic tic disorder has been reported with a comprehensive behavioral intervention compared with supportive Rx and education.
- Important components of Rx are appropriate evaluation and Rx of coexisting conditions (e.g., ADHD, OCD).
- DBS has shown some promising results as an alternative Rx in some pts with medically refractory disease.

9 WILSON'S DISEASE

Wilson's disease is a disorder of copper transport with inadequate biliary copper excretion, leading to an accumulation of the metal in liver, brain, kidneys, and corneas. The gene for Wilson's disease is located on chromosome 13.

Diagnosis
H&P
- Chronic liver disease/cirrhosis with hepatosplenomegaly, ascites, ↓ serum alb, prolonged prothrombin time, portal HTN
- Neurologic presentation
  - Movement disorder: tremors, ataxia
- Ocular: The Kayser-Fleischer ring is a gold-yellow ring seen at the periphery of the iris; these should be sought with slit-lamp examination by a skilled examiner.
- Stigmata of acute or chronic liver disease

Labs
- ↓ Serum ceruloplasmin level (<200 mg/L)
- ↓ Serum copper (<65 µg/L)
- 24-hr urinary copper excretion > 100 µg (nl <30 µg) to support dx; ↑ to > 1200 µg/24 hr after 500 mg of D-penicillamine (nl <500 µg/24 hr)
- Liver bx (to confirm bx): hepatic copper content (>250 µg/g of dry weight) (nl is 20-50 µg)

Treatment
- Penicillamine, trientine (chelator Rx)
- Zinc: inhibits intestinal copper absorption
- Liver transplantation for severe hepatic failure unresponsive to chelation
- Family screening of first-degree relatives necessary

10 RESTLESS LEGS SYNDROME (RLS)

Autosomal dominant disorder common among first-degree relatives that manifests as an awake phenomenon consisting of an urge to move legs, usually associated with feeling of discomfort in legs

Classification
- Primary RLS is without any obvious cause, with no associated disorder.
- Secondary RLS is associated with other medical conditions. The most common associations are pregnancy, iron deficiency anemia, ESRD, and PD.

Diagnosis
- Polysomnography to document periodic limb movements during sleep

Labs
- Iron status: serum ferritin, total iron binding capacity, percent saturation
- CBC for anemia, in case of iron deficiency
- Metabolic panel: BUN and serum Cr for renal insufficiency

Treatment
- Rx options for RLS
  - Dopamine agonists, pramipexole and ropinirole, are first-line agents.
  - Anticonvulsants: Gabapentin was shown to be effective in multiple studies.

F. DEMENTIA

Dementia is a syndrome characterized by progressive loss of previously acquired cognitive skills including memory, language, insight, and judgment. Alzheimer's disease is believed to account for the majority (50% to 75%) of all cases of dementia.

Diagnosis
- There is no definitive imaging or lab test for the dx of Alzheimer's disease and most forms of dementia; rather, dx depends on clinical history, a thorough physical and neurologic exam, and use of reliable and valid diagnostic criteria (i.e., DSM-V or NINDCS-ADRDA) such as the following:
  - Loss of memory and one or more additional cognitive abilities (aphasia, apraxia, agnosia, or other disturbance in executive functioning)
  - Impairment in social or occupational functioning that represents a decline from a previous level of functioning and results in significant disability
  - Deficits that do not occur exclusively during the course of delirium
  - Insidious onset and gradual progression of symptoms
  - Cognitive loss documented by neuropsychologic tests
  - No physical signs, neuroimaging, or laboratory evidence of other diseases that can cause dementia (i.e., metabolic abnlities, medication or toxin effects, infection, stroke, PD, subdural hematoma, or tumors)

H&P
- Spouse or other family member, usually not the pt, notes insidious memory impairment.
- Pts have difficulties learning and retaining new information and handling complex tasks (e.g., balancing the checkbook), and they have impairments in reasoning, judgment, spatial ability, and orientation (e.g., difficulty driving, getting lost away from home).
- Behavioral changes, such as mood changes and apathy, may accompany memory impairment. In later stages pts may develop agitation and psychosis.
- Atypical presentations include early and severe behavioral changes, focal findings on examination, parkinsonism, hallucinations, falls, or onset of symptoms younger than the age of 65.
- Pts with isolated memory loss who lack functional impairment at home or work do not meet criteria for dementia but may have mild cognitive impairment (MCI). Identifying pts with MCI is important because pts with MCI may have a slightly higher rate of progression to dementia.
- The diagnostic evaluation should include the following:
  - An attempt at the Folstein Mini-Mental State Examination to screen for dementia and to document the progression of disease over time by repeating the test at 3- to 6-mo intervals (Table 10-14)
  - One venipuncture for a profile of blood values: glucose, CBC, electrolytes, ALT, AST, BUN, Cr, VDRL, Ca, Mg, TSH, HIV (selected pts), B_{12} level, RBC folate
  - Depending on PE and hx findings, other tests may include brain MRI, PET scan, and LP.

TABLE 10-14 ■ The Mini-Mental State Examination (MMSE)	
Parameter	**Score**
Orientation: What is the month, day, date, year, season? Where are you? What floor, city, country, state? (Score 1 point for each item correct.)	10
Registration: State three items (ball, flag, tree). (Score 1 point for each item that the pt registers *without* your having to repeat the words. You may repeat the words until the pt is able to register the words, but do not give the pt credit. You must also tell the pt that he/she should memorize those words and that you will ask him/her to recall those words later.)	3
Attention: Can you spell the word WORLD forward, then backward? Can you subtract 7 from 100, and keep subtracting 7? (100-93-86-79-72) (Do both items but give credit for the best of the two performances.)	5
Memory: Can you remember those three words I asked you to memorize? (Do not give clues or multiple choice.)	3
Language:	
Naming: Can you name (show) a pen and a watch?	2
Repetition: Can you repeat "No ifs, ands, or buts"?	1
Comprehension: Can you take this piece of paper in your right hand, fold it in half, then put it on the floor? (Score 1 point for each item done correctly.)	3
Reading: Read and obey "Close your eyes."	1
Writing: Can you write a sentence?	1
Visuospatial: Have pt copy intersecting pentagons.	1
Total	30

Interpretation: Traditionally, with use of a cutoff score of 23 of 30, the sensitivity and specificity of the MMSE have been reported to be 87% and 82%, respectively, for detection of delirium or dementia in hospitalized pts. However, cognitive performance as measured by the MMSE varies within the population by age and education. To adjust for these variables, it has been proposed that a cutoff score of 19 is appropriate for pts with 0 to 4 years of education and will identify those individuals performing below the level of 75% of their peers; the cutoff score should be 23 for those with 5 to 8 years of education and 27 for those with 9 to 12 years of education. A score <29 would be abnl in 75% of individuals with a college education.
Modified from Folstein MR, Folstein SE, McHugh PR: "Mini-mental state": A practical method for grading the cognitive state of patients for the clinician. J Psychiatr Res 12:189, 1975.

- Of great importance is the identification of treatable causes of dementia:
  - Drug induced
  - Depression
  - Hypothyroidism
  - Hyperthyroidism
  - Hypoglycemia
  - Vitamin B_{12} or folate deficiency
  - Subdural hematoma
  - Liver failure
  - NPH
  - Stroke
  - CNS infections
  - Other infection
  - Cerebral neoplasm
  - Renal failure
  - Ethanol abuse
  - Hypoxia
  - Hypercalcemia
  - Vasculitis
  - Cardiopulmonary disorders
  - Severe anemia
- Table 10-15 describes distinguishing features of common progressive dementias.

Treatment

- Pursue the causes.
- Avoid restraints, but use them for safety if necessary.
- Control hyperactivity of delirium w/haloperidol. Administer 0.5 to 1 mg IM, IV, or PO initially and the observe pt for 20 to 30 min. If the pt remains unmanageable but has not had any adverse reactions to haloperidol, double the dose and continue monitoring. Lorazepam 1 mg IM qh may also be administered if needed, but it often has a paradoxical effect in elderly pts.
- Neuropsychiatric sx of dementia are common and associated w/poor outcomes for pts and caregivers. Nonpharmacologic interventions include counseling the

TABLE 10-15 ■ Distinguishing Features of Common Progressive Dementias				
Disease	Symptoms and Signs	Age Affected	Duration of Illness	Neurologic Signs
Alzheimer's disease	Amnestic memory loss early Getting lost Lack of awareness of one's illness Sleep-wake cycle disturbance Apathy	>65 yr	Years, up to a decade	Normal until advanced stage
Familial Alzheimer's disease	Same as Alzheimer's disease	From the 30s	Years	Normal until advanced stage
Frontotemporal dementia	Personality change Disinhibition Obsessions and compulsions "Alien stare" Amnestic memory loss later Visuospatial intact	45-65 yr	Years	Normal until advanced stage
Lewy body dementia	Early falls Visual hallucinations Neuroleptic sensitivity Fluctuating course	>50 yr	Months to years	Early extrapyramidal signs, with rigidity greater than tremor
Corticobasal ganglionic degeneration	Limb apraxia "Alien hand" Visual spatial deficits	>60 yr	Years	Apraxia Rigidity Myoclonus
Vascular dementia	Retrieval memory loss Depression Slowness Stepwise progression	>65 yr	Years	Focal neurologic deficits Rigidity and cogwheeling Gait abnlity
Normal-pressure hydrocephalus	Retrieval memory loss Urinary incontinence Progressive gait difficulty Slowness Visuospatial infarct	Any age	Months	Gait abnlity Hyperreflexia (legs > arms) Babinski's signs

From Goldman L, Ausiello D (eds): Cecil Textbook of Medicine, 22nd ed. Philadelphia, Saunders, 2004.

caregiver about the nonintentional nature of the psychotic features, behavior modification, maintenance of routines, and environmental safety. Effective medications for long-term use in pts w/behavioral problems associated w/dementia are risperidone and olanzapine.

■ Donepezil, rivastigmine, and galantamine are reversible acetylcholinesterase inhibitors approved for Rx of mild to moderate dementia of Alzheimer's type. They may be helpful in delaying the progression of Alzheimer's disease if used in the early stages. They can provide modest improvement of sx and temporary stabilization of cognition by lengthening the time from assisted community living to nursing home placement. Memantine is an N-methyl-D-aspartate (NMDA) receptor blocker indicated for the Rx of moderate to severe Alzheimer's disease. It can produce slight improvements in cognitive performance. The clinical significance of these improvements is small. Memantine can be used in combination w/anticholinesterase inhibitors.

G. MULTIPLE SCEROSIS (MS)

Chronic autoimmune demyelinating disease of the CNS characterized by clinical attacks (relapses) correlated w/lesions separated in time and space. A relapse is the subacute onset of neurologic dysfunction that lasts for ≥24 hr. Subtypes of MS include the following: *relapsing-remitting MS (RRMS)*, relapses followed by complete or nearly complete recovery; *secondary progressive MS (SPMS)*, progression of disability w/few or no relapses; and *primary progressive MS (PPMS)*, progression from onset. Rare MS variants include the following: *Balo's concentric sclerosis*, alternating rings of myelination and demyelination; *Marburg's disease*, tumor-like lesion w/significant edema; and *Schilder's diffuse sclerosis*, childhood onset w/one to two large, symmetric lesions. *Neuromyelitis optica* (Devic's disease) involves primarily the optic nerves and spinal cord and is considered a separate disease.

Table 10-16 summarizes the McDonald criteria for MS.

TABLE 10-16 ■ **Summary of Revised 2005-2010 McDonald Criteria for Diagnosis of MS**

Clinical Attacks	Clinical Lesions	Paraclinical Testing Needed
2	2	None
2	1	MRI dissemination in space *or* two lesions on MRI consistent with MS plus positive CSF
1	2	MRI dissemination in time
1	1	MRI dissemination in space *or* two MRI lesions consistent with MS and positive CSF *and* MRI dissemination in time

Evidence of clinical lesions by physical examination or evoked potentials.

Diagnosis of PPMS: 1 year evidence of disease progression and two of the following:

(1) evidence for dissemination in space, (2) evidence for dissemination in time, or (3) positive CSF

MRI dissemination in space, by either (1) one or more T2 lesion in two of the four typical areas for MS lesions (periventricular, juxtacortical, infratentorial, or spinal cord) or (2) awaiting further clinical attack implicating a distinctly separate CNS region. *MRI dissemination in time,* a new enhancing lesion ≥3 mo or a new nonenhancing lesion ≥6 mo after the initial attack; *positive CSF,* positive oligoclonal bands or elevated immunoglobulin G index ≥6.

Modified from Degenhardt A: Ferri's Clinical Advisor, 2013. St. Louis, Mosby, 2012, p. 700. Incorporates 2010 Revisions to Diagnostic criteria of MS (for details, please see original article: Polman CH, Reingold SC, Banwell B, et al: Diagnostic criteria for multiple sclerosis: 2010 revisions to McDonald's criteria. Ann Neurol 69:292-302, 2011).

Diagnosis

- MS: based on revised 2005 McDonald criteria (see Table 10-16)
- RRMS: at least two relapses—two clinical lesions distinctly separated in space and time or one clinical lesion plus paraclinical testing
- PPMS: insidious progression of disability with a positive CSF and either dissemination in both space and time or ongoing progression for ≥1 yr

H&P
- Visual abnlities
  - Paresis of medial rectus muscle on lateral conjugate gaze (internuclear ophthalmoplegia) and horizontal nystagmus of the adducting eye
  - Central scotoma, ↓ visual acuity (optic neuritis)
  - A *Marcus Gunn pupil* (pupil that paradoxically dilates w/direct light), indicating damage to the optic nerve anterior to the chiasm, is frequently present.
  - Nystagmus
- Abnlities of reflexes
  - ↑ DTRs
  - (+) Hoffmann's sign, (+) Babinski's reflex
  - ↓ Abd skin reflex, ↓ cremasteric reflex
- *Lhermitte's sign:* flexion of the neck while the pt is lying down elicits an electrical sensation extending bilaterally down the arms, back, and lower trunk.
- *Unthoff's phenomenon:* exercise- or heat-induced deterioration of function
- *Charcot's neurologic triad:* nystagmus, scanning speech, and intention tremor
- Impaired recognition of objects by touch alone (astereognosis)

Imaging
- MRI of brain w/gadolinium can identify lesions as small as 3 to 4 mm and is used to assess disease load, activity, and progression.
- MRI reveals multiple, predominantly periventricular plaques; however, normal MRI cannot be used to exclude MS.
- MRI of the cervical spine can also be helpful.

Labs
- LP for all first relapses when the dx of MS is not definite. Possible CSF abnlities include ↑ protein and mononuclear WBCs (both usually only mild). CSF IgG index and (+) oligoclonal bands are seen in 70% and 90%, respectively, of clinically definite MS cases. False(+) results occur w/IgG index in CNS infections and inflammation but rarely w/oligoclonal bands.
- Serum: CBC, ESR, CRP, CHEM 7, LFTs, ANA, vitamin B_{12}, Lyme titer, TSH
- Consider evoked potentials (VEP, SSEP, BAER): Demyelination will slow conduction velocities.

Treatment

Acute General Rx

- Relapses: high-dose IV methylprednisolone (3-5 days of 1 g/day; alternative dose is 15 mg/kg/day), often followed by a 7- to 10-day prednisone taper. No evidence suggests that high-dose corticosteroids alter the long-term course of disease.
- If pt has marked acute disability and acute corticosteroid therapy has failed, plasma exchange (5 to 7 exchanges on alternate days) have shown benefit.

Chronic Treatment

- Disease-modifying therapy: includes interferon-β1a, interferon-β1b, and glatiramer acetate. Interferons require routine CBC and LFT checks (initially in 1 mo, q3mo thereafter), occasionally TSH. None are needed with glatiramer acetate. Interferons can frequently cause flulike symptoms.
- Fingolimod, a sphingosine-1-phosphate receptor modulator, is approved as the first oral disease-modifying agent. Common side effects are liver toxicity, bradycardia with the first dose only, and pancytopenia. Its use may be reasonable in pts who cannot tolerate or do not benefit from alternative disease-modifying therapies and in those who have had one or more relapses or new white-matter lesions on MRI within the past year.
- Dalfampridine is a potassium channel blocker approved to improve walking speed in patients with MS.
- Cytotoxic: Methotrexate or azathioprine is occasionally used in RRMS or PPMS. Consider cyclophosphamide or mitoxantrone (causes dose-dependent cardiotoxicity) for frequent relapses with significant disability progression and for early secondary progressive MS. Emerging potential agents with long-term immunosuppressive effects include cladribine, alemtuzumab, daclizumab, laquinimod, and teriflunomide.
- Monoclonal antibodies: Natalizumab is approved for treatment of RRMS in the form of monthly infusions. It has been associated with an increased risk of developing progressive multifocal leukoencephalopathy (rare and fatal brain infection). Pts taking natalizumab must enter into a registry for monitoring.
- Spasticity: Onabotulinum toxin type A injection is FDA approved as first-line therapy for upper limb spasticity. Baclofen, tizanidine, dantrolene diazepam, lorazepam, and intrathecal baclofen are other alternatives.
- Pain: carbamazepine, gabapentin, or amitriptyline
- Spastic bladder: oxybutynin, tolterodine, or propantheline; prazosin for spastic sphincter
- Fatigue: Consider amantadine 100 mg bid, modafinil (most effective for somnolence), or fluoxetine.
- Tremor: clonazepam, carbamazepine, propranolol, or gabapentin. Wrist splints may be helpful.

H. DISORDERS OF THE SPINAL CORD

1 COMPRESSIVE MYOPATHIES

- Spinal cord compression is the neurologic loss of spine function. Lesions may be complete or incomplete and develop gradually or acutely. Incomplete lesions often are manifested as distinct syndromes, as follows:
  - Central cord syndrome
  - Anterior cord syndrome
  - Brown-Séquard syndrome
  - Conus medullaris syndrome
  - Cauda equina syndrome

Etiology

- Trauma
- Tumor
- Infection
- Inflammatory processes
- Degenerative disk conditions w/spinal stenosis
- Acute disk herniation
- Cystic abnlities

Diagnosis

H&P

- Clinical features reflect the amount of spinal cord involvement:
  - Motor loss and sensory abnlities

- (+) Babinski's reflex
- Clonus
- Gradual compression: manifested by progressive difficulty walking, clonus w/ weight bearing, and involuntary spasm; development of sensory sx; bladder dysfunction (late)
  - Central cord syndrome: variable quadriparesis, w/UEs more severely involved than the LEs; some sensory sparing
  - Anterior cord syndrome: motor, pain, and temperature loss below the lesion
  - Brown-Séquard syndrome
    - Caused by injury to either half of the spinal cord and resulting in the loss of motor function, position, vibration, and light touch on the affected side
    - Pain and temperature sense loss on the opposite side
  - Conus medullaris syndrome: variable motor loss in the LEs w/loss of bowel and bladder function
  - Cauda equina syndrome: typical low back pain, weakness in both LEs, saddle anesthesia, and loss of voluntary bladder and bowel control

Imaging
- MRI

Treatment
- Urgent surgical decompression

2 INFECTIOUS MYOPATHIES
- HIV infection
- Viral myositis
- Trichinosis
- Toxoplasmosis
- Cysticercosis
- Bacterial infections

3 INFLAMMATORY MYOPATHIES
- SLE, RA
- Sarcoidosis
- Paraneoplastic syndrome
- Polymyositis, dermatomyositis
- Polyarteritis nodosa
- MCTD
- Scleroderma
- Inclusion body myositis
- Sjögren's syndrome
- Cimetidine, D-penicillamine

4 ENDOCRINE-RELATED MYOPATHIES

Corticosteroid-Induced Myopathy
- Proximal limb weakness (mostly legs) in chronic corticosteroid pts

Demographics
- Women affected ×2 as men
- ↑ Risk use high-dose (≥30 mg/day) prednisone

Diagnosis
- Cushingoid body habitus
- Neurologic exam: intact ocular, facial, distal extremity strength; nl sensory exam and DTRs
- Labs: serum CK and EMG results nl (↑ CK or abnl EMG suggests recurrence of partly Rx myositis or another myopathy)
- Muscle biopsy: non-dx, only shows atrophy type IIb muscle fibers

Treatment
- Slow tapering of corticosteroid Rx with discontinuation

Thyrotoxic Myopathy
- Symmetric muscle weakness in pts with classic hyperthyroidism or hypothyroidism

Clinical and Presentation and Treatment
- If hyperthyroidism (muscle atrophy/fasciculations) VS hypothyroidism (muscle hypertrophy)
  - Serum CK level and EMG usually nl
  - Correct endocrine disorder to resolve myopathy

Toxic Myopathies
- Clinical presentation of proximal muscle weakness, myalgia, and cramps should prompt review of current medications (statins) as a recent ↑ dosage, switch, or addition can ↑ myopathy risk.
- Concomitant use of drugs that inhibit CYP3A4 (macrolides, cyclosporine, itraconazole, protease inhibitors) will ↑ risk myopathies in pts taking lovastatin, simvastatin, atorvastatin. In these pts, pravastatin, rosuvastatin, or fluvastatin (differently metabolized) may be preferable.

5 IDIOPATHIC TRANSVERSE MYELITIS
Demyelination in a transverse region of the spinal cord due to an inflammatory process leading to sensory and motor changes below the lesion

Etiology
- Demyelination due to the body's immune response to infection, post-vaccination, may be onset of multiple sclerosis (MS), or may be idiopathic (15%30% of cases).
  - About 50% of pts have had a recent URI.
  - EBV and CMV are most common viral infections.
  - Hepatitis B, varicella, enterovirus, rhinovirus, mycoplasma, syphilis, measles, Lyme disease are less common.

Diagnosis
- Transverse myelitis should be suspected in pts with a hx of rapid (hr to days) onset of motor weakness, sensory abnlities referable to the spinal cord, and bladder or bowel dysfunction. The dysfunction is bilateral (not necessarily symmetric) and there is a clearly defined sensory level.
- LP looking for oligoclonal bands for MS or infection
- MRI of brain and MRI of spine at level of suspected involvement

H&P
- The clinical signs are caused by an interruption in ascending and descending neuroanatomic pathways in the transverse plane of the spinal cord and a resulting sensory level is characteristic of transverse myelitis.
- Rapid onset of symmetric or asymmetric paraparesis or paraplegia of the lower extremities over a few days, ascending paresthesia, trunk sensory level, back pain, sphincter dysfunction, and (+) Babinski with upgoing toes bilaterally. The arms may also be involved but < the legs in most cases.
- One third to one half of pts present with localizing back pain.
- There is progression to nadir of clinical deficits between 4 hr and 21 days after symptom onset.

Labs
- CSF: ↑ protein/nl protein, lymphocytes, and nl glucose
- Serum NMO-IgG to w/up neuromyelitis optica, which should be ruled out.
- Oligoclonal bands should be absent in CSF in transverse myelitis and (+) in MS.
- Liver enzymes may help to differentiate if it is postinfectious transverse myelitis versus MS.
- Consider autoimmune w/up for lupus.

Treatment
- High-dose IV corticosteroid (e.g., methylprednisolone 1000 mg/day for 3-5 days)
- Rescue Rx with plasma exchange may be helpful in pts who do not respond to corticosteroids.
- Combination Rx with plasmapheresis and immunosuppressive agents (e.g., cyclophosphamide) may also be effective.
- Naproxen, ibuprofen for pain

I. PERIPHERAL NEUROPATHIES

1 GENERAL APPROACH
Figure 10-4 describes a systematic approach to evaluate neuropathy.

2 MONONEUROPATHIES

a Carpal Tunnel Syndrome
Compressive neuropathy of the median nerve as it passes under the transverse carpal ligament at the wrist. It is the most common entrapment neuropathy.

Diagnosis
- Pain, paresthesia in the first, second, and third fingers and the lateral half of the fourth finger, worse at night

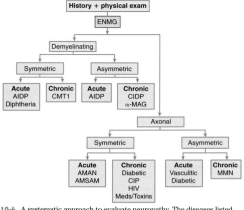

FIGURE 10-4. A systematic approach to evaluate neuropathy. The diseases listed are examples of neuropathies associated with specific neurophysiologic and clinical findings. Diabetic distal, predominantly sensory neuropathies are manifested as chronic axonal neuropathies; acute asymmetric neuropathies can also occur with diabetes. Most neuropathies caused by toxins or by side effects of medication are chronic, symmetric axonal neuropathies. Acute inflammatory demyelinating polyradiculoneuropathy (AIDP), acute motor axonal neuropathy (AMAN), and acute motor and sensory axonal neuropathy (AMSAN) are subtypes of Guillain-Barré syndrome. These and other examples are discussed in more detail in the text. *CIDP,* chronic inflammatory polyradiculoneuropathy; *CIP,* chronic illness polyneuropathy; *CMT1,* Charcot-Marie-Tooth disease type 1, a genetic disorder; *ENMG,* electroneuromyography; *HIV,* human immunodeficiency virus–related neuropathy; *α–MAG,* anti–myelin-associated glycoprotein; *MMN,* multifocal motor neuropathy. *(From Goldman L, Schafer AI [eds]: Goldman's Cecil Medicine, 24th ed. Philadelphia, Saunders, 2012.)*

- **Tinel's sign** at wrist: Tapping lightly over the median nerve on the volar surface of the wrist produces a tingling sensation radiating from the wrist to the hand.
- **Phalen's sign:** reproduction of sx after 1 min of gentle, unforced wrist flexion
- EMG: impaired sensory conduction across the carpal tunnel

Treatment
- Activity modification
- Nocturnal wrist splint
- Corticosteroid injection of carpal canal on ulnar side of palmaris longus tendon proximal to wrist crease
- Short-term benefit from U/S Rx
- Ergonomic keyboards (vs standard keyboards)
- Surgery in refractory cases

b Bell's Palsy

Acute peripheral facial (seventh) nerve palsy

Etiology
- HSV is thought to be the most common viral pathogen, followed by herpes zoster.

Diagnosis
- Onset is usually acute to subacute over hours of unilateral facial paralysis with maximal weakness at 3 wk. One third of pts demonstrate incomplete paralysis, whereas the remaining two thirds have complete paralysis. Recovery is present within the first 6 mo.

Treatment
- Glucocorticoid Rx: prednisone 60 to 80 mg/day for 1 wk
- Started at ≤72 hr shortens recovery time and ↑ % of pts with complete recovery. Use of valacyclovir not recommended (Rx efficacy did not differ from placebo). No added benefit was seen with combination Rx.

- 71% of pts: complete recovery
- Recurrence rate is 7%. Average time to recurrence is 10 yr.

3 POLYNEUROPATHIES

a Diabetic Neuropathy

Diagnosis
- EMG can be helpful in confirming the presence, extent, and severity of neuropathy.

H&P
- Distal symmetric polyneuropathy (DSPN)
  - Pts most commonly experience numbness and tingling but may also experience feelings of tightness or a sensation of heat or cold.
  - Pain is not uncommon, is often worst at night, and can be burning, aching, shooting, or lancinating.
  - These sx begin in the feet and may slowly ascend over months to years. Sx in the hands do not generally occur until sx in the lower extremities have reached the level of the knees. In more severe cases, the sx can spread to the trunk and head.
  - Neurologic examination reveals early loss of small-fiber modalities resulting in ↓ pinprick and temperature sensation with later involvement of large-fiber modalities leading to a reduction in vibratory and proprioceptive sensation. Ankle reflexes are usually ↓ or absent, and more proximal reflexes may also become involved as the neuropathy progresses. Strength is usually nl, but there can be some motor involvement leading to mild weakness and atrophy, which are usually limited to intrinsic foot muscles and ankle dorsiflexors.
- Autonomic neuropathy
  - GI sx are common and can include early satiety, bloating, vomiting, constipation, or diarrhea.
  - Cardiovascular complications include cardiac arrhythmias and postural hypotension.
  - Pts may also have sx related to dysfunction of the GU (erectile dysfunction and incontinence) or thermoregulatory (excessive or ↓ sweating, intolerance of cold or heat) systems.
- Regional diabetic polyneuropathy
  - The most common presentation is diabetic lumbosacral radiculoplexus neuropathy, which is also known as diabetic amyotrophy or *Bruns-Garland syndrome.* Pts usually report acute or subacute onset of severe pain involving the lower back, hip, and thigh.
  - Weakness and atrophy of the affected leg progress over the course of days to weeks, often predominantly in the anterior thigh.
- Focal diabetic neuropathy
  - Diabetic pts are at ↑ risk for common limb mononeuropathies, particularly median neuropathy at the wrist and ulnar neuropathy at the elbow, but other nerves (femoral, sciatic, or peroneal) can be involved as well.

Treatment
- Topical agents: Lidocaine 5% patch can be applied to painful areas for 12 hr a day.
- Anticonvulsants: gabapentin (100-1200 mg tid) and pregabalin (50-100 mg tid)
- Antidepressants: amitriptyline (10-100 mg qhs), nortriptyline (25-150 mg qhs), and duloxetine (60-120 mg daily)

b Charcot-Marie-Tooth Disease (CMT)

Heterogeneous group of noninflammatory inherited peripheral neuropathies characterized by chronic motor and sensory polyneuropathy. It is the most common inherited neuromuscular disorder. Transmission may be autosomal dominant, autosomal recessive, or X-linked, with some sporadic cases reported.

Diagnosis
- Symmetric, slowly progressive distal motor neuropathy resulting in weakness and atrophy in legs, often progresses to involve hands
- High-arched feet (pes cavus), claw toe deformities, and hammer toes
- Atrophy of the lower legs producing a storklike appearance (muscle wasting does not involve the upper legs)
- ↓ Proprioception and weakness of ankle dorsiflexors often interfere with balance and gait (steppage gait)

Treatment
- Symptomatic and supportive care is managed by a multidisciplinary team including physical and occupational Rx.

- Musculoskeletal pain may respond to acetaminophen or NSAIDs; neuropathic pain may respond to tricyclic antidepressants or drugs such as carbamazepine or gabapentin.
- Occasionally, orthopedic surgery is required to correct severe pes cavus deformity or hip dysplasia.

c Guillain-Barré Syndrome (GBS)

Acute inflammatory demyelinating polyradiculopathy predominantly affecting motor function. GBS is the most common cause of acute ascending flaccid paralysis.

Etiology

- Most pts give h/o respiratory (mycoplasma)/GI illness (*Campylobacter jejuni*) within 30 days of neurologic sx onset.

Diagnosis

History

- Rapid progression of acute symmetric progressive weakness, usually > distally than proximally and > in the legs than in the arms
- The pt often reports difficulty in ambulating, getting up from a chair, or climbing stairs.
- The ascending paralysis affects motor nerves more than sensory nerves. Sensory loss (predominantly position and vibration senses) is variable but usually mild.
- In some pts, the initial manifestations may involve the cranial musculature or the UEs (e.g., tingling of the hands).
- As a general rule, weakness reaches its max within 14 days.

Physical Exam

- Symmetric weakness, initially involving proximal muscles, subsequently both proximal and distal muscles
- ↓ Or absent reflexes bilaterally early in the disease
- Minimum to moderate glove and stocking anesthesia
- Ataxia and pain in a segmental distribution possible in some pts (caused by involvement of posterior nerve roots)
- Autonomic abnlities (bradycardia or tachycardia, hypotension or HTN) also possible
- Respiratory insufficiency (caused by weakness of intercostal muscles)
- Facial paresis, difficulty swallowing (secondary to cranial nerve involvement)

Labs

- LP: Typical findings include ↑ CSF protein (especially IgG) and presence of few mononuclear leukocytes (albuminocytologic dissociation).

EMG/NCS

- Slowed conduction velocities; motor, sensory, and F wave latencies. EMG may be nl in first 7 to 10 days.

Treatment

- Close monitoring of respiratory function (frequent [q1h initially] bedside measurements of FVC and (−) inspiratory force to assess pulmonary muscle strength) because respiratory failure is the major potential problem in GBS.
- Infusion of IVIG (0.4 g/kg/day for 5 days). Always check serum IgA levels before infusion to prevent anaphylaxis in deficient pts.
- Plasma exchange: 200 to 250 mL/kg during five sessions qod
- IVIG and plasma exchange are equally effective. The selection of one or the other is determined by availability and risk of particular complications. For example, plasma exchange should be avoided in pts w/prominent autonomic dysfunction.
- There is no proven benefit of combining IVIG and plasma exchange.
- Ventilatory support may be necessary in 10% to 20% of pts. Adequate fluid/electrolyte support and nutrition are necessary, especially in pts w/dysautonomia or bulbar dysfunction.
- Aggressive nursing care is required to prevent decubitus ulcers, infections, fecal impactions, and pressure nerve palsies and for mouth care to prevent ventilator-associated pneumonias.
- Monitor and treat autonomic dysfunction (bradyarrhythmias or tachyarrhythmias, orthostatic hypotension, systemic HTN, altered sweating).
- Treat back pain and dysesthesia w/low-dose tricyclic antidepressants, gabapentin, and the like. Opiate narcotics can be used cautiously in the short term but may compound dysautonomia.
- DVT prophylaxis

d Chronic Inflammatory Demyelinating Polyneuropathy (CIDP)

Symmetric proximal and distal weakness with associated sensory loss along with ↓ or absent reflexes for >2 mo

- NCS: features of demyelination including prolonged distal latencies and F-waves, slowed velocities, and at least one nerve demonstrating partial conduction block (feature of acquired demyelination)

H&P

- Characterized by occurrence of symmetric weakness in both proximal and distal muscles that progressively ↑ over 2 mo
- Associated with impaired sensation, postural instability, ↓ or absent DTRs, and variable craniofacial-bulbar involvement

Labs

- CSF analysis to assess for albumin-cytologic dissociation (i.e., ↑ protein with nl cell count), along with appropriate laboratory studies to exclude associated conditions

Treatment

- IVIG, plasmapheresis/plasma exchange, and corticosteroids. There is no difference in efficacy among these three modalities of Rx.
- Azathioprine, mycophenolate mofetil, cyclophosphamide, rituximab, and cyclosporine may be used as secondary agents.

J. AMYOTROPHIC LATERAL SCLEROSIS (ALS)

Progressive, degenerative neuromuscular condition of undetermined etiology affecting corticospinal tracts and anterior horn cells and resulting in dysfunction of both UMN and LMN, respectively

Etiology

- 90% to 95% sporadic
- Of the familial cases, 10% to 20% associated w/genetic defect in copper-zinc superoxide dismutase enzyme

Diagnosis

- EMG and NCS (El Escorial criteria)
- Assessment of respiratory function (forced vital capacity [FVC], [−] inspiratory force)

H&P

- LMN signs: weakness, hypotonia, wasting, fasciculations, hyporeflexia or areflexia
- UMN signs: loss of fine motor dexterity, spasticity, extensor plantar responses, hyperreflexia, clonus
- Preservation of extraocular movements, sensation, bowel and bladder function
- Dysarthria, dysphagia, pseudobulbar affect, frontal lobe dysfunction
- Respiratory insufficiency, typically late in the disease
- ALS comprises approximately 90% of adult-onset motor neuron diseases. Other presentations of motor neuron disease include progressive muscular atrophy, primary lateral sclerosis, progressive bulbar palsy, progressive pseudobulbar palsy, and ALS-parkinsonism-dementia complex.

Labs

- Vitamin B_{12}, thyroid function, parathyroid hormone, HIV may be considered.
- Serum protein and immunofixation electrophoresis
- DNA studies for SMA or bulbospinal atrophy, hexosaminidase levels in pure LMN syndrome
- 24-hour urine for heavy metals if indicated

Imaging

- MRI to r/o brain and spinal cord disorders
- Modified barium swallow to evaluate aspiration risk

Treatment

- PEG tube placement improves nutritional intake, promotes weight stabilization, and eases medication administration.
- Nutrition, speech Rx, physical and occupational Rx services are indicated.
- Suction device is used for sialorrhea.
- Communication may be eased with computerized assistive devices.
- Early discussion should cover living will, resuscitation orders, desire for PEG and tracheostomy, potential long-term care options.
- Encourage contact with local support groups.

- Riluzole, a glutamate antagonist, is the only FDA-approved medication known to extend tracheostomy-free survival in pts with ALS.
- Spasticity may be treated pharmacologically with baclofen, tizanidine, clonazepam.
- Pseudobulbar affect may improve with amitriptyline, sertraline, or dextromethorphan/quinine.

Disposition
- Mean duration of sx is 3 to 5 yr.
- Approximately 20% of pts survive >5 yr.

K. NEUROMUSCULAR JUNCTION DISORDERS

1 MYASTHENIA GRAVIS (MG)
Acquired autoimmune disorder of neuromuscular transmission characterized by the presence of a γ-globulin Ab (AChR-Ab) directed against postsynaptic acetylcholine receptor or against muscle-specific tyrosine kinase (MuSK) receptors

Diagnosis

H&P
- The hallmark of MG is weakness made worse w/exercise and improved by rest. Sx fluctuate and are often better in the morning.
- >50% of pts present initially w/ptosis, ocular muscle weakness, or both.
- Pts have difficulty in chewing, abnl smile, dysarthria, dysphagia.
- Involvement of the respiratory muscles may require intubation and assisted ventilation.
- Pain may occur in fatigued muscles (e.g., neck muscles).
- Clinical manifestations reproducible w/exercise. Observation of the pt performing repetitive muscle contractions of involved muscles will demonstrate rapidly developing weakness.
- PE may be nl at rest.
- Pts w/h/o ptosis will demonstrate fatigue weakness and ptosis when asked to sustain upward gaze for >3 min w/o interruption.

Labs and Other Tests
- Edrophonium test: improvement of sx after use of anticholinesterase medications (edrophonium)
- EMG: single-fiber electromyography: sensitivity >90 % but nonspecific
- MRI or CT of anterior mediastinum: thymoma found in 12%
- TSH: thyroid disease found in 30% of pts
- Vitamin B_{12} level: r/o pernicious anemia
- ANA, RF (association w/SLE, RA)
- (+) Ab against MuSK receptors

Treatment
- Acetylcholinesterase inhibitors: Pyridostigmine is first-line Rx.
- Immunosuppressants: corticosteroids, azathioprine, mycophenolate mofetil, rituximab for more severe or generalized disease
- Plasmapheresis and IVIG in refractory cases
- Thymectomy in thymomatous MG

2 LAMBERT-EATON MYASTHENIC SYNDROME
Disorder of neuromuscular transmission caused by Ab against presynaptic voltage-gated P/Q Ca channels on motor and autonomic nerve terminals. The two forms are paraneoplastic (most common, small cell lung cancer 50-70%) and nonparaneoplastic (autoimmune).

Diagnosis

H&P
- Weakness w/↓ or absent muscle stretch reflexes
- Proximal LE muscles affected most
- Transient strength improvement w/brief exercise
- Autonomic dysfunction common (dry mouth in 75%, sexual dysfunction, blurred vision, constipation, orthostasis)

EMG/NCS
- ↓ Motor amplitudes w/nl sensory studies
- Labs: ↑ titers of P/Q-type calcium channel Ab

Treatment

- Acute: plasma exchange (200-250 mL/kg over 10-14 days) or IVIG (2 g/kg over 2-5 days)
- Chronic Rx: anticholinesterase agents (pyridostigmine)

L. HEAD INJURY

1 EPIDURAL HEMATOMA

Collection of blood between the skull and dura mater (Fig. 10-5)

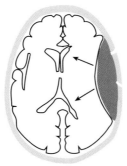

FIGURE 10-5. Epidural hematoma. The *arrows* show the pattern of brain displacement. *(From Weissleder R, Wittenberg J, Harisinghani M, Chen JW [eds]: Primer of Diagnostic Imaging, 5th ed. St. Louis, Mosby, 2011.)*

Etiology

- Head trauma causing temporal bone fracture resulting in middle meningeal artery tear
- Neoplasms that have spread into the epidural space

Diagnosis

H&P

- Lucid interval after the head trauma is followed by progressive reduction in the level of consciousness as the hematoma enlarges and the underlying brain is displaced inward.
- The initial injury causes brain concussion and loss of consciousness from which the pt awakens and may have some headache but seems otherwise to have recovered.
- Downward transtentorial herniation may develop rapidly, causing third nerve compression and an ipsilateral hemiparesis.

Imaging

- Brain CT

Treatment

- Emergency surgical evacuation

2 SUBDURAL HEMATOMA

Bleeding into the subdural space, caused by rupture of bridging veins between the brain and venous sinuses (especially where stretched by underlying cerebral atrophy). Figure 10-6 illustrates subdural hematoma and compares it with epidural hematoma.

Diagnosis

H&P

- Vague headache, often worse in morning than evening
- Some apathy, confusion, and clouding of consciousness is common, although frank coma may complicate late cases. Chronic subdural hematomas may cause a dementia picture.
- Neurologic sx may be transient, simulating TIA.
- Almost any sign of cortical dysfunction may occur, including hemiparesis, sensory deficits, and language abnlities, depending on which part of the cortex is compressed by the hematoma.
- New-onset seizures should raise the index of suspicion.

	Epidural hematoma	Subdural hematoma
Incidence	In <5% of TBIs	In 10%–20% of TBIs
Cause	Fracture	Tear of cortical veins
Location	Between skull and dura	Between dura and arachnoid
Shape	Biconvex	Crescentic
CT	70% hyperintense, 30% isointense	Variable depending on age
TIW MRI	Isointense	

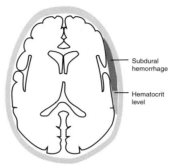

FIGURE 10-6. Subdural hematoma and comparison with epidural hematoma. *(From Weissleder R, Wittenberg J, Harisinghani M, Chen JW [eds]: Primer of Diagnostic Imaging, 5th ed. St. Louis, Mosby, 2011.)*

Labs
- Hct, Plt count, PTT, and PT/INR

Imaging
- CT of brain

Treatment
- Small subdural hematomas may be left untreated and the pt observed; but if there is an underlying cause, such as anticoagulation, this should be rapidly corrected to prevent further accumulation of blood.
- Neurosurgical drainage of blood from subdural space through burr hole is the definitive procedure, although it is common for the hematoma to reaccumulate.

3 CONCUSSION
- Complex pathophysiologic process affecting the brain. When traumatic biomechanical rotational/angular acceleration forces are applied to the brain, they cause shear strain of underlying neural elements. Although not required, it may be associated with direct trauma.
- Concussions typically result in rapid onset of a short-lived neurologic functional deficit that spontaneously resolves. Chronic injury may result in long-term neuropathologic changes.
- Concussion results in a graded set of clinical syndromes that may or may not involve loss of consciousness. Table 10-17 describes commonly used grading scales for concussion. Resolution of the clinical sx typically follows a sequential course. It is typically associated with grossly nl structural neuroimaging.

Diagnosis

Workup
- Sideline assessment
  - Neurologic assessment uses a standardized tool, such as SCAT2 (Sport Concussion Assessment Tool) or SAC (Standardized Assessment of Concussion).
  - Monitor for deterioration; no athlete should be left alone.
- Neurocognitive testing
  - Computer-based programs, such as ImPACT, ANAM, CogSport
  - Neuropsychiatric testing administered by a neuropsychologist
- Gait/balance testing with a tool such as the Balance Error Scoring System (BESS)

	Grade of Concussion		
TABLE 10-17 ■ Grading Scales for Concussion			
Scale	I	II	III
Colorado	Confusion; no LOC; PTA <30 min	LOC <5 min; confusion; PTA >30 min	LOC >5 min; PTA >24 h
Cantu	PTA <30 min; no LOC	LOC <5 min; PTA 30 min to 24 h	LOC >5 min; PTA >24 h
AAN	Transient confusion; symptoms <15 min; no LOC	No LOC; transient confusion; symptoms >15 min	Any LOC

AAN, American Academy of Neurology; *LOC*, loss of consciousness; *PTA*, posttraumatic amnesia.

Modified from Vincent JL, Abraham E, Moore FA, et al (eds): Textbook of Critical Care, 6th ed. Philadelphia, Saunders, 2011.

- When used in combination, symptom assessment, balance assessment, and neurocognitive testing provide a sensitivity of >90% for the identification of concussion.

Imaging
- Head CT or MRI for grade II or III concussion with persistent abnlities on exam or symptoms lasting >1 wk

Treatment
- Immediate removal of athlete from game/athletic activity
- Physical rest: no return to play until asymptomatic for atleast 24 hours
- Cognitive rest to limit sx
  - Modifications at school
  - Modifications at home/recreation
  - Sleep encouraged

11 Pulmonary and Critical Care

A. CHEST X-RAY

1 EVALUATING THE CHEST X-RAY

- Figure 11-1 illustrates the location of various pulmonary and cardiac structures seen on a CXR (PA view). The following is a short guide to reading a CXR.
  1. Check exposure technique for lightness or darkness.
  2. Verify left and right by looking at the heart shape and stomach bubble, respectively.
  3. Check for rotation. Does the thoracic spine shadow align in the center of the sternum between the clavicles?
  4. Make sure the CXR is taken in full inspiration (10 posterior or 6 anterior ribs should be visible).
  5. Is the film a portable, AP, or PA film? (The heart size cannot be accurately judged from an AP film.)
  6. Check the soft tissues for foreign bodies or SC emphysema.
  7. Check all visible bones and joints for osteoporosis, old fxs, metastatic lesions, rib notching, or presence of cervical ribs.
  8. Look at the diaphragm for tenting, free air, and position.
  9. Check hilar and mediastinal areas for the following: size and shape of the aorta, presence of hilar nodes, prominence of hilar blood vessels, elevation of vessels (left slightly higher), and elevation of the left main stem bronchus indicating left atrial enlargement.
  10. Look at the heart for size, shape, calcified valves, and enlarged atria.
  11. Check the costophrenic angles for fluid or pleural scarring.
  12. Check the pulmonary parenchyma for infiltrates, ↑ interstitial markings, masses, absence of nl margins, air bronchograms, or ↑ vascularity and "silhouette" signs.
  13. Look at the lateral film for the following: confirmation and position of questionable masses or infiltrates, size of retrosternal air space, AP chest diameter, vertebral bodies for bony lesions or overlying infiltrates, and posterior costophrenic angle for small effusion.

2 CALCIFICATIONS ON CHEST X-RAY

- Lung neoplasm (primary or metastatic)
- Silicosis
- Idiopathic pulmonary fibrosis (IPF)
- Tuberculosis
- Histoplasmosis
- Disseminated varicella infection
- Mitral stenosis (end-stage)
- Secondary hyperparathyroidism

3 CARDIAC ENLARGEMENT

Cardiac Chamber Enlargement
- Chronic volume overload
- Mitral or aortic regurgitation
- Left-to-right shunt (PDA, VSD, AV fistula)
- Cardiomyopathy
- Ischemic
- Nonischemic
- Decompensated pressure overload
- AS
- HTN
- High-output states
- Severe anemia
- Thyrotoxicosis
- Bradycardia
- Severe sinus bradycardia
- Complete heart block

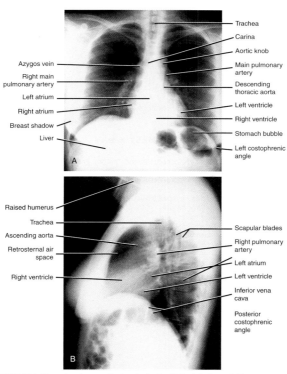

FIGURE 11-1. Normal anatomy on the female chest radiograph in the upright posteroanterior projection (**A**) and in the lateral projection (**B**). *(From Mettler FA: Primary Care Radiology. Philadelphia, Saunders, 2000.)*

Left Atrium
- LV failure of any cause
- Mitral valve disease
- Myxoma

Right Ventricle
- Chronic LV failure of any cause
- Chronic volume overload
- Tricuspid or pulmonic regurgitation
- Left-to-right shunt (ASD)
- Decompensated pressure overload
- Pulmonic stenosis
- Pulmonary HTN
- Primary
- Secondary (PE, COPD)
- Pulmonary veno-occlusive disease

Right Atrium
- RV failure of any cause
- Tricuspid valve disease
- Myxoma
- Ebstein's anomaly

Multichamber Enlargement
- Hypertrophic cardiomyopathy
- Acromegaly
- Severe obesity

Pericardial Disease
- Pericardial effusion w/ or w/o tamponade
- Effusive constrictive disease
- Pericardial cyst, loculated effusion

Pseudocardiomegaly
- Epicardial fat
- Chest wall deformity (pectus excavatum, straight back syndrome)
- Low lung volumes
- AP CXR

4 CAVITARY LESION ON CHEST X-RAY

Necrotizing Infections
- Bacteria: anaerobes, *Staphylococcus aureus*, enteric gram(–) bacteria, *Pseudomonas aeruginosa*, *Legionella* species, *Haemophilus influenzae*, *Streptococcus pyogenes*, *Streptococcus pneumoniae*, *Rhodococcus*, *Actinomyces*
- Mycobacteria: *Mycobacterium tuberculosis*, *Mycobacterium kansasii*, *Mycobacterium avium-intracellulare*
- Bacteria-like: *Nocardia* species
- Fungi: *Coccidioides immitis*, *Histoplasma capsulatum*, *Blastomyces hominis*, *Aspergillus* species, *Mucor* species
- Parasitic: *Entamoeba histolytica*, *Echinococcus*, *Paragonimus westermani*

Cavitary Infarction
- Bland infarction (w/ or w/o superimposed infection)
- Lung contusion

Septic Embolism
- *Staphylococcus aureus*
- Anaerobes
- Others

Vasculitis
- Wegener's granulomatosis
- Periarteritis

Neoplasms
- Bronchogenic carcinoma
- Metastatic carcinoma
- Lymphoma

Miscellaneous Lesions
- Cysts, blebs, bullae, or pneumatocele w/ or w/o fluid collections
- Sequestration
- Empyema w/air-fluid level
- Bronchiectasis

5 MEDIASTINAL MASSES OR WIDENING ON CHEST X-RAY

- Lymphoma: Hodgkin's disease and non-Hodgkin's lymphoma
- Sarcoidosis
- Vascular: aortic aneurysm, ectasia or tortuosity of aorta or bronchocephalic vessels
- Carcinoma: lungs, esophagus
- Esophageal diverticula
- Hiatal hernia
- Achalasia
- Prominent pulmonary outflow tract: pulmonary HTN, PE, right-to-left shunts
- Trauma: mediastinal hemorrhage
- Pneumomediastinum
- Lymphadenopathy caused by silicosis and other pneumoconioses
- Leukemias
- Infections: TB, viral (rare), mycoplasmal (rare), fungal, tularemia
- Substernal thyroid

- Thymoma
- Teratoma
- Bronchogenic cyst
- Pericardial cyst
- Neurofibroma, neurosarcoma, ganglioneuroma

B. USE AND INTERPRETATION OF PULMONARY FUNCTION TESTS

- Basic spirometry: Figure 11-2
- PFTs in common lung diseases: Table 11-1
- Flow volume curves: Figure 11-3

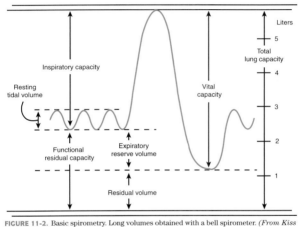

FIGURE 11-2. Basic spirometry. Long volumes obtained with a bell spirometer. *(From Kiss GT: Diagnosis and Management of Pulmonary Disease in Primary Practice. Menlo Park, Calif, Addison-Wesley, 1982.)*

TABLE 11-1 ■ Pulmonary Function Test Patterns in Common Lung Diseases

Disorder	FVC	FEV$_1$	FEV$_1$/FVC	RV	TLC	Diffusion (D$_{LCO}$)	Bronchodilator Response
Asthma	↓	↓	↓	NI, ↑	NI, ↑	NI	+
Chronic obstructive bronchitis	↓	↓	↓	NI, ↑	NI, ↑	NI	−
Chronic obstructive bronchitis w/ broncho-spasm	↓	↓	↓	NI, ↑	NI, ↑	NI	+
Emphysema	↓	↓	↓	NI, ↑	NI, ↑	NI, ↓	−
Interstitial fibrosis	↓	NI, ↓	NI, ↑	NI, ↓	↓	↓	−
Obesity, kyphosis	↓	NI, ↓	NI, ↑	NI, ↑	↓	NI	−

↑, greater than predicted; ↓, less than predicted.

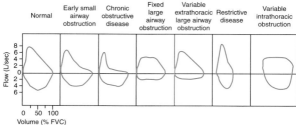

FIGURE 11-3. Flow-volume curves of restrictive disease and various types of obstructive diseases compared with normal curves.

C. PULMONARY FORMULAS

- Lung volumes: Box 11-1
- Alveolar-arterial O_2 gradient (A-a gradient): Box 11-2
- Evaluation of pt in respiratory failure: Box 11-3

Box 11-1 • Lung Volumes: Normal Volumes in Upright Subjects

Volume or Capacity	Approximate Value in Upright Subjects
Total lung capacity (TLC)	6 L
Vital capacity (VC)	4.5 L
Residual volume (RV)	1.5 L
Inspiratory capacity (IC)	3 L
Functional residual capacity (FRC)	3 L
Inspiratory reserve volume (IRV)	2.5 L
Expiratory reserve volume (ERV)	1.5 L
Tidal volume (VT)	0.5 L

The VC is calculated as:

$$VC = IRV + ERV + VT$$

The RV is calculated as the difference between the FRC and the ERV:

$$RV = FRC - ERV$$

Alternatively, if the TLC and VC are known, the following formula can be used:

$$RV = TLC - VC$$

Box 11-2 • Alveolar-Arterial Oxygen Gradient (A-a Gradient)

$$A - a\ gradient = \left[713\ (FIO_2) - \left(\frac{PaCO_2}{0.8} \right) \right] - PaO_2$$

Normal A-a gradient = 5-15 mm
FIO_2, fraction of inspired oxygen (normal = 0.21-1.0)
$PaCO_2$, arterial carbon dioxide tension (normal = 35-45 mm Hg)
PaO_2, arterial partial pressure of oxygen (normal = 70-100 mm Hg)
Ddx of A-a gradient:

Abnormality	15% O_2	100% O_2
Diffusion defect	Increased gradient	Correction of gradient
V/Q mismatch	Increased gradient	Partial or complete correction of gradient
Right-to-left shunt (intra-cardiac or pulmonary)	Increased gradient	Increased gradient (no correction)

Age-predicted Pao_2 = Expected Pao_2 − 0.3(age − 25) [expected Pao_2 at sea level is 100 mg/Hg]
As a rough rule of thumb: Expected Pao_2 ≈ Fio_2 (%) × 5
$AaDO_2$ = (Fio_2 × [BP^* − 47]) − (Pao_2 + $Paco_2$), where BP = barometric pressure
Pao_2/Fio_2 ratio

Oxygenation index = [(mean airway pressure × FIO_2)/Pao_2] × 100

V_D/V_T = ($Paco_2$ − $PEco_2$) /$Paco_2$ (N = 0.2 − 0.4)

From Vincent JL, Abraham E, Moore FA, et al (eds): Textbook of Critical Care, 6th ed. Philadelphia, Saunders, 2011.

$AaDO_2$, Alveolar-arterial gradient; V_D, dead space.

D. MECHANICAL VENTILATION

INDICATIONS (Please see section "M" for Respiratory Failure Classification)
1. Clinical assessment: presence of apnea, tachypnea (>40 bpm), or respiratory failure that cannot be adequately corrected by any other means
2. Clinical instability, failure to protect the airway—usually from declining mental status
3. ABGs: severe hypoxemia despite high-flow O_2 or significant CO_2 retention (e.g., Po_2 <50, Pco_2 >50)
4. Physiologic parameters are of limited use because many pts w/respiratory insufficiency are unable to perform PFTs, and their respiratory failure mandates immediate intervention. Some of the commonly accepted physiologic parameters for intubation and respiratory support are as follows:
   a. VC <10 mL/kg
   b. Inspiratory force ≤25 cm H_2O
   c. FEV_1 <10 mL/kg
   d. V_T <5 mL/kg BW
   e. $\dot{V}_E$ >10 L/min
   f. Ratio of RR (breaths/min) to V_T (L) >105
   Note: The clinical assessment is the most important determinant of the need for mechanical ventilation because neither physiologic parameters nor ABGs distinguish between acute and chronic respiratory insufficiency (e.g., a Pco_2 >60 mm Hg and an RR >30/min may be the "norm" for a pt w/COPD, whereas the same values in a young, otherwise healthy adult are indications for intubation and mechanical ventilation).

ICU SEDATION
Commonly used agents are GABA agonists such as propofol and benzos. These agents can cause respiratory depression and delirium. The α-adrenoreceptor agonist dexmedetomidine is as effective for sedation but significantly better in pts at risk for delirium.

COMMON MODES OF MECHANICAL VENTILATION
Invasive mechanical ventilation is defined as ventilatory support supplied through endotracheal intubation. The use of devices that apply intermittent (−) extrathoracic pressure or furnish intermittent positive pressure through a tight-fitting nasal or face mask w/o an artificial airway in place is known as *noninvasive ventilation*. The delivery of gas under positive pressure into the airways and the lungs is known as *positive-pressure ventilation* (Table 11-2).
1. **IMV:** The pt is allowed to breathe spontaneously, and the ventilator delivers a number of machine breaths at a preset rate and volume.
   a. Advantages and indications
      i. IMV is indicated in the majority of spontaneously breathing pts because it maintains respiratory muscle tone and results in less depression of cardiac output than with ACV.
      ii. It is useful for weaning because as the IMV rate is ↓, the pt gradually assumes the bulk of the breathing work.
   b. Disadvantages
      i. The ↑ work of breathing results in ↑ O_2 consumption (deleterious to pts w/ myocardial insufficiency).
      ii. IMV is not useful in pts w/depressed respiratory drive or impaired neurologic status.

TABLE 11-2 ■ Modes of Positive-Pressure Ventilation

Mode	Description	Advantages and Disadvantages
Controlled mechanical ventilation (CMV)	Ventilator f, inspiratory time, and V_T (and thus $\dot{V}_E$) preset	Can be used in patients w/sedation or paralysis; ventilator cannot respond to ventilatory needs
Assisted mechanical ventilation (AMV) or assist-control ventilation (ACV)	Ventilator V_T and inspiratory time preset, but patient can f (and thus $\dot{V}_E$)	Ventilator may respond to ventilatory needs; ventilator may undertrigger or overtrigger, depending on sensitivity
Intermittent mandatory ventilation (IMV)	Ventilator delivers preset V_T, f, and inspiratory time, but patient also can breathe spontaneously	May ↓ asynchronous breathing and sedation requirements; ventilator cannot respond to ventilatory needs
Synchronized intermittent mandatory ventilation (SIMV)	Same as IMV, but ventilator breaths delivered only after patient finishes inspiration	Same as IMV, and patient not over-inflated by receiving spontaneous and ventilator breaths at same time
High-frequency ventilation (HFV)	Ventilator f is and V_T may be smaller than V_D	May reduce peak airway pressure; may cause auto-PEEP
Pressure support ventilation (PSV)	Patient breathes at own f; V_T determined by inspiratory pressure and C_{RS}	↑ comfort and ↓ work of breathing; ventilator cannot respond to ventilatory needs
Pressure control ventilation (PCV)	Ventilator peak pressure, f, and respiratory time preset	Peak inspiratory pressures may be ↓; hypoventilation may occur
Inverse ratio ventilation (IRV)	Inspiratory time exceeds expiratory time to facilitate inspiration	May improve gas exchange by ↑ time spent on inspiration; may cause auto-PEEP
Airway pressure release ventilation (APRV)	Patient receives CPAP at high and low levels to simulate V_T	May improve oxygenation at lower airway pressure; hypoventilation may occur
Proportional assist ventilation (PAV)	Patient determines own f, pressures, and flows	May amplify spontaneous breathing; depends entirely on patient's respiratory drive

Modified from Goldman L, Schafer AI (eds): Goldman's Cecil Medicine, 22nd ed. Philadelphia, Saunders, 2004.
C_{RS}, Respiratory system compliance; f, respiratory rate; V_D, dead space.

    iii. It was previously assumed that the degree of respiratory muscle rest was proportional to the level of machine assistance. However, more recent evidence indicates that respiratory-sensor output does not adjust to breath-to-breath changes in respiratory load, and IMV may therefore contribute to the development of respiratory muscle fatigue or prevent recovery from it.

2. **ACV:** The pt breathes at his or her own rate, and the ventilator senses the inspiratory effort and delivers a preset V_T w/each pt effort; if the pt's RR ↓ past a preset rate, the ventilator delivers tidal breaths at the preset rate.

    a. Advantages and indications: ACV is useful in pts w/neuromuscular weakness or CNS disturbances.

    b. Disadvantages

      i. Tachypnea may result in significant hypocapnia and respiratory alkalosis.

      ii. Improper setting of sensitivity to the (−) pressure necessary to trigger the ventilator may result in "fighting the ventilator" when the sensitivity is set too low.

      iii. ↑ Sensitivity may result in hyperventilation; sensitivity is generally set so that an inspiratory effort of 2 to 3 cm will trigger ventilation.

      iv. The respiratory muscle tone is not well maintained in pts on ACV, and this may result in difficulty w/weaning.

3. **CMV:** The pt does not breathe spontaneously; the RR is determined by the physician; the ventilator assumes all respiratory work by delivering a preset volume of gas at a preset rate.

    a. Advantages and indications

      i. CMV is useful in pts who are unable to make an inspiratory effort (e.g., severe CNS dysfunction) and in pts w/excessive agitation or breathing effort.

      ii. Pts w/excessive agitation are often sedated w/morphine or benzos and paralyzed w/pancuronium bromide; adequate sedation is necessary to eliminate awareness of paralysis.

      iii. Initial pancuronium dose is 0.08 mg/kg IV in adults.

      iv. Later incremental doses starting at 0.01 mg/kg may be used as necessary to maintain paralysis; pancuronium should be administered only by or under the supervision of experienced clinicians; a combination of neostigmine and atropine may be used to reverse the action of the pancuronium.

b. Disadvantages: Paralyzed pts on CMV must be closely monitored because ventilator malfunction or disconnection is rapidly fatal.

4. **SIMV:** A hybrid of ACV and IMV, the ventilator delivers a number of specified breaths/min (as w/IMV). However, at the appropriate interval (e.g., q6sec if machine rate is 10 breaths/min), the machine waits for an ETT pressure deflection to signal pt effort and then delivers a positive-pressure breath; ventilator breaths are thus synchronized w/pt respiratory efforts, as w/assist features of ACV.

5. Other useful ventilation modes are as follows:

a. **Pressure control ventilation (PCV):** A ventilatory mode in which inspiratory pressure, RR, and inspiratory time (T_I) are determined by the ventilator settings. Because inspiratory pressure is the controlled variable, V_T during PCV is influenced by the mechanical properties of the respiratory system (resistance and compliance).

b. **Pressure support ventilation (PSV):** A ventilatory mode in which the pt's inspiratory effort is supported by a set level of inspiratory pressure. This pressure is maintained until respiratory flow falls below a threshold value, signaling the onset of expiration. V_T during PSV is determined by pt effort and the mechanical properties of the lung. PSV differs from PCV in that the RR and the T_I are determined by the pt.

c. **Inverse ratio ventilation (IRV):** A ventilatory strategy in which the inspiratory-to-expiratory ratio is prolonged to 1:1 or greater. In pts w/ARDS, IRV is used to improve oxygenation by increasing mean airway pressure. This modality is used as a salvage Rx when adequate oxygenation cannot be achieved w/ conventional ventilation in ARDS. When used, pressure cycled IRV is preferred because of ↓ barotrauma risk.

d. **Noninvasive positive-pressure ventilation (NPPV), Continuos positive airway pressure (CPAP), Bi-level positive airway pressure (BiPAP):** In NPPV, ventilatory support is delivered by use of a mechanical ventilator connected to a mouthpiece or mask instead of an ETT. It is very useful in pts w/chronic respiratory failure caused by neuromuscular disease or thoracic deformities and in pts w/idiopathic hypoventilation. It improves the pt's well-being and may eliminate the need for tracheostomies. It is also used in pts as a short-term bridge to avoid intubation and mechanical ventilation, when possible, in conditions that are rapidly reversible, such as hypercarbic respiratory failure in COPD and, importantly, acute pulmonary edema in heart failure. It is also sometimes used as salvage Rx in pts w/any of the indications for intubation who do not want to be intubated. **CPAP** is applied with an oxygen source connected to either a tight-fitting nasal or full-face mask or via nasal prones. It delivers high concentration of oxygen and maintains (+) airway pressure in the spontaneously breathing patient. It offers the benefit of maintaining alveolar expansion and decreases work of breathing. **BiPAP,** like CPAP can be provided by mask, but it requires a ventilator to assist with flow delivery. The patients inspiratory effort triggers the BiPAP machine to deliver decelerating flow in order to reach a preset pressure, defined as inspiratory positive airway pressure. When a pt's own inspiratory flow falls below a preset amount, ventilatory assistance ceases and maintains airway pressure at a predetermined value (usually 5-10 mmHg).

SELECTION OF VENTILATOR SETTINGS

1. V_T is 10 to 15 mL/kg of ideal BW. Low volume ventilation = 6-8 ml/kg w/ARDS
2. Rate (number of tidal breaths delivered per minute) is 8 to 16, depending on the desired $Paco_2$ or pH (↑ rate = ↓ $Paco_2$).
3. Mode is IMV, ACV, CMV (or PCV or PSV, depending on what is available at one's institution).
4. O_2 concentration (Fio_2): The initial Fio_2 should be 100% unless it is evident that a lower Fio_2 will provide adequate oxygenation. The Fio_2 should be calibrated down as quickly as possible to prevent O_2 toxicity.
5. Obtain ABGs 15 to 30 minutes after initiation of mechanical ventilation.
6. Immediate CXR is indicated after intubation to evaluate for correct placement of ETT.
7. Sedation orders (e.g., morphine, diazepam) are necessary in most pts.
8. PEEP:

a. The application of PEEP may prevent the closure of edematous small airways; it is indicated when arterial oxygenation is inadequate (saturation <90%) despite an Fio_2 >50%; it is useful in pts w/diffuse lung edema and

TABLE 11-3 ■ Effects of Ventilator Setting Changes

Ventilator Setting Changes	Typical Effects on Blood Gases	
	Paco$_2$	Pao$_2$
↑ PIP	↓	↑
↑ PEEP	↑	↑
↑ Rate (IMV)	↓	Minimal ↑
↑ I/E ratio	No change	↑
↑ Fio$_2$	No change	↑
↑ Flow	Minimal ↓	Minimal ↑
↑ Power (in HFOV)	↓	No change
↑ $\overline{PAW}$ (in HFOV)	Minimal ↓	↑

From Tschudy MM, Arcara KM: The Harriet Lane Handbook, 19th ed. Philadelphia, Mosby, 2012.

HFOV, High-frequency oscillatory ventilation; *I/E,* inspiratory/expiratory ratio; $\overline{PAW}$, mean airway pressure; *PIP,* peak inspiratory pressure.

TABLE 11-4 ■ Common Ventilator Machine Settings for Various Disorders

Condition	Mode	Vt, V̇E	PEEP (cm H$_2$O)	Pressure Targets	Fio$_2$
Depressed CNS drive	Mandatory ACV, SIMV	Vt = 10 mL/kg V̇E = 6-8 L/min	0-5	Peak usually <35 cm H$_2$O	Minimum for Sao$_2$ >90%
Neuromuscular insufficiency	Acute: mandatory ACV, SIMV	Vt = 8-10 mL/kg V̇E = 6-8 L/min	0-5	Peak usually <35 cm H$_2$O	As above
	Mild, recovering: SIMV and PSV, PSV alone	Guarantee VT >350 mL w/PSV breaths	0-5		
COPD	Early: ACV, SIMV Late: see text	Vt = 8 mL/kg V̇E: minimize, usually 8-10 L/min Peak flow ≥60 L/min	0*	Plateau <30 cm H$_2$O; monitor for intrinsic PEEP (auto-PEEP)	As above

*PEEP added to obstructive disease only in special circumstances.

From Noble J (ed): Textbook of Primary Care Medicine, 2nd ed. St. Louis, Mosby, 1996.

refractory hypoxemia caused by intrapulmonary shunting (e.g., ARDS). It is also useful to ↓ the needed Fio$_2$ to ↓ O$_2$ toxicity. In reality, ≥5 mm PEEP is used on virtually everyone, but it can be ↓ if oxygenation is not a problem but intubation-associated hypotension is.

  b. PEEP is generally started at 5 cm H$_2$O and by increments of 2 to 5 cm to maintain the Pao$_2$ at 60 mm Hg or greater.

  c. The use of PEEP can result in pulmonary barotrauma and hemodynamic compromise (secondary to ↓ right ventricular filling).

  d. Pts receiving PEEP should have their cardiac output frequently monitored; the measurement of mixed venous O$_2$ sat is useful to evaluate the effect of PEEP on cardiac output. The surrogate of cardiac output (BP) is fine in most pts.

9. Adjust the initial ventilator setting according to results of the ABGs and clinical response.

  a. Use the lowest Fio$_2$ necessary to maintain a Pao$_2$ >60 mm Hg (90% Hgb saturation in pts w/nl pH).

  b. Adjust V̇E (VT time rate) to nlize the pH and the Paco$_2$.

    i. The VT or the rate will ↓ Paco$_2$ and ↑ pH.

    ii. Do not lower the Paco$_2$ below the "norm" for that pt (e.g., some pts w/ COPD should be allowed to maintain their usual mildly ↑ Paco$_2$ to avoid alkalosis and to provide stimulus for breathing).

348 10. Effects of ventilator setting changes are described in Table 11-3. Common ventilator machine settings for various disorders are described in Table 11-4 and Box 11-4.

Box 11-4 • Steps and Guidelines for Initiating Mechanical Ventilation*

1. Ventilatory mode
Unintubated patients:
- NIV for patients with COPD and acute hypercapnic respiratory failure if alert, cooperative, and hemodynamically stable
- NIV not routinely recommended for acute hypoxemic respiratory failure

Intubated patients:
- Assist/control with volume-limited ventilation as initial mode
- Consider specific indications for PCV or HFOV (see text) in acute lung injury
- SIMV: consider if some respiratory effort, dyssynchrony
- PSV: consider if patient's effort good, ventilatory needs moderate to low, and patient more comfortable during PSV trial

2. Oxygenation
- If infiltrates on chest radiograph, then
- Fio_2: begin with 0.8-1.0, reduce according to Spo_2
- PEEP: begin with 5 cm H_2O, increase according to Pao_2 or Spo_2, Fio_2 requirements, and hemodynamic effects; consider PEEP/Fio_2 "ladder"; goal of Spo_2 >90%, Fio_2 ≤0.6
- No infiltrates on chest radiograph (COPD, asthma, PTE), Fio_2: start at 0.4 and adjust according to Spo_2 (consider starting higher if PE is strongly suspected)

3. Ventilation
- V_T: begin with 8 mL/kg PBW; decrease to 6 mL/kg PBW over a few hours if acute lung injury present
- Rate: begin with 10-20 breaths/min (10-15 if not acidotic; 15-20 if acidotic); adjust for pH; goal pH >7.3 with maximal rate of 35; may accept lower goal if V_E high

4. Secondary modifications
- Triggering: in spontaneous modes, adjustment of sensitivity levels to minimize effort
- Inspiratory flow rate of 40-80 L/min; higher if tachypneic with respiratory distress or if auto-PEEP present, lower if high pressure in ventilator circuit leads to a high-pressure alarm
- Assessment of auto-PEEP, especially in patients with increased airways obstruction (e.g., asthma, COPD)
- I/E ratio: 1:2, either set or as function of flow rate; higher (1:3 or more) if auto-PEEP present
- Flow pattern: decelerating ramp reduces peak pressure

5. Monitoring
- Clinical: blood pressure, ECG, observation of ventilatory pattern including assessment of dyssynchrony, effort or work by the patient; assessment of airflow throughout expiratory cycle
- Ventilator: V_T, V_E, airway pressures (including auto-PEEP), total compliance
- ABGs, pulse oximetry

Modified from Goldman L, Schafer AI (eds): Goldman's Cecil Medicine, 24th ed. Philadelphia, Saunders, 2012.
Decisions within this algorithm will be influenced by the specific conditions of the individual patient. HFOV, high-frequency oscillatory ventilation; I/E ratio, inspiratory-to-expiratory ratio; NIV, noninvasive ventilation; PBW, predicted body weight; PTE, pulmonary thromboembolism.

MAJOR COMPLICATIONS

1. Pulmonary barotrauma (e.g., pneumomediastinum, pneumothorax, SC emphysema, pneumoperitoneum) is generally secondary to high levels of PEEP, excessive V_T, high peak airway pressures, and coexistence of significant lung disease.
2. Pulmonary thromboemboli can be prevented by vigorous leg care, antiembolic stockings, and use of prophylactic LMWH.
3. GI bleeding: Prophylaxis w/IV ranitidine 50 mg q8h, PPIs, or sucralfate suspension, 1 g q6h through NG tube, is indicated in most pts on mechanical ventilators.
4. Arrhythmias: Avoid the use of arrhythmogenic drugs and prevent rapid acid-base shifts.
5. Accumulation of large amount of secretions: Frequent respiratory toilet is necessary in all pts on mechanical ventilators. Consider mouth care with chlorhexidine.
6. Others include nosocomial infections, laryngotracheal injury, malnutrition, hypophosphatemia, O_2 toxicity, and psychosis. Risk factors for pneumonia are severe illness, old age (>60 years), prior administration of abx, and supine head position. Respiratory ICU pts who are managed in the semirecumbent (30- to 45-degree head-up) position have a lower incidence of nosocomial pneumonia. Use of sucralfate rather than H_2 antagonists is also associated w/lower incidence

of nosocomial pneumonia. Extubation as rapidly as possible is important to help prevent ventilator-associated pneumonia.

WITHDRAWAL OF MECHANICAL VENTILATORY SUPPORT

Common Criteria for Ventilator Weaning

1. Improved clinical status (the pt is alert and hemodynamically stable); the process that required mechanical ventilation is reversed.
2. Adequate oxygenation (Pao_2 >60 mm Hg w/inspired O_2 concentration of 40%)
3. pH 7.33 to 7.48 w/acceptable $Paco_2$
4. RR ≤25 breaths/min
5. VC ≥10 mL/kg
6. Resting $\dot{V}_E$ <10 L/min, w/ability to double the resting $\dot{V}_E$
7. Peak pressure more (−) than −25 cm H_2O
8. V_T >5 mL/kg
9. The ratio of respiratory frequency to V_T during 1 minute of spontaneous breathing, also known as the ***rapid shallow breathing index (f/Vt)***, is a good predictor of a pt's readiness for weaning; a value of <100 breaths/min/L indicates that weaning probably will be successful, especially if it is confirmed by serial measurements.

Note: The preceding criteria are only guidelines; significant variation may be present (e.g., an RR of 30 breaths/min may be acceptable in a pt w/COPD). Failure to meet these criteria does *not* mean that the pt will not be weaned successfully. Figure 11-4 is an algorithm for discontinuing ventilation and for extubation.

APPROACH TO DISCONTINUING VENTILATION/EXTUBATION

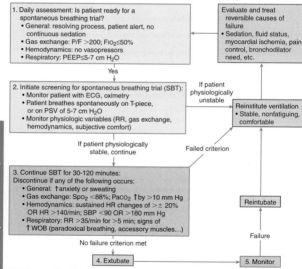

FIGURE 11-4. Algorithm for assessing whether a patient is ready to be liberated from mechanical ventilation and extubated. *P/F,* Pao_2/Fio_2 ratio; *WOB,* work of breathing. *(From Goldman L, Schafer AI [eds]: Goldman's Cecil Medicine, 24th ed. Philadelphia, Saunders, 2012.)*

Methods of Weaning

1. Weaning by IMV
   a. Gradually ↓ the IMV as tolerated (e.g., two breaths q3-4h), monitoring ABGs PRN. Monitoring of clinical signs (RR, pt's comfort, and V_T) is usually sufficient to avoid repeated ABGs.

    b. Do not change more than one parameter at a time.

    c. When the pt is tolerating an IMV of 4 to 6, a trial w/T tube can be attempted. The T tube is attached to the ETT and delivers humidified O_2 (FIO_2 40%).

    d. If the pt tolerates the T tube well, extubation may be attempted.

       i. Have adequate equipment and personnel available if reintubation is necessary (start early in the day).

       ii. Suction airway and oropharynx.

       iii. Deflate cuff and extubate.

       iv. Administer O_2 by face mask (FIO_2 40%-100%).

       v. Auscultate the lungs for adequate air movement.

       vi. Closely monitor VS.

       vii. Obtain ABGs approximately 15 to 30 minutes after extubation.

    e. Reintubate if extubation is poorly tolerated.

2. Stable pts w/o pulmonary disease and w/good probability of quick extubation (e.g., after uncomplicated cardiac surgery) may be given a direct trial of T tube (bypassing gradual ↓ of IMV).

3. PSV

    a. Titrate pressure to achieve a frequency of ≤25 breaths/min; allow a CPAP of ≤cm H_2O.

    b. Set pressure support initially at 18.0 ± 6.1 cm H_2O, and attempt to reduce this level of support by 2 to 4 cm H_2O at least bid.

    c. Extubate pts who tolerate a pressure support setting of 5 cm H_2O for 2 hr w/ no apparent ill effects.

4. Intermittent trials of spontaneous breathing

    a. Disconnect the stable pt from the ventilator and allow the pt to breathe spontaneously through either a T-tube circuit or a continuous-flow circuit designed to provide a CPAP of ≤5 cm H_2O.

    b. Attempt the trial at least bid and gradually ↑ the duration of the trial.

    c. Provide ACV for ≥1 hour between the trials.

    d. Extubate pts who are able to breathe on their own for ≥2 hr w/o signs of distress.

5. Once-daily trial of spontaneous breathing

    a. Disconnect the stable pt from the ventilator and allow him or her to breathe spontaneously through a T-tube circuit for ≤2 hr each day.

    b. Extubate pts who tolerate a 2-hour trial w/o signs of distress.

    c. Reinstitute ACV for 24 hr if signs of intolerance develop.

Failure to Wean from Mechanical Ventilator

Failure usually results from premature attempts at weaning (e.g., pt is hemodynamically unstable). Other common, reversible causes of failure to wean are as follows:

1. Hypophosphatemia, hypomagnesemia, hypokalemia
2. Drug toxicity (e.g., excessive CNS depression from analgesics, sedatives). Continuous infusions of sedative drugs may prolong the duration of mechanical ventilation. Daily interruption of sedative infusions until the pt is awake ↓ the duration of mechanical ventilation.
3. Bronchospasm
4. Excessive secretions
5. Significant acid-base disturbances (e.g., metabolic alkalosis depresses respiratory drive)
6. Hypothyroidism
7. Malnutrition
8. Small-bore ETT (tube >8 mm is preferred)
9. Interference w/chest wall (e.g., chest tube, restraints)

VENTILATOR-ASSOCIATED PNEUMONIA

1. Ventilator-associated pneumonia occurs in 9% to 24% of pts intubated >48 hr.
2. The etiology of ventilator-associated pneumonia varies w/the following factors:

    a. Onset <5 days after hospital admission or intubation

    b. Presence of risk factors (previous recent abx Rx, corticosteroid use, structural lung disease, and immunosuppression)

3. Pts w/pneumonia diagnosed <5 days after hospital admission or intubation and w/no risk factors can be empirically treated w/one of the following abx:

    a. Second- or third-generation cephalosporin

    b. β-Lactam w/ or w/o β-lactamase inhibitors

    c. Quinolones

4. Pts w/risk factors or those diagnosed 5 days or more after hospital admission or intubation can be empirically treated w/two abx from the following classes:
    a. Antipseudomonal lactam agents (e.g., imipenem, meropenem, cefepime, ceftazidime, piperacillin-tazobactam)
    b. Quinolones with w/reliable antipseudomonal activity
    c. Aminoglycoside
5. Consider addition of vancomycin in institutions w/MRSA.
6. Recommended duration of Rx is 7 days, longer if *Pseudomonas* infection is diagnosed.

E. ACUTE RESPIRATORY DISTRESS SYNDROME (ARDS)

This form of noncardiogenic pulmonary edema results from acute damage to the alveoli. The definition of ARDS includes the following components: a ratio of Pao_2 to the Fio_2 ≤200, regardless of the level of PEEP; the detection of bilateral pulmonary infiltrates on the frontal CXR; PAWP ≤18 mm Hg or no clinical evidence of diminished LV function.

Etiology
- Sepsis (>40%)
- Aspiration: near-drowning, aspiration of gastric contents (>30%)
- Trauma (>20%)
- Multiple transfusions, blood products
- Drugs (OD of morphine, methadone, heroin; reaction to nitrofurantoin)
- Noxious inhalation (chlorine gas, high O_2 concentration)
- Post resuscitation
- Cardiopulmonary bypass
- Pneumonia
- TB
- Burns
- Pancreatitis

Diagnosis

Labs
- ABGs: initially, varying degrees of hypoxemia, generally resistant to supplemental O_2; subsequently, respiratory alkalosis, ↓ Pco_2, and widened alveolar-arterial gradient. Hypercapnia occurs as the disease progresses.
- Hemodynamic monitoring (when indicated): Although no hemodynamic profile is *diagnostic* of ARDS, the presence of pulmonary edema, CO, and ↓ PAWP is characteristic of ARDS.

Imaging
- CXR: Bilateral interstitial infiltrates are usually seen within 24 hr; they are often more prominent in the bases and periphery. Near-total "whiteout" of both lung fields can be seen in advanced stages.

Treatment
- Identification and Rx of the precipitating condition
    - Blood and urine cultures and trial of abx in presumed sepsis (routine administration of abx in all cases of ARDS is not recommended)
    - Stabilization of bone fx in pts w/major trauma
    - Bowel rest and crystalloid resuscitation in pancreatitis
- Ventilatory support: A ventilator strategy for pts with ARDS is described in Figure 11-5.
- Fluid management: Optimal fluid management is pt specific. Swan-Ganz catheterization may be indicated and is useful to guide fluid replacement. A PCWP of approximately 12 mm Hg is ideal.
- DVT prophylaxis
- Stress ulcer prophylaxis w/sucralfate suspension (by NG tube) or IV PPIs or IV H_2 blockers
- An algorithm for the initial management of ARDS is described in Figure 11-6.

F. ASTHMA

DEFINITION

The National Asthma Education and Prevention Program (NAEPP) guidelines define asthma as "a chronic inflammatory disease of the airways in which many cells

VENTILATORY STRATEGY FOR PATIENTS WITH ARDS*

Goal 1: Low Vt/Pplat	Goal 2: Adequate Oxygenation	Goal 3: Arterial pH
Initiation: Calculate PBW —Male: 50 + 2.3 (height [inches]−60) —Female: 45.5 + 2.3 (height [inches]−60) Initiate volume assist control —Start with 8 mL/kg, and ↓ to 6 mL/kg over a few hours	*Specific goal:* Pao₂ 55-80 mm Hg or Spo₂ 88-95% Use only Fio₂/PEEP combinations shown below to achieve this target • if oxygenation is low, choose Fio₂/PEEP combination (from Fio₂/PEEP table) below • if oxygenation is high, choose Fio₂/PEEP combination to the left	*Goal:* pH: 7.30-7.45 Acidosis algorithm If pH 7.15−7.30 • ↑set rate until pH >7.30 or Paco₂ <25 mm Hg (max RR = 35) • if RR = 35 & pH <7.30 NaHCO₃ may be given If pH <7.15 • ↑set RR to 35 • if set RR = 35 & pH <7.15, Vt may be ↑in 1 mL/kg steps until pH >7.15 (Pplat target may be exceeded) Alkalosis algorithm If pH >7.45 • ↓set RR until patient RR > set RR (minimum set RR = 6/min)

Keep Pplat (based on 0.5-sec pause) <35 cm H₂O
If Pplat >30 cm H₂O, ↓Vt by 1 mL/kg to 5 or 4 mL/kg
If Pplat <25 AND Vt <6 mL/kg, ↑Vt by 1 mL/kg until Pplat > 25 cm H₂O OR Vt = 6 mL/kg
If patient severely distressed and/or breath stacking, consider ↑Vt to 7 or 8 mL/kg, as long as Pplat≤30 cm H₂O †

Fio₂/PEEP Table

Fio₂	0.3	0.4	0.4	0.5	0.5	0.6	0.7	0.7	0.7	0.8	0.9	0.9	0.9	1.0
PEEP	5	5	8	8	10	10	10	12	14	14	14	16	18	20–24

*Based on ARDS Network Algorithm

† If compliance of the chest wall is markedly decreased (e.g., massive ascites), it may not be reasonable or necessary (if the patient is very hypoxemic) to allow a Pplat >30 cm H₂O.

FIGURE 11-5. Ventilatory strategy for patients with ARDS. Several caveats should be considered when using the low Vt strategy: (1) Vt is based on predicted body weight (PBW), not actual body weight; PBW tends to be about 20% lower than actual BW; (2) the protocol mandates decreases in the Vt lower than 6 mL/kg of PBW if the plateau pressure (Pplat) is greater than 30 cm H₂O and allows for small increases in Vt if the patient is severely distressed and/or if there is breath stacking, as long as Pplat remains at 30 cm H₂O or lower; (3) because arterial CO₂ levels will rise, pH will fall; acidosis is treated with increasingly aggressive strategies dependent on the arterial pH; (4) the protocol has no specific provisions for the patient with a stiff chest wall, which in this context refers to the rib cage and abdomen; in such patients, it seems reasonable to allow Pplat to increase to more than 30 cm H₂O, even though it is not mandated by the protocol; in such cases, the limit on Pplat may be modified based on analysis of abdominal pressure, which can be estimated by measuring bladder pressure. *(From Goldman L, Schafer AI [eds]: Goldman's Cecil Medicine, 24th ed. Philadelphia, Saunders, 2012.)*

and cellular elements play a role: in particular mast cells, neutrophils, eosinophils, T lymphocytes, macrophages, and epithelial cells. In susceptible individuals, this inflammation causes recurrent episodes of coughing (particularly at night or early in the morning), wheezing, breathlessness, and chest tightness. The episodes are usually associated w/widespread but variable airflow obstruction that is reversible either spontaneously or as a result of Rx." Exposure to relevant allergens precedes symptoms. Other triggers include viral VRIs, cold air, stress, and exercise.

Status asthmaticus can be defined as a severe continuous bronchospasm.

Diagnosis

■ For symptomatic adults and children aged >5 yr who can perform spirometry, asthma can be dx after H&P documenting an episodic pattern of respiratory sx and from spirometry that indicates partially reversible airflow obstruction (>12% and 200 mL in 1 FEV₁ after inhaling a short bronchodilator or receiving a short [2-3 wk] course of PO corticosteroids).

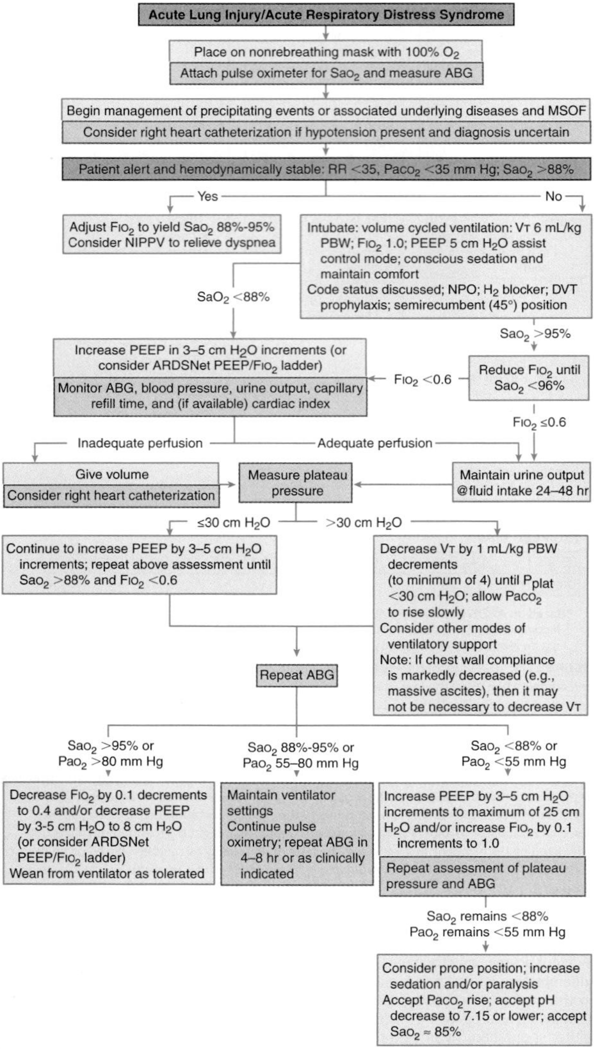

FIGURE 11-6. Algorithm for the initial management of ARDS. *MSOF,* Multisystem organ failure; *NIPPV,* noninvasive intermittent positive-pressure ventilation; *PBW,* predicted body weight. (From Goldman L, Schafer AI [eds]: Goldman's Cecil Medicine, 24th ed. Philadelphia, Saunders, 2012.)

Test	Predicted Value (%)	Severity of Asthma
PEFR	>80	
FEV₁	>80	No spirometric abnormalities
MMEFR	>80	
PEFR	>80	
FEV₁	>70	Mild asthma
MMEFR	55-75	
PEFR	>60	
FEV₁	45-70	Moderate asthma
MMEFR	30-50	
PEFR	<50	
FEV₁	<50	Severe asthma
MMEFR	10-30	

From Goldman L, Schafer AI (eds): Goldman's Cecil Medicine, 24th ed. Philadelphia, Saunders, 2012. In Ferri F: Ferri's Clinical Advisor: 5 Books in 1. 2013 edition. Philadelphia, Mosby, 2012.

- The degree of reversibility measured by spirometry correlates w/airway obstruction. Table 11-5 describes the relative severity of an asthmatic attack as indicated by PEFR, FEV₁, and MMEFR.
- Physical exam findings vary w/the stage and severity of asthma and may reveal only inspiratory and expiratory phases of respiration. Exam during **status asthmaticus** may reveal
  • Tachycardia and tachypnea
  • Use of accessory respiratory muscles
  • **Pulsus paradoxus** (inspiratory decline in systolic BP >10 mm Hg)
- PFT's show obstructive pattern
- Normal spirometry and high suspicion for asthma → bronchial challenge testing.
- Wheezing: Absence of wheezing (silent chest) or ↓ wheezing can indicate worsening obstruction.
- ΔMS is generally secondary to hypoxia and hypercapnia and constitutes an indication for urgent intubation.
- Paradoxical abd and diaphragmatic movement on inspiration (detected by palpation over the upper part of the abd in a semirecumbent position) is an important sign of impending respiratory crisis and indicates diaphragmatic fatigue.
- The following abnlities in VS are indicative of severe asthma exacerbation:
  • Pulsus paradoxus >18 mm Hg
  • RR >30 breaths/min
  • Tachycardia w/HR >120 bpm

Labs
- ABGs can be used in staging the severity of an asthmatic attack:
  • Mild: ↓ Pao₂ and Paco₂, ↑ pH
  • Moderate: ↓ Pao₂, nl Paco₂, nl pH
  • Severe: marked ↓ Pao₂, Paco₂, and ↓ pH
- Peak flow <40% or 40%-69% of patients personal best warrants increased frequency of scheduled and PRN SABA Rx as well as systemic steroids (quick taper preferred)

Imaging
- CXR is usually nl but may show evidence of thoracic hyperinflation (e.g., flattening of the diaphragm, volume over the retrosternal air space).
- ECG: Tachycardia and nonspecific ST-T wave changes are common during an asthmatic attack; may also show cor pulmonale, RBBB, RAD, and counterclockwise rotation.

Treatment
- Table 11-6 describes the classification of asthma severity and therapeutic considerations. A stepwise approach for managing asthma in youths >12 yr and adults is described in Figure 11-7.
- The differentiation of asthma from COPD can be challenging. An hx of atopy and intermittent, reactive sx points toward a dx of asthma, whereas smoking and advanced age are more indicative of COPD. Spirometry is useful to distinguish asthma from COPD. Table 11-7 summarizes differentiating features of asthma and COPD.

III

DISEASES AND DISORDERS
11. Pulmonary and Critical Care

TABLE 11-6 ■ Classifying Asthma Severity and Initiating Treatment in Youths ≥12 Yr and Adults*

		Classification of Asthma Severity (≥12 yr)			
			Persistent		
Components of Severity		Intermittent	Mild	Moderate	Severe
Impairment Normal FEV_1/FVC: 8-19 yr, 85%; 20-39 yr, 80%; 40-59 yr, 75%; 60-80 yr, 70%	Symptoms	≤2 days/wk	>2 days/wk but not daily	Daily	Throughout the day
	Night time awakenings	≤2×/mo	3-4×/mo	>1×/wk but not nightly	Often 7×/wk
	Short-acting β_2-agonist use for symptom control (not prevention of EIB)	≤2 days/wk	>2 days/wk but not daily, and not more than 1× on any day	Daily	Several times per day
	Interference with normal activity	None	Minor limitation	Some limitation	Extremely limited
	Lung function	Normal FEV_1 between exacerbations			
		FEV_1 >80% predicted	FEV_1 >80% predicted	FEV_1 >60% but <80% predicted	FEV_1 <60% predicted
		FEV_1/FVC normal	FEV_1/FVC normal	FEV_1/FVC reduced 5%	FEV_1/FVC reduced >5%
Risk	Exacerbations requiring oral systemic corticosteroids	0-1/yr	≥2/yr →		
		← Consider severity and interval since last exacerbation. Frequency and severity may fluctuate → over time for patients in any severity category. Relative annual risk of exacerbations may be related to FEV_1.			
Recommended Step for Initiating Therapy		Step 1	Step 2	Step 3	Step 4 or 5
				Also, consider short course of oral systemic corticosteroids.	
			In 2-6 wk, evaluate level of asthma control that is achieved and adjust therapy accordingly.		

*Assessing severity and initiating treatment for patients who are not currently taking long-term control medications. The stepwise approach is meant to assist, not replace, the clinical decision making required to meet individual patient needs.

Level of severity is determined by assessment of both impairment and risk. Assess impairment domain by patient's/caregiver's recall of previous 2-4 wk and spirometry. Assign severity to the most severe category in which any feature occurs.

At present, data are inadequate to correlate frequencies of exacerbation with different levels of asthma severity. In general, more frequent and intense exacerbations (e.g., requiring urgent, unscheduled care, hospitalization, or ICU admission) indicate greater underlying disease severity. For treatment purposes, patients who had ≥2 exacerbations requiring oral systemic corticosteroids in the past year may be considered the same as patients who have persistent asthma, even in the absence of impairment levels consistent with persistent asthma.

To access the complete *Expert Panel Report 3: Guidelines for the Diagnosis and Management of Asthma,* go to www.nhlbi.nih.gov/guidelines/asthma/asthgdln.pdf.

EIB, Exercise-induced bronchospasm

From National Asthma Education and Prevention Program: Expert Panel Report 3: Guidelines for Diagnosis and Management of Asthma. NIH publication 08-4051. Bethesda, Md, National Institutes of Health, 2007.

G. CHRONIC OBSTRUCTIVE PULMONARY DISEASE (COPD)

DEFINITION

COPD is an inflammatory respiratory disease caused by exposure to tobacco smoke. It is characterized by the presence of airflow limitation that is not fully reversible. Traditionally, COPD was described as encompassing *emphysema,* characterized by loss of lung elasticity and destruction of lung parenchyma w/enlargement of air spaces,

Stepwise Approach for Managing Asthma in Youths ≥12 Yr and Adults

Intermittent Asthma	Persistent Asthma: Daily Medication
	Consult with asthma specialist if step 4 care or higher is required.
	Consider consultation at step 3.

Step 6
Preferred:
High-dose ICS + LABA + oral corticosteroid

AND

Consider omalizumab for patients who have allergies

Step 5
Preferred:
High-dose ICS + LABA

AND

Consider omalizumab for patients who have allergies

Step 4
Preferred:
Medium-dose ICS + LABA

Alternative:
Medium-dose ICS + either LTRA, theophylline, or zileuton

Step 3
Preferred:
Low-dose ICS + LABA
OR
Medium-dose ICS

Alternative:
Low-dose ICS + either LTRA, theophylline, or zileuton

Step 2
Preferred:
Low-dose ICS

Alternative:
Cromolyn, LTRA, nedocromil, or theophylline

Step 1
Preferred:
SABA PRN

Step up if needed
(first, check adherence, environmental control, and comorbid conditions)

Assess control

Step down if possible
(and asthma is well controlled at least 3 months)

Each step: Patient education, environmental control, and management of comorbidities
Steps 2–4: Consider subcutaneous allergen immunotherapy for patients who have allergic asthma

Quick-Relief Medication for All Patients
• SABA as needed for symptoms. Intensity of treatment depends on severity of symptoms: up to 3 treatments at 20-minute intervals as needed. Short course of oral systemic corticosteroids may be needed.
• Use of SABA >2 days a week for symptom relief (not prevention of EIB) generally indicates inadequate control and the need to step up treatment.

FIGURE 11-7. Stepwise approach for managing asthma in youth ≥12 yr old and in adults. *EIB,* Exercise-induced bronchospasm; *ICS,* inhaled corticosteroid; *LABA,* inhaled long-acting β₂-agonist; *LTRA,* leukotriene receptor antagonist; *SAEA,* inhaled short-acting β₂-agonist. *(From National Asthma Education and Prevention Program: Expert Panel Report 3: Guidelines for Diagnosis and Management of Asthma. NIH publication 08-4051. Bethesda, Md, National Institutes of Health, 2007.)*

TABLE 11-7 ■ Differentiating Features of COPD and Asthma

	COPD	Asthma
Smoker or ex-smoker	Most	Possibly
Symptoms <35 yr of age	Rare	Common
Atopic features (rhinitis, eczema)	Uncommon	Common
Cellular infiltrate	Macrophages, neutrophils, CD8+ T cells	Eosinophils, CD4+ T cells
Cough and sputum	Daily/common	Intermittent
Breathlessness	Persistent and progressive	Variable
Night time symptoms	Uncommon	Common
Significant diurnal or day-to-day variability of symptoms	Uncommon	Common
Bronchodilator response (FEV₁ and PEFR)	<15%	>20%
Corticosteroid response	Poor	Good

From Ballinger A: Kumar & Clark's Essentials of Clinical Medicine, 5th ed. Edinburgh, Saunders, 2012.

TABLE 11-8 ■ Classification of COPD Severity (GOLD Criteria)		
Stage	Function	Symptoms
Stage I: mild	FEV_1/FVC <70% FEV_1 ≥80% predicted	Chronic cough, none/mild breathlessness
Stage II: moderate	FEV_1/FVC <70% 50% ≤ FEV_1 <80% predicted	Breathlessness on exertion
Stage III: severe	FEV_1/FVC <70% 30% ≤ FEV_1 <50% predicted	Breathless on minimal exertion; possible weight loss and depression
Stage IV: very severe	FEV_1/FVC <70% FEV_1 <30% predicted or FEV_1 <50% predicted plus respiratory failure	Breathless at rest

Modified from Global Strategy for the Diagnosis, Management and Prevention of COPD. Available at: www.goldcopd.com

and *chronic bronchitis,* characterized by obstruction of small airways and productive cough >3 mo in duration for >2 successive years. These terms are no longer included in the formal definition of COPD, although they are still used clinically.

Etiology
- Tobacco exposure
- Occupational exposure to pulmonary toxins (e.g., dust, noxious gases, vapors, fumes, cadmium, coal, silica). The industries w/the highest exposure risk are plastics, leather, rubber, and textiles.
- Atmospheric pollution
- AAT deficiency (<1% of pts w/COPD)

Diagnosis
H&P
- Peripheral cyanosis, productive cough, tachypnea, tachycardia
- Dyspnea, pursed-lip breathing w/use of accessory muscles for respiration, ↓ breath sounds, wheezing
- Acute exacerbation of COPD is mainly a clinical dx and generally is manifested w/ worsening dyspnea, sputum purulence, and volume.

Classification
- Table 11-8 describes the classification of COPD based on the GOLD criteria.

Imaging
- CXR: hyperinflation w/flattened diaphragm, tenting of the diaphragm at the rib, and retrosternal chest space, ↑ AP diameter
- ↓ Vascular markings and bullae in pts w/"emphysema"
- Thickened bronchial markings and enlarged right side of the heart in pts w/"chronic bronchitis"

Treatment
- Guideline recommendations for hospital management of COPD exacerbations are provided in Table 11-9.

H. PULMONARY VASCULAR DISEASE

1 PULMONARY EMBOLISM (PE)

Definition
Lodging of a thrombus or other embolic material from a distant site in the pulmonary circulation

Etiology
- Risk factors for PE:
  - Hematologic disease (e.g., factor V Leiden mutation, antithrombin III deficiency, protein C deficiency, protein S deficiency, lupus anticoagulant, PV, dysfibrinogenemia, PNH, acquired protein C resistance w/o factor V Leiden, G20210A prothrombin mutation)
  - Prolonged immobilization, ↓ mobility
  - Postoperative state, major surgery
  - Trauma to lower extremities, immobilizer or cast
  - Estrogen-containing birth control pills, hormone replacement Rx
  - Prior h/o DVT or PE

	Global Initiative for Chronic Obstructive Lung Disease[*]	American Thoracic Society/European Respiratory Society[†]	National Institute for Clinical Excellence[‡]
Date of statement	2010	2004	2010
Diagnostic testing	Chest radiograph, oximetry, ABGs, and ECG. Other testing as warranted by clinical indication.	Chest radiograph, oxygen saturation, ABGs, ECG, sputum Gram stain, and culture	Chest radiograph, ABG, ECG, complete blood count, sputum smear and culture, blood cultures if febrile
Bronchodilator therapy	Inhaled short-acting β_2-agonist is recommended. Consider ipratropium if inadequate clinical response. Consider theophylline or aminophylline as second-line intravenous therapy.	Inhaled short-acting β_2-agonist and/or ipratropium with spacer or nebulizer, as needed	Administer inhaled drugs by nebulizer or handheld inhaler. Specific agents and dosing regimens are not specified. Consider theophylline if response to inhaled bronchodilators is inadequate.
Antibiotics	Recommended if (1) increases in dyspnea, sputum volume, and sputum purulence all are present; (2) increase in sputum purulence along with increase in either dyspnea or sputum volume; or (3) need for assisted ventilation. See original document for complex treatment algorithm.	Base choice on local bacterial resistance patterns. Consider amoxicillin/clavulanate or respiratory fluoroquinolones. If *Pseudomonas* species and/or other Enterobacteriaceae are suspected, consider combination therapy.	Administer only if history of purulent sputum. Initiate with an aminopenicillin, a macrolide, or a tetracycline, taking into account local bacterial resistance patterns. Adjust therapy according to sputum and blood cultures.
Systemic corticosteroids	Daily prednisolone 30-40 mg (or its equivalent) orally for 7-10 days	Daily prednisone 30-40 mg orally for 10-14 days; equivalent dose intravenously if unable to tolerate oral intake Consider inhaled corticosteroids.	Daily prednisolone 30 mg (or its equivalent) orally for 7-14 days
Supplemental oxygen	Maintain oxygen saturation >90%. Monitor ABGs for hypercapnia and acidosis.	Maintain oxygen saturation >90%. Monitor ABGs for hypercapnia and acidosis.	Maintain oxygen saturation within the individualized target range. Monitor ABGs.
Assisted ventilation	Indications for NPPV include severe dyspnea, acidosis (pH ≤7.35) and/or hypercapnia (P_{CO_2} >45 mm Hg), and RR >25 breaths/min. Contraindications to NPPV include respiratory arrest, hemodynamic instability, impaired mental status, copious bronchial secretions, and extreme obesity. Intubate if contraindication to NPPV or failure of NPPV (worsening ABGs or clinical status). Consider likelihood of recovery and patient's wishes and expectations before intubation.	Consider with pH <7.35 and P_{CO_2} >45-60 mm Hg and RR >24 breaths/min. Institute NPPV in a controlled environment, unless there are contraindications (e.g., respiratory arrest, hemodynamic instability, impaired mental status, copious bronchial secretions, and extreme obesity). Intubate if contraindication to NPPV or failure of NPPV (worsening ABGs or clinical status).	NPPV treatment of choice for persistent hypercapnic respiratory failure. Consider functional status, body mass index, home oxygen, comorbidities, prior ICU admissions, age, and FEV_1 when assessing suitability for intubation and ventilation.

From Goldman L, Schafer AI (eds): Goldman's Cecil Medicine, 24th ed. Philadelphia, Saunders, 2012.

[*]Data from http://www.goldcopd.com.

[†]Data from MacNee W: Standards for the diagnosis and treatment of patients with COPD: a summary of the ATS/ERS position paper. Eur Respir J 23:932-946, 2004.

[‡]Data from http://www.nice.org.uk.

TABLE 11-10 ■ Wells Clinical Prediction Rule for Likelihood of Pulmonary Embolism	
Variable	Points
Predisposing Factors	
Previous VTE	1.5
Recent surgery or immobilization	1.5
Cancer	1
Symptoms	
Hemoptysis	1
Signs	
HR >100 bpm	1.5
Clinical signs of DVT	3
Clinical Judgment	
Alternative diagnosis less likely than PE	3
Clinical Probability	**Total Points**
Low	<2
Moderate	2-6
High	>6

Modified from Wells PS, Ginsberg JS, Anderson DR, et al: Use of a clinical model for safe management of patients with suspected pulmonary embolism. Ann Intern Med 129:997-1005, 1998.

- CHF
- Pregnancy and early puerperium
- Visceral cancer (lung, pancreas, alimentary and GU tracts)
- Spinal cord injury
- Prolonged air travel
- Central venous catheterization
- Advanced age
- Obesity, smoking
- COPD, DM, acute medical illness

Diagnosis

H&P

- The likelihood of PE can be estimated using Wells clinical prediction rule (Table 11-10).
- Most common physical finding: tachypnea
- Chest pain: may be nonpleuritic or pleuritic (infarction)
- Syncope (massive PE)
- Hemoptysis, cough
- Evidence of DVT: may be present (e.g., swelling and tenderness of extremities)
- Cardiac exam: tachycardia, pulmonic component of S_2, murmur of tricuspid insufficiency, RV heave, right-sided S_3
- Pulmonary exam: rales, localized wheezing, friction rub

Labs

- ABGs: ↓ Pao_2 and $Paco_2$, ↑ pH
- A-a O_2 gradient (measure of the difference in O_2 concentration between alveoli and arterial blood): An nl A-a gradient makes the dx of PE unlikely.
- Plasma D-dimer by ELISA: An nl plasma D-dimer level is useful to r/o PE in pts w/ nondiagnostic lung scan and a low pretest probability of PE. However, it cannot "rule in" PE because it is ↑ w/many other disorders (e.g., metastatic cancer, trauma, sepsis, postoperative state).

Imaging

- CXR: ↑ diaphragm, pleural effusion, dilation of pulmonary artery, infiltrate or consolidation, abrupt vessel cutoff, or atelectasis. A wedge-shaped consolidation in the middle and lower lobes suggests a pulmonary infarction and is known as *Hampton's hump*.
- Spiral CT: excellent modality for dx PE (Fig. 11-8). It can also detect other pulmonary disease that can mimic PE.
- Lung scan (in pt w/nl CXR):
  - An nl lung scan does r/o PE.
  - A V/Q mismatch suggests PE, and a lung scan interpretation of high probability is confirmatory.
- Figure 11-9 is a diagnostic algorithm incorporating the Wells criteria, D-dimer testing, and V/Q scan.

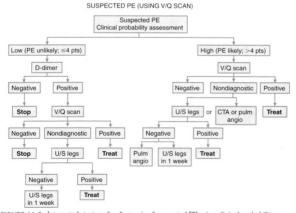

SUSPECTED PE (USING CTA)

Suspected PE
Clinical probability assessment

Low (PE unlikely; ≤4 pts) — High (PE likely; >4 pts)

Low branch:
D-dimer → Negative → **Stop**; Positive → CTA → Negative → **Stop**; Nondiagnostic → U/S legs → Negative → U/S legs in 1 week; Positive → **Treat**; CTA Positive → **Treat**

High branch:
CTA → Negative / Nondiagnostic / Positive
Negative or Nondiagnostic → U/S legs or Pulm angio; U/S legs → Negative → Pulm angio or U/S legs in 1 week; Positive → **Treat**; CTA Positive → **Treat**

FIGURE 11-8. Integrated strategy for diagnosis of pulmonary embolism (PE) using clinical probability assessment, measurement of D-dimer, and computer tomography angiography (CTA) as primary imaging test. Patients with low clinical probability (i.e., PE unlikely, negative D-dimer) need no further testing, but if D-dimer is positive, they should proceed to CTA, and if this is nondiagnostic, to ultrasonography of legs. Then either treat or repeat ultrasound in 1 week. Patients with high clinical probability (i.e., PE likely) need not have D-dimer measure but should proceed directly to CTA. If CTA is not diagnostic, options are to perform ultrasonography of legs or proceed to pulmonary angiography. If ultrasound of legs is negative, options are to repeat in 1 week or proceed to pulmonary angiography. *(From Vincent JL, Abraham E, Moore FA, et al [eds]: Textbook of Critical Care, 6th ed. Philadelphia, Saunders, 2011.)*

SUSPECTED PE (USING V/Q SCAN)

FIGURE 11-9. Integrated strategy for diagnosis of suspected PE using clinical probability assessment, measurement of D-dimer, and V/Q scan as primary imaging test. Patients with low clinical probability (i.e., PE unlikely, negative D-dimer) need no further investigation. If D-dimer is positive, V/Q scan performed; if not diagnostic, proceed to ultrasound. Then either treat or repeat ultrasound in 1 week. Patients with high probability (i.e., PE likely) need not have D-dimer measured but should proceed directly to V/Q scan. If V/Q scan not diagnostic, options are to perform CTA, pulmonary angiography, or ultrasonography of legs. If ultrasonography is negative, either repeat in 1 week or perform pulmonary angiogram. *(From Vincent JL, Abraham E, Moore FA, et al [eds]: Textbook of Critical Care, 6th ed. Philadelphia, Saunders, 2011.)*

- Angiography: Pulmonary angiography is the gold standard; however, it is invasive, expensive, and not readily available in some clinical settings. False(+) pulmonary angiograms may result from mediastinal disorders such as radiation fibrosis and tumors.
- CTA is an accurate, noninvasive tool in the dx of PE at the main, lobar, and segmental pulmonary artery levels. A major advantage of CTA over standard pulmonary angiography is its ability to dx intrathoracic disease other than PE that may account for the pt's clinical picture. It is also less invasive, less costly, and more widely available. Its major shortcoming is its poor sensitivity for subsegmental emboli. It is contraindicated in patients with GFR<30/renal failure.
- Gadolinium-enhanced MRA of the pulmonary arteries has a moderate sensitivity and high specificity for the dx of PE; MRA is best reserved for selected pts when CT scan and lung scan are inconclusive and the risk of pulmonary angiography is high.
- ECG: abnl in 85% of pts w/acute PE. Frequent abnlities are sinus tachycardia; S_1,Q_3,T_3 pattern (10% of pts); S_1,S_2,S_3 pattern; T wave inversion in V_1 to V_6; acute RBBB; new-onset AF; ST-segment depression in lead II; RV strain.

Treatment
- See the section on venous thromboembolism in Chapter 7 for Rx of PE.
- Acute pulmonary artery embolectomy may be indicated in a pt w/massive PE and refractory hypotension.

2 PULMONARY HYPERTENSION

Definition
Mean PAP >25 mm Hg at rest or >30 mm Hg w/exercise. Sustained ↑ in PAP secondary to pulmonary venous pressure, hypoxic pulmonary vasoconstriction, or flow is referred to as secondary pulmonary HTN.

Etiology and Classification
- Table 11-11 describes an updated classification of pulmonary HTN.

Diagnosis
H&P
- Exertional dyspnea: most common presenting sx (60%)
- Fatigue and weakness
- Syncope, classically exertion related or after a warm shower w/peripheral vasodilation
- Chest pain
- Hoarse voice from compression of recurrent laryngeal nerve by an enlarged pulmonary artery (*Ortner's syndrome*)
- Loud P_2 component of the second heart sound and paradoxical splitting of second heart sound
- Right-sided S_4
- JVD
- Abd distention/ascites
- Prominent parasternal (RV) impulse
- Holosystolic TR murmur heard best along the left fourth parasternal line that ↑ in intensity w/inspiration
- Peripheral edema

Labs
- CBC: nl or may show secondary polycythemia
- ANA (r/o connective tissue disease), HIV, LFTs, antiphospholipid Abs
- ABGs: ↓ Po_2 and Sao_2
- PFTs: r/o obstructive or restrictive lung disease
- Overnight sleep study: r/o sleep apnea/hypopnea

Imaging
- ECG: RA enlargement (tall P wave >2.5 mV in leads II, III, aVF) and RV enlargement (RAD >100 and R wave > S wave in lead V_1)
- CXR: enlargement of the main and hilar pulmonary arteries w/rapid tapering of the distal vessels, described as peripheral oligemia. RV enlargement may be evident on lateral films.
- Spiral CT or V/Q scan: r/o PE
- Doppler echo: assesses ventricular function, excludes significant valvular disease, and visualizes abnl shunting of blood between heart chambers if present. It also provides an estimate of the pulmonary artery systolic pressure.

TABLE 11-11 ■ Updated Clinical Classification of Pulmonary Hypertension
Group 1
Pulmonary Arterial Hypertension (PAH)
Idiopathic PAH
Heritable
BMPR2
ALK1, endoglin (with or without hereditary hemorrhagic telangiectasia)
Unknown
Drug- and toxin-induced
Associated with
Connective tissue diseases
HIV infection
Portal hypertension
Congenital heart diseases
Schistosomiasis
Chronic hemolytic anemia
Persistent Pulmonary Hypertension of the Newborn
Pulmonary Veno-occlusive Disease with Left-to-Right Shunts and/or Pulmonary Capillary Hemangiomatosis
Group 2
Pulmonary Hypertension Secondary to Left-Sided Heart Disease
Systolic dysfunction
Diastolic dysfunction
Valvular disease
Group 3
Pulmonary Hypertension Secondary to Lung Diseases and/or Hypoxia
COPD
Interstitial lung disease
Other Pulmonary Diseases with Mixed Restrictive and Obstructive Pattern
Sleep-disordered breathing
Alveolar hypoventilation disorders
Chronic exposure to high altitude
Developmental abnormalities
Group 4
Chronic Thromboembolic Pulmonary Hypertension (50% have no hx of DVT/PE)
Group 5
Pulmonary Hypertension with Unclear Multifactorial Mechanisms
Hematologic disorders: myeloproliferative disorders, splenectomy
Systemic disorders: sarcoidosis, pulmonary Langerhans cell histiocytosis: lymphangioleiomyomatosis, neurofibromatosis, vasculitis
Metabolic disorders: glycogen storage disease, Gaucher's disease, thyroid disorders
Others: tumoral obstruction, fibrosing mediastinitis, chronic renal failure on dialysis

Modified From Simonneau G et al: Updated clinical classification of pulmonary hypertension. J Am Coll Cardiol 54:S43-S54, 2009.

ALK1, Activin receptor-like kinase type 1; *BMPR2*, bone morphogenetic protein receptor type 2.

Treatment

Acute Rx

- Diuretics (e.g., furosemide 40-80 mg qd)
- Digoxin in pts w/AF
- Short-acting vasodilators: IV adenosine, epoprostenol, or inhaled nitric oxide

Chronic Rx

- CCB (diltiazem, amlodipine, or nifedipine)
- Prostanoids (epoprostenol, treprostinil, and iloprost) act as potent vasodilators of pulmonary arteries and inhibitors of Plt aggregation.
- Endothelin receptor antagonists: bosentan, ambrisentan, and sitaxsentan
- Phosphodiesterase inhibitors: sildenafil and tadalafil
- Warfarin Rx w/goal INR 1.5 to 2.0 is recommended for all pts w/PPH and although not proven may be indicated in secondary pulmonary HTN.
- Lung transplantation and heart-lung transplantation are other options in pts w/ end-stage class IV disease. Atrial septostomy may be performed as a bridge to transplantation.

TABLE 11-12 ■ **Overview of Idiopathic Interstitial Pneumonias**

Diagnosis	Clinical Findings	HRCT Features	Differential Diagnosis
UIP/IPF	40-70 yr, M>F; >6-mo dyspnea, cough, crackles, clubbing; poor response to steroids	Peripheral, basal, subpleural reticulation and honeycombing, ± ground-glass opacity	Collagen vascular disease, asbestosis, CHP, scleroderma, drugs (bleomycin, methotrexate)
NSIP	40-50 yr, M = F; dyspnea, cough, fatigue, crackles; may respond to steroids	Bilateral, patchy, subpleural ground-glass opacity, ± reticulation	Collagen vascular disease, CHP, DIP
RB-ILD	30-50 yr, M > F; dyspnea, cough	Ground-glass, centrilobular nodules, ± centrilobular emphysema	Hypersensitivity pneumonitis
AIP/diffuse alveolar damage	Any age, M = F; acute-onset dyspnea, diffuse crackles and consolidation	Ground-glass consolidation, traction bronchiectasis, and architectural distortion	ARDS, infection, edema, hemorrhage
COP	Mean 55 yr, M = F; <3-mo hx of cough, dyspnea, fever; may respond to steroids	Subpleural and peribronchial consolidation, ± nodules in lower zones; atoll sign (ring-shaped opacity)	Collagen vascular disease, infection, vasculitis, sarcoidosis, lymphoma, alveolar carcinoma
DIP	30-54 yr, M > F; insidious onset weeks to months of dyspnea, cough	Ground-glass opacity, lower zone, peripheral	Hypersensitivity pneumonitis, NSIP
LIP	Any age, F > M	Ground-glass opacity, ± poorly defined centrilobular nodules, thin-walled cysts, and air trapping	DIP, NSIP, hypersensitivity pneumonitis

From Ferri F: Ferri's Clinical Advisor: 5 Books in 1. 2013 edition. Philadelphia, Mosby, 2012.

AIP, Acute interstitial pneumonia; *CHP*, chronic hypersensitivity pneumonitis; *COP*, cryptogenic organizing pneumonia; *DIP*, desquamative interstitial pneumonitis; *IPF*, idiopathic pulmonary fibrosis; *LIP*, lymphoid interstitial pneumonia; *NSIP*, nonspecific interstitial pneumonia; *RB-ILD*, respiratory bronchiolitis–associated interstitial lung disease; *UIP*, usual interstitial pneumonia.

I. DIFFUSE PARENCHYMAL LUNG DISEASE

1 INTERSTITIAL LUNG DISEASE (ILD)

ILD includes a large group of nonmalignant disorders characterized by diffuse damage to the lung parenchyma by inflammation and fibrosis or granulomatous reaction in interstitial or vascular areas. Table 11-12 provides an overview of idiopathic interstitial pneumonias.

Diagnosis

H&P

- Dyspnea
- Tachypnea
- Bibasilar end-inspiratory dry crackles
- Pulmonary HTN
- Cyanosis, clubbing

Labs

- ABGs: nl or may show respiratory alkalosis
- ANA, ANCA, ACE level, RF, LDH
- Bronchoscopy and BAL may help identify type of ILD. However, their role in defining the stage of disease and the response to Rx is controversial.
- Bx is the most effective method for confirming dx and assessing disease activity.

Imaging (Box 11-5)

- CXR, HRCT: bibasilar reticular pattern
- PFTs: Well-defined patterns in PFTs are usually consistent w/restrictive defect (↓ FRC, RV, and TLC) resulting from ↓ lung compliance caused by alveolar wall thickening from inflammation and fibrosis. Diffusing capacity ↓ from inflammation and thickening of alveolar walls, although nonspecific. FEV_1/FVC is usually nl or because lung stiffness keeps small airways open, although some conditions (e.g., sarcoidosis) may ↓ airflow.

Treatment
- Prednisone 0.5 to 1 mg/kg qd × 4 to 12 wk, then re-evaluate; if stable, taper; if not, maintain × another 4 to 12 wk; if still not improved, add cyclophosphamide or azathioprine.
- Supplemental O_2 PRN in pts w/hypoxemia; avoidance of tobacco and occupational exposures

J. GRANULOMATOUS LUNG DISEASE

1 SARCOIDOSIS

Chronic systemic granulomatous disease of unknown cause, characterized histologically by the presence of nonspecific, noncaseating granulomas

Diagnosis

H&P

- Clinical manifestations often vary w/stage of the disease and degree of organ involvement; pts may be asymptomatic, but CXR may demonstrate findings consistent w/sarcoidosis (see the later section on imaging). Nearly 50% of pts w/ sarcoidosis are dx by incidental findings on CXR. Frequent manifestations:
  - Pulmonary manifestations: dry, nonproductive cough; dyspnea; chest discomfort
  - Constitutional sx: fatigue, weight loss, anorexia, malaise
  - Visual disturbances: blurred vision, ocular discomfort, conjunctivitis, iritis, uveitis (65% of pts)
  - Dermatologic manifestations: erythema nodosum (10% of pts), macules, papules, SC nodules, hyperpigmentation, lupus pernio (indurated violaceous lesions on the nose, lips, ears, cheeks that can erode into underlying cartilage and bone)
  - Myocardial disturbances (5% of pts): arrhythmias, cardiomyopathy

- Splenomegaly, hepatomegaly
- Rheumatologic manifestations: arthralgias have been reported in up to 40% of pts
- Neurologic and other manifestations: cranial nerve palsies, diabetes insipidus, meningeal involvement, parotid enlargement, hypothalamic and pituitary lesions, peripheral adenopathy

Labs
- Hypergammaglobulinemia, anemia, leukopenia
- LFT abnlities
- Hypercalcemia (11% of pts), hypercalciuria (40% of pts): secondary to GI absorption, abnl vitamin D metabolism, and calcitriol production by sarcoid granuloma
- ACE in 60% of pts; nonspecific and generally not useful as a dx tool and in following the course of the disease

Imaging
- CXR and chest CT
  - Adenopathy of the hilar and paratracheal nodes
  - Parenchymal changes may also be present, depending on the stage of the disease: stage 0, nl x-ray; stage I, bilateral hilar adenopathy; stage II, stage I plus pulmonary infiltrate; stage III, pulmonary infiltrate w/o adenopathy; stage IV, advanced fibrosis w/evidence of honeycombing, hilar retraction, bullae, cysts, and emphysema.
- PFTs (spirometry and diffusing capacity of the lung for CO): may be nl or may reveal a restrictive pattern or obstructive pattern
- ^{18}FDG-PET: useful in identifying sites for dx bx in pts w/o apparent lung involvement
- ^{18}FDG-PET and MRI w/gadolinium: useful in pts w/suspected cardiac and neurologic involvement

Treatment
- Most pts will not require any Rx.
- Corticosteroids should be considered in pts w/severe sx (e.g., dyspnea; chest pain; hypercalcemia; ocular, CNS, or cardiac involvement; and progressive pulmonary disease).
- MTX 7.5 to 15 mg once/wk: in pts w/progressive disease refractory to corticosteroids
- Hydroxychloroquine: effective for chronic disfiguring skin lesions, hypercalcemia, and neurologic involvement
- NSAIDs: useful for musculoskeletal sx and erythema nodosum

Prognosis
- Most pts w/sarcoidosis have spontaneous remission within 2 yr and do not require Rx. Their course can be followed by periodic clinical evaluation, CXR, and PFTs.
- However, 25% to 33% of pts have unrelenting disease leading to clinically significant organ impairment. Adverse prognostic factors are age at onset >40 yr, cardiac involvement, neurosarcoidosis, progressive pulmonary fibrosis, chronic hypercalcemia, chronic uveitis, involvement of nasal mucosa, nephrocalcinosis, and presence of cystic bone lesions and lupus pernio.

2 GRANULOMATOSIS WITH POLYANGIITIS (WEGENER'S GRANULOMATOSIS)
- Multisystem disease generally consisting of the classic triad of:
  - Necrotizing granulomatous lesions in the upper or lower respiratory tracts
  - Generalized focal necrotizing vasculitis involving both arteries and veins
  - Focal GN of the kidneys
- "Limited forms" of the disease can also occur and may evolve into the classic triad. Granulomatosis with polyangiitis can be classified by the "ELK" classification, which identifies the three major sites of involvement: E, ears, nose, and throat or respiratory tract; L, lungs; K, kidneys.

Diagnosis

H&P
- Clinical manifestations often vary w/the stage of the disease and degree of organ involvement.
- Frequent manifestations:
  - Upper respiratory tract: chronic sinusitis, chronic otitis media, mastoiditis, nasal crusting, obstruction and epistaxis, nasal septal perforation, nasal lacrimal duct stenosis, saddle nose deformities (resulting from cartilage destruction)

- Lung: hemoptysis, multiple nodules, diffuse alveolar pattern
- Kidney: renal insufficiency, GN
- Skin: necrotizing skin lesions
- Nervous system: mononeuritis multiplex, cranial nerve involvement
- Joints: monarthritis or polyarthritis (nondeforming), usually affecting large joints
- Mouth: chronic ulcerative lesions of the oral mucosa, "mulberry" gingivitis
- Eye: proptosis, uveitis, episcleritis, retinal and optic nerve vasculitis

Labs
- (+) test result for cytoplasmic pattern of ANCA (cANCA)
- Other labs: anemia, leukocytosis, hematuria, RBC casts, and proteinuria; ↑ serum Cr, ↓ CrCl, ↑ ESR, (+) RF, and ↑ CRP
- Bx of one or more affected organs should be attempted; the most reliable source for tissue dx is the lung. Lesions in the nasopharynx (if present) can be easily sampled.

Imaging
- CXR: bilateral multiple nodules, cavitated mass lesions, pleural effusion (20%)
- PFTs: useful in detecting stenosis of the airways

Treatment
- Prednisone 60 to 80 mg/day and cyclophosphamide 2 mg/kg. Once the disease is under control, prednisone is tapered and cyclophosphamide is continued. Other potentially useful agents in pts intolerant of cyclophosphamide are azathioprine, MTX, and mycophenolate mofetil.
- TMP-SMX: useful alternative in pts w/lesions limited to the upper or lower respiratory tracts in absence of vasculitis or nephritis. Rx w/TMP-SMX (160 mg/800 mg bid) also ↓ the incidence of relapses in pts w/Wegener's granulomatosis in remission. It is also useful in preventing *Pneumocystis* pneumonia, which occurs in 10% of pts receiving induction Rx. When used for prophylaxis, dose of TMP-SMX (160 mg/800 mg) is 1 tablet 3×/wk.

K PLEURAL DISEASE

1 Pleural Effusion/Thoracentesis
Indications
1. Presence of any pleural effusion of unknown cause
2. Relief of dyspnea caused by large pleural effusion

Contraindications
1. Clotting abnlities
2. Thrombocytopenia
3. Uncooperative pt or pt w/severe cough or hiccups

Localization of Pleural Effusion
1. Physical examination: dullness to percussion, loss of tactile fremitus
2. CXR: PA view is usually sufficient in identifying the fluid collection; but in case of equivocal effusions, a lateral decubitus CXR can demonstrate layering out of the pleural fluid. Effusions >1 cm on a lateral decubitus film are usually sufficiently large to be removed at the bedside w/o additional imaging.
3. Fluoroscopy, ultrasonography, or CT guidance in performing thoracentesis if the fluid collection has the following qualities:
   a. <10 mm thick
   b. Not freely movable on the lateral decubitus x-ray view

Procedure
1. Position pt in a sitting position w/arms and head supported on a bedside adjustable table.
2. Identify the area of effusion by gentle percussion.
3. Clean the area w/povidone-iodine solution and maintain strict aseptic technique.
4. Insert the needle in the posterior chest (≈5 to 10 cm lateral to the spine, in the midpoint between the spine and the posterior axillary line) in one to two interspaces below the point of dullness to percussion.
5. Anesthetize the skin and SC tissues w/1% to 2% lidocaine, using a 25-gauge needle.
6. Make sure that the needle is positioned and advanced above the superior margin of the rib (the intercostal nerve and the blood supply are located near the inferior margin). "Walk" the needle over the superior margin of the rib and deeper into the interspace, to anesthetize the intercostal muscle layers.

7. Apply (–) pressure as the needle is advanced. In thin pts, this needle is often sufficiently long to reach the pleural space. If pleural fluid is withdrawn, anesthetize the pleura adequately and note the depth at which it was reached. If it is not reached, use a longer, 20- to 22-gauge syringe w/1% to 2% lidocaine, advance it slowly w/(–) pressure along the same tract as the prior needle, anesthetize the pleura adequately, and advance the needle into the pleural space. If the purpose of the thoracentesis is for dx only, a 30- to 50-mL syringe may then be attached and pleural fluid withdrawn for diagnostic studies. If the purpose of the thoracentesis is fluid removal, proceed further as below. Place a clamp on the needle at skin level to mark the depth, then remove the needle and note the depth of insertion needed for the thoracentesis needle.

8. In the previous puncture site, insert a 17-gauge needle (flat bevel) attached to a 30-mL syringe via a three-way stopcock connected to a drainage tube.

9. Slowly advance the needle (above the superior margin of the rib) and gently aspirate while advancing.

10. Keep a clamp or a hemostat on the needle at the level previously marked to prevent it from inadvertently advancing forward. Many thoracentesis kits have a catheter that may be advanced over the needle to remove the risk of a sharp needle within the pleural space.

11. Remove the necessary amount of pleural fluid (usually 100 mL for diagnostic studies), but do not remove >1000 mL of fluid at any one time because of risk of pulmonary edema or hypotension (pneumothorax from needle laceration of the visceral pleura is also much more likely to occur if an effusion is completely drained).

12. Gently remove the needle.

13. Obtain measurements of serum LDH, alb, glucose, and total protein levels.

14. Process the pleural fluid; the initial laboratory studies should be aimed only at distinguishing an exudate from a transudate (Fig. 11-10).
    a. Tube 1: protein, LDH, alb
    b. Tubes 2, 3, 4: Save the fluid until further notice. In selected pts w/suspected empyema, ascertaining a pH level may be useful (generally <7.0).

15. Table 11-13 subdivides pleural effusions based on Light's criteria.

TABLE 11-13 ■ Evaluation of Pleural and Peritoneal Effusions

Test	Exudate	Transudate
Fluid LDH	>200 IU/dL	<200 IU/dL
Fluid protein	>3 g	<3 g
Fluid-to-serum LDH ratio	>0.6 IU/dL	<0.6 IU/dL
Fluid-to-serum protein ratio	>0.5 IU/dL	<0.5 IU/dL
Specific gravity	>1.016	<1.016
Appearance	Cloudy	Clear, thin
	Viscous	Nonclotting

From Weissleder R, Wittenberg J, Harisinghani M, Chen JW (eds): Primer of Diagnostic Imaging, 5th ed. St. Louis, Mosby, 2011.

L. LUNG CANCER

The WHO distinguishes 12 types of pulmonary neoplasms. Among them, the major types are *squamous cell carcinoma, adenocarcinoma, small cell carcinoma,* and *large cell carcinoma.* However, the crucial difference in the dx of lung cancer is between small cell (SCLC) and non–small cell lung cancer (NSCLC) types because the prognosis and therapeutic approach are different. NSCLC consists of 3 main histologic subtypes (adenocarcinoma, squamous cell, and large cell carcinoma) compromising >80% of all lung cancers. Bronchoalveolar carcinoma, another type of lung cancer, accounts for ≈5% of all lung cancers. Table 11-14 describes selected characteristics of lung carcinomas.

Diagnosis

H&P

- Cough, hemoptysis, dyspnea, wheezing
- Chest, shoulder, and bone pain
- Weight loss, fatigue, fever, anorexia, dysphagia

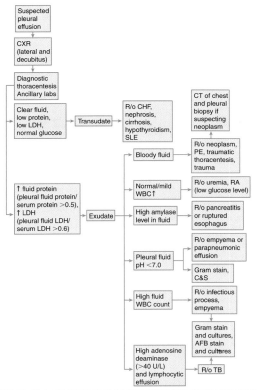

FIGURE 11-10. Diagnostic thoracentesis algorithm. *(From Ferri FF: Ferri's Best Test: A Practical Guide to Clinical Laboratory Medicine and Diagnostic Imaging, 2nd ed. Philadelphia, Mosby, 2010.)*

TABLE 11-14 ■ Selected Characteristics of Lung Carcinomas				
Histologic Cell Type	Percentage of Total (%)	Frequent Location	Initial Metastases	Comments
Adenocarcinoma	35	Midlung and periphery	Lymphatics	Associated w/peripheral scars
Squamous cells (epidermoid)	20-30	Central	Local invasion	Frequent cavitation and obstructive phenomena
Small cell (oat cell)	20	Central	Lymphatics	Cavitation rare Associated w/deletion of short arm of chromosome 3
Large cell	15-20	Periphery	CNS, mediastinum	Rapid growth rate w/ early metastases
Bronchioloalveolar	5	Periphery, may be bilateral	Lymphatics, hematogenous, and local invasion	No correlation w/ cigarette smoking Cavitation rare

- Paraneoplastic syndromes:
  - **Lambert-Eaton syndrome:** myopathy involving proximal muscle groups
  - Endocrine manifestations: hypercalcemia, ectopic ACTH, SIADH
  - Neurologic: subacute cerebellar degeneration, peripheral neuropathy, cortical degeneration
  - Musculoskeletal: polymyositis, clubbing, hypertrophic pulmonary osteoarthropathy
  - Hematologic or vascular: migratory thrombophlebitis, marantic thrombosis, anemia, thrombocytosis, or thrombocytopenia
  - Cutaneous: acanthosis nigricans, dermatomyositis
- Pleural effusion (10% of pts), recurrent pneumonias (secondary to obstruction), localized wheezing
- SVC syndrome
- **Horner's syndrome:** constricted pupil, ptosis, facial anhidrosis caused by spinal cord damage between C8 and T1 secondary to a superior sulcus tumor (bronchogenic carcinoma of the extreme lung apex). A superior sulcus tumor associated w/ipsilateral Horner's syndrome and shoulder pain is known as a **Pancoast tumor.**

Procedures

- *Flexible fiberoptic bronchoscopy:* Brush and bx specimens are obtained from any visualized endobronchial lesions and other abnormal areas identified through endobronchial ultrasonography guidance.
- *Transthoracic FNAB w/fluoroscopic or CT scan guidance* is used to evaluate peripheral pulmonary nodules.
- *Mediastinoscopy and anteromedial sternotomy* is indicated in suspected tumor involvement of the mediastinum.
- *Bone marrow aspiration* is performed in selected pts w/SCLC w/LDH or cytopenia.
- *PFTs* are performed determine whether the pt can tolerate any loss of lung tissue. The postop predicted pulmonary function = preop function – calculated % of lung function to be lost with surgery. Pneumonectomy is possible if the pt has a preoperative FEV_1 >2 L, or if the maximal voluntary ventilation is >50% of predicted capacity. Individuals w/FEV_1 >1.5 L are suitable for lobectomy w/o further evaluation unless there is evidence of ILD or undue dyspnea on exertion. In that case, D_{LCO} should be measured. If the D_{LCO} is <80% predicted nl, the pt is not clearly operable; if the postop predicted FEV_1 and D_{LCO} are >40%, surgery is possible.
- *Genetic mutations testing of lung specimen:* detection of epidermal growth factor receptor (EGFR) and anaplastic lymphoma kinase (ALK)

Imaging

- CXR
- CT chest
- PET w/^{18}F-fluorodeoxyglucose ([18]FDG-PET): for preop staging of NSCLC
- CT of liver and brain; bone scan in all pts w/SCLC and pts w/NSCLC suspected of involving these organs

Staging

NSCLC

- The international staging system for NSCLC: Stage I is N0 (no lymph node involvement). Stage II (N1 [spread to ipsilateral bronchopulmonary or hilar lymph nodes]) includes localized tumors for which surgical resection is the preferred Rx. Stage III is subdivided into IIIA (potentially resectable) and IIIB. The surgical management of stage IIIA disease (N2 [involvement of ipsilateral mediastinal nodes]) is controversial. Only 20% of N2 disease is considered minimal disease (involvement of only one node) and technically resectable. Stage IV indicates metastatic disease. The pathologic staging system uses a tumor–nodal involvement–metastasis system.
- In pts w/SCLC, the staging system from the Veterans Administration Lung Cancer Study Group contains two stages:
  - Limited stage disease: confined to the regional lymph nodes and to one hemithorax (excluding pleural surfaces)
  - Extensive stage disease: spread beyond the confines of limited-stage disease

Treatment

NSCLC

- Surgical resection (lobectomy, pneumonectomy)
  - Indicated in pts w/limited disease (stage I or II). This represents 15% to 30% of diagnosed cases. Lobectomy can be performed by VATS with less morbidity and shorter hospitalization.

- Preoperative chemoRx: consider in pts w/more advanced disease (stage IIIA) who are being considered for surgery. Gene expression profiles that predict the risk of recurrence in pts w/early-stage (IA) NSCLC have been identified. These pts are at high risk for recurrence and may also benefit from adjuvant chemoRx.
- Postoperative adjuvant chemoRx (chemoRx given after surgical resection of an apparently localized tumor to eradicate occult mets) w/vinorelbine plus cisplatin: consider in pts w/completely resected stage IB or stage II NSCLC and good performance status. Adjuvant chemoRx is generally indicated for pts w/resected tumors that are stages IIA through IIIA.

- Rx of unresectable NSCLC
  - RadioRx can be used alone or in combination w/chemoRx; it is used primarily for Rx of CNS and skeletal mets, SVC, and obstructive atelectasis. Although thoracic radioRx is generally considered standard Rx for stage III disease, it has limited effect on survival. Palliative radioRx should be delayed until sx occur because immediate Rx offers no advantage over delayed Rx and results in more adverse events from the radioRx.
  - ChemoRx: Current drugs of choice are paclitaxel + either carboplatin or cisplatin; cisplatin + vinorelbine; gemcitabine + cisplatin; carboplatin or cisplatin + docetaxel. The overall results are disappointing, and none of the standard regimens for NSCLC is clearly superior to the others. The addition of bevacizumab to paclitaxel + carboplatin results in significant survival benefit but carries a risk of Rx-related death. Gefitinib and erlotinib are PO inhibitors of EGFR tyrosine kinase. Both agents are approved only for pts in whom at least one prior chemoRx regimen has failed. The inhibition of ALK in lung tumors with crizotinib, an orally available small-molecule inhibitor of the ALK tyrosine kinase, has resulted in tumor shrinkage and significantly prolonged progression-free survival.
  - The addition of chemoRx to radioRx improves survival in pts w/locally advanced, unresectable NSCLC. The absolute benefit is relatively small, however, and should be balanced against the toxicity associated w/the addition of chemoRx.

SCLC
- Limited stage disease: standard Rxs include thoracic radioRx and chemoRx (cisplatin and etoposide)
- Extensive stage disease: standard Rxs include combination chemoRx (cisplatin or carboplatin + etoposide or combination of irinotecan and cisplatin)
- Prophylactic cranial irradiation: for pts in complete remission to ↓ the risk of CNS metastasis

M. RESPIRATORY FAILURE CLASSIFICATION

A. HYPOXEMIC ("TYPE I") RESPIRATORY FAILURE
- ↓ in oxyhemoglobin that does not correct with supp. O_2
- PaO_2 (ambient air) ≤ 60 mmHg
- PCO_2 typically normal or < 40 mmHg
- Hypoxemia is the result of persistent perfusion of lung units that are not ventilating as a result of fluid (pus, blood, edema) or alveolar collapse => intrapulmonary shunt physiology results in inability to correct with supp. O_2. Hypoxemia can be corrected with administration of PEEP which "results" and opens up collapsed/fliud-filled alveoli.
  - Examples: ARDS, CHF, Atelectasis, Pneumonia

B. HYPERCAPNIC ("TYPE II") RESPIRATORY FAILURE
- Occurs as a result of insufficient alveolar ventilation from ↑CO_2
- PaO_2 ↓
- PCO_2 ↑ as a result of ↑CO_2 production and/or decreased alveolar ventilation (secondary to respiratory muscle weakness/excessive mechanical work of breathing, decreased respiratory drive, and lung diseases with impaired gas exchange such as: COPD)
  - Examples: COPD/Asthma (obstructive lung disease), Neuromuscular disease (Myasthenia Gravis, GBS when VC < 15-20 cc/kg and NIF < 30). Restrictive Lung Disease (Extrapulmonary – kyphoscoliosis, ascites, and Intrapulmonary – Fibrotic Lung disease)

12 Rheumatology

A. ARTHOCENTESIS

INDICATIONS
1. Presence of effusion of unexplained etiology
2. Steroid injection
3. Decompression of a hemorrhagic effusion in traumatized joints
4. Evaluation of abx response in pts w/infectious arthritis
5. Removal of purulent fluid in distended infected joints

CONTRAINDICATIONS
1. Cellulitis or broken skin over the intended entry site
2. Coagulopathy
3. Unstable joint

PROCEDURE
1. Palpate the joint and identify the extensor surface (vessels and nerves are less commonly found here).
2. With firm pressure, use a ballpoint pen that has the writing portion retracted to mark the specific area of the joint to be aspirated.
3. Clean the skin w/an antiseptic solution.
4. Use a 25-gauge needle to infiltrate the skin w/1% to 2% lidocaine.
5. Gently insert an 18- or 20-gauge needle connected to a 20- to 30-mL syringe; a slight "pop" may be felt as the needle penetrates the capsule.
6. Apply gentle suction to the syringe to aspirate the fluid.
7. Gently remove the needle, and apply slight pressure to the puncture site.
8. Process the aspirated synovial fluid:
   a. Tube 1 (no heparin): viscosity, mucin clot
   b. Tube 2 (containing heparin): glucose level
   c. Tube 3 (containing heparin): Gram stain, C&S, cytology, CBC w/diff
   d. Glass slide: Place a drop of fluid and examine under polarized light.
   e. Plate w/Thayer-Martin medium (used in cases of suspected gonococcal arthritis); assessment for Lyme titer, cultures for anaerobes, *Mycobacterium tuberculosis,* and fungi should be ordered only when clearly indicated.
9. Draw samples for measurement of serum glucose level.

INTERPRETATION OF RESULTS
1. Color: Normally it is clear or pale yellow; cloudiness indicates an inflammatory process or presence of crystals, cell debris, fibrin, or TGs.
2. Viscosity is high because of hyaluronate; when fluid is placed on a slide, it can be stretched to a string longer than 2 cm before separating (low viscosity indicates breakdown of hyaluronate [lysosomal enzymes from leukocytes] or the presence of edema fluid).
3. Mucin clot: Add 1 mL of fluid to 5 mL of a 5% acetic acid solution, and allow 1 min for the clot to form; a firm clot (does not fragment on shaking) is nl and indicates the presence of large molecules of hyaluronic acid (this test is nonspecific and infrequently done).
4. Glucose level: nl is approximately = serum glucose level; a difference of >40 mg/dL suggests infection.
5. Total protein concentration is <2.5 g/dL in nl synovial fluid; it is ↑ in cases of inflammatory and septic arthritis.
6. Microscopic examination for crystals:
   a. Gout: monosodium urate crystals
   b. Pseudogout: Ca^{2+} pyrophosphate dihydrate crystals

Figure 12-1 is an algorithm for analysis of joint fluid.

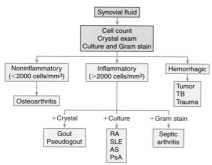

FIGURE 12-1. Algorithm for analysis of joint fluid. Examples of inflammatory arthritis are indicated, although many conditions can produce these findings. AS, ankylosing spondylitis; PsA, psoriatic arthritis. *(From Goldman L, Schafer AI [eds]: Goldman's Cecil Medicine, 24th edition. Philadelphia, Saunders, 2012.)*

B. ARTHRITIS, MONARTICULAR AND OLIGOARTICULAR

- Septic arthritis (*Staphylococcus aureus, Neisseria gonorrhoeae,* meningococci, streptococci, *Streptococcus pneumoniae,* enteric gram(–) bacilli)
- Crystalline-induced arthritis (gout, pseudogout, Ca oxalate, hydroxyapatite, and other basic Ca/phosphate crystals)
- Traumatic joint injury
- Hemarthrosis
- Monarticular or oligoarticular flare of an inflammatory polyarticular rheumatic disease (RA, psoriatic arthritis, Reiter's syndrome, SLE)

C. ARTHRITIS, POLYARTICULAR

- RA, juvenile (rheumatoid) polyarthritis
- SLE, other connective tissue diseases, erythema nodosum, palindromic rheumatism, relapsing polychondritis
- Psoriatic arthritis, ankylosing spondylitis
- Sarcoidosis
- Lyme arthritis, bacterial endocarditis, *Neisseria gonorrhoeae* infection, rheumatic fever, Reiter's disease
- Crystal deposition disease
- Hypersensitivity to serum or drugs
- Hepatitis B, HIV infection, rubella, mumps
- Other: serum sickness, leukemias, lymphomas, enteropathic arthropathy, Whipple's disease, Behçet's syndrome, Henoch-Schönlein purpura, familial Mediterranean fever, hypertrophic pulmonary osteoarthropathy

D. VASCULITIC SYNDROMES

See Table 12-1.

E. SYSTEMIC LUPUS ERYTHEMATOSUS (SLE)

Chronic multisystemic disease characterized by production of antibodies and protean clinical manifestations

TABLE 12-1 ■ Systemic Vasculitis*

Large-Vessel	Pathophysiology	Clinical Features/Dx	Management
Giant Cell Arteritis (Temporal Arteritis)	Affects large-caliber vessels that contain internal elastic membranes Multinucleated giant cells w/in vessel wall or adventitia Age >50 yr Women 2:1	New-onset headache (temporal or occipital) in pt >50 yr Visual changes/loss (ischemia of optic nerve ± inflammation of ophthalmic artery) Jaw claudication (± ischemia of masseter or temporalis mm) PMR (pain in hip/shoulder girdle) UE limb claudication, subclavian steal Aortic regurgitation **Dx:** ↑↑↑ ESR and CRP Anemia + thrombocytosis Established via temporal artery bx	Prednisone 1 mg/kg/day gives rapid response Treat **immediately** when dx is suspected; temporal artery biopsy findings will **not** change w/steroid administration until at least 4 wk Taper prednisone over 4–6 wk, guided by ESR and CRP Flares commonly occur during tapering and are managed by increasing the prednisone dose by 10 mg over dose that initially controlled the disease Low-dose aspirin to ↓ risk of CVA
Polymyalgia Rheumatica	Pain and stiffness in the proximal limbs associated w/elevated acute phase reactants Associated w/giant cell and late-onset RA	Pain, stiffness, and limitation in passive ROM of the shoulder and hip girdle muscles **No** peripheral joint swelling **Dx:** ↑ ESR and CRP Mild normochromic, normocytic anemia	Low-dose prednisone Tapered over a 6-mo period Can use MTX as steroid-sparing agent
Takayasu Arteritis	Affects aorta and its major branches, pulmonary arteries 2nd–4th decade of life Women 8:1	*Inflammatory Phase* Fever, arthralgias, myalgias, malaise, wt loss for several months Audible bruits over carotid, subclavian, renal, iliac vessels *Pulseless Phase* UE/LE claudication ± vascular insufficiency Pulse deficits and differential systolic BP's HTN ± RAS **Dx:** ↑ ESR and CRP CTA or MRA or aorta and branches to show narrowing	*Inflammatory Phase* High-dose corticosteroids Can use MTX or TNF-α blockers as corticosteroid-sparing agents *Pulseless Phase* Difficult to Rx because active vessel inflammation may be absent ⇒ Look for inflammation w/contrast MRI and PET scans Low-dose aspirin Treat lipids aggressively to prevent atherosclerosis

TABLE 12-1 ■ Systemic Vasculitis—cont'd

Medium-Vessel	Pathophysiology	Clinical Features/Dx	Management
Polyarteritis Nodosa	Inflammation and necrosis of medium-sized and small muscular artery walls Age of onset: 40-60 yr **50%** cases associated with Hep B	Fever, arthralgia, myalgia, abd pain, wt. loss Peripheral nerve: mononeuritis multiplex HTN ± renoarteriolar involvement Testicular pain, painful cutaneous nodules/skin ulcers/palpable purpura/livedo reticularis Spares lungs **Dx:** P-ANCA Necrotizing arteritis on bx specimens of involved skin, sural nerve (do not use kidney given risk of hemorrhage) Aneurysms and stenoses on CTA	High-dose corticosteroids x several weeks w/slow taper following Use cyclophosphamide in patients who do not respond In Hep B(+) patients, give **short** course (1-2 wk) of steroids w/antiviral Rx (entecavir) [>50% HBeAg(+)] Pts w/polyarteritis nodosa respond w/resolution of arteritis and seroconversion to hep B e-antibody positivity
Kawasaki's Disease	Usually occurs in children Seen in adults w/HIV	Fever >5 days + nonexudative conjunctivitis, erythema of oral mucosa Edema of extremities w/desquamation ACS or peripheral vascular occlusion Coronary aneurysms (MC in children) **Dx:** made by clinical features	High-dose salicylates and early administration of IVIG TTE to r/o coronary artery aneurysm

Small-Vessel	Pathophysiology	Clinical Features/Dx	Management
Wegener's Granulomatosis (Granulomatosis w/Polyangiitis)	Involvement of small to medium-sized arteries and can be associated w/a "pauci-immune" (no immune complexes) GN	Upper airway disease (70%): sinusitis, epistaxis, and nasal septal perforation/saddle nose deformity ± cartilage erosion Pulmonary: cough, hemoptysis, pleurisy, multifocal infiltrates or nodules on CXR Ocular symptoms: scleritis, uveitis, keratitis Purpura, ulcers on skin Pauci-immune GN (80%) **Dx:** C-ANCA Established by kidney or lung bx Antiproteinase-3 Abs⁺	High-dose corticosteroids w/3-6-mo course of cyclophosphamide B-cell depletion Rx w/rituximab has been shown to be equally as effective as cyclophosphamide Following remission: steroids are tapered and cyclophosphamide is stopped ⇒ Rx is continued for **18 mo w/azathioprine** or wkly **MTX** (90% achieve remission, relapses are frequent w/MTX) Bactrim for PCP prophylaxis

Continued

TABLE 12-1 ■ Systemic Vasculitis—cont'd

Small-Vessel	Pathophysiology	Clinical Features/Dx	Management
Microscopic Polyangitis	Necrotizing vasculitis that predominantly affects the lungs and kidneys Age of onset: 30-50 yr	Fever, arthralgia, purpuric skin rash, mononeuritis multiplex Rapidly progressive GN or pulmonary hemorrhage **Dx:** P-ANCA Antimyeloperoxidase Ab (60%-80%) Confirm w/bx of affected tissue (skin, lung, kidney): lung: pulmonary capillaritis; kidney: pauci-immune or diffuse necrotizing GN similar to Wegener's; skin: necrotizing arteritis of arterioles	High-dose corticosteroids + cyclophosphamide OR rituximab Following remission, those treated w/cyclophosphamide should transition to azathioprine or wkly MTX
Churg-Strauss Syndrome	Systemic vasculitis in the spectrum of hypereosinophilic disorders	Most often occurs in setting of antecedent asthma, allergic rhinitis, sinusitis Eosinophilia (>10%) Migratory pulmonary infiltrates Fever, arthralgias, myalgias, purpura **Dx:** P-ANCA (50%); usually have pauci-immune GN and mononeuritis Established by bx and confirmed eosinophilic tissue infiltration	High-dose corticosteroids allow full remission in 80-90% Oral or IV cyclophosphamide is recommended in pts w/neuro, GI, renal, or cardiac involvement Maintenance Rx w/azathioprine or MTX for 12-18 mo following remission
Henoch-Schönlein Purpura	"Systemic" IgA nephropathy Usually occurs in children In men >50 yr old, look out for association w/ solid tumors or MDS	Palpable purpura affecting distal LEs Abdominal pain, arthritis Hematuria/proteinuria Usually self-limiting **Dx:** Confirm w/bx of affected tissue (skin, lung, kidney): skin: shows presence of leukocytoclastic vasculitis w/IgA deposits; kidney: GN w/IgA deposition	Short course of moderate-dose steroids (20-40 mg/day of prednisone) Decreases duration and severity of skin and joint symptoms associated w/HSP In patients w/proliferative GN give high-dose steroids and monthly cyclophosphamide

TABLE 12-1 ■ Systemic Vasculitis—cont'd			
Small-Vessel	Pathophysiology	Clinical Features/Dx	Management
Essential Cryoglobulinemic Vasculitis	Immunoglobulins that precipitate from serum in the cold Type I cryoglobulins: monoclonal, self-aggregate, associated w/Waldenström's and MM; associated w/hyperviscosity Type II cryoglobulins: monoclonal IgM or IgA rheumatoid factors that bind to Fc of IgG, associated w/hep C and HIV Type II cryoglobulins: seen in setting of auto-immune disorders (SLE, Sjögren's, RA)	Palpable purpura, mononeuritis multiplex LAD, HSM Renal failure ± GN **Dx:** ↓C3, C4 (immune-complex GN) **80%** of type-II cryoglobulinemic vasculitis is associated w/hep C	Hep C–associated cryoglobulinemia responds to antiviral therapy w/interferon alfa + ribavirin Short course of corticosteroids In patients with renal failure, digital gangrene, neuro disease, 2-3-wk course of plasma exchange recommended
Cutaneous Leukocytoclastic Vasculitis	Seen in pts w/connective tissue diseases and as a reaction to drugs/viruses 40% idiopathic 60% ± autoimmune disease (SLE), drugs, infection, hematologic malignancy	Palpable purpura, tender nodules, persistent urticaria, or shallow ulcers Lesions seen most commonly on distal LEs **Dx:** Neutrophils and mononuclear cells invading the walls of dermal capillaries, arterioles, and venules seen on bx	Removal of offending drugs or treatment of the infectious etiology Favorably responds to NSAIDs, colchicine, or dapsone Manage urticarial lesions w/combining antihistamines (H_1 and H_2 blockers)

*Vasculitis: Inflammation of blood vessel walls that causes vessel narrowing/occlusion, aneurysm, or rupture.

Etiology

■ The exact etiology and pathogenesis are uncertain.
■ Genetic susceptibility to lupus is likely inherited as a polygenic trait. Multiple genetic linkages including 1q23, 2q35-37, 6p21-11, and 12q24 show strong associations with SLE. Environmental factors such as ultraviolet light exposure and Epstein-Barr virus infection may have a triggering role. Autoantibodies can be present years before the diagnosis of SLE. Evidence supports the improper processing of nuclear proteins and nucleic acid from programmed cell death. This leads to the presentation of self-DNA to plasmacytoid dendritic cells. Plasmacytoid dendritic cells propagate antibody and immune complex production and other arms of specific autoimmunity.

Diagnosis

H&P

■ Constitutional: unexplained fever, fatigue, malaise
■ Skin: malar rash sparing nasolabial folds (**acute cutaneous lupus**), annular or papulosquamous rash (**subacute cutaneous lupus**), raised erythematous patches with subsequent edematous plaques and adherent scales (**discoid cutaneous lupus**); alopecia, nasal, or oropharyngeal ulcerations; Raynaud's phenomenon; petechiae, palpable purpura, skin ulceration, or digital ischemia (**vasculitis**); livedo reticularis or livedo racemosa (secondary antiphospholipid antibody syndrome)
■ Musculoskeletal: arthritis (tenderness, swelling, effusion) typically affecting peripheral joints; myositis
■ Cardiac: pericardial rub (pericarditis), heart murmur (**Libman-Sachs endocarditis** and other valvular heart disease), congestive heart failure (myocarditis), premature atherosclerotic heart disease
■ Pulmonary: pleuritis, pneumonitis, diffuse alveolar hemorrhage
■ Gastrointestinal: abdominal pain, intestinal vasculitis, ascites
■ Neurologic: headache, psychosis, seizure, acute confusional states, peripheral or cranial neuropathy, transverse myelitis, CVA, chronic cognitive impairment
■ Hematologic: anemia (hemolytic, anemia of chronic disease, aplastic anemia), thrombocytopenia, leukopenia, lymphadenopathy, secondary antiphospholipid antibody syndrome
■ Renal: ARF, proteinuria, nephritic syndrome, nephrotic syndrome

W/Up

■ The diagnosis of SLE is suspected when any *four or more* of the following 1997 American College of Rheumatology criteria are present:
  • Malar rash
  • Discoid rash
  • Photosensitivity (recurrence of unusual skin rash in sun exposed areas)
  • Oral or nasopharyngeal painless ulceration
  • Arthritis
  • Serositis (pleuritis, pericarditis)
  • Renal disorder (persistent proteinuria >0.5 g/day, or 3+ on dipstick if quantitation not performed; cellular casts)
  • Neurologic disorder (seizures, psychosis [in absence of offending drugs or metabolic derangement])
  • Hematologic disorder:
    ■ Hemolytic anemia with reticulocytosis
    ■ Leukopenia (<4000/mm³ total on two or more occasions)
    ■ Lymphopenia (<1500/mm³ on two or more occasions)
    ■ Thrombocytopenia (<100,000/mm³ in the absence of offending drugs)
  • Immunologic disorder:
    ■ Anti–double-stranded DNA antibody (Anti-dsDNA)
    ■ Anti-Smith antibody (Anti-Sm)
    ■ Antiphospholipid antibodies (anticardiolipin IgM or IgG, lupus anticoagulant, or false(+) fluorescent treponemal antibody absorption test or *Treponema pallidum* immobilization for 6 mo)
    ■ Antinuclear antibody (ANA): an abnormal titer of ANA by immunofluorescence or equivalent assay at any time in the absence of drugs known to be associated with drug-induced lupus syndrome

Labs

■ Suggested initial laboratory evaluation of suspected SLE:
  • CBC w/diff, BUN, creat, urinalysis, ESR, PT, PTT, complements (C3, C4, CH50)
  • ANA

- Consider additional laboratory testing:
  - Anti-dsDNA, anti-Sm, anti-SSA, anti-SSB, anti-RNP antibodies
  - Lupus anticoagulant, anticardiolipin antibodies especially in pts with thrombotic events
  - Random spot urine protein–to–urine creatinine ratio, 24-hour urine protein collection if proteinuria

Imaging
- CXR for evaluation of pulmonary involvement (pleural effusion, pulmonary infiltrates)
- ECG for complaint of unexplained chest pain
- Echo if unexplained murmur, evidence of new or unexplained congestive heart failure, or suspected pericarditis

Treatment
- Defined courses of corticosteroids are useful for a variety of SLE symptoms.
- Immunosuppressive drugs such as MTX or azathioprine are used as steroid-sparing drugs.
- Joint pain and mild serositis are generally well controlled with NSAIDs or low-dose corticosteroids. Hydroxychloroquine and MTX are also effective for arthritis. Leflunomide or anti-TNF agents may be considered for difficult arthritis.
- Cutaneous manifestations
  - Topical or intradermal corticosteroids are helpful for individual discoid lesions, especially in the scalp.
  - Hydroxychloroquine is efficacious. Some studies support a combination of quinacrine and hydroxychloroquine for refractory skin disease.
- Hematologic manifestations
  - Corticosteroids are first-line Rx.
  - Azathioprine can be used for thrombocytopenia or hemolytic anemia.
  - IV immunoglobulin and rituximab may be considered for severe leukopenia, autoimmune hemolytic anemia, or autoimmune thrombocytopenia.
- Central nervous system manifestations
  - Headaches are treated symptomatically.
  - Anticonvulsants and antipsychotics may be indicated.
  - Standard Rx for other neuropsychiatric SLE symptoms is not established.
- Renal disease (class III, IV, V lupus nephritis)
  - The use of high doses of IV cyclophosphamide with corticosteroids given at monthly intervals is more effective in preserving renal function than is treatment with glucocorticoids alone.
  - Increasingly, mycophenolate mofetil at higher doses has become the induction treatment of choice because of its improved tolerability and better fertility profile. Studies show that pts treated with mycophenolate mofetil as induction Rx have similar renal and nonrenal outcomes as compared with high-dose IV cyclophosphamide.
- Mycophenolate mofetil or azathioprine is used for maintenance Rx.
- Severe nonrenal organ disease
  - Evidence from systematic RCTs for nonrenal lupus treatment is comparatively limited.
  - High-dose IV cyclophosphamide is used as induction treatment. Azathioprine or mycophenolate mofetil may be used as maintenance drugs.
  - IV immunoglobulin may be considered in severe disease when concomitant infection is present.
  - Plasmapheresis may be considered in critical situations, but efficacy is not proven in controlled trials, and infectious complication is a substantial consideration.
- New Rx
  - Rituximab: RCTs for rituximab as an adjunct induction agent were (–) in terms of both renal and nonrenal outcomes. Other clinical trials have shown an improvement in certain SLE parameters with rituximab.
  - Belimumab: approved for Rx of active autoantibody(+) SLE in adults. It can modestly reduce disease activity and appears to have a glucocorticoid-sparing effect. Cost is a limiting factor (≈$35,000/yr).

III

DISEASES AND DISORDERS
12. Rheumatology

F. RHEUMATOID ARTHRITIS (RA)

Systemic autoimmune disease characterized by inflammatory polyarthritis, which affects peripheral joints, especially the small joints of the hands and feet. Chronic untreated inflammation may lead to joint erosions and joint destruction.

Etiology

- Unknown. It is likely that a combination of genetic and environmental factors lead to aberrant immune activation and inflammatory response in the joint. Stages of disease development presumably include:
  - Initiation of immune response. The trigger is unknown.
  - Perpetuation of inflammatory response involves migration of inflammatory cells into joint space, activation of macrophage-like and fibroblast-like synoviocytes, and development of "synovial pannus," a thickened synovial membrane.
  - The pannus releases proinflammatory cytokines (TNF-α, IL-1, IL-6, IL-8), as well as proteases, which erode cartilage and bone.
  - Many of the newer "biologic" DMARDs are engineered to target these cytokines.

Genetics

- Genetic factors account for more than 50% of risk of disease. RA is polygenic; identified genetic associations include *HLA-DRB1*, *PTPN22*, and *PADI4*.

Diagnosis

- The American College of Rheumatology and the European League Against Rheumatism developed newer classification criteria for RA. Four variables constitute these criteria.
  - The number and size of involved joints (score 0 to 5, with higher scores for a larger number of small joints affected)
  - Results of RF and anti–citrullinated protein antibody testing (score 0 to 3, with more points for a high (+) RF or anti-CCP)
  - Abnormal ESR or elevated CRP (1 point)
  - Symptom duration >6 wk (1 point)
  - Scores ≥6 points are considered to have "definite RA." Max score is 10 points.

H&P

- Initial presentation:
  - Pts have >6 wk of pain, swelling, warmth in one or more peripheral joints, frequently with symmetric joint involvement involving wrists, hands and/or feet, and often associated with >1 hr of morning stiffness.
  - Most commonly involved joints include MCP, PIP, wrists, MTP, and ankles.
  - The elbows, shoulders, hips, and knees are also affected.
  - DIP joints are spared.
  - Sacroiliac and vertebral joints are spared except for C1 to C2.
- Chronic long-standing disease:
  - "*Swan-neck*" (DIP flexion and PIP hyperextension) and "*boutonniere*" (PIP flexion and DIP hyperextension) deformities occur, as well as MCP subluxation resulting in ulnar drift.
  - C1 to C2 inflammation can lead to odontoid erosion and transverse ligament laxity, resulting in atlantoaxial subluxation and cord compression.
  - Joint damage of wrists, elbows, shoulders, hips, and knees can lead to severe osteoarthritis, necessitating joint surgery and/or replacement.
- Extra-articular manifestations:
  - Secondary Sjögren's syndrome (~35%): immune-mediated inflammation of lacrimal and salivary glands resulting in dry mouth and eyes (*sicca syndrome*)
  - Rheumatoid nodules (25%): on extensor surfaces and pressure points, in RF(+) disease. Histopathology demonstrates palisading histiocytes surrounding fibrinoid necrosis.
  - Normocytic normochromic anemia
  - **Felty's syndrome:** RA with splenomegaly and leukopenia
  - Pulmonary disease
  - Pleural disease (effusions, pleuritis)
  - Interstitial lung disease (up to 10% clinically significant)
  - Vasculitis
- Cardiac disease
  - Pericarditis
  - ↑ Risk cardiovascular disease

- Ocular disease
  - Keratoconjunctivitis sicca (dry eye, without dry mouth/secondary Sjögren's syndrome) (10%)
  - Episcleritis, scleritis
  - Amyloidosis: long-standing RA; can affect heart, kidney, liver, spleen, intestines, and skin

Labs
- RF: an immunoglobulin directed against the Fc region of the IgG
  - Sensitivity <60%
  - Specificity <80%. False(+) results are seen with hep C, subacute bacterial endocarditis, sarcoidosis, malignancy, Sjögren's syndrome, SLE, increasing age
- Anti–cyclic citrullinated peptide (anti-CCP) antibodies. More specific than RF for rheumatoid arthritis (up to 95% to 98%). Sensitivity similar to RF. The presence of either RF or anti-CCP ("sero[+] RA") is associated with more severe RA.
- ↑ ESR, ↑ CRP
- CBC w/diff: possible mild anemia and leukocytosis
- Synovial fluid: inflammatory, with >2000 PMNs

Imaging
- Plain radiography:
  - Earlier changes include soft tissue swelling, joint space narrowing, and periarticular osteopenia.
  - Later changes include periarticular erosions, especially in MCPs, PIPs, MTPs, and wrist. This reflects cartilage and bone destruction secondary to pannus.
- MRI and musculoskeletal ultrasound are more sensitive for detecting erosive disease and joint effusion/synovitis.

Treatment
- Early identification and treatment of RA with DMARDs are crucial. More than half of pts have radiographic joint damage within 2 yr of disease onset, but early aggressive treatment (with DMARDs) is associated with less damage.
- NSAIDs: sometimes used initially to relieve pain and mild inflammation; may also be used later in the disease course for additional control of pain and inflammation. NSAIDs are *not* disease modifying.
- Corticosteroids: oral or intra-articular, frequently used initially to reduce inflammation rapidly until oral DMARD treatments take effect. They may also be used during acute flares or in low doses for additional control of inflammation. They have many side effects, including but not limited to weight gain and increased risk of diabetes, osteoporosis, and avascular necrosis.
- DMARDs can be classified into "nonbiologic" and "biologic" treatments.
- Nonbiologic DMARDs: commonly used agents are MTX, hydroxychloroquine, sulfasalazine, and leflunomide. Most of these are associated with potential toxicity and require close monitoring. They are also slow-acting drugs that require >8 wk to become fully effective.
- MTX is the most commonly used DMARD worldwide for the treatment of RA.
- "Triple Rx"(MTX, hydroxychloroquine, and sulfasalazine) is superior to MTX alone.
- Biologic DMARDs: newer biologically engineered therapies that target cytokines and cells involved in the RA inflammatory response. Major side effects include an increased risk of severe infection, most notably reactivation of TB with anti-TNF agents. A (–) PPD is prerequisite to initiate Rx. Biologic DMARDs are most effective when used in combination with a nonbiologic DMARD, usually MTX.
- TNF-α inhibitors (TNFIs): include infliximab, etanercept, adalimumab, certolizumab pegol, and golimumab
- Abatacept (CTLA-4Ig): a recombinant protein that prevents costimulatory binding of antigen presenting cell to T cell, thus preventing T-cell activation
- Tocilizumab (anti-IL6): a monoclonal antibody against the IL-6 receptor
- Rituximab (anti-CD20): a monoclonal antibody against CD20 antigen on B lymphocytes

G. SPONDYLOARTHROPATHIES

Table 12-2 compares spondyloarthropathies with RA.

Feature	Rheumatoid Arthritis	Ankylosing Spondylitis	Enteropathic Arthritis	Psoriatic Arthritis	Reactive Arthritis
Male-to-female ratio	1:3	3:1	1:1	1:1	10:1
HLA association	DR4	B27	B27 (axial)	B27 (axial)	B27
Joint pattern	Symmetric, peripheral	Axial	Axial and peripheral	Axial and asymmetric peripheral	Axial and asymmetric peripheral
Sacroiliac	0	Symmetric	Symmetric	Asymmetric	Asymmetric
Syndesmophyte	0	Smooth, marginal	Smooth, marginal	Coarse, non-marginal	Coarse, nonmarginal
Eye	Scleritis	Iritis	±	0	Iritis and conjunctivitis
Skin	Vasculitis	0	0	Psoriasis	Keratoderma
Rheumatoid factor	>80%	0	0	0	0

From Goldman L, Schafer AI (eds): Goldman's Cecil Medicine, 24th edition. Philadelphia, Saunders, 2012.

H. SYSTEMIC SCLEROSIS

Scleroderma (systemic sclerosis [SSc]) is a connective tissue disorder that is characterized by thickening and fibrosis of the skin and variably severe involvement of diverse internal organs. It can be subdivided into two major subgroups: (1) *limited cutaneous SSc (lcSSc),* which involves mainly the face, neck, arms, and hands, and (2) *diffuse cutaneous SSc (dcSSc),* which affects the skin in a more generalized distribution including the entire extremities, face, neck, and trunk. Both subgroups typically have characteristic internal organ involvement.

Etiology
- The etiology of this condition is unknown. Genetic profiles show clustering of different alleles according to the subtype of SSc. There is abnormal selection of fibroblasts and aberrant control of connective tissue synthesis by fibroblasts and other cells. Although there are characteristic autoantibodies detected, it is not clear that they directly participate in the pathogenesis of the disease.
- Extracellular connective tissue activation
- Frequent immunologic abnormalities including autoantibodies
- Inflammation in the early stages of disease
- Vasoconstriction

Diagnosis
Physical Findings
- Skin
  - Tightening of the skin begins on the hands and then progresses to the forearms, face, and neck; the skin is shiny, taut, and sometimes red, with a loss of creases and hair.
  - Later, skin tightening may limit movement by causing flexion contractures of the fingers, wrists, and elbows.
  - Pigmentary changes may occur.
  - Skin atrophy and digital gangrene of fingertips occurs during later stages.
- Musculoskeletal
  - Joint pain and swelling
  - Symmetric inflammatory arthritis
  - Myopathy
- Gastrointestinal involvement
  - Esophageal dysmotility with heartburn, dysphagia, and odynophagia
  - Delayed gastric emptying
  - Small bowel dysmotility with abdominal cramps and diarrhea
  - Colon dysmotility with constipation
  - Primary biliary cirrhosis

- Pulmonary manifestations
  - Pulmonary fibrosis with symptoms of dyspnea and nonproductive cough, as well as fine inspiratory crackles on examination
  - Pulmonary HTN
- Cardiac involvement
  - Myocardial fibrosis that leads to congestive heart failure
- Renal involvement
  - Malignant HTN
  - Rapidly progressive renal failure
- Other organ involvement
  - Hypothyroidism
  - Erectile dysfunction
  - Sjögren's syndrome
  - Entrapment neuropathies
- CREST syndrome (term now replaced by lcSSc)
  - **C**alcinosis, **R**aynaud's syndrome, **e**sophageal dysmotility, **s**clerodactyly, **t**elangiectasias—with CREST syndrome, scleroderma is limited to the distal extremities. This acronym is now considered obsolete by many because it does not accurately reflect the burden of internal organ involvement.

Clinical Presentation
- Raynaud's phenomenon: initial complaint in 70% of pts (The prevalence of Raynaud's phenomenon is 5% to 10% in the general population; most cases do not progress to scleroderma.)
- Finger or hand swelling that is sometimes associated with carpal tunnel syndrome
- Arthralgias/arthritis
- Internal organ involvement

Labs
- (+) Anti-Th/To antibodies with lcSSC (associated with PAH)
- Antinuclear antibodies (homogeneous, speckled, or nucleolar patterns) in both lcSSC and dcSSC
- (−) antibody to native DNA
- (−) anti–smooth muscle antibody
- Autoantibodies against ribonucleoprotein (+) in 20% of pts, anti-U3RNP with dcSSC (associated with PAH, myositis)
- RF (+) in 20% of pts
- Anticentromere antibodies in one third of pts with lcSSc
- (+) extractable nuclear antibody to Scl-70 in 40% of pts with dcSSc (also called anti-topoisomerase Ab, associated with ILD)
- Routine biochemistry tests may indicate specific organ involvement (e.g., liver, kidney, muscle)

Imaging
- Arthritis: joint radiographs
- Gastrointestinal
  - Endoscopy (diagnostic procedure of choice; may be therapeutic)
  - Cine-esophagography (in rare circumstances)
  - Barium swallow (occasionally indicated)
  - Esophageal manometry (almost never necessary)
- Pulmonary
  - CXR
  - PFTs (especially single-breath diffusion capacity for CO)
  - Chest CT
  - Bronchoscopy with biopsy
  - Gallium lung scan
  - Bronchoalveolar lavage
- Heart
  - ECG
  - Ambulatory (Holter) ECG monitoring
  - Echocardiography
  - Cardiac catheterization
- Kidney: renal biopsy
- Skin: skin biopsy

Treatment
- No disease-modifying Rx available. Immunosuppressive agents used in individual pts. Prednisone should be used with extreme caution, especially in doses >20 mg/day

- Raynaud's syndrome:
  - Ca^{2+} channel blockers (i.e., long-acting dihydropyridines)
  - Peripheral α_1-adrenergic blockers
  - Angiotensin II receptor blockers
  - Pentoxifylline
  - Phosphodiesterase inhibitors
  - Stellate ganglionic blockades
  - Digital sympathectomy
- Arthralgias: nonsteroidal anti-inflammatory drugs
- Skin: For extensive skin fibrosis, immunomodulatory drugs have been used such as MTX, mycophenolate, and cyclophosphamide but have not been proved to be beneficial.
- Esophageal reflux
  - H_2RB
  - PPIs
- Pulmonary HTN and fibrosis
  - O_2
  - Diuretics (with caution)
  - Endothelin-1 receptor inhibitors (bosentan, ambrisentan)
  - Sildenafil, tadalafil
  - Prostacyclin analogues (epoprostenol, iloprost, treprostinil)
  - Lung transplantation
  - Cyclophosphamide chemoRx for symptomatic scleroderma-related interstitial lung disease
- Renal involvement
  - ACEIs
  - Dialysis
  - Renal transplantation

I. ENTEROPATHIC ARTHRITIS

See Table 12-3.

TABLE 12-3 ■ Enteropathic Arthritis		
Feature	Peripheral Arthritis	Sacroiliitis, Spondylitis
Crohn's Disease (CD)		
Frequency in CD	10%-20%	2%-7%
HLA-B27 associated	No	Yes
Pattern	Transient, symmetric	Chronic
Course	Related to activity of CD	Unrelated to activity of CD
Effect of surgery	Remission of arthritis uncommon	No effect
Effect of anti-TNF therapy	Effective	Effective
Ulcerative Colitis (UC)		
Frequency in UC	5%-10%	2%-7%
HLA-B27 associated	No	Yes
Pattern	Transient	Chronic
Course	More common in pancolitis than proctitis; related to activity of UC	Unrelated
Effect of surgery	Remission of arthritis	No effect

From Goldman L, Schafer AI (eds): Goldman's Cecil Medicine, 24th edition. Philadelphia, Saunders, 2012.

J. CRYSTAL-INDUCED ARTHRITIDES

See Table 12-4.

1 GOUT

Disease characterized by deposition of monosodium urate crystals in and about joints, w/subsequent acute or chronic arthritis

Diagnosis

H&P

- The typical presentation is monarticular and characterized by sudden severe pain involving the first metatarsophalangeal joint (**podagra**), although the midtarsal and ankle are also frequently affected; any joint may be involved, but acute polyarthritis is uncommon.

TABLE 12-4 ■ Comparison of Crystal-Induced Arthritides

Crystal-Induced Arthritis	Characteristics of Crystals (from Joint Aspiration)	Commonly Involved Joints	Comments and Therapy
Gouty arthritis	Monosodium urate crystals	First metatarso-phalangeal, ankles, midfoot	See text
Ca²⁺ pyrophosphate deposition disease (pseudogout)	Ca²⁺ pyrophosphate dihydrate crystals Rhomboid or polymorphic, weakly positive, birefringent crystals	Knees, wrists	X-ray films of involved joint may reveal linear calcifications (chondrocalcinosis) on articular cartilage Possible associated conditions must be ruled out: Hyperparathyroidism Hypothyroidism Hemochromatosis Hypomagnesemia Therapy: NSAIDs, joint immobilization, intra-articular steroids
Hydroxyapatite arthropathy	Ca²⁺ hydroxyapatite crystals Crystals form nonbirefringent clumps w/synovial fluid when placed on slide Dx often requires microscopy because of the small size of the crystals	Knees, hips, shoulders	Usually affects younger pts than the other crystal-induced arthritides do Therapy: NSAIDs, joint immobilization, intra-articular steroids
Ca²⁺ oxalate–induced arthritis	Ca²⁺ oxalate crystals Bipyramidal, positive birefringent crystals	DIP, PIP joints of hands	Often seen in pts undergoing dialysis who take large doses of ascorbic acid (metabolized to oxalate) Therapy: NSAIDs, joint immobilization, intra-articular steroids

- PE reveals a warm, tender, swollen, erythematous joint; fever may be present, particularly if several joints are involved. Extensive soft tissue swelling, heat, and erythema extending to above and below the affected joint are frequently present and may be confused w/cellulitis.

Labs
- Serum uric acid level may be ↑, but it is often nl during the acute attack, later rising when the sx resolve.
- Aspiration and analysis of synovial fluid from the inflamed joint confirm the dx; examination of the fluid w/a polarized light microscope w/compensator reveals monosodium urate crystals (needle-shaped, strongly (–) birefringent crystals) w/ synovial fluid leukocytes.

Treatment
- NSAIDs: PO: indomethacin, naproxen, ibuprofen. Ketorolac may be given IM in NPO pts.
- Colchicine can be given PO or IV; PO dose is 1.2 mg followed by a second dose of 0.6 mg 1 hr later. IV administration has been associated w/risk of bone marrow suppression and renal or hepatic cell damage. Extravasation can also cause tissue necrosis.
- Glucocorticoids (triamcinolone acetonide or ACTH): reserved for pts w/ contraindications to NSAIDs or colchicine or if PO medication is precluded (e.g., postop). Triamcinolone acetonide, 60 mg IM; or ACTH, 40 IM or 25 by slow IV infusion. Intra-articular steroids may be used to treat a single inflamed joint (dexamethasone PO₄⁻³ 1-6 mg).
- Prednisone 20 to 40 mg PO qd can be used short term in pts refractory or intolerant to NSAIDs/colchicine or responding poorly to these agents.

- Xanthine oxidase inhibitors (allopurinol, febuxostat) are used in pts w/frequent recurrent attacks. Hypouricemic Rx should not be started for at least 4 wk after the acute attack has resolved because it may prolong the acute attack and can also precipitate new attacks by rapidly lowering the serum uric acid level.
- Colchicine, 0.6 mg PO bid, is indicated for acute gout prophylaxis before hypouricemic Rx is started. It is generally discontinued 6-8 wk after normalization of serum urate levels. Long-term colchicine Rx (0.6 mg qd or bid) may be necessary in pts w/frequent gout attacks despite the use of uricosuric agents. It can also be used as an alternative to uricosuric agents.

K. IDIOPATHIC INFLAMMATORY MYOPATHIES

See Table 12-5.

TABLE 12-5 ■ Classification of the Idiopathic Inflammatory Myopathies

Classification Group	Associated Clinical Features	Severity of Myositis	Response of Myositis to Therapy	Prognosis (5-yr Survival)
Clinical Groups				
Polymyositis	None of the features below	Variable	Variable	Moderate (~80%)
Dermatomyositis	Gottron's papules or heliotrope rash	Mild to moderate	Good	Moderate (~85%)
Connective tissue myositis	Overlap with other connective tissue diseases	Mild	Excellent	Good (~90%)
Cancer-associated myositis	Cancer diagnosed within 2 yr of idiopathic inflammatory myopathy	Variable	Moderate to poor	Poor, secondary to cancer (~60%)
Juvenile myositis	Dx before age 18 yr Dermatomyositis >> polymyositis Subcutaneous calcifications GI vasculitis	Variable	Moderate to good	Good (>95%)
Inclusion body myositis	Insidious onset in older white men Distal involvement, atrophy, and asymmetric weakness Poor response to therapy	Mild but progressive	Poor	Few deaths, but significant morbidity (>85%)
Serologic Groups				
Antisynthetases	Acute onset in polymyositis or dermatomyositis Interstitial lung disease, fever, dyspnea on exertion, arthritis, mechanic's hands, Raynaud's phenomenon	Moderate to severe	Moderate, but flares with taper	Poor (~75%)
Anti–signal recognition particle	Acute onset in black female pts Palpitations, cardiac disease, severe weakness No rash (clinically polymyositis)	Severe	Poor	Very poor (~30%)
Anti–Mi-2	Classic dermatomyositis "V" and "shawl" rashes, cuticular changes	Mild	Good	Good (>90%)

From Goldman L, Schafer AI (eds): Goldman's Cecil Medicine, 24th edition. Philadelphia, Saunders, 2012.

A. RHABDOMYOLYSIS

Acute or subacute event resulting in damage or necrosis of striated muscle

Etiology

- Trauma (e.g., crush syndrome, burns, electrical shock)
- Muscle ischemia (e.g., thrombosis, embolism, vasculitis, sickle cell disease, pressure necrosis, tourniquet shock)
- Drugs: Drug-induced rhabdo can occur through several mechanisms.
  - Primary, toxin induced (e.g., ethanol, methadone, ethylene glycol, isopropyl alcohol, CO poisoning)
  - Long-term intake of drugs associated w/hypokalemia (e.g., thiazides)
  - OD of certain drugs (e.g., barbiturates, heroin, cocaine)
  - Malignant hyperthermia (usually seen in genetically predisposed individuals, after exposure to halothane, succinylcholine, or pancuronium)
  - NMS (associated w/use of phenothiazines, butyrophenones, antipsychotics, cocaine, or diphenhydramine, usually in pts w/dehydration and electrolyte imbalance)
  - Use of certain lipid-lowering agents (e.g., combination of statins and gemfibrozil, or erythromycin and simvastatin; and amiodarone; amphetamines, haloperidol)
  - Direct myotoxicity (e.g., colchicine, zidovudine, cyclosporine, itraconazole)
- Infections
  - Bacterial (e.g., *Streptococcus, Salmonella, Clostridium, Legionella, Leptospira, Shigella*)
  - Viral (e.g., echo, coxsackie, influenza, CMV, herpes, EBV, hepatitis)
  - Parasites (trichinosis)
- Excessive muscle stress (e.g., marathon runners, status epilepticus, delirium tremens)
- Genetic defects (carnitine deficiency, phosphorylase deficiency, glucosidase deficiency, cytochrome disturbances)
- Miscellaneous: brown recluse spider bite, snake bite, hornet sting, polymyositis, dermatomyositis, heat stroke, DKA, hyponatremia, hypophosphatemia, myxedema, thyroid storm, RMSF, hypothermia, CO, cyclic antidepressants, phenylpropanolamine, codeine, phencyclidine (PCP), amphetamines, LSD, Reye's syndrome

Diagnosis

H&P

- Variable muscle tenderness. Rhabdo apart from statin use is manifested w/muscle sx only 50% of the time.
- Weakness
- Muscle rigidity
- Fever
- Altered consciousness
- Muscle swelling
- Malaise, fatigue. In statin-induced rhabdo, fatigue (74%) is nearly as common as muscle pain (88%).
- Dark urine (secondary to myoglobin in urine, will make dipstick false (+) for RBC's)

Labs

- ↑↑ CK: Elevations may exceed 100,000 U/L in fulminant rhabdo; the development of renal failure is not directly related to the threshold level of CK; isoenzyme fractionation is useful: if CK-MB >5% of the total CK, involvement of the myocardium is likely.
- ↑Serum Cr: The etiology of the renal failure is uncertain and probably multifactorial (renal tubular obstruction by precipitated myoglobin, direct myoglobin toxicity, hypotension, dehydration, ↓ GFR, intravascular coagulation).
- Serum K+: Preexisting hypokalemia is a contributing factor to rhabdo; fulminant rhabdo can result in life-threatening hyperkalemia secondary to ↑ K+ release from damaged muscle and impaired renal excretion.

- Ca^{2+} and PO_4^{-3}: Initially, pts have hyperphosphatemia from muscle necrosis, secondary hypocalcemia from Ca^{2+} deposition in the injured muscle, and ↓ 1,25-dihydroxycholecalciferol; later (in the diuretic phase of renal failure), hypercalcemia is present as a result of remobilization of the deposited Ca^{2+} and secondary hyperparathyroidism.
- Myoglobin: This is present in the serum and urine; the urine is brownish, has granular casts, and is O-toluidine(+); a quick visual method to separate myoglobinuria from hemoglobinuria is to examine the urine and serum simultaneously: reddish brown urine and pink serum indicate hemoglobinuria, whereas brown urine and clear serum suggest myoglobinuria; ↑ in serum myoglobin precedes the ↑ in CK level and is useful to estimate the risk of renal failure (serum myoglobin levels >2000 μg/L may be associated w/renal insufficiency).

Treatment
- Vigorous fluid replacement is given to maintain a good urinary output, at least until myoglobin disappears from the urine. Initially NS should be given at a rate of 1.5 L/hr w/close monitoring of cardiac, pulmonary, and electrolyte status. Maintain ↑ rate of IV fluids at least until CPK <1000 U/L. Pts may require >15 L of fluid in the initial 24 hr to achieve urine flow rates of 200 to 300 mL/hr.
- Administration of a single dose of mannitol (100 mL of a 25% solution IV during 15 min) remains controversial. Mannitol acts as an osmotic diuretic, renal vasodilator, and intravascular volume expander and may convert oliguric renal failure to nonoliguric.
- Alkalinization of the urine w/addition of 44 mEq/L of $NaHCO_3$ is advocated by some experts. The goal is to maintain urine pH >6.5. $NaHCO_3$ may ↑ solubility of uric acid and myoglobulin; however, it may promote Ca deposition.
- Hyperkalemia caused by rhabdo is most severe 10 to 40 hr after injury; initial treatment w/sodium polystyrene sulfonate may be indicated; hyperkalemia caused by rhabdo responds poorly to treatment w/glucose and insulin; attempts to correct hyperkalemia and initial hypocalcemia w/Ca infusion may result in metastatic calcifications and severe hypercalcemia in the recovery period; hemodialysis may be necessary in pts w/severe hyperkalemia, volume overload, uremic pericarditis, or uremic encephalopathy.

Clinical Pearls
- The average length of time on statin Rx before rhabdo is 1 yr. The average time to onset of rhabdo after addition of fibrate to statin Rx is 32 days.
- Statin-induced rhabdo is 12× more frequent when statins are combined w/fibrates compared w/statin monoRx.

B. SHOCK

- Figure 13-1 defines shock and its various causes.
- Box 13-1 describes the physical exam and selected lab signs in shock.
- Table 13-1 illustrates the physiologic response and basic Rx of shock.
- Figure 13-2 is an algorithmic approach to the general hemodynamic management of shock.
- Table 13-2 describes the action of various vasopressor agents used in shock.

C. HYPOTHERMIA

DEFINITION
Rectal temperature <35° C (95.8° F). *Accidental hypothermia* is unintentionally induced in ↓ core temperature in absence of preoptic anterior hypothalamic conditions.
Diagnosis
H&P
- The clinical presentation varies w/the severity of hypothermia; shivering may be absent if body temperature is <33.3° C (92° F) or in pts taking phenothiazines.
- Hypothermia may masquerade as CVA, ataxia, or slurred speech, or the pt may appear comatose or clinically dead.
- Physiologic stages of hypothermia:
  - Mild hypothermia (32.2° C-35° C [90° F-95° F]): arrhythmias, ataxia
  - Moderate hypothermia (28° C-32.2° C [82.4° F-90° F]): progressive ↓ of level of consciousness, pulse, CO, and respiration; fibrillation, dysrhythmias (susceptibility to VT); elimination of shivering mechanism for thermogenesis

Shock	Hypovolemic	Cardiogenic	Extracardiac/Obstructive	Distributive	Dissociative
Definition	Blood or fluid loss, both leading to a decreased circulating blood volume, diastolic filling pressure, and volume.	Severe reduction in cardiac function resulting from direct myocardial damage or a mechanical abnormality of the heart.	Obstruction to flow in the cardiovascular circuit that leads to inadequate diastolic filling or decreased systolic function because of increased afterload.	Arterial and venous dilation leads to a decrease in preload, with decreased, normal, or elevated cardiac output, depending on the presence of myocardial depression. Inflammatory causes produce microcirculatory dysfunction, hypotension, and multiple organ system dysfunction without a decrease in cardiac output.	Impairment of oxygen utilization or impairment of the cellular machinery.
Etiologies	**Hemorrhagic:** Trauma Gastrointestinal Retroperitoneal Postoperative surgical procedures **Fluid depletion (non-hemorrhagic):** External fluid loss Dehydration Vomiting Diarrhea Polyuria **Interstitial fluid redistribution:** Thermal injury Trauma Anaphylaxis **Increased vascular capacitance (venodilation):** Sepsis Anaphylaxis Toxins/drugs	**Myopathic:** Myocardial infarction Left ventricle Right ventricle **Myocardial contusion (trauma):** Myocarditis Cardiomyopathy Postischemic myocardial stunning Septic myocardial depression Pharmacologic Anthracycline cardiotoxicity Calcium channel blockers **Mechanical:** Valvular failure (stenotic or regurgitant) Hypertrophic cardiomyopathy Ventricular septal defect **Arrhythmias:** Bradycardia Tachycardia	**Impaired diastolic filling (decreased ventricular preload):** Direct venous obstruction (vena cava) Intrathoracic obstructive tumors **Increased intrathoracic pressure:** Tension pneumothorax Mechanical ventilation (with excessive pressure or volume depletion) Asthma **Decreased cardiac compliance:** Constrictive pericarditis Cardiac tamponade **Impaired systolic contraction (increased ventricular afterload):** Right ventricle Pulmonary embolus (massive) Air embolus Acute pulmonary hypertension Left ventricle occlusion or aortic dissection	Septic (bacterial, fungal, viral, rickettsial) Toxic shock syndrome Anaphylactic anaphylactoid Neurogenic (spinal shock) Endocrinologic Adrenal crisis Thyroid storm	Toxic (e.g., nitroprusside, bretylium, cyanide) End-stage sepsis Catecholamine toxicity

FIGURE 13-1. Shock. *(From Goldman L, Schafer AI [eds]: Goldman's Cecil Medicine, 24th ed. Philadelphia, Saunders, 2012.)*

Central nervous system	Acute delirium, restlessness, disorientation, confusion, and coma, which may be secondary to decreased cerebral perfusion pressure (mean arterial pressure minus intracranial pressure). Pts with chronic hypertension or increased intracranial pressure may be symptomatic at normal blood pressures. Cheyne-Stokes respirations may be seen with severe decompensated heart failure. Blindness can be a presenting complaint or complication.
Temperature	Hyperthermia results in excess tissue respiration and greater systemic oxygen delivery requirements. Hypothermia can occur when decreased systemic oxygen delivery or impaired cellular respiration decreases heat generation.
Skin	Cool distal extremities (combined low serum bicarbonate and high arterial lactate levels) aid in identifying pts with hypoperfusion. Pallor, cyanosis, sweating, and decreased capillary refill and pale, dusky, or clammy extremities indicate systemic hypoperfusion. Dry mucous membranes and decreased skin turgor indicate low vascular volume. Low toe temperature correlates with the severity of shock.
General cardio-vascular	Neck vein distention (e.g., heart failure, pulmonary embolus, pericardial tamponade) or flattening (e.g., hypovolemia), tachycardia, and arrhythmias. Decreased coronary perfusion pressures can lead to ischemia, decreased ventricular compliance, and increased left ventricular diastolic pressure. A "mill wheel" heart murmur may be heard with an air embolus.
Heart rate	Usually elevated. However, paradoxical bradycardia can be seen in pts with preexisting cardiac disease and severe hemorrhage. Heart rate variability is associated with poor outcomes.
Systolic blood pressure	May actually increase slightly when cardiac contractility increases in early shock and then fall as shock advances. A single episode of undifferentiated hypotension with a systolic blood pressure <80 mm Hg carries an in-hospital mortality of 18%.
Diastolic blood pressure	Correlates with arteriolar vasoconstriction and may rise early in shock and then fall when cardiovascular compensation fails
Pulse pressure	Defined as systolic minus diastolic pressure and related to stroke volume and the rigidity of the aorta. It increases early in shock and decreases before systolic pressure decreases.
Pulsus para-doxus	An exaggerated change in systolic blood pressure with respiration (systolic blood pressure declines >10 mm Hg with inspiration) seen in asthma, cardiac tamponade, and air embolus
Mean arterial blood pressure	Diastolic blood pressure + [pulse pressure/3]
Shock index	Heart rate/systolic blood pressure. Normal = 0.5 to 0.7. A persistent elevation of the shock index (>1.0) indicates impaired left ventricular function (as a result of blood loss and/or cardiac depression) and is associated with increased mortality.
Respiratory	Tachypnea, increased minute ventilation, increased dead space, bronchospasm, hypocapnia with progression to respiratory failure, acute lung injury, and adult respiratory distress syndrome
Abdomen	Low-flow states may result in abdominal pain, ileus, gastrointestinal bleeding, pancreatitis, acalculous cholecystitis, mesenteric ischemia, and shock liver
Renal	Because the kidney receives 20% of cardiac output, low cardiac output reduces the glomerular filtration rate and redistributes renal blood flow from the renal cortex toward the renal medulla, leading to oliguria. Paradoxical polyuria in sepsis may be confused with adequate hydration.
Metabolic	Respiratory alkalosis is the first acid-base abnormality, but metabolic acidosis occurs as shock progresses. Hyperglycemia, hypoglycemia, and hyperkalemia may develop.

From Goldman L, Schafer AI (eds): Goldman's Cecil Medicine, 24th ed. Philadelphia, Saunders, 2012.

TABLE 13-1 ■ Types of Shock, Physiologic Response, and Basic Treatment

Type of Shock	HR	Preload	Contractility	SVR	Treatment
Hypovolemic	↑	↓↓	±	↑	■ High-flow oxygen ■ Fluid resuscitation: evaluate perfusion after 60 mL/kg total volume bolused, then consider pressors
Septic (early, warm)	↑	↓↓	±	↓	■ High-flow oxygen ■ Fluid resuscitation ■ Antibiotics ■ Pressors (dopamine, norepinephrine, phenylephrine)
Septic (late, cold)	↑	↓↓	↓	↑	■ High-flow oxygen ■ Fluid resuscitation ■ Antibiotics ■ Pressors (dopamine, norepinephrine, phenylephrine)
Anaphylactic	↑	↓↓	↓	↓	■ High-flow oxygen ■ Epinephrine (IM) ■ Fluid resuscitation
Neurogenic	↑	↓↓	±	↓↓	■ Fluid resuscitation ■ Pressors (norepinephrine)
Cardiogenic	↑	↑	↓↓	↑	■ High-flow oxygen ■ Fluid resuscitation (5-10 mL/kg) ■ CHF management (CPAP/BiPAP, diuretics, ACE inhibitors) ■ Inotropes (milrinone, dobutamine)
Obstructive	Cause dependent	Cause dependent	Cause dependent	Cause dependent	■ Therapy directed at primary etiology of shock

From Tschudy MM, Arcara KM: The Harriet Lane Handbook, 19th ed. Philadelphia, Mosby, 2012.

- Severe hypothermia (<28° C [82.4° F]): absence of reflexes or response to pain, ↓ cerebral blood flow, ↓ CO_2, risk of VF or asystole

Labs
- Metabolic acidosis and respiratory acidosis are usually present. ↓ K+ initially, then ↑ K+ w/↓ temp; extreme hyperkalemia indicates a poor prognosis; ↓ Hct (caused by hemoconcentration), ↓ leukocytes, ↓ Plt (caused by splenic sequestration), ↑ clotting time

Imaging
- CXR: generally not helpful; may reveal evidence of aspiration (e.g., intoxicated pt w/aspiration pneumonia)
- ECG (Fig. 13-3): ↑ PR, QT, and QRS segments; ↑ ST segments, inverted T waves, AV block; hypothermic J waves (*Osborn waves*), characterized by notching of the junction of the QRS complex and ST segments, may appear at 25° C to 30° C.

Treatment
- Secure an airway before warming all unconscious pts; precede ETT w/oxygenation (if possible) to ↓ the risk of arrhythmias during the procedure.
- Peripheral vasoconstriction may impede placement of a peripheral IV catheter; consider femoral venous access as an alternative to the jugular or subclavian sites to avoid ventricular stimulation.
- A Foley catheter should be inserted, and urinary output should be monitored and maintained >0.5 to 1 mL/kg/hr w/intravascular volume replacement.
- Continuous ECG monitoring of pts is recommended; consider ventricular arrhythmia Rx w/bretylium; lidocaine is generally ineffective, and procainamide is associated w/incidence of VF in hypothermic pts.

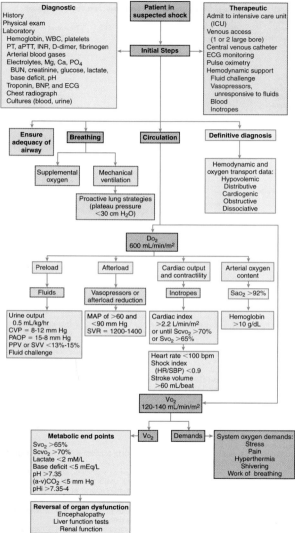

FIGURE 13-2. General hemodynamic management. Do₂, (system) oxygen delivery; PAOP, pulmonary artery occlusion pressure; pHi, intestinal mucosal pH; PPV, pulse pressure variation; SVV, stroke volume variation; Vo₂, (systemic) oxygen consumption. *(From Goldman L, Schafer AI [eds]: Goldman's Cecil Medicine, 24th ed. Philadelphia, Saunders, 2012.)*

TABLE 13-2 ■ Vasopressor Agents							
		Peripheral Vasculature			Cardiac Effects		
Agent	Dose Range	Vasoconstriction	Vasodilation	HR	Contractility	Dysrhythmias	Typical Use
Dopamine	1-4 μg/kg/min	0	1+	1+	1+	1+	"Renal dose" does not improve renal function; may be used with bradycardia and hypotension
	5-10 μg/kg/min	1-2+	1+	2+	2+	2+	
	11-20 μg/kg/min	2-3+	1+	2+	2+	3+	Vasopressor range
Vasopressin	0.04-0.1 U/min	3-4+	0	0	0	1+	Septic shock, post-cardiopulmonary bypass shock state; no outcome benefit in sepsis
Phenylephrine	20-200 μg/min	4+	0	0	0	1+	Vasodilatory shock; best for supraventricular tachycardia
Norepinephrine	1-20 μg/min	4+	0	2+	2+	2+	First-line vasopressor for septic shock, vasodilatory shock
Epinephrine	1-20 μg/min	4+	0	4+	4+	4+	Refractory shock, shock with bradycardia, anaphylactic shock
Dobutamine	1-20 μg/kg/min	1+	2+	1-2+	3+	3+	Cardiogenic shock, septic shock
Milrinone	37.5-75 μg/kg bolus followed by 0.375-0.75 μg/min	0	2+	1+	3+	2+	Cardiogenic shock, right heart failure; dilates pulmonary artery; caution in renal failure

From Goldman L, Schafer AI (eds): Goldman's Cecil Medicine. 24th ed. Philadelphia, Saunders, 2012.

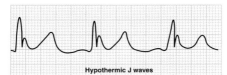

FIGURE 13-3. Hypothermic J waves. *(From Ferri F, Practical Guide to the Care of the Medical Patient, 8th ed, St. Louis, Mosby 2011)*

- Correct severe acidosis and electrolyte abnlities.
- Hypothyroidism, if present, should be promptly treated (refer to the section on myxedema coma in Chapter 5).
- If clinical evidence suggests adrenal insufficiency, administer IV methylprednisolone.
- In pts unresponsive to verbal or noxious stimuli or w/ΔMS, 100 mg of thiamine, 0.4 mg of naloxone, and 1 ampule of 50% dextrose may be given.
- Warm (104° F-113° F [40° C-45° C]), humidified O_2 should also be given if it is available.
- Specific treatment:
  - Mild hypothermia (rectal temperature <32.3° C [90° F]): Passive external rewarming is indicated. Place the pt in a warm room (temperature >21° C [69.8° F]) and cover w/insulating material after gently removing wet clothing; recommended rewarming rates vary between 0.5° C and 20° C/hr but should not exceed 0.55° C/hr in elderly pts.
  - Moderate to severe hypothermia: delivery of heat through fluids: Methods include warm GI irrigation (w/saline enemas and by NG tube), IV fluids (usually D_5NS w/o K^+) warmed to 104° F to 107.6° F (40° C-42° C), peritoneal dialysis w/dialysate heated to 40.5° C to 42.5° C, and inhalation of heated humidified O_2. Consider immersion in a bath of warm water (40° C-41° C); active external rewarming may produce shock because of excessive peripheral vasodilation. Ideal candidates are previously healthy, young pts w/acute immersion hypothermia. Extracorporeal blood warming w/cardiopulmonary bypass appears to be an efficacious rewarming technique in young, otherwise healthy pts.

D. HEAT STROKE

DEFINITION

Life-threatening heat illness characterized by extreme hyperthermia, dehydration, and neurologic manifestations (core temperature >40° C [104° F])

Diagnosis

H&P

- Neurologic manifestations (seizures, tremor, hemiplegia, coma, psychosis, and other bizarre behavior)
  - Evidence of dehydration (poor skin turgor, sunken eyeballs)
  - Tachycardia, hyperventilation
  - Hot, red, and flushed skin
  - Sweating often (not always) absent, particularly in elderly pts

Labs

- ↑ BUN, Cr, Hct
- Hyponatremia or hypernatremia, hyperkalemia or hypokalemia
- ↑ LDH, AST, ALT, CPK, bili
- Lactic acidosis, respiratory alkalosis (secondary to hyperventilation)
- Myoglobinuria, hypofibrinogenemia, fibrinolysis, hypocalcemia

Treatment

- Remove the pt's clothes, and place the pt in a cool and well-ventilated room.
- If the pt is unconscious, position the pt on his/her side and clear the airway. Protect the airway and augment oxygenation (e.g., nasal O_2 at 4 L/min to keep Sao_2 >90%).
- Monitor body temperature q5min. Measurement of the pt's core temperature w/ rectal probe is recommended. Goal is to ↓ the body temperature to 39° C (102.2° F) in 30 to 60 min.

- Spray the pt w/cool mist, and use fans to enhance airflow over the body (rapid evaporation method).
- Immersion of the pt in ice water, stomach lavage w/iced saline solution, IV administration of cooled fluids, and inhalation of cold air are advisable only when the means for rapid evaporation are not available. Immersion in tepid water (15° C [59° F]) is preferred to ice water immersion to minimize risk of shivering.
- Use of ice packs on axillae, neck, and groin is controversial because the resulting peripheral vasoconstriction may induce shivering.
- Antipyretics are ineffective because the hypothalamic set point during heat stroke is nl despite the body temperature.
- Intubate a comatose pt, insert a Foley catheter, and start nasal O_2.
- Continuous ECG monitoring is recommended.
- Insert at least two large-bore IV lines, and begin IV hydration w/NS or lactated Ringer's solution.
- Treat complications as follows:
  - Hypotension: Administer vigorous hydration w/NS or lactated Ringer's solution.
  - Convulsions: Give diazepam 5 to 10 mg IV (slowly).
  - Shivering: Give chlorpromazine 10 to 50 mg IV.
  - Acidosis: Use bicarbonate judiciously (only in severe acidosis).
  - Observe for evidence of rhabdo, hepatic, renal, or cardiac failure and treat accordingly.

E. MALIGNANT HYPERTHERMIA

DEFINITION

Muscle rigidity and elevated temperature in the setting of recently administered anesthetic agents, most commonly halogenated inhalation agents (halothane) or depolarizing muscle relaxants (succinylcholine)

Etiology

In genetically susceptible individuals, administration of anesthetic agents results in release of Ca^{2+} from the sarcoplasmic reticulum of skeletal muscles that causes muscle rigidity and hypermetabolism. This leads to significant heat production that overwhelms the body's normal ability to dissipate heat.

Diagnosis

H&P
- Within minutes to hours after anesthetic is given, the pt develops muscle rigidity (especially masseter spasm), hyperthermia (≤45° C), tachycardia that may progress to other dysrhythmias, and hypotension. Skin initially reddens but then becomes cyanotic and mottled. There is also increased CO_2 production.
- Rhabdomyolysis, acute renal failure, and DIC may soon follow.

Labs
- CBC, TSH, electrolytes (especially K^+, Ca^{2+}, and phosphorus), PT, PTT, BUN, creat, ALT, AST, and CK

Treatment
- The most important measures for treatment include stopping the anesthetic agents, starting dantrolene, ensuring physical cooling, and preventing sequelae. Antipyretics are not useful because the hypothalamic set point is not altered by cytokines.
- Cool the pt w/an ice bath, ice packs in the groin and axillae, cool spray with fans, or cooling blankets. In severe instances extracorporeal partial bypass or iced peritoneal lavage may be used. Stop cooling when core temperature reaches 38° C to prevent overcooling.
- Carefully monitor the pt's cardiovascular and respiratory status with constant core temperature measurements.
- Dantrolene is the mainstay of treatment, starting with a bolus of 5 mg/kg IV, which should be repeated every 5 min until symptoms abate or a maximum of 10 to 20 mg/kg is reached. Then 24 hr of 10 mg/kg/day IV should be given.
- β-Blockers or lidocaine may be useful for dysrhythmias, but verapamil should be avoided because its use with dantrolene has been shown to depress cardiac function.
- $NaHCO_3$ may be necessary to reverse acidosis.
- Aggressive hydration with forced diuresis and urine alkalinization should be instituted as treatment for rhabdomyolysis.

F. NEUROLEPTIC MALIGNANT SYNDROME (NMS)

Disorder characterized by hyperthermia, muscle rigidity, autonomic dysfunction, and depressed/fluctuating levels of arousal that evolve during 24 to 72 hr

Etiology
- Neuroleptic drugs have different potencies for inducing NMS:
  - Typical neuroleptics: high potency, haloperidol; medium potency, chlorpromazine, fluphenazine; low potency, levomepromazine, loxapine
  - Atypical neuroleptics: low potency, risperidone, olanzapine, clozapine, quetiapine

Diagnosis
H&P
- Muscle rigidity (hypertonia, cogwheeling, or "lead pipe" rigidity)
- Hyperthermia (38.6° C-42.3° C, usually <40° C)
- Autonomic sx: diaphoresis, sialorrhea, skin pallor, urinary incontinence
- Tachycardia, tachypnea
- Labile BP (HTN or postural hypotension)
- ΔMS (agitation, catatonia, fluctuating consciousness, obtundation)

Labs
- ↑ CPK (>71% of pts, w/mean value of 3700 U/L)
- Urinary myoglobin
- Leukocytosis, usually 10,000 to 40,000/mm^3
- Electrolytes and renal function
- ABGs
- Drug levels

Treatment
- Stop all neuroleptic agents, and reinstitute any recently discontinued dopaminergic agents.
- Initiate active cooling (cooling blanket and antipyretics).
- IV benzos (e.g., diazepam 2-10 mg, w/total daily dose of 10-60 mg) are given to relax muscles and to control agitation.
- Bromocriptine 2.5 to 10 mg IV q8h and by 5 mg/day is given until clinical improvement is seen. The drug should be continued for ≥10 days after the syndrome has been controlled and then tapered slowly.
- Dantrolene 0.25 mg/kg IV q6-12h is followed by a maintenance dose up to 3 mg/kg/day. After 2 to 3 days, pts may be given the drug PO (25-600 mg/day in divided doses). Oral dantrolene Rx (50-600 mg/day) may be continued for several days afterward.
- Electroconvulsive Rx w/neuromuscular blockage is indicated in pharmacologically refractory cases. Succinylcholine should not be used because it may cause hyperkalemia and cardiac arrhythmias in pts w/rhabdo or dysautonomia.

G. ANAPHYLAXIS

Sudden-onset, life-threatening event characterized by respiratory, cardiovascular, GI, and cutaneous manifestations, as well as vasodilatory hemodynamic changes in response to a particular allergen

Etiology
- Caused by sudden systematic release of histamine and other inflammatory mediators from basophils and mast cells → swelling of the mucous membranes and urticarial rash on the skin. Virtually any substance may induce anaphylaxis.
- Foods and food additives: peanuts, tree nuts, eggs, shellfish, fish, cow's milk, fruits, soy
- Medications: antibiotics, especially penicillins, insulin, allergen extracts, opiates, vaccines, NSAIDs, contrast media, streptokinase
- Bee or wasp sting, snake venom, fire ant venom
- Blood products, plasma, immunoglobulin, cryoprecipitate, whole blood
- Latex

Diagnosis
H&P

- Urticaria, pruritus, skin flushing, angioedema
- Dyspnea, cough, wheezing, shortness of breath

- Nausea, vomiting, diarrhea, difficulty swallowing
- Hypotension, tachycardia, weakness, dizziness, malaise, vascular collapse

Differential Diagnosis
- Endocrine disorders (carcinoid, pheochromocytoma)
- Globus hystericus, anxiety disorder
- Systemic mastocytosis
- PE, serum sickness, vasovagal reactions
- Severe asthma (the key clinical difference is the abrupt onset of symptoms in anaphylaxis versus a history of progressive worsening of symptoms)
- Septic shock or other form of vasodilatory shock
- Airway foreign body

Labs
- Generally tests are not helpful because anaphylaxis is typically diagnosed clinically.
- ABG analysis may be useful to exclude PE, status asthmaticus, and foreign body aspiration.
- ↑ Serum and urine histamine levels and serum tryptase levels can be useful for dx of anaphylaxis, but these tests are not commonly available in the emergency setting.

Imaging
- Imaging is generally not helpful.
- CXRs for evaluation of foreign body aspiration or pulmonary disease are indicated in pts with acute respiratory compromise.
- Consider ECG in all pts with sudden loss of consciousness, chest pain, dyspnea and in any elderly pt. ECG in anaphylaxis usually reveals sinus tachycardia.

Treatment
- Establish and protect the airway. Provide supplemental O_2 if indicated.
- IV access should be rapidly established, and IV fluids (i.e., NS) should be administered. The pt should be placed supine or in Trendelenburg's position if hemodynamically unstable.
- Cardiac monitoring is recommended.
- Epinephrine: IM injection at a dose of 0.3 mg of aqueous epinephrine for adults and children >30 kg. Epinephrine 0.15 mg should be given for children <30 kg (1:1000 concentration). IM is preferred because it provides more reliable and quicker rise to effective plasma levels. The dose may be repeated after ≈5 to 15 min if symptoms persist.
- Adjunct therapies: These include H_1 and H_2 receptor antagonists, diphenhydramine 25 to 50 mg IV or IM, or PO in mild cases, and famotidine 20 to 40 mg IV, or PO in mild cases.
- Corticosteroids are not useful in the acute episode because of their slow onset of action; however, they should be administered in most cases to prevent prolonged or recurrent anaphylaxis. Commonly used agents are prednisone, methylprednisolone 40 to 250 mg IV in adults (1-2 mg/kg in children), or longer-acting dexamethasone.
- Aerosolized β-agonists (e.g., albuterol, 2.5 mg, repeat PRN 20 min) are useful to control bronchospasm.
- Vasopressor therapy with epinephrine (1:10,000), or dopamine is indicated in pts with refractory hypotension after crystalloid resuscitation.

H. ALCOHOL WITHDRAWAL

Syndrome that occurs when a person stops ingesting alcohol after prolonged consumption. Sx vary according to the severity of the pt's alcohol abuse and the time interval from the pt's previous alcohol ingestion.

Diagnosis
- *Tremulous state* (early alcohol withdrawal, "impending delirium tremens," "shakes," "jitters")
  • Time interval: usually occurs 6 to 8 hr after the last drink or 12 to 48 hr after reduction of alcohol intake; becomes most pronounced at 24 to 36 hr
  • Manifestation: tremors, mild agitation, insomnia, tachycardia; sx relieved by alcohol
- *Alcoholic hallucinosis:* Hallucinations are usually auditory but occasionally are visual, tactile, or olfactory; usually there is no clouding of sensorium as in delirium (clinical presentation may be mistaken for an acute schizophrenic episode). Disordered perceptions become most pronounced after 24 to 36 hr of abstinence.
- *Withdrawal seizures ("rum fits")*
  • Time interval: usually occur 7 to 30 hr after cessation of drinking, w/a peak incidence between 13 and 24 hr.

- Manifestations: generalized convulsions w/loss of consciousness. Focal signs are usually absent; consider further investigation w/CT scan of head and EEG if clearly indicated (e.g., presence of focal neurologic deficits, prolonged postictal confusion state). In addition, in a febrile pt who is having *a seizure or ΔMS, an LP may be necessary.*

■ *Delirium tremens (DTs)*
  - Time interval: variable. It usually occurs within 1 wk after reduction or cessation of heavy alcohol intake and persists for 1 to 3 days. Peak incidence is 72 and 96 hr after the cessation of alcohol consumption.
  - Manifestations: profound confusion, tremors, vivid visual and tactile hallucinations, autonomic hyperactivity. This is the most serious clinical presentation of alcohol withdrawal (mortality is ≈15% in untreated pts).

Treatment
Inpatient
■ Admit to medical ward (private room); monitor VS q4h; institute seizure precautions; maintain adequate sedation.
■ Labs: serum electrolytes, BUN, Cr, Mg^{2+}, PO_4^{-3}, Ca^{2+} levels, glucose, CPK
■ Administer oxazepam or lorazepam as follows:
  - In pts w/DTs, initially lorazepam 2 to 5 mg IM/IV repeated PRN. In stable pts, PO administration may be sufficient: day 1, 2 mg PO q4h while awake and not lethargic; day 2, 1 mg PO q4h while awake and not lethargic; day 3, 0.5 mg PO q4h while awake and not lethargic. Hospital protocols may include oxazepam or chlordiazepoxide (cation if ↑ LFTs) for sedation.
  - In pts w/mild to moderate withdrawal and w/o h/o seizures, individualized benzo administration (rather than a fixed-dose regimen) results in lower benzo administration and avoids unnecessary sedation. The *Clinical Institute Withdrawal Assessment—Alcohol (CIWA-A) scale* can be used to measure the severity of alcohol withdrawal. It consists of the 10 following items: nausea; tremor; autonomic hyperactivity; anxiety; agitation; tactile, visual, and auditory disturbances; headache; and disorientation. The maximum score is 67. When the CIWA-A score is >8, pts are usually given 2 to 4 mg of lorazepam hourly.
  - Vitamin replacement: thiamine 100 mg IV or IM for at least 5 days, plus PO multivitamins. The IV administration of glucose can precipitate Wernicke's encephalopathy in alcoholic pts w/thiamine deficiency; therefore, thiamine administration should precede IV dextrose.
  - Hydration PO or IV (high-calorie solution); if IV: glucose w/Na^+, K^+, Mg^{2+}, and PO_4^{-3} replacement PRN. Hypomagnesemia is very common in alcoholism and can lead to arrhythmias if left untreated.
  - Withdrawal seizures can be treated w/diazepam 2.5 mg/min IV until seizures are controlled (check for respiratory depression or hypotension); IV lorazepam 1 to 2 mg q2h can be used in place of diazepam. Generally, withdrawal seizures are self-limited and Rx is not required. The use of phenytoin or other anticonvulsants for short-term Rx of alcohol withdrawal seizures is not recommended.
  - β-Blockers: useful for controlling BP and tachyarrhythmias. However, they do not prevent progression to more serious sx of withdrawal and, if used, should not be administered alone but in conjunction w/benzos. β-Blockers should be avoided in pts w/contraindications to their use (e.g., bronchospasm, bradycardia).

Clinical Pearl
Blood ethanol level ↓ by 20 mg/dL/hr in a nl 70-kg person.

I. ACUTE POISONING

1 ACETAMINOPHEN POISONING
The amount of acetaminophen necessary for hepatic toxicity varies with the pt's body size and hepatic function. It is recommended that APAP intake should not exceed 4 g for adults and 90 mg/kg in children within a 24-hr period.

Diagnosis
H&P
■ Clinical presentation varies by dose ingested and time from ingestion.
  - Phase I (0-24 hr): initial symptoms possibly mild or absent and consisting of anorexia, diaphoresis, malaise, nausea, vomiting and a subclinical rise in transaminase levels
  - Phase II (24-72 hr): right upper quadrant pain, vomiting, somnolence, tachycardia, hypotension, and continued increase in transaminases

- Phase III (72-96 hr): hepatic necrosis with abdominal pain, jaundice, hepatic encephalopathy, coagulopathy, hypoglycemia, renal failure fatality from multiorgan failure
- Phase IV (4 days-3 wk): complete resolution of symptoms and complete resolution of organ failure

Labs

- Initial labs should include a STAT plasma acetaminophen level with a second level drawn approximately 4 hr after the initial ingestion. Subsequent levels can be obtained every 2 to 4 hr until the levels stabilize or decline. These levels should be plotted on the Rumack-Matthew nomogram (Fig. 13-4) to calculate potential hepatic toxicity. The nomogram cannot be used with pts who present >24 hr after ingestion, extended-release preparations, long-term ingestions, or when the time of ingestion is unknown.
- Transaminases (AST, ALT), bilirubin level, INR, BUN, and creat should be initially obtained on all pts.
- Serum and urine toxicology screen for other potential toxic substances is also recommended on admission. Screening for infectious hepatitis should also be considered. β-hCG should be obtained in all women of childbearing age.

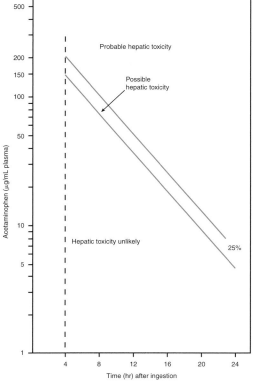

FIGURE 13-4. Rumack-Matthew nomogram for acetaminophen poisoning. *(From Rumack BH, Matthew H: Pediatrics 55:871, 1975. In Rosen P [ed]: Emergency Medicine, 4th ed. St. Louis, Mosby, 1998.)*

Treatment

- Consultation with a Poison Control Center is recommended for pts who have ingested a large amount of acetaminophen and/or other toxic substances. A single toxic dose of acetaminophen usually exceeds 7 g or 150 mg/kg in the adult.
- Hepatotoxicity is defined as any ↑ ALT or AST >1000 IU/L, and hepatic failure is hepatotoxicity with hepatic encephalopathy. For those who cannot be risk stratified using the nomogram, the American College of Emergency Physicians recommends that N-acetylcysteine be administered without delay to those >12 yr and >8 hr after ingestion at presentation.
- Administer activated charcoal 1 g/kg PO if the pt is seen within 1 hr of ingestion or the clinician suspects polydrug ingestion that delays gastric emptying.
- Determine blood levels 4 hr after ingestion; if in the toxic range, start N-acetylcysteine (NAC) either IV (Acetadote) or PO (Mucomyst). Acetylcysteine IV loading dose is 150 mg/kg ×1 diluted in 200 mL D_5W over 15 to 60 min. Maintenance dose is 50 mg/kg diluted in 500 mL D_5W over 4 hr, followed by 100 mg/kg diluted in 1000 mL D_5W over 16 hr. The dose does not require adjustment for renal or hepatic impairment or for dialysis. Total administration time is 21 hours.
- Oral administration is 140 mg/kg PO as a loading dose, followed after 4 hr by 70 mg/kg PO q4h for a total of 17 doses. N-acetylcysteine Rx should be started within 24 hr of acetaminophen overdose. Total administration time is 72 hours.
- Advantages of IV administration include more reliable absorption, fewer doses, and shorter duration of treatment.
- Monitor acetaminophen level; use a graph to plot possible hepatic toxicity. Repeat AST/ALT and APAP levels after 12 to 14 hr of IV acetylcysteine infusion and continue infusion for >16 hr if transaminases are elevated, if acetaminophen concentration is measurable, or if coagulopathy exists (INR >1.5-2.0).
- Provide adequate IV hydration ($D_{5½}NS$ at 150 mL/hr).
- In pts on IV N-acetylcysteine who have liver failure, frequent monitoring of VS, O_2sat by pulse ox, AST, Cr, hypoglycemia, and infection is essential.
- If acetaminophen level is nontoxic, N-acetyl-cysteine Rx may be d/c.

2 AMPHETAMINE OVERDOSE

Diagnosis
H&P
- Tachycardia, HTN, mydriasis, agitation, seizures, diaphoresis, psychosis, hyperthermia

Labs
- Lytes, BUN, Cr, CPK

Treatment
- Activated charcoal
- Gastric lavage for acute large ingestion
- Sedation w/benzos (diazepam)
- Haloperidol for hallucinations and psychosis
- Propranolol or lidocaine for arrhythmias

Clinical Pearl
Induction of emesis is contraindicated.

3 BARBITURATE OVERDOSE

Diagnosis
H&P
- Lethargy, respiratory depression, coma
- ↓ DTRs, extensor plantar response

Labs
- BMP, LFTs, Ca, Mg, PO_4
- Serum and urine toxicology screen; ethanol, ASA, and acetaminophen level

Imaging
- CXR, ECG

Treatment
- IV bolus $NaHCO_3$, 2 mEq/kg IV push, then maintenance infusion begun (132 mEq $NaHCO_3$ in 1 L D_5W at 250 mL/hr)
- Administration of activated charcoal (0.5-1 g/kg; max: ≤50 g PO) in water or sorbitol by NG tube
- Gastric lavage w/early presentation
- Hemoperfusion

4 COCAINE OVERDOSE

Diagnosis

H&P

■ Phase I
  • CNS: euphoria, agitation, headache, vertigo, twitching, bruxism, nonintentional tremor
  • N/V, fever, HTN, tachycardia
■ Phase II
  • CNS: lethargy, hyperreactive DTRs, seizures (status epilepticus)
  • Sympathetic overdrive: tachycardia, HTN, hyperthermia
  • Incontinence
■ Phase III
  • CNS: flaccid paralysis, coma, fixed dilated pupils, loss of reflexes
  • Pulmonary edema
  • Cardiopulmonary arrest
■ Psychological dependence manifested w/habituation, paranoia, hallucinations (cocaine "bugs")
■ CNS: cerebral ischemia and infarction, cerebral arterial spasm, cerebral vasculitis, cerebral vascular thrombosis, subarachnoid hemorrhage, intraparenchymal hemorrhage, seizures, cerebral atrophy, movement disorders
■ Cardiac: acute myocardial ischemia and infarction, arrhythmias and sudden death, dilated cardiomyopathy and myocarditis, infective endocarditis, aortic rupture
■ Pulmonary (secondary to smoking crack cocaine)
  • Inhalation injuries: cartilage and nasal septal perforation, oropharyngeal ulcers
  • Immunologically mediated diseases: hypersensitivity pneumonitis, bronchiolitis obliterans; pulmonary vascular lesions and hemorrhage, pulmonary infarction, pulmonary edema secondary to LV failure, pneumomediastinum, and pneumothorax
■ GI: gastroduodenal ulceration and perforation; intestinal infarction or perforation, colitis
■ Renal: AKI secondary to rhabdo and myoglobinuria; renal infarction; focal segmental glomerulosclerosis
■ Obstetric: placental abruption, low infant weight, prematurity, microcephaly
■ Psychiatric: anxiety, depression, paranoia, delirium, psychosis, suicide

Labs

■ Toxicology screen (urine): Cocaine is metabolized within 2 hr by the liver to major metabolites, benzoylecgonine and ecgonine methyl ester, that are excreted in the urine. Metabolites can be identified in urine within 5 min of IV use and ≤48 hr after PO ingestion.
■ Blood: CBC, lytes, glucose, BUN, Cr, Ca
■ ABGs
■ Serum CK and troponins

Treatment

■ Inhalation: Wash nasal passages.
■ Agitation:
  • Check STAT glucose.
  • Diazepam 15 to 20 mg PO or 2 to 10 mg IM or IV for severe agitation
■ Hyperthermia:
  • Check rectal temperature, CK, electrolytes.
  • Monitor w/continuous rectal probe; bring temperature down to 101° F within 30 to 45 min.
■ Rhabdo:
  • Vigorous hydration w/urine output ≥2 mL/kg
  • Mannitol or bicarbonate for rhabdo resistant to hydration
■ Seizure management (status epilepticus):
  • Diazepam 5 to 10 mg IV over 2 to 3 min; may be repeated every 10 to 15 min PRN
  • Lorazepam 2 to 3 mg IV over 2 to 3 min can be used instead of diazepam.
  • Phenytoin loading dose 15 to 18 mg/kg IV at a rate not to exceed 25 to 50 mg/min under cardiac monitoring
  • Phenobarbital loading dose 10 to 15 mg/kg IV at a rate of 25 mg/min. An additional 5 mg/kg may be given in 30 to 45 min if seizures are not controlled.

- Refractory seizures, consider:
  - Pancuronium 0.1 mg/kg IV
  - Halothane general anesthesia
  - Both require EEG monitoring to determine brain seizure activity.

■ HTN:
- Cocaine-induced HTN usually responds to benzos. If this fails:
  - Consider A-line for continuous BP monitoring.
  - Avoid the use of CCBs (may potentiate the incidence of seizures and death, especially in body packers).
  - The use of β-blockers may exacerbate cocaine-induced vasoconstriction.
  - Phentolamine (unopposed adrenergic effects) or NTG may be required.
- If diastolic pressure >120 mm Hg: hydralazine hydrochloride 25 mg IM or IV; may repeat q1h
- If HTN uncontrolled or hypertensive encephalopathy is present: sodium nitroprusside initially at 0.5 μg/kg/min not to exceed 10 μg/kg/min

■ Chest pain:
- CXR, ECG, cardiac enzymes
- Benzos for agitation
- ASA and NTG for ischemic pain
- Percutaneous transluminal coronary angioplasty may be preferred over thrombolysis for cocaine-associated MI.
- The use of β-adrenergic blockers remains controversial because of the unopposed α-adrenergic effects of cocaine. Thus consider using β-blockers w/alpha blocking properties (eg. Labetalol).
- The combination of nitroprusside and a β-adrenergic blocking agent or phentolamine alone or in addition to a β-adrenergic blocking agent may successfully treat myocardial ischemia and HTN.

■ Ventricular arrhythmias:
- Antiarrhythmia agents should be used w/caution during the early period after cocaine exposure as a result of their proarrhythmic and proconvulsant effects.
- Propranolol 1 mg/min IV for up to 6 mg is given (may result in unopposed α-adrenergic effects).
- Lidocaine 1.5 mg/kg IV bolus is followed by IV infusion (controversial: may be proarrhythmic and proconvulsant).
- Termination of ventricular arrhythmias may be resistant to lidocaine and even cardioversion.

5 ETHANOL POISONING

Diagnosis

H&P

■ Alcohol inhibits the conversion of lactate to glucose in the liver. Alcoholic ketoacidosis usually follows binge drinking.

■ Abd pain, vomiting, starvation, volume depletion

Labs

■ AG metabolic acidosis

■ ↑ Osmolal gap (difference between the measured and calculated serum osmolality)

■ N/↓ blood glucose

■ ↑ BUN, Cr, hypophosphatemia, hypokalemia, hypomagnesemia

Treatment

■ Volume repletion, thiamine and glucose administration

■ Correction of hypophosphatemia, hypokalemia, and hypomagnesemia if present

Clinical Pearl

Metabolic acidosis is also associated w/ingestion of ethylene glycol and methanol in addition to ethanol. Direct measurement of these substances should be performed whenever possible.

6 ETHYLENE GLYCOL, ISOPROPYL ALCOHOL, AND METHANOL POISONING

Diagnosis

H&P

■ Ethylene glycol is a component of antifreeze and industrial solvents. It has a sweet taste and may be ingested accidentally or in suicide attempts. Methanol is a component of wood alcohol (moonshine liquor), copy machines, embalming fluid, paint removers, and windshield wiper fluid. Isopropyl alcohol is found in rubbing alcohol.

- CNS sx (lethargy, seizures, coma), renal failure, pulmonary, cardiac failure
- Dehydration
- Optic papillitis leading to blindness from metabolism of methanol to formaldehyde and formic acid

Labs
- AG acidosis in ethylene glycol and methanol poisoning. Isopropyl alcohol does not cause ↑ AG or ketoacidosis because the metabolite is acetone, but test results are (+) for ketones.
- ↑ Osmolal gap (difference between the measured and calculated serum osmolality)
- Ca oxalate crystals in the urine in ethylene glycol poisoning
- Toxicology screen and quantification

Treatment*
- Competitive inhibition of alcohol dehydrogenase w/fomepizole (preferred) or ethanol (when fomepizole is not available) and hemodialysis (in all cases when ethanol is used as Rx and in fomepizole Rx and profound acidemia and signs of optic or renal injury)
- Criteria for initiation of Rx: ethylene glycol plasma concentration ≥20 mg/dL (3.2 mmol/L) or methanol plasma concentration >20 mg/dL (6.2 mmol/L); suspected ethylene glycol or methanol ingestion and two or more of the following criteria: arterial pH <7.3, Osmo gap >10 mOsm/L, serum CO_2 level <20 mmol/L
- Dosing of fomepizole:
  - Pts not undergoing hemodialysis: Loading dose is 15 mg/kg BW, followed by 10 mg/kg q12h; after 48 hr, 15 mg/kg q12h.
  - Pts undergoing hemodialysis use the same dose except the drug is given 6 hr after the first dose and q4h thereafter.
  - Continue fomepizole Rx until the plasma ethylene glycol or methanol concentration is <20 mg/dL.
- IV rehydration is indicated in all pts, with $NaHCO_3$ administration in pts w/pH <7.3.
- In methanol poisoning, administer folinic acid (leucovorin) 1 mg/kg BW IV (≤50 mg) or stereospecific levoleucovorin at one-half dose of leucovorin. The administration of folate is beneficial because formic acid is catabolized to CO_2 and water by tetrahydrofolate synthetase (enzyme dependent on stored folate).
- Pyridoxine may be beneficial in ethylene glycol poisoning (pyridoxine is a cofactor in metabolism of glycolic acid to glycine).

Clinical Pearls
- The CNS dysfunction is primarily the result of the keto aldehyde metabolites.
- Intratubular obstruction and ARF may be caused by oxalate crystals in ethylene glycol poisoning.

7 CARBON MONOXIDE POISONING

Etiology
- Exposure to smoke from fires; motor vehicle exhaust; or the burning of wood, charcoal, or natural gas for cooking or heating in poorly ventilated areas. CO is a colorless, odorless, tasteless, nonirritating gas. When inhaled, it produces toxicity by causing cellular hypoxia.

Diagnosis
H&P
- Mild to moderately severe poisoning may manifest w/headache, fatigue, dizziness, nausea, dyspnea, confusion, or blurry vision.
- Severe poisoning may manifest w/arrhythmias, myocardial ischemia, pulmonary edema, lethargy, ataxia, syncope, seizure, coma, or cherry-red skin.

Labs
- ↑ Carboxyhemoglobin (COHgb) level. Note: COHgb level >5% in nonsmokers confirms exposure. Heavy smokers may have levels of 10%.
- Direct measurement of Sao_2. Note: Pulse oximetry and ABG may be falsely nl because neither measures Sao_2 directly. Pulse oximetry is inaccurate because of the similar absorption characteristics of oxyhemoglobin and COHgb. ABG is inaccurate because it measures O_2 dissolved in plasma (which is not affected by CO) and then calculates Sao_2.
- Lytes, glucose, BUN, Cr, CPK, ABG (because lactic acidosis and rhabdo may develop)
- Pregnancy test in women of childbearing age (fetus at high risk)
- Consider toxicology screen

*Data from Brent J: N Engl J Med 360:21, 2009.

Treatment

- Removal from site of CO exposure
- Ensuring of adequate airway
- Continuous ECG monitoring
- Fetal monitoring if pregnant
- 100% O_2 by tight-fitting nonrebreather mask or ETT for 6 to 12 hr ($\downarrow$ half-life of COHgb from 4-6 hr to 60-90 min)
- Hyperbaric O_2 (2.5-3 atm)
- Half-life of COHgb to 20 to 30 min, amount of O_2 dissolved in plasma
- Questionable whether there is any beneficial effect over normobaric O_2
- May prevent the delayed neurologic sequelae of CO poisoning by $\downarrow$ cellular hypoxia and toxicity
- Consider for individuals with:
  - Severe intoxication (COHgb >25%, h/o loss of consciousness, neurologic sx or signs, CV compromise, severe metabolic acidosis)
  - Persistent sx after 2 to 4 hr of normobaric O_2
  - Pregnant women w/COHgb >15% or signs of fetal distress: CO elimination slower in fetus than in mother; fetal Hgb has greater affinity for CO than does adult Hgb
  - Should be instituted quickly if deemed necessary
  - Consider concomitant poisoning w/other toxic/irritant gases that may be present in smoke (e.g., cyanide) or thermal injury to airway. Toxic effects of CO and cyanide are synergistic.
  - Identify source of exposure and determine whether the poisoning was accidental.

Clinical Pearls

- Survivors of severe poisoning are at 14% to 40% risk for neurologic sequelae ranging from parkinsonism to neuropsychiatric sx (personality and memory disorders). Neurologic deficits are usually apparent within 3 wk of poisoning (but may manifest months later). Brain MRI may show changes in the white matter and basal ganglia.
- Sx of toxicity and prognosis do not correlate well w/COHgb levels.

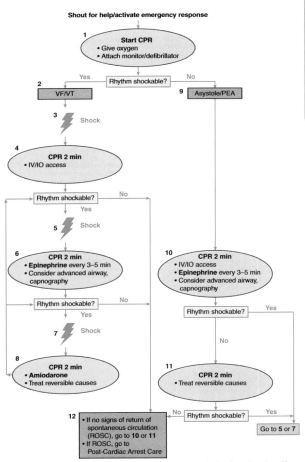

Shout for help/activate emergency response

1
Start CPR
• Give oxygen
• Attach monitor/defibrillator

Rhythm shockable?
— Yes → **2** VF/VT
— No → **9** Asystole/PEA

3 Shock

4
CPR 2 min
• IV/IO access

Rhythm shockable? — No
— Yes

5 Shock

6
CPR 2 min
• **Epinephrine** every 3–5 min
• Consider advanced airway, capnography

Rhythm shockable? — No
— Yes

7 Shock

8
CPR 2 min
• **Amiodarone**
• Treat reversible causes

10
CPR 2 min
• IV/IO access
• **Epinephrine** every 3–5 min
• Consider advanced airway, capnography

Rhythm shockable? — Yes
— No

11
CPR 2 min
• Treat reversible causes

Rhythm shockable? — Yes → Go to **5** or **7**
— No

12
• If no signs of return of spontaneous circulation (ROSC), go to **10** or **11**
• If ROSC, go to Post–Cardiac Arrest Care

FIGURE A1 **Cardiac arrest algorithm.** *(Reprinted with permission from American Heart Association: Advanced Cardiovascular Life Support [ACLS] Pocket Reference Card Set. © Channing Bete Company, Inc.)*

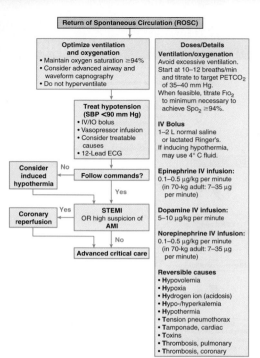

FIGURE A2 Immediate post–cardiac arrest care algorithm. PETCO₂, End tidal carbon dioxide tension. (*Reprinted with permission from American Heart Association: Advanced Cardiovascular Life Support [ACLS] Pocket Reference Card Set. © Channing Bete Company, Inc.*)

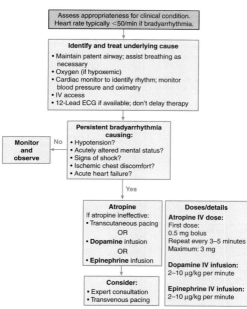

FIGURE A3 Bradycardia with a pulse algorithm. *(Reprinted with permission from American Heart Association: Advanced Cardiovascular Life Support [ACLS] Pocket Reference Card Set. © Channing Bete Company, Inc.)*

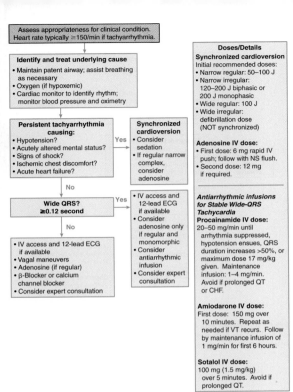

FIGURE A4 **Tachycardia with a pulse algorithm.** *(Reprinted with permission from American Heart Association: Advanced Cardiovascular Life Support [ACLS] Pocket Reference Card Set. © Channing Bete Company, Inc.)*

Page numbers followed by *f* indicate figures; *t*, tables; and *b*, boxes.

Ferri's Practical Guide: Fast Facts for Patient Care, 9th Edition
Expert Consult - Online and Print

Fred F. Ferri, MD, FACP

For nearly 25 years, Ferri's **concise, pocket-sized resource** has served as **the go-to reference for practical, clinical information** among students, residents, and other medical professionals. Formerly known as *Practical Guide to the Care of the Medical Patient*, this volume continues to provide a **fast, effective, and efficient** way to identify the important clinical, laboratory, and diagnostic imaging information you need to get through your internal medicine clerkship or residency.

- **Apply the latest knowledge and techniques** with this updated and streamlined title, which still stays true to the Ferri name.

- **Quickly find important information** with content organized into three major sections: **Section I**, titled "**Surviving the Wards**", contains information on charting, laboratory evaluation and formulary; **Section II** provides the differential diagnosis of common signs and symptoms likely to be encountered in the acute care setting; **Section III** has been completely revised and subdivided into 11 specialty specific diseases and disorders.

- **Carry just the sections you need**, add personalized materials, and keep everything together and safe with an improved ring binder and design.

- **Access the full text and procedural videos online** at expertconsult.com.

An **Expert Consult** title
expertconsult.com

Don't miss all the advantages of consulting this title online. **Activate your access** at **expertconsult.com** today!

- Access the **full text online** from any computer or mobile device

- Perform **rapid searches** on any topic

- Follow links to **PubMed abstracts** for most bibliographical references

Look for your **activation instructions** on the **inside front cover**!

Recommended Shelving Classification
Internal Medicine